ANAC's
Core Curriculum *for*
HIV/AIDS Nursing

THIRD EDITION

Association of Nurses in AIDS Care

Edited by

Barbara Swanson, PhD, RN, ACRN

Associate Professor
Rush University College of Nursing
Chicago, Illinois

JONES AND BARTLETT PUBLISHERS
Sudbury, Massachusetts
BOSTON   TORONTO   LONDON   SINGAPORE

World Headquarters
Jones and Bartlett Publishers
40 Tall Pine Drive
Sudbury, MA 01776
978-443-5000
info@jbpub.com
www.jbpub.com

Jones and Bartlett Publishers
Canada
6339 Ormindale Way
Mississauga, Ontario L5V 1J2
Canada

Jones and Bartlett Publishers
International
Barb House, Barb Mews
London W6 7PA
United Kingdom

Jones and Bartlett's books and products are available through most bookstores and online booksellers. To contact Jones and Bartlett Publishers directly, call 800-832-0034, fax 978-443-8000, or visit our website www.jbpub.com.

Substantial discounts on bulk quantities of Jones and Bartlett's publications are available to corporations, professional associations, and other qualified organizations. For details and specific discount information, contact the special sales department at Jones and Bartlett via the above contact information or send an email to specialsales@jbpub.com.

The authors, editor, and publisher have made every effort to provide accurate information. However, they are not responsible for errors, omissions, or for any outcomes related to the use of the contents of this book and take no responsibility for the use of the products and procedures described. Treatments and side effects described in this book may not be applicable to all people; likewise, some people may require a dose or experience a side effect that is not described herein. Drugs and medical devices are discussed that may have limited availability controlled by the Food and Drug Administration (FDA) for use only in a research study or clinical trial. Research, clinical practice, and government regulations often change the accepted standard in this field. When consideration is being given to use of any drug in the clinical setting, the health care provider or reader is responsible for determining FDA status of the drug, reading the package insert, and reviewing prescribing information for the most up-to-date recommendations on dose, precautions, and contraindications, and determining the appropriate usage for the product. This is especially important in the case of drugs that are new or seldom used.

Production Credits
Publisher: Kevin Sullivan
Acquisitions Editor: Emily Ekle
Acquisitions Editor: Amy Sibley
Associate Editor: Patricia Donnelly
Editorial Assistant: Rachel Shuster
Associate Production Editor: Katie Spiegel
Senior Marketing Manager: Barb Bartoszek
V.P., Manufacturing and Inventory Control: Therese Connell
Composition: Atlis Graphics, Inc.
Cover Design: Scott Moden
Cover Image: © Gualberto Becerra/ShutterStock, Inc.
Printing and Binding: Malloy, Inc.
Cover Printing: Malloy, Inc.

Library of Congress Cataloging-in-Publication Data
ANAC's core curriculum for HIV/AIDS nursing / Association of Nurses in AIDS Care ; edited by Barbara Swanson. — 3rd ed.
  p. ; cm.
 Includes bibliographical references and index.
 ISBN 978-0-7637-5459-4
 1. AIDS (Disease)—Nursing. I. Swanson, Barbara, 1958- II. Association of Nurses in AIDS Care. III. Title: Association of Nurses in AIDS Care's core curriculum for HIV/AIDS nursing. IV Title: Core curriculum for HIV/AIDS nursing.
 [DNLM: 1. Acquired Immunodeficiency Syndrome—nursing—Outlines. 2. HIV Infections—nursing—Outlines. WY 18.2 A532 2010]
 RC606.6.A533 2010
 616.97'920231—dc22

2009010234

6048
Printed in the United States of America
13 12 11 10 09   10 9 8 7 6 5 4 3 2 1

Dedication

In Memory of Leslie Schor

Contents

Association of Nurses in AIDS Care

The Association of Nurses in AIDS Care (ANAC) is a nonprofit professional nursing organization committed to fostering the individual and collective professional development of nurses involved in the delivery of health care to persons infected or affected by the human immunodeficiency virus (HIV) and to promoting the health, welfare, and rights of all HIV-infected persons.

The members of ANAC strive to achieve the mission by:

- Creating an effective network among nurses in HIV/AIDS care
- Studying, researching, and exchanging information, experiences, and ideas leading to improved care for persons with HIV/AIDS infection
- Providing leadership to the nursing community in matters related to HIV/AIDS infection
- Advocating for HIV-infected persons
- Promoting social awareness concerning issues related to HIV/AIDS

Inherent in these goals is an abiding commitment to the prevention of further HIV infection.

Preface

Since its founding, ANAC has shown a singular commitment to improving the lives of those affected by HIV/AIDS. Nowhere is this commitment more fully articulated than in *ANAC's Core Curriculum for HIV/AIDS Nursing*. Drawing from the expertise of frontline clinicians and scholars, the first two editions of the *Core Curriculum* provided nurses with the evidence-based knowledge to provide quality care to the diverse groups that comprise the HIV/AIDS population. In this third edition, we have endeavored to uphold the standard of excellence set by the editors of the first two editions. The clinical management of HIV/AIDS is constantly evolving, thus the third edition of the *Core Curriculum* has evolved to keep pace. Toward that end, the reader will notice that some topics contained in the first two editions are gone, replaced by new topics that the editors believe represent the current salient clinical issues in HIV/AIDS nursing. Additionally, we have added case studies with test questions to assist nurses to apply the *Core Curriculum's* content to the management of patients in a variety of settings.

For the past 13 years, *ANAC's Core Curriculum for HIV/AIDS Nursing* has been an indispensable resource for nurses who care for persons with HIV/AIDS. The editors and I believe that the third edition continues this tradition of excellence. I welcome your comments.

Barbara Swanson
barbara_a_swanson@rush.edu

Chapter Editors

Chapter 1
Janice Zeller, PhD, RN, FAAN, Professor, Rush University College of Nursing, Chicago, Illinois

Chapter 2
Richard S. Ferri, PhD, ANP, ACRN, FAAN, HIV/Hepatitis Nurse Practitioner Specialist, Crossroads Medical, Harwich, Massachusetts; Freelance Medical Writer and Editor

Chapter 3
F. Patrick Robinson, PhD, RN, ACRN, Assistant Professor and Executive Assistant Dean, College of Nursing, University of Illinois at Chicago

Chapter 4
Joyce K. Keithley, DNSc, RN, FAAN, Professor, Rush University College of Nursing, Chicago, Illinois

Chapter 5
Barbara Swanson, PhD, RN, ACRN, Associate Professor, Rush University College of Nursing, Chicago, Illinois

Chapter 6
Christine Balt, MS, RN, FNP, BC, AACRN, Nurse Practitioner, Indiana University School of Medicine Division of Infectious Diseases, Wishard Health Services Infectious Disease Clinic, Indianapolis, Indiana

Chapters 7, 8, 9, and 10
Barbara Kiernan, PhD, APRN, Interim Department Chair and Associate Professor, Medical College of Georgia School of Nursing, Augusta, Georgia

Chapter 11 and Appendices
Sande Gracia Jones, PhD, ARNP, ACRN, CS, BC, FAAN, Associate Professor, College of Nursing and Health Sciences, Florida International University, Miami, Florida

Contributing Authors

Tony Adinolfi, MSN, RN, ANP, Senior Scientific Liaison, Infectious Diseases, Astellas Pharma US, Inc., Deerfield, Illinois
Candidiasis, Herpes Simplex Virus (HSV)

Michele Agnoli, BSN, RN, ACRN, Clinical Program Coordinator, Midwest AIDS Training and Education Center, Jane Addams College of Social Work, University of Illinois at Chicago
Psoriasis

Sarah Ailey, PhD, RNC, Associate Professor, Rush University College of Nursing, Chicago, Illinois
Individuals with Intellectual and Developmental Disabilities (I/DD)

Michelle Alexander, MN, RN, Instructor, Rush University College of Nursing, Chicago, Illinois
Vision Loss/Visual Impairment

Joyce K. Anastasi, PhD, DrNP, RN, FAAN, LAc, Professor, School of Nursing, Columbia University, New York, New York
Diarrhea, Nausea and Vomiting

Christine Balt, MS, RN, FNP, BC, AACRN, Nurse Practitioner, Indiana University School of Medicine Division of Infectious Diseases, Wishard Health Services Infectious Disease Clinic, Indianapolis, Indiana
HIV-Infected Healthcare Workers, Incarcerated Persons, Lesbians and Bisexual Women

Emily A. Barr, MSN, RN, CPNP, CNM, Senior Faculty, The Children's Hospital Immunodeficiency Program, The Department of Infectious Disease, The Children's Hospital, Aurora, Colorado
Case Study: Pediatrics

Kathleen Barrett, MSN, RN, Project Consultant in QA and Infection Control, Oak Park, Illinois
Hepatitis A, Hepatitis B, Hepatitis C

Julie Barroso, PhD, ANP, APRN, BC, FAAN, Associate Professor and Specialty Director, Adult Nurse Practitioner Program, Research Development Coordinator, Office of Research Affairs, Duke University School of Nursing, Durham, North Carolina
Fatigue

Jo Anne Bennett, PhD, RN, ACRN, Research Scientist, New York City Department of Health, New York, New York
Historical Overview of HIV Pandemic, Epidemiology of HIV Disease, Prevention of HIV Disease, HIV Testing

Marsha J. Bennett, DNS, APRN, ACRN, Associate Professor and Associate Dean for Nursing Research, Scholarship & Science, Louisiana State University Health Sciences Center School of Nursing, New Orleans, Louisiana
Case Study: Psychiatric Issues

Bernadette Capili, DNSc, NP-C, Assistant Professor, School of Nursing, Columbia University, New York, New York
Diarrhea, Nausea and Vomiting

Joseph P. Colagreco, MS, ANP-BC, NP-C, Research Nurse Practitioner, Department of Medicine, Beth Israel Deaconess Medical Center, Boston, Massachusetts
Pathophysiology of HIV Infection

Michele Crespo-Fierro, MS/MPH, RN, AACRN, Clinical Instructor, New York University College of Nursing, New York, New York; Nurse Consultant, Private Practice, Fresh Meadows, New York
Migrant/Seasonal Farm Workers and Day Laborers, Recent Immigrants, Latinos, Cervical Neoplasia, Kaposi's Sarcoma (KS), Non-Hodgkin's Lymphoma, Cardiomyopathy

Sheila Davis, DNP, ANP, FAAN, Nurse Practitioner, Infectious Diseases, Massachusetts General Hospital; Assistant Professor, MGH Institute of Health Professions, Boston, Massachusetts
Coccidioidomycosis, Cryptococcosis, Histoplasmosis, Toxoplasmosis, Cytomegalovirus (CMV)

Carol Davison, MSN, RN, FNP-BC, Family Nurse Practitioner, University of Medicine and Dentistry of New Jersey, Francois-Xavier Bagnoud Center for Children, Newark, New Jersey
Adherence to Medical Regimens for Children and Families

Joseph DeSantis, PhD, ARNP, ACRN, Assistant Professor, University of Miami School of Nursing and Health Studies, Coral Gables, Florida
Preventing Transmission of HIV in Patient Care Settings, End-of-Life Issues

Joanne Despotes, MPH, RN, ACRN, Tuberculosis Nurse Case Manager, Division of Pulmonary and Critical Care Medicine, Stroger Hospital of Cook County, Chicago, Illinois
Mycobacterium Avium Complex (MAC), Mycobacterium Tuberculosis

Marion Donohoe, MSN, RN, CPNP, Pediatric Nurse Practitioner, Infectious Disease Services, St. Jude Children's Research Hospital, Memphis, Tennessee
Disclosure, Case Study: Pediatrics

Anna M. S. Duloy, BS, Research Assistant, Rush University College of Nursing, Chicago, Illinois
Cognitive Impairment

Margaret Dykeman, PhD, NP, Faculty of Nursing, University of New Brunswick, Canada
Commercial Sex Workers, Homeless Persons

Tom Emanuele, BSN, RN-BC, ACRN, Case Management Manager, Parkland Health and Hospital System, Dallas, Texas
Case Management

Maithe Enriquez, PhD, APRN-BC, Assistant Professor, Schools of Nursing and Medicine, University of Missouri, Kansas City
Case Study: Pathophysiology

Mary Faut Rodts, DNP, CNP, ONC, FAAN, Associate Professor, Rush University College of Nursing, Chicago, Illinois
Impaired Mobility

Kelly Fugate, ND, RN, Associate Project Director, Specialist, Division of Standards and Survey Methods, The Joint Commission, Oakbrook Terrace, Illinois
Bacterial Pneumonia, Pneumocystosis, Cough, Dyspnea

Susan W. Gaskins, MPH, DSN, ACRN, Professor, Capstone College of Nursing, University of Alabama, Birmingham, Alabama
Rural Communities

Brian K. Goodroad, CNP, AACRN, Nurse Practitioner, Infectious Clinic, Abbot Northwestern Hospital, Minneapolis, Minnesota
Managing Antiretroviral Therapy

Kristin M. Grage, MA, CNP, Certified Nurse Practitioner, Positive Care Center, Hennepin County Medical Center, Minneapolis, Minnesota
Healthcare Follow-Up

Vicki Hannemann, BSN, RN, Nurse Clinician, Hemophilia and Thrombosis Center, University of Minnesota Medical Center, Fairview, Minnesota
People with Hemophilia

Connie Highsmith, BSN, RN, ACRN, Clinical Supervisor Sub-Specialty, Medical Associates Health Centers, Menomonee Falls, Wisconsin
Case Management

Barbara J. Holtzclaw, PhD, RN, FAAN, Nurse Scientist/Professor, College of Nursing and Graduate College, University of Oklahoma Health Sciences Center, Oklahoma City, Oklahoma
Fever

Sande Gracia Jones, PhD, ARNP, ACRN, CS, BC, FAAN, Associate Professor, College of Nursing and Health Sciences, Florida International University, Miami, Florida
Case Study: Medical-Surgical Nursing

Clair Kaplan, MSN, RN, APRN(WHNP), MHS, MT(ASCP), Assistant Professor of Nursing, Adult, Family, Gerontologic, and Women's Health Program, Yale University School of Nursing, New Haven, Connecticut
Case Study: Obstetrics

Joyce K. Keithley, DNSc, RN, FAAN, Professor, Rush University College of Nursing, Chicago, Illinois
Anorexia and Weight Loss, Dysphagia and Odynophagia, Cognitive Impairment, Oral Hairy Leukoplakia, HIV-Related Wasting Syndrome, Fat Redistribution Syndrome

Barbara Kiernan, PhD, APRN, Interim Department Chair and Associate Professor, Medical College of Georgia School of Nursing, Augusta, Georgia
Symptomatic Conditions in Infants and Children with Advancing Disease

Carl A. Kirton, DNP, RN, ANP-BC, ACRN, Vice President of Nursing and Nurse Practitioner, North General Hospital, New York, New York; Clinical Associate Professor of Nursing, New York University; President, ANAC
Immunizations, The African American Community

Kandace Landreneau, PhD, RN, CCTC, Associate Professor, College of Nursing and Health Sciences, University of Texas at Tyler
Case Study: Pathophysiology

Eric G. Leach, MSN, RN, FNP, Private Practice, New York, New York
Transgender/Transsexual Persons

Wade Leon, MA, ANP, PMHNP, APRN, BC, Regional Medical Scientist, Boehringer-Ingelheim, Ridgefield, Connecticut; Instructor, New York Medical College, Valhalla, New York
Depression, Bipolar Disorder, Anxiety Disorders, Delirium, HIV-Associated Dementia Complex, Mental Illness and Substance Use, Nephropathy

Martin C. Lewis, MEd, MSN, APRN-BC, ANP, CLNC, Alpha Dog Health Consultants, LLC, Lambertville, New Jersey
Selected Laboratory Values

Debra E. Lyon, PhD, RN, FNP-BC, Associate Professor, Virginia Commonwealth University, School of Nursing, Richmond, Virginia
Impaired Glucose Tolerance (IGT), Dyslipidemia

Richard C. MacIntyre, PhD, RN, FAAN, Professor and Robert Wood Johnson Executive Nurse Fellow, Samuel Merritt University, Sacramento, California
Ethical and Legal Concerns

Hanna Major-Wilson, MSN, ARNP, CPN, Faculty, University of Miami Miller School of Medicine, Coral Cables, Florida
Adolescents

R. Kevin Mallinson, PhD, RN, AACRN, FAAN, Assistant Professor, Department of Nursing, Georgetown University School of Nursing & Health Studies, Washington, DC
The Gay and Bisexual Male Community, The Deaf Community

Linda Manfrin-Ledet, DNS, APRN, BC, Associate Professor of Nursing, Nicholls State University, College of Nursing, Thibodaux, Louisiana
Case Study: Psychiatric Issues

Shean Marley, ASN, COE, RN, ACRN, CEN, Staff Nurse, Internal Medicine, Massachusetts General Hospital, Boston, Massachusetts
Herpes Zoster

Donna Maturo, MSN, ARNP, PNP, BC, Division of Adolescent Medicine, University of Miami Miller School of Medicine, Coral Gables, Florida
Adolescents

Tanya Melich-Munyan, BSN, RN, Community/Public Health Supervisor, Faculty Practice Services, Rush University College of Nursing, Chicago, Illinois
Vision Loss/Visual Impairment

Nora A. Merriam, MSN, MPH, RN, Ruskin, Florida
The Blind and Visually Impaired Community

Bonnie Minter, MS, RN, CPNP, Nurse Practitioner, Pediatric HIV Clinic, Grady Health System, Atlanta, Georgia
Clinical Manifestations and Management of the HIV-Infected Infant and Child

Angela Moss, MS, RN, ANP, Assistant Professor, Rush University College of Nursing, Chicago, Illinois
Individuals with Intellectual and Developmental Disabilities (I/DD)

Gayle Newshan, PhD, NP, RN, BC, Director, Department of Holistic Care, Pain and Stress Management, St. John's Riverside Hospital, Yonkers, New York
Pain

Summer S. Nijem, APRN, CPNP-PC, Pediatric Nurse Practitioner, Grady Infectious Disease Program, Atlanta, Georgia
Managing Antiretroviral Therapy in HIV-Infected Infants and Children, Pain, Anorexia and Weight Loss

Kathleen M. Nokes, PhD, RN, FAAN, Professor and Director of the Graduate Nursing Program, Hunter College, CUNY and Hunter-Bellevue School of Nursing, New York, New York
Older Adults, Sleep Disturbances

Patricia M. O'Kane, MA, RN, NP, Nurse Practitioner, Department of Psychiatry, The Brookdale University Hospital & Medical Center, Brooklyn, New York
Spirituality and Related Concepts

Kristin Kane Ownby, PhD, RN, ACHPN, ACRN, AOCN, Associate Professor of Clinical Nursing, The University of Texas Health Science Center School of Nursing at Houston
Idiopathic Thrombocytopenia Purpura, Cryptosporidiosis, Thrombocytopenia

J. Craig Phillips, PhD, LLM, RN, PMHCNS-BC, ACRN, Assistant Professor, School of Nursing, University of British Columbia, Vancouver, British Columbia
Selected Laboratory Values

Norma Rolfsen, MS, AACRN, Program Director, HIV Care Program, Research and Education Foundation of the Michael Reese Medical Staff, Chicago, Illinois
Giardia, Syphilis

Helen C. Rominger, MSN, RN, FNP, CCRC, AACRN, Nurse Practitioner and Clinical Research Coordinator, Division of Infectious Diseases, Indiana University School of Medicine, Wishard Memorial Hospital, Indianapolis, Indiana
Adolescents, Pregnant Women, Women

Neal Rosenburg, MSN, RN, Faculty, Goldfarb School of Nursing at Barnes-Jewish College, St. Louis, Missouri
Substance Users

Leslie Schor, MSN, RN, ACRN, Jacksonville, Florida
Preventing Transmission of HIV in Patient Care Settings

Craig R. Sellers, PhD, RN, APRN, ANP-BC, Director of Adult Nurse Practitioner Program and Senior Teaching Associate, University of Rochester School of Nursing, Rochester, New York
Progressive Multifocal Leukoencephalopathy (PML), Ethical and Legal Concerns

Judy K. Shaw, PhD, ANP-C, Healthcare Service Provider, Infectious Disease Section, Samuel S. Stratton VA Medical Center, Albany, New York
Case Study: Pharmacology

Sarah Shelton, PsyD, MS, MPH, Licensed Clinical Psychologist and Director, Pediatric Psychological Services, Assistant Professor, Psychiatry and Health Behavior, Assistant Professor, Pediatrics, Medical College of Georgia Children's Medical Center, Augusta, Georgia
Decision Making and Family Autonomy, Stress Reduction in Pediatric HIV, Social Isolation and Stigma, Surrogate Caregivers

Rebekah Shepard, DNP, RN, ANP, Assistant Professor, Rush University College of Nursing, Chicago, Illinois
Response to an HIV Diagnosis: Infected Person, Response to an HIV Diagnosis: Family and Significant Other, Caregiver Burden/Strain, Depression, Bipolar Disorder, Anxiety Disorders, Delirium, HIV-Associated Dementia Complex, Male Sexual Dysfunction, Female Sexual Dysfunction

David J. Sterken, MN, CNS, CPNP, Pediatric Infectious Disease Nurse Practitioner, Clinical Nurse Specialist, DeVos Children's Hospital, Grand Rapids, Michigan
Fever, Teaching for Health Promotion, Wellness, and Prevention of Transmission

Barbara Swanson, PhD, RN, ACRN, Associate Professor, Rush University College of Nursing, Chicago, Illinois
Leukopenia, Osteopenia, Osteoporosis, Avascular Necrosis, Lactic Acidosis, Oral Lesions, Perinatal Transmission of HIV Infection, Cognitive Impairment and Developmental Delay

Donna Taliaferro, PhD, RN, Associate Dean for Research, Goldfarb School of Nursing at Barnes-Jewish College, St. Louis, Missouri
Anemia, Substance Users

Gail B. Williams, PhD, RN, PMHCNS-BC, Professor, Department of Family Nursing Care, The University of Texas Health Science Center at San Antonio School of Nursing
Substance Users

Thomas P. Young, MS, NP, AAHIVS, Assistant Clinical Professor, Community Health Systems, Adult Nurse Practitioner Program, University of California, San Francisco; Senior Clinical Science Manager, Global Pharmaceutical Research & Development, Virology, Abbott Laboratories
Baseline Assessment

Janice M. Zeller, PhD, RN, FAAN, Professor, Rush University College of Nursing, Chicago, Illinois
Peripheral Neuropathy, HIV-Related Encephalopathy

CHAPTER 1

HIV Infection, Transmission, and Prevention

1.1 HISTORICAL OVERVIEW OF HIV PANDEMIC

1. The acquired immunodeficiency syndrome (AIDS) pandemic was one of the key international health and demographic events of the late 20th century.
   a. When AIDS first appeared in 1980–1981, few would have predicted the worldwide burden of disease, death, and orphanhood it would precipitate by the turn of the millennium, particularly in sub-Saharan Africa.
   b. By the turn of the century, in some countries, over 30% of adults were living with human immunodeficiency virus (HIV) infection, a situation that has raised concerns about its potential to destabilize regional and global security.
   c. The impact of HIV/AIDS has always been greatest in the poorest countries, where over 95% of new infections currently occur.i.
2. HIV/AIDS has become a major political issue, both nationally and globally, that challenges government decision making and the medical establishment's authority about healthcare research and delivery.
   a. Many governments were slow to respond, in large part through failure to recognize the magnitude of the problem and its potential impact, along with, many believe, a lack of concern for the disenfranchised groups that were most affected.
      i) In the United States, AIDS emerged during a decade of reduced federal funding for numerous government programs, including public health programs, leaving cities with few resources to deal with the growing crisis.
         (1) Some U.S. government officials held the view that it was not a broad societal threat and suggested that the public health community and others were exaggerating its magnitude and potential impact to get government spending to fund gay organizations; some opposed using government funds to address sexuality in any way other than extramarital abstinence and heterosexual monogamy.
         (2) Fall 1986—Surgeon General's Report on Acquired Immune Deficiency
      ii) In Africa, HIV's unique characteristics influenced sociopolitical responses to the epidemic (Iliffe, 2006).
         (1) Because many AIDS manifestations were already endemic, leaders were slow to grasp the scale of the new problem.
         (2) There was reluctance to be identified as the source of a problem that the Western developed world associated with marginalized groups, and the well-publicized

epidemiologic association with monkeys and investigations into distinctive sexual practices were perceived to have racist connotations.

(3) The epidemic's parallel to an expansion of Western medicine in Africa, including immunization programs, fueled perceptions of exploitation and conspiracy.

b. International collaboration:

i) In spring 1985, following the first International AIDS Conference, an international network, Collaborating Centres on AIDS, formed.

ii) In 1986, WHO published a global AIDS strategy.

iii) In 1996, the UN Joint Program on HIV/AIDS (UNAIDS) was established to advocate global action and to coordinate HIV-related efforts across UN agencies.

iv) In the 1990s, global public–private partnerships became an increasingly popular approach for addressing health and welfare problems in the developing world. These partnerships emphasize collaboration among civil communities, local and national governments, and the multinational commercial and philanthropic private sector.

3. HIV/AIDS may be the most complex health challenge humanity has ever confronted.

a. AIDS has led to the emergence of a more concerted and higher level political leadership.

b. In April 2001, the UN established the Global AIDS and Health Fund, later referred to as the Global Fund to Fight AIDS, Tuberculosis, and Malaria (GFATM).

c. In June 2001, the UN General Assembly held a Special Session on AIDS (UNGASSA), at which delegates endorsed a Global Strategy Framework for simultaneously reducing risk, vulnerability, and impact. They unanimously adopted a Declaration of Commitment that specified accelerating and raising spending.

d. In December 2003, WHO/UNAIDS launched the "3 X 5" initiative, which specified universal access to antiretroviral (ARV) therapy as a long-term goal, with a shorter term target for getting 3 million people on ARV therapy by the end of 2005.

e. In 2003, the United States launched the President's Emergency Plan for AIDS Relief (PEPFAR)—the largest international initiative ever to address a single disease.

4. HIV had a silent beginning (Buve et al., 2002; Quinn, 2001; UNAIDS, 2005).

a. The human immunodeficiency viruses (HIV-1 and HIV-2) are of zoonotic origin in Africa (Korber et al., 2000; Zhu et al., 1998).

i) The virus probably emerged around 1930, and although the earliest evidence of isolated cases of HIV-1 infection dates from the late 1950s, the epidemic did not arise until the mid-1970s around Kinshasa. Within 10 years, a generalized epidemic had emerged across the continent, with 1 to 2 million Africans infected.

ii) HIV-2, likely emerging 10 or more years earlier than HIV-1, has been associated with many fewer cases and has been largely confined to West Africa.

b. HIV spread to the western hemisphere (Cohen, 2007; Gilbert et al., 2007).

i) Haiti appears to have the oldest epidemic outside sub-Saharan Africa.

(1) The earliest documented U.S. HIV-1 infection appeared in 1977; first known case in Haiti, 1978.

(a) Contrary to previous theories suggesting that the Haitian epidemic was seeded by gay American tourists in the 1970s, recent molecular analyses of viral isolates from Haitian patients treated in Miami in the early 1980s confirmed that

HIV-1 spread to Haiti from Central Africa around 1966, and then to the United States around 1969 (Gilbert et al., 2007).

(2) The first HIV-2 case in the United States was diagnosed in 1987; fewer than 100 cases were diagnosed over the next decade.

c. From the United States, HIV-1 spread via homosexual contact from one northern hemisphere country to another, but the European epidemic did not gain momentum until several years after it became widespread in the United States.

d. Viral spread among injection drug users (IDUs) in both North America and Europe lagged several years behind the epidemic in homosexual populations (Des Jarlais et al., 1992).

   i) Spread among IDUs in Europe reflected travel and multiple introductions, rather than bridging from local homosexual communities.

e. Continuing epidemic waves over the next 2 decades extended the pandemic to Latin America, Eastern Europe, South and Southeast Asia, Australia, and the Western Pacific region.

   i) At the end of the 1st decade, Asia accounted for < 1% of AIDS cases worldwide.

   ii) Despite widespread poverty, gender inequality, injection drug use, hidden male homosexuality, and extensive commercial sex, the epidemic did not become generalized in Latin America.

5. Tracking the early epidemic:

a. The world first became aware of the clinical entity that would become known as AIDS with a June 1981 report by the CDC, which described clusters of fatal *Pneumocystis carinii* pneumonia (PCP) and Kaposi's sarcoma (KS) cases over the previous 6 months in relatively young men in California and New York (CDC, 1981a, 1981b).

   i) The CDC established a task force in June 1981, asked health departments to report PCP and KS, and began compiling weekly surveillance reports.

   ii) Within months, similar cases were reported in Europe and the United States among women, children, people with hemophilia, injecting drug users, infants, and people from Haiti and Central Africa (Zaire).

   iii) The label AIDS (acquired immunodeficiency syndrome) was adopted by CDC in the summer of 1982.

b. The causal pathogen (HIV-1), a T-lymphotropic retrovirus, was recovered from people with AIDS in Europe, California, and other locations in 1983. A second, less infective and less virulent virus (HIV-2), was identified in 1985.

c. In 1985, a test to screen for antibody to the virus was approved by the FDA, primarily to screen the blood supply.

6. Treatment:

a. In May 1987, zidovudine (ZDV, AZT), a nucleoside reverse transcriptase inhibitor, became the first antiretroviral approved by the FDA.

b. As additional ARVs became available, the limitations of monotherapy quickly became apparent (e.g., resistance, side effects).

c. Highly active antiretroviral therapy (HAART) regimens, popularly called ARV cocktails or combination therapy, were introduced in 1995 and transformed HIV disease into a chronic condition requiring long-term treatment.

   d. The availability of fixed-dose combination pills in the 2000s has made the regimens easier and more convenient.

   e. In 2005, generic antiretrovirals became available.

7. Societal responses to the epidemic have been wide-ranging and include activism, fear, empathy, denial, blame, discrimination, exceptionalism, grief, guilt, optimism, complacency, myths, and conspiracy theories (Bayer, 1991; Bayer & Oppenheimer, 2000; Bennett, 1988, 1995a, 1995b, 1998; Dalton, 1989; Iliffe, 2006; Kinsella, 1989; Valdiserri, 2004).

   a. In some U.S. communities, entire families, social networks, and neighborhoods confronted devastating tolls of suffering and death, whereas in others, few knew of any affected persons.

   b. Terminology referring to risk groups inadvertently focused attention on the people affected rather than the modes of transmission of the infectious pathogen. This focus had the effect of both stigmatizing those affected and confusing people's perceptions of the nature of the risk.

   c. Recognizing behavioral risk factors also served to make distinctions, at least in some media, between those who had become infected as a result of their own actions as being "deserving of" suffering and those who had become infected passively through receiving blood or blood products or by vertical transmission as being "innocent victims."

   d. Community mobilization, self-help, and advocacy efforts, including political activism, were seen worldwide.

      i)   In the United States, the epidemic galvanized gay consciousness and pride, community spirit, political activism, volunteerism, and eventually coalition building with other disenfranchised groups.

      ii) People with AIDS (PWAs) attending the Second National AIDS Forum at the Lesbian and Gay Health Foundation conference drafted a consensus statement that came to be known as the Denver Principles. At its core was insistence on the semantic rejection of the terms *patient* and *victim*.

      iii) The gay community's unprecedented response to the urgent needs brought by the epidemic shaped an entirely new social service network and invigorated healthcare consumer activism, and grassroots AIDS service organizations (ASOs) spread across the country and around the globe.

         (1) These community initiatives played a major role in calling media attention to the epidemic and pressured government agencies for a more aggressive response.

   e. The California Nurses Association was a leading advocate. Its train-the-trainer model for instructing nurses and health professionals about AIDS became an exemplar used, copied, and adapted by many others.

   f. The first nursing article about AIDS was published in the *American Journal of Nursing* in November 1982 by two staff nurses at a New York City hospital (Allen & Mellin, 1982).

REFERENCES

Allen, J., & Mellin, G. (1982). The new epidemic: Immune deficiency, opportunistic infections, and Kaposi's sarcoma. *American Journal of Nursing, 82*(11), 1718–1722.

Bayer, R. (1991). *Private acts, social consequences: AIDS and the politics of public health.* New Brunswick, NJ: Rutgers University Press.

Bayer, R., & Oppenheimer, G. M. (2000). *AIDS doctors: Voices from the epidemic.* New York: Oxford University Press.

Bennett, J. A. (1988). *Heroism and activism: Nurses battle AIDS.* Kansas City, MO: American Nurses Association.

Bennett, J. A. (1995a). AIDS and social disease. *Holistic Nursing Practice, 10*(1), 77–89.

Bennett, J. A. (1995b). Nurses' attitudes about acquired immunodeficiency syndrome care: What research tells us. *Journal of Professional Nursing 11*(6), 339–350.

Bennett, J. A. (1998). Fear of contagion: A response to stress? *Advances in Nursing Science, 21*(1), 76–87.

Buve, A., Bishikwabo-Nsarhaza, K., & Mutangadura, G. (2002). The spread and effect of HIV-1 infection in sub-Saharan Africa. *Lancet, 359*(9322), 2011–2017.

Centers for Disease Control and Prevention (CDC). (1981a). Kaposi's sarcoma and pneumocystis pneumonia among homosexual men—New York City and California. *Morbidity and Mortality Weekly Report, 30*(25), 305–308.

Centers for Disease Control and Prevention (CDC). (1981b). Pneumocystis pneumonia—Los Angeles. *Morbidity and Mortality Weekly Report, 30*(21), 250–252.

Cohen, J. (2007, October 29). How HIV took the world by storm. *Science NOW Daily News.* Retrieved February 4, 2009, from http://sciencenow.sciencemag.org/cgi/content/full/2007/1029/1

Dalton, H. L. (1989). AIDS in blackface. *Daedalus, 118,* 205–227.

Des Jarlais, D. C., Friedman, S. R., Choopanya, K., Vanichseni, S., & Ward, T. P. (1992). International epidemiology of HIV and AIDS among injecting drug users. *AIDS, 6*(10), 1053–1068.

Gilbert, M. T. P., Rambaut, A., Wlasiuk, G., Spira, T. J., Pitchenik, A. E., & Worobey, M. (2007). The emergence of HIV/AIDS in the Americas and beyond. *Proceedings of the National Academy of Sciences, Early Edition.* Retrieved February 4, 2009, from www.pnas.org/cgi/doi/10.1073/pnas.0705329104

Iliffe, J. (2006). *The African AIDS epidemic: A history.* Oxford, UK: James Currey.

Joint United Nations program on HIV/AIDS (UNAIDS). (2005). *AIDS in Africa: Three scenarios to 2025.* Retrieved March 7, 2005, from http://www.unaids.org

Kinsella, J. (1989). *Covering the epidemic: AIDS and the American media.* New Brunswick, NJ: Rutgers University Press.

Koop, C. E. (1987). *Surgeon general's report on acquired immune deficiency syndrome.* Washington, DC: U.S. Public Health Service.

Korber, B., Muldoon, M., Theiler, J., et al. (2000). Timing the ancestor of the HIV-1 pandemic strain. *Science, 288*(5472), 1789–1796.

Quinn, T. C. (2001). AIDS in Africa: A retrospective. *Bulletin of the World Health Organization, 79*(12), 1156–1158.

Valdiserri, R. O. (2004). Mapping the roots of HIV/AIDS complacency: Implications for program and policy development. *AIDS Education and Prevention, 16*(5), 426–439.

World Health Organization (WHO). (1986). *Global strategy for the prevention and control of acquired immunodeficiency syndrome: Projected needs for 1986–1987.* Geneva, Switzerland: Author.

Zhu, T., Korber, B. T., Nahmias, A. J., Hooper, E., Sharp, P. M., & Ho, D. D. (1998). An African HIV-1 sequence from 1959 and implications for the origin of the epidemic. *Nature, 391*(6667), 594–597.

1.2 EPIDEMIOLOGY OF HIV DISEASE

1. The epidemiology of any disease is its distribution among diverse population groups.

    a. The systematic study of the epidemiology of a disease—including the personal and environmental characteristics associated with it—provides the evidence base for planning control measures and evaluating their impact.

        i)   Knowing both incidence and prevalence is essential for program development and assessing needs for services and resources.

            (1) HIV incidence counts reflect reported diagnoses. If infected persons do not access care or are not correctly diagnosed, or if reporting is incomplete, incidence

will be undercounted. Systems must also be in place to preclude duplicate counting (i.e., reporting by name with birthplace and date).

(2) The timing of incidence peaks and how many people are infected will depend on both transmission dynamics and the size of the susceptible population. Transmission will slow when a population is saturated with infection. Thus, in some areas, HIV incidence in adolescents and young adults (15–24 years) may rise compared with older groups, although risk behavior may not have declined in the older group nor risen in the younger group.

(3) HIV prevalence is estimated from the combination of cumulative incidence (case occurrences) and deaths of people with HIV infection, regardless of cause.

(a) Rising prevalence may reflect greater incidence and/or lower mortality.

(4) HIV prevalence in the United States is currently higher than ever before despite declining incidence because mortality has declined while the annual number of new cases remains stable.

(5) Percentages or proportions: Denominators are key to interpreting the implications of changes.

(a) Apparently slowing rates of increase may not reflect plateauing, much less declining, morbidity or mortality. This is because as the incidence rate climbs, the denominator on which the rate of increase is calculated becomes larger, so the rate of increase drops.

(i) There may even be need to expand prevention efforts despite a falling percentage increase in new cases.

(b) Changes or differences in percentages may reflect trends in the epidemiologic pattern(s) of other, associated diseases.

(i) For example, incidence of active tuberculosis (TB) among PWAs will reflect both the prevalence of advanced immunodeficiency in the HIV population and the prevalence of untreated latent TB infection (LTBI), which will reflect, in turn, the background prevalence of active TB in the population at large and access to TB treatment.

b. To track how HIV is spread in the United States and detect changes in transmission dynamics, the U.S. Centers for Disease Control and Prevention (CDC) categorizes the transmission risk associated with each reported case of HIV (and AIDS) using a hierarchical system that places each adult and adolescent case in a single category according to the person's whole history of transmission risk:

i) When a person's history of possible exposures indicates that s/he could have been infected in more than one way, the transmission is not classified according to either a specific exposure incident or the most frequent exposures the person has experienced. Rather, it is counted in the highest category in the hierarchy.

(1) The transmission categories for adults, in hierarchical order, are as follows:

(a) Men who have sex with men (MSM). This category includes men who report sexual contact with both men and women (i.e., bisexual men).

(b) Those who engage in injecting drug use

(c) Men who have sex with men and also inject drugs

(d) People with hemophilia/coagulation disorder

        (e) Those who engage in heterosexual contact

        (f) Recipients of blood transfusion, blood components, or tissue allograph

        (g) Those with no identified risk (NIR). This category includes the following:

            (i) Cases in persons who report no history of possible exposure

            (ii) Cases for which risk data are unavailable or have not been reported

            (iii) Cases for which epidemiologic follow-up is still ongoing

    ii) Cases in children < 13 years are classified in 2 major categories:

        (1) Those with hemophilia/coagulation disorder

        (2) Mother with, or at risk for, HIV infection

2. Counting cases of infection versus cases of AIDS

    a. AIDS morbidity and mortality have been the most consistent measures of the pattern and volume of HIV in a community because both are visible events, not dependent on whether a person sought or was offered testing.

      i) Case definition for HIV/AIDS surveillance:

        (1) The current U.S. surveillance case definition (CDC, 2008) requires laboratory confirmation of HIV infection; diagnosis of an AIDS-defining condition in the absence of laboratory-confirmed HIV infection is not sufficient to classify an individual as having HIV infection or AIDS. The 2007 World Health Organization surveillance case definition also requires laboratory confirmation (WHO, 2007).

      ii) With HAART delaying progression to symptomatic disease and AIDS, AIDS surveillance provides, at best, a decade-old picture of the epidemic. Thus, a surveillance system that monitors only AIDS is not effective. So in 1998, CDC proposed that all states track HIV infection, not just AIDS (CDC, 1999).

    b. Future AIDS incidence depends not only on HIV prevalence, but also on the epidemiology of utilization of treatment and the impact of current and future treatments on disease progression.

      i) Access, adherence, treatment costs, and viral resistance will influence use and efficacy of treatments and, in turn, their impact on AIDS incidence and mortality trends.

      ii) WHO/UNAIDS reports that $< 2\%$ of infected people are receiving antiretroviral therapy, and over 70% of those with such treatment live in high-income countries where $< 0.1\%$ of AIDS deaths have occurred (UNAIDS, 2005).

      iii) The long-term consequences, beneficial and adverse, of prolonged survival with antiretroviral regimens are not yet known.

3. Surveillance is the routine, ongoing systematic collection and analysis of epidemiologic data to detect both extent of disease spread and also changes in the trends or distribution of all aspects of the natural history of disease occurrence, including the use of resources to alter them.

    a. Both passive and active surveillance are used to monitor HIV/AIDS.

    b. Passive surveillance is accomplished through case reporting by clinicians and laboratories.

      i) Mandatory reporting systems

        (1) The Centers for Disease Control and Prevention (CDC) compile national data for the United States from aggregate reports provided without names by states and territorial health departments.

        (a) Named reporting has been a central part of AIDS surveillance since it began.

(i)   Named reporting does not preclude anonymous testing: Because anonymous test sites do not collect personal identifying information—either pretest or following a positive result—they do not have names to report.

(ii)   Surveys have shown that named reporting does not deter testing (Hecht et al., 2000).

c. Active surveillance takes place when investigators review clinical, laboratory, and other records or conduct population surveys to ascertain occurrence of health events and their sequellae.

   i)   Registries: systems of keeping a data file for all cases of a particular condition or experience in order to facilitate follow-up so that sequelae can be monitored, including disease course and interventions.

     (1)   Since 1981, the national HIV/AIDS reporting system (HARS) has provided data to track the progression of the AIDS epidemic, detect patterns of transmission, assess prevention programs, provide an epidemiological basis for planning, and allocate federal resources.

       (a)   HARS includes only HIV cases from states that follow its surveillance guidelines, which include standards for tracking that can link HIV and AIDS diagnoses, and also for verification to avert double counting (i.e., named reporting).

       (b)   Linkages between HIV registries and TB registries or between HIV and STD registries are not automatic or standard, but depend on state and local health regulations regarding use of the respective data.

   ii)   Medical record reviews

   iii)   Death certificates

   iv)   Sentinel hospital, clinic, and laboratory networks

   v)   Hospital admission and discharge data

   vi)   Aggregate insurance records

   vii)   Disease outbreak investigations

   viii)   Case finding: concerted public health search efforts to identify previously unidentified cases

     (1)   Contact tracing: efforts to identify individuals who have been exposed to an infected person

     (2)   Partner notification

     (3)   Network analysis

   ix)   Screening: efforts to detect previously unrecognized disease by offering testing to selected populations

   x)   Behavioral surveillance

     (1)   Behavioral risk factor surveillance survey (BRFSS)

     (2)   National Survey of Family Growth (NSFG) and General Social Survey (GSS)

     (3)   National HIV Behavioral Surveillance System (NHBS) started in 2002 to help state and local health departments monitor selected behaviors and access to prevention services among groups at highest risk for infection.

     (4)   HIV Testing Survey (HITS) is an anonymous periodic cross-sectional interview survey that monitors testing behaviors.

xi) Cohort studies, although not fully representative of the population of interest, provide an opportunity to measure the impact of interventions on a population over time.

    (1) Seroprevalent cohorts

        (a) With over 5,500 male enrollees in four U.S. cities, the multicenter AIDS cohort study (MACS), begun in 1983, is one of the largest prospective HIV studies in the world. It provides an observational database for the study of disease natural history and treatment outcome in real world clinical practice (i.e., outside research trials).

        (b) A women's cohort study (WIHS) was started in 1994.

        (c) The Centers for AIDS Research Network of Integrated Clinical Systems (CFAR CNICS) cohort includes 15,000 adults who started primary care for HIV after January 1, 1995 (with about 1,400 new enrollees each year).

        (d) The North American AIDS Cohort Collaboration on Research and Design (NA-ACCORD) integrates data of > 90,000 patients from > 50 sites in the United States and Canada that have been collecting data for up to 20 years (i.e., since before the multisite collaboration began).

    (2) Seroincident cohort

        (a) The European CASCADE cohort started in 1997 and follows people with a known date of seroconversion.

d. HIV surveillance has expanded from an emphasis on transmission risks to ensure ascertainment of new areas of epidemic spread, to addressing the changing epidemiology of HIV-associated illness, and to evaluating access to care and the impact of prevention and treatment interventions.

  i) The availability of effective therapies presents new public health challenges and roles for surveillance.

    (1) Epidemiological studies are important for characterizing provider and patient characteristics and identifying the factors associated with, or potential barriers to, the use of HAART.

        (a) Patient factors consistently associated with lower utilization of therapy are younger age, use of illicit drugs, and nonwhite race.

        (b) Providers' practice style, which may determine regimen switching or discontinuation and influence patient adherence, can influence HAART effectiveness within a population.

    (2) The potential effects of long-term exposure to HIV and HAART on cardiovascular disease (CVD) and diabetes are of increasing concern.

        (a) Involves examining the epidemiology of HAART complications, such as CVD and diabetes, as well as related risk behaviors and other risk factors.

        (b) So far, there is no evidence that CVD risks are reversing the major gains in quality and duration of life associated with HAART.

    (3) Heart disease and stroke are now among the leading causes of death in people with HIV, as they are in the general population not infected by HIV.

    (4) Validity data are needed to determine if risk assessment/prediction tools developed for noninfected populations are valid for the HIV-infected population.

(5) With longer survival of infected persons, there is need for age-specific mortality data.

    (a) Anticipate a rise in non-AIDS deaths from the competing risks of aging.

(6) HIV-negative infants of infected mothers in Africa experience high morbidity and mortality, including low birth weight and slow growth.

    (a) Understanding the biological and/or social bases of this association may help develop interventions that could complement programs to prevent mother-to-child HIV transmission (PMCT), such as adult HIV treatment services targeting childbearing women both preconception and antenatally.

        (i) Impact of maternal immunosuppression, advanced disease progression, and/or opportunistic illnesses on unborn and newborns is substantial.

        (ii) Reduced passive immunity from transplacental and cord blood, and nutrient and micronutrient deficiencies in breast milk may diminish infant's capacity to fight common infections.

        (iii) Higher risk of early measles has been related to low mother-to-infant antibody levels.

        (iv) Congenital infections may occur due to increased maternal shedding, which would not have been apparent in the United States and Europe before perinatal prophylaxis was available because the background coinfection burden is much lower.

        (v) Impact on infants' immune development or on their capacity for an adequate immunogenic response to vaccines is not known.

4. HIV-1 epidemiology

  a. The HIV-1 pandemic today comprises multiple epidemics that differ in scale, timing, and etiologic determinants.

    i) HIV-1 distribution is characterized by a marked heterogeneity across continents.

    ii) Even within single countries, there are mixed low- and high-prevalence populations.

    iii) WHO and UNAIDS identify three types of HIV epidemics for HIV planning purposes, and a fourth has been proposed:

      (1) Low-level: Despite its presence for many years, largely confined to groups with higher risk behaviors, HIV incidence has never reached significant levels in any subpopulation.

        (a) Prevalence has been consistently < 5% in all subgroups.

      (2) Concentrated: Despite its rapid spread in a specified subpopulation, HIV is not well established in the general population.

        (a) Prevalence: Although consistently ≥ 5% in at least one subpopulation, reflecting active networks of risk within the subpopulation(s), remains < 1% in pregnant women in urban areas.

        (b) Continuing course of epidemic will depend on the frequency and nature of links between highly infected subpopulations and the general population.

      (3) Generalized: HIV is firmly established in the general population, in which sexual networking is sufficient to sustain an epidemic independent of higher risk subpopulations that may contribute disproportionately to growing prevalence.

        (a) Prevalence: Consistently over 1% in pregnant women.

(4) Hyperendemic (proposed): Prevalence greater than 15% in the general population. In seven countries today, 1 of 5 adults is HIV-infected.

b. Transmission

   i) There has been little change in the modes of HIV transmission in the United States since the beginning of the epidemic, but the distribution of cases across risk categories and demographic groups has shifted.

     (1) Most cases have resulted from sexual contact.

       (a) From the beginning of the epidemic, men with male sexual contact accounted for the largest number of AIDS cases. Incidence of transmission declined over the first decade, but in the HAART era, annual MSM incidence rose 37%.

          (i) This increase is attributable to increasing risky behavior offsetting HAART's effect on reducing transmission.

       (b) Heterosexual contact accounts for about a third of new cases (80% of cases in women, 15% of cases in men).

       (c) Although there are no confirmed cases of female-to-female transmission, sexual transmission between women is possible.

     (2) From the beginning of the epidemic, drug abuse has played an important role in HIV transmission, and injecting drug use is currently driving HIV transmission in many areas of the world. Injecting drug users (IDUs) are at risk from sharing needles and from sex.

       (a) The majority of infection transmission among IDUs may actually occur via sexual exposure, not by sharing needles (Mathias, 2002).

     (3) Perinatal (vertical) transmission: Before effective prophylactic intervention became routine in the United States in the mid-1990s, AIDS had become the first and second leading causes of death, respectively, in Hispanic and black children under 5 years old, with the majority of deaths occurring in the first year. An estimated 1,000 to 2,000 HIV-infected infants were born each year.

       (a) After the 1994 Public Health Service prevention recommendations for antiretroviral treatment of pregnant women, perinatally acquired pediatric HIV in the United States declined by over half within 5 years. Since 2000, it has almost disappeared.

     (4) Transfusion-related HIV transmission was effectively halted in the United States following the implementation in 1985 of routine HIV antibody screening of blood.

     (5) Occupational exposure of healthcare and laboratory workers cumulatively account for about 5% of adults with reported AIDS diagnoses in the United States, although most of these persons have also reported other risk factors.

     (6) Transmission to patients during invasive procedures is rarely reported.

   ii) Adolescent girls are at higher risk of infection, in part due to sexual mixing of older men with young girls, lack of knowledge among adolescents, cultural norms that prevent women from protecting themselves during sexual activity, myths among men that having sex with a virgin can cure HIV, and adolescent female biology (greater risk of vaginal tearing in young girls).

iii) Transmission dynamics in Africa have led to a different epidemiologic profile.
  (1) Modes of transmission in Africa
    (a) Heterosexual intercourse
    (b) Perinatal mother-to-child transmission
      (i) In Africa, the absolute number of reproductive-aged women with HIV infection continues to increase.
      (ii) Breastfeeding accounts for one-third to one-half of the estimated 600,000 mother-to-child transmissions that occur each year.
    (c) Parenteral exposure from transfusion of unscreened blood and reused, un-sterilized needles
    (d) Scarification practices
  (2) Risk factors in Africa
    (a) Young age at first marriage
    (b) Young age of women at sexual debut
    (c) Large age differences between spouses and between sexual partners
    (d) Lack of male circumcision in context of high rates of sexually transmitted infections (STIs).
c. In 2000, WHO projected that the epidemic would peak in 2010, but others suggested the peak might come as late as 2030–2040. Most recently, UNAIDS (2007) estimates that global incidence peaked in the 1990s and stabilized in 2001, with downward trends in some countries, including sub-Saharan Africa, as a result of natural epidemic trends and scaled-up prevention. Overall prevalence continues to rise, although the proportion of seroprevalence is stable.
  i) Between 30 and 36 million people are living with HIV.
    (1) This estimate is 9 to 17% lower than the number estimated a year earlier (UNAIDS, 2006a, 2006b). The lower estimate does not imply a sharp decline in incidence or prevalence, however; rather it is the artifact of improved surveillance systems in some countries, especially India.
  ii) More than half of all new infections occur in 15- to 24-year-olds, and about 10% of new infections occur in children under 15.
  iii) With infection prevalence > 20% in some countries, sub-Saharan Africa is the most severely affected region of the world (Iliffe, 2006; UNAIDS, 2005).
    (1) More than two-thirds of the world's infected adults and > 90% of infected children are in this region.
    (2) Over three-fourths of AIDS deaths have occurred here.
    (3) The central reason Africa has had the worst epidemic is most likely because HIV arose there first, and did not arise in any particular subpopulation, nor did incidence predominate in any population segment.
      (a) Local epidemics of diverse illnesses, including STIs, were easily attributed to the rapid expansion of transportation over the same period and to population disruptions caused by civil strife in the decade following the birth of newly independent countries.
      (b) Characteristics of HIV disease that made silent expansion possible:
        (i) Mildly infectious

(ii) Slow, asymptomatic disease course

(iii) Manifested by multiple diseases, many of which were common in sub-Saharan Africa—so it was not perceived as a single entity

(c) It is possible that the higher rates of risk behavior that precipitated initial transmission dynamics did not persist, but the resulting high prevalence in the absence of effective treatment sustained continuing disease spread.

iv) Although 90% of European cases have been in Western Europe, the epidemic has been rising most sharply in Central and Eastern Europe since 1995.

v) In the United States, HIV incidence peaked around 1985 (CDC, 2007).

(1) The South is the only region where the AIDS rate continues to rise.

(2) The largest proportion ($>$ 80%) of reported cases is in larger urban areas.

(3) Women account for $>$ 25% new cases each year.

(a) Greater than 75% of new cases in women occur among African Americans.

(4) The disproportionately high rate of HIV infection and AIDS among black and Hispanic men, women, and children has been a constant pattern throughout the epidemic—and the disparity is growing.

(a) This overrepresentation initially reflected the higher prevalence in drug users, their sexual partners, and offspring, but it is now seen in nearly every transmission category.

(b) Although African American and Hispanic women together represent less than one-fourth of women in the United States, they account for more than three-fourths of AIDS cases.

(c) Although African Americans represent only 13% of the population, they account for about 50% of new infections.

(i) A disproportionate number are unaware that they are infected; the highest prevalence ($\sim$ 64%) of unrecognized infection is in African American MSM.

d. Mortality

i) In 1992, HIV became the leading cause of death in U.S. men between 25 and 44 years of age (which it remains for African American men).

(1) The annual HIV death rate peaked in 1995, declined through 1997, and leveled off after 1998.

(2) Over two-thirds of HIV-related deaths have occurred in people between 25 and 44 years old.

ii) In 2002, it had become the leading cause of death worldwide in people under 60, and in adults 15 to 60 years old.

(1) Mortality continued to climb steadily in most developing countries with high HIV prevalence until 2005.

iii) Declines are attributed to more people receiving antiretroviral treatment.

(1) Although HAART reduces the percentages of deaths caused by AIDS, HIV-infected persons continue to die from both HIV- and non-HIV-related causes, and there is substantial HIV-related morbidity.

(a) Contributors to HIV-related morbidity, either singly or in combination, include the following:

             (i)   Late presentation

             (ii) Late or no initiation of HAART

             (iii) Drug-related toxicities

             (iv) Coinfection, such as with hepatitis B or C virus

   (2) Potential implications of longer survival

      (a) Possible excess incidence of many diseases in the HIV population over the general or background population might occur as a result of the following:

         (i)   Long-term immunocompromise

         (ii) Coinfections, such as hepatitis C virus

      (b) Morbidity due to cumulative adverse effects of long-term antiretroviral treatment

      (c) New AIDS-defining or HIV-related illnesses may evolve. Rarer, slower developing diseases may become evident, such as lymphomas and other non-AIDS-defining cancers.

      (d) Development of strains of HIV that are resistant to currently available HIV therapy

      (e) Increasing prevalence of other exposures that could negatively impact health, such as smoking

5. HIV-2 epidemiology

   a. HIV-2 infections occur predominantly in 18 West African countries, about half of which have > 1% prevalence.

     i)   Prevalence is declining.

   b. Modes of transmission are the same, but HIV-2 is less infectious than HIV-1; mother-to-child transmission is rare. Infectiousness seems to increase as disease advances.

   c. HIV-2 is less virulent than HIV-1: Disease is milder and progresses more slowly.

REFERENCES

Centers for Disease Control and Prevention (CDC). (1999). Guidelines for national human immunodeficiency virus case surveillance, including monitoring of human immunodeficiency virus infection and acquired immunodeficiency syndrome. *Morbidity and Mortality Weekly Report, 48*(RR-13), 11–17.

Centers for Disease Control and Prevention (CDC). (2007). Cases of HIV infection and AIDS in the United States and dependent areas, 2005. *HIV/AIDS Surveillance Report,* Volume 17, Revised Edition.

Centers for Disease Control and Prevention (CDC). (2008). Revised surveillance case definitions for HIV infection among adults, adolescents, and children aged < 18 months and for HIV infection and AIDS among children aged 18 months to < 13 years—United States, 2008. *Morbidity and Mortality Weekly Report, 57*(RR-10), 1–13.

Hecht, F. M., Chesney, M. A., Lehman, J. S., Osmond, D., Vranizqn, K., Colman, S., et al. (2000). Does HIV reporting by name deter testing? *AIDS, 14*(12), 1801–1808.

Iliffe, J. (2006). *The African AIDS epidemic: A history*. Athens, OH: Ohio University Press.

Joint United Nations program on HIV/AIDS (UNAIDS). (2005). *AIDS in Africa: Three scenarios to 2025*. Retrieved March 7, 2005 from http://www.unaids.org

Joint United Nations program on HIV/AIDS (UNAIDS)/World Health Organization (WHO). (2006a). *Report on the global AIDS epidemic*. Geneva, Switzerland: Author.

Joint United Nations program on HIV/AIDS (UNAIDS)/World Health Organization (WHO). (2006b). *AIDS epidemic update*. Geneva, Switzerland: Author.

Joint United Nations program on HIV/AIDS (UNAIDS)/World Health Organization (WHO). (2007). *AIDS epidemic update*. Geneva, Switzerland: Author.

Mathias, R. (2002). High-risk sex is main factor in HIV infection for men and women who inject drugs. *NIDA Notes, 17*(2), 5, 10.

World Health Organization (WHO). (2007). *WHO case definitions of HIV for surveillance and revised clinical staging and immunological classification of HIV-related disease in adults and children.* Retrieved March 3, 2009, from http://www.who.int/hiv/pub/guidelines/hivstaging/en/index.html

1.3 PREVENTION OF HIV DISEASE

1. Prevention comprises any activity or effort undertaken to reduce the risk of an undesirable health event or process from starting, continuing, or worsening.
2. Prevention activities are directed at a range of risk factors, in other words, personal, environmental, or situational characteristics that are associated with occurrences of particular health events.
3. Prevention messages target audiences' differential information needs.
   a. It is equally important to target infected persons with a spectrum of interventions to reduce their infectiousness as targeting the uninfected to reduce their exposure and infection risk.
   b. Universal prevention activities aim to reach entire populations or subpopulations. Examples include the following:
      i) Universal blood and body fluid precautions in clinical settings
      ii) Routine risk screening as a "vital sign" for people ≥ 15 years old during medical and nursing assessments in all healthcare settings
      iii) Provider-initiated HIV counseling and testing (PICT) at primary care visits
      iv) Sex education in schools—at all levels
         (1) Sex education in schools does not result in sex at younger age and may even delay onset of sexual activity (Mueller, Gavin, & Kulkarni, 2008).
         (2) Sexual activity is more likely to be safe among those who received education compared with those who did not.
         (3) Programs that teach only abstinence are not as effective as those that include explicit information about sexual activity and risk reduction in addition to encouraging abstinence and delaying sex until marriage.
         (4) Programs that focus on pregnancy prevention and do not address sexually transmitted infections (STIs) identify activities that may allow transmission (e.g., oral sex) as safe.
      v) World AIDS Day
   c. Selected prevention activities differentially target population segments and design specific messages according to group-level variables, such as known risks. Examples include the following:
      i) Risk-based testing, including mandatory PICT for pregnant women
      ii) Incorporating primary prevention into medical care of people already infected
      iii) Incorporating HIV prevention into addiction prevention and treatment programs
      iv) Street and community outreach
      v) Peer education programs
      vi) Prevent transition to injecting drug use among both HIV-positive and HIV-negative noninjecting drug users (both never injectors and former injectors)

    vii) Relapse prevention for those who have changed risky sexual or drug use behavior

  d. Indicated prevention activities are personalized based on individual-level variables, such as the individual's specifically appraised risk or specific difficulties with particular risk situations or risk-reduction efforts. For example,

    i) Brief motivational interviewing is focused, goal-directed, client-centered, directive counseling aimed at eliciting behavioral change by helping individuals examine and resolve ambivalence.

    ii) Tailoring creates or adapts customized interventions, including teaching and counseling for a specific individual, based on data collected from the individual, including both personal goals and feedback about previous counseling or teaching.

      (1) Suggest course of action based on person's own stated perspective about recommended preventive actions.

      (2) Focus on how person has handled specific problem situations, reinforcing what succeeded and discussing alternatives to unsuccessful efforts.

    iii) Prevention case management provides in-depth, ongoing intensive counseling with specific behavioral objectives for individuals at high risk whose behavior is not being effectively influenced by other shorter term or less intense strategies.

4. Prevention interventions can be delivered at different levels of the population: individual, family, community, and system.

  a. Universal and selected interventions may be administered to individuals, groups, or in community-level campaigns.

  b. Indicated interventions can be administered individually or in groups.

  c. Community-level interventions also address social, organizational, political, and economic determinants of risky behavior, such as the following:

    i) Domestic and intimate partner violence (IPV)

    ii) Gender relations

    iii) Sex trafficking

    iv) Education of healthcare and social service professions, clergy, and so forth

    v) Stigma and discrimination

  d. Human rights aspects of prevention and treatment access

  e. Systems-level interventions

    i) Ensuring health care and social service infrastructure

      (1) STI control programs

      (2) Syringe and needle exchange programs

      (3) Testing sites, including PICT and anonymous testing

      (4) Lowering cost to purchase syringes and needles

      (5) Expanding condom availability and accessibility

      (6) Training healthcare workers and outreach workers, including peer educators

    ii) Ensuring that the introduction of new prevention methods does not inadvertently lead to complacency and disinhibit risky behavior

    iii) Church leaders have a key role in developing opinions within faith-based organizations as well as larger communities. They can have a strong influence on acceptance of people with HIV and attitudes about prevention initiatives.

    iv) Drug laws and enforcement

(1) Legal purchase of hypodermic syringes and/or needles without a prescription

(2) Arresting persons for carrying drug paraphernalia promotes sharing

5. Risk screening and prevention counseling can be incorporated in adult and adolescent primary care, and should be considered an integral component of the medical care of the following persons:

   a. Those with addictions

   b. People with active tuberculosis

   c. Those seeking contraception, fertility, or other reproductive healthcare services

   d. Women who are pregnant

   e. People with HIV infection or other STIs

   f. Those with history of possible exposures to STIs or blood-borne pathogens

6. Prevention counseling is an interactive process aimed at assisting individuals to make healthier decisions so that they can avoid acquiring and/or transmitting infection.

   a. Voluntary HIV counseling and testing (VCT) and routine provider-initiated counseling and testing (PICT) are both essential.

   i) A negative test result does not mean that a person has not been engaging in risky behavior.

       (1) Review history of potential exposures and establish risk-reduction plan.

           (a) Address possible underestimation of current and future risk due to misperception that the negative result is an indicator of low susceptibility.

       (2) If continuing potential risk of exposure exists, refer person for follow-up prevention counseling and/or for prevention risk management.

   ii) Prevention counseling for HIV-positive persons begins with and is an integral part of posttest counseling when the result is positive. It must be personalized and repeated over time as a routine part of their continuing primary care.

7. Risk screening versus risk assessment

   a. Risk screening is a brief evaluation of risk factors used to determine if a person needs counseling and testing. It can be administered by a written self-report checklist or other questionnaire, face-to-face interview, or computer-assisted interview (CAI).

   b. Risk assessment is a fundamental part of client-centered prevention counseling sessions. It involves encouraging a person to identify, acknowledge, and discuss in detail his/her personal risk for acquiring or transmitting HIV.

   i)   Use open-ended questions.

   ii) Avoid asking, "Have you ever . . . ?" Instead ask, for both risky behavior and precautions, "How often . . . ?" "When was the last time?"

   iii) Ask about partners' infection status, risk history, HIV testing history.

   c. Avoid being technical, clinical, or general. Be as concrete and explicit as possible.

8. Three levels of prevention are distinguished by their respective focus on different stages in the natural history of a disease process:

   a. Primary prevention efforts are implemented prepathogenesis and aim to avert infection, by reducing or eliminating the risks of exposure and transmission.

   i) Eliminate reservoir of infection (e.g., provide sterile injection equipment, screen blood supply, and provide safe alternatives to breastfeeding, which is the primary route of mother-to-child transmission).

ii) Biologic and chemoprophylaxis
  (1) Preexposure prophylaxis to alter susceptibility of an uninfected person (potential host)
    (a) Vaccine
      (i) To date, trials of potential vaccines have been unsuccessful and there is no promising candidate in the pipeline, suggesting that an effective vaccine is > 10 years away.
    (b) Male circumcision (surgical removal of some or the entire foreskin from the penis) reduces, but does not eliminate, risk.
      (i) Because the foreskin may be more vulnerable to traumatic tearing during intercourse, providing a portal of entry, uncircumcised men are more likely to contract virus from an infected partner.
    (c) Prevention and treatment of STIs
    (d) Preexposure prophylaxis (PREP) with once-daily administration of a long-acting antiretroviral agent or combination pill to reduce infection after exposure is being tested in Asia, Africa, South America, and the United States.
  (2) Preexposure prophylaxis to reduce the infectiousness of infected person
    (a) Male circumcision (CDC, 2007): In addition to being more susceptible to infection, uncircumcised men may also be more efficient transmitters. Lower male-to-female transmission rate compared with uncircumcised men could, however, reflect lower viral shedding from circumcised men, or it could be related to lower prevalence of ulcerative STIs in the female partners of the circumcised men studied.
    (b) Antiretroviral treatment for HIV-positive persons
      (i) During pregnancy, labor, and delivery to prevent perinatal transmission.
      (ii) An extended nevirapine regimen is being tested in Africa to reduce risk from breastfeeding.
      (iii) Suppression of viral load below 1,500 copies/ml has been shown to reduce risk of heterosexual transmission (Quinn et al., 2001).
      (iv) The relative lack of treatment access may have contributed to the rising HIV incidence in African American and Hispanic American communities since the late 1990s.
  (3) Chemical barriers
    (a) Microbicide—an antimicrobial gel, cream, or other formulation that can be applied topically into the vagina and/or rectum to kill, block, or inactivate HIV
      (i) The different mechanisms of action of the microbicides being tested include the following:
        1. Breaking down outer viral membrane
        2. Maintaining vaginal acidity (an environment not supportive to HIV)
        3. Inhibiting viral attachment to cells in vaginal wall
        4. Interfering with the process by which HIV enters cells and establishes infection
        5. Strengthening the body's natural mucosal defenses

          (ii) Other methods of administration are also being explored, such as delivering via vaginal rings or cervical barriers.

          (iii) Oral formulations may also be possible.

iii) Mechanical or physical barriers to transmission may act at exit portal(s) of an infected host and at entry portal(s) of an uninfected host.

    (1) Condoms (male or female), made of latex, polyurethane, or other synthetic material may be correctly and consistently used during intercourse and with insertive sex toys.

        (a) Condoms made of natural membranes, called skins or lambskins, are not effective barriers.

    (2) No barrier methods have been determined by the FDA to be effective protection against oral-genital or oral-anal HIV transmission. However, there is some limited protection from natural rubber latex sheets, dental dams, condoms that have been cut and spread open, and plastic wrap.

    (3) Cervical barriers that are currently used for contraception, such as diaphragms, may be protective.

    (4) Gloves for handling contaminated materials:

        (a) Although latex and polyurethane gloves are effective barriers to patient-to-caregiver and caregiver-to-patient transmission, they can be—and often are—sources of nosocomial cross-contamination.

          (i) Gloves are not a substitute for hand washing.

          (ii) Gloves must be changed between patients.

          (iii) Gloves are not routinely needed for giving bed baths or basic skin care, changing bed linens, and so forth. Wear gloves when there is visible blood, feces, or drainage.

          (iv) Personal care and personal service workers (e.g., hairdressers, barbers, cosmetologists, massage therapists, physical therapists) do not routinely need to wear gloves.

        (b) Infected and uninfected persons should cover exposed cuts, sores, and broken skin.

        (c) Plastic goggles and eyeglasses (with large lenses) and masks should be used when there is likelihood of splash.

iv) Postexposure prophylaxis with antiretroviral administration may be given within hours after exposure to interrupt process of infection.

    (1) Newborns of HIV-infected mothers without prenatal prophylaxis

    (2) Accidental occupational exposures

v) Drug treatment for opioid dependence to reduce exposure risk

vi) Cognitive-behavioral interventions address the knowledge, attitudes, decision making processes, and skills involved in reducing risk, such as the following:

    (1) Blood and body fluid isolation precautions, universally applied, to break the chain of infection

    (2) Continuum of safer sexual activity (CDC, 1998, 2000, 2006a, 2006b, 2007a, 2007b)

        (a) Abstinence

(b) Delaying age of first sexual intercourse

(c) Mutual monogamy between uninfected partners

(d) Limiting the number of sexual partners and the frequency of partner change, particularly casual partnering (i.e., liaisons, hookups) and anonymous partnering

    (i)   Know one's own and partner's status.

(e) Always and correctly using barrier protection; avoiding slippage and breakage

(f) Not sharing sex toys

(g) Using condoms with sex toys

(h) Open-mouth ("French") kissing, a potential transmission route, albeit low risk

(3) Factors that may enhance or inhibit transmission:

(a) STIs can increase the risks of acquisition and transmission of HIV to others (i.e., increase both susceptibility and infectiousness).

(b) Alterations of normal mucosal barriers, such as genital ulcers or other lesions (due to trauma or disease) on either the infected person or the uninfected exposed person may increase the risks of transmission.

(c) Mechanical contraceptive barriers may traumatize the vagina or alter the integrity of the uterine cervix.

(d) The spermicide Nonoxynol-9 enhances transmission (despite previous recommendations for its use to inhibit transmission).

(4) Ensuring informed decision making: Assess how individuals make sense of the explanations and instructions they have received from different sources, and identify and correct misconceptions. For example,

(a) Definitions of "having sex" and "casual contact" are not universal, potentially leading to risky behavior when safe behavior is intended.

    (i)   Some people, often younger people, do not consider anal or oral intercourse to be sex—either because these activities are not procreative or because physical virginity may be preserved.

    (ii) Some have misinterpreted the phrase *casual contact* to mean casual sex and infer or believe that HIV and other sexually transmitted pathogens won't be spread during a casual or one-time *hookup* (i.e., outside an established or steady relationship).

(b) People with HIV/AIDS who are taking antiretroviral treatment (or their sexual partners) may stop using condoms, accepting the reduced, but continuing, risk or erroneously thinking that taking antiretrovirals or having an undetectable viral load eliminates the possibility of viral transmission.

(c) Ineffective condom-avoidant sexual risk-reduction strategies may be adopted (e.g., withdrawal, serosorting, negotiated safety as an alternative to monogamy in established relationships, strategic positioning between discordant male sexual partners, negotiating protection strategies around partner's viral load).

      (i)   Although not so effective as consistent condom use, it is possible that a combination of these strategies could be more effective in an unprotected (*barebacking*) encounter than any one of them.

      (ii)   It is also possible that these strategies could contribute to reducing infection spread on a population level, which would depend on whether they were used to replace higher risk activity.

(5) Conception planning for discordant couples and HIV-infected women

(6) Safer needle use:

    (a) Stop injecting drugs that have not been prescribed by a medical provider, or do not start.

    (b) Seek treatment for substance abuse, and seek assistance to prevent relapse.

    (c) Always use a new, sterile syringe and needle for each injection and to prepare drug for injection; do not reuse or share.

      (i)   Use only syringes and needles obtained from a reliable source (e.g., pharmacies, syringe exchange programs).

      (ii)   If new, sterile equipment is not available, clean and disinfect used equipment by boiling or flushing with fresh, full-strength bleach—this reduces, but does not eliminate, infection.

    (d) Any item that is contaminated with blood containing the virus can contaminate all the other items. Therefore,

      (i)   Always use new or disinfected container (cooker) and new filter (cotton) to prepare drug.

      (ii)   Use sterile diluents; if not available, use fresh tap water.

      (iii)   Do not share diluents or drug preparation equipment (containers, cookers, filters/cotton).

    (e) Clean injection site with new alcohol swab before injection.

    (f) Do not recap needles after use.

    (g) Safely dispose of syringes and needles after one use.

(7) Syringe and needle exchange programs have a dual function: They not only provide drug injectors access to sterile works, but by removing used works from circulation, they also reduce the reservoir of infection.

(8) Harm reduction steps for both injecting and noninjecting drug users is an approach to prevention that meets the users "where they're at."

    (a) Although the ultimate goal is to prevent drug use, harm reduction recognizes that people change incrementally.

    (b) Expanding access to harm reduction strategies may be essential for curbing the epidemic in countries with recent and sometimes explosive outbreaks of HIV and/or HCV among drug injectors.

(9) Tattooing has not resulted in documented transmission of HIV, although it has been a mechanism for transmitting hepatitis viruses.

b. Secondary prevention efforts are implemented after infection has begun and aim to avert or delay disease progression by stopping or slowing pathologic processes.

   i)   Therapeutic vaccine to slow disease progression: Traditionally, vaccines have been used to prevent infection, but AIDS vaccine research is also investigating vaccines that would not completely prevent infection, but would improve the immune system's ability (cellular immunity) to fight HIV once infection has occurred.

    ii)   Timely access to antiretroviral therapy and other psychosocial interventions, including substance abuse and mental health treatment

    iii) Confidential partner notification, also called contact tracing, as part of infected persons' ongoing care in conjunction with assessing their continuing risk

        (1) Purpose: Notify sexual and/or needle-sharing partners of their exposure and assist them in gaining access to counseling, testing, and other secondary and tertiary prevention or treatment services, as needed (or primary prevention if contact is uninfected). This happens at two levels:

            (a) Staff from public health department notifies contact of possible exposure history, and recommends HIV testing.

               (i)   Research has found this approach to be more effective compared with self-disclosure by infected person or partner notification by clinician.

               (ii) Such notification maintains the infected person's confidentiality.

            (b) Infected person voluntarily discloses to past and current partners, who receive referral for testing. This can be done with assistance of healthcare provider(s) or other social support person(s).

  c. Tertiary prevention efforts aim to avert the complications of disease and its treatment—in other words, opportunistic illnesses and other HIV-related problems, and also adverse effects of antiretroviral agents (e.g., antiretroviral resistance, lipodystrophy, metabolic syndrome) and other interventions.

    i)   Adherence counseling and support to avert drug resistance

    ii)   Risk assessment and prophylaxis for opportunistic infections

    iii) Immunization boosters, if indicated, when immunity is compromised

9. Evaluation is an essential component of prevention programs and begins in the planning.

  a. Appropriateness: good program-to-audience match, goals based on needs assessment

  b. Implementation (process evaluation): planned activities carried out as planned

  c. Effectiveness (outcome evaluation):

    i)   Immediate: target audience remembers the message

    ii)   Short-tem:

        (1) Changes in knowledge, attitudes, and behaviors

        (2) Trends in STI rates indicative of safer behavior

        (3) Greater condom availability and uptake

        (4) Greater social support and expanded community response, including preparation of healthcare providers to provide prevention counseling and PICT, participation by schools, and so forth

    iii) Long-term:

        (1) Sustained changes in HIV/STI-related risk behaviors

        (2) Reductions in HIV transmission rates

        (3) Decline in AIDS-related mortality rates

        (4) Reduced individual and societal vulnerability to HIV/AIDS

        (5) Sustained changes in societal norms

  d. Cost-effectiveness

REFERENCES

Centers for Disease Control and Prevention (CDC). (1998). *HIV partner counseling and referral services: Guidance.* Atlanta, GA: Author.

Centers for Disease Control and Prevention (CDC). (2000). *Preventing the sexual transmission of HIV, the virus that causes AIDS: What you should know about oral sex. HIV/AIDS.* Atlanta, GA: Author.

Centers for Disease Control and Prevention (CDC). (2006a). *Fact sheet: HIV/AIDS among women who have sex with women.* Atlanta, GA: Author.

Centers for Disease Control and Prevention (CDC). (2006b). Revised recommendations for HIV testing of adults, adolescents, and pregnant women in health-care settings. *Morbidity and Mortality Weekly Report, 55*(RR-14), 1–17.

Centers for Disease Control and Prevention (CDC). (2007a). *Are you at risk?* Retrieved March 3, 2009, from http://www.cdc.gov/hiv/resources/brochures/at-risk.htm

Centers for Disease Control and Prevention (CDC). (2007b). *HIV/AIDS science facts: Male circumcision and risk for HIV transmission—implications for the United States.* Atlanta, GA: Author.

Mueller, T. E., Gavin, L. E., & Kulkarni, A. (2008). The association between sex education and youth's engagement in sexual intercourse, age at first intercourse, and birth control use at first sex. *Journal of Adolescent Health, 42*(1), 89–96.

Quinn, T. C. (2001). AIDS in Africa: A retrospective. *Bulletin of the World Health Organization, 79*(12), 1156–1158.

U.S. National Institute of Drug Abuse (NIDA). (no date). Principles of HIV prevention in drug-using populations. Retrieved September 4, 2007, from http://drugabuse.gov/POHP/FAQ_1.html

1.4 PATHOPHYSIOLOGY OF HIV INFECTION

1. Retroviruses, RNA viruses (taxonomy; Butler et al., 2007)
   a. Retroviruses can be classified into subgroups based on their pathogenic potential.
      i) Oncovirus (induces neoplastic disease in vivo)
         (1) Human T-lymphotrophic virus-I (HTLV-I)
            (a) Etiologic agent of adult T-cell leukemia (ATL), T-cutaneous lymphoma, and HTLV-I associated myelopathy
            (b) Endemic to southern islands of Japan, parts of the United States, most of the Caribbean, northern South America, and Africa
         (2) Human T-lymphotrophic virus-II (HTLV-II): not known to cause disease, but there have been reports of myelopathy and tropical spastic paraparesis in HTLV-II-infected persons (Blankson, 2008).
         (3) Human T-lymphotrophic virus-V (HTLV-V): associated with mycosis
         (4) Feline leukemia virus (FeLV): animal retrovirus found only in cats
         (5) Simian T-lymphotrophic virus (STLV): animal retrovirus found in Japanese macaque and Asian and African monkeys and apes
      ii) Lentiretrovirus (*Lentiviridae*) subgroup or slow virus
         (1) HIV type 1 (HIV-1)
            (a) HIV-1 is the most prevalent human retrovirus in the world.
            (b) HIV-1 comprises three distinct virus groups: M, N, and O.
            (c) M is the predominant (main) group, and it consists of 11 clades. These subtypes are denoted A through K.
         (2) HIV type 2 (HIV-2)
            (a) HIV-2 is primarily localized to Western Africa.
            (b) There are eight groups of HIV-2, denoted A through H.

      (3) Simian immunodeficiency virus (SIV) and feline immunodeficiency virus (FIV): animal retroviruses that are linked to AIDS-like disease in Asian macaques and domestic cats, respectively.

  b. Unique properties of retroviruses

    i)   Genes are encoded as two single-stranded RNA molecules (RNA viruses).

    ii) Transcription of genetic message is reversed: RNA to DNA versus DNA to RNA.

    iii) Reverse transcriptase enzyme is responsible for transcribing RNA into DNA.

    iv) Three common genes are *env, pol, gag.*

    v) Able to incorporate viral DNA into genome of host target cells

      (1) Incorporated retroviral DNA can be transcribed to produce exogenous budding viruses.

      (2) Internal core proteins are most conserved proteins among viruses within the group.

      (3) Envelope glycoproteins are least conserved proteins for viruses within the group.

2. Human immunodeficiency virus (HIV; Gomez & Hope, 2005)

  a. The structure of HIV

    i)   Retrovirus is slightly $>$ 100 nm in diameter.

    ii) General appearance is of a dense cylindrical viral core surrounded by a lipid envelope.

    iii) Principle components of the viral core are two strands of HIV RNA, reverse transcriptase (p51), protease (p11), and integrase (p32).

    iv) The lipid envelope contains the glycoproteins gp120 and gp41.

    v) The HIV genome contains three genes called *env, pol,* and *gag* and six additional regulatory genes called *nef, vpr, vpu, vif, tat,* and *rev.*

      (1) Env codes for gp 120 and gp 41 (precursor gp 160)

      (2) Pol codes for reverse transcriptase (RT), integrase, and protease

      (3) Gag codes for p24, p6, p7, and p17

      (4) Each of the regulatory genes code for a single protein whose name is the same as the name of the gene

  b. Two phases of HIV life cycle

    i)   Establishing infection in a host T cell (T-lymphocyte)

      (1) Attachment

        (a) Attachment occurs via binding of viral gpl20 to the CD4 surface molecule expressed on CD4-positive T-lymphocytes, monocytes, and macrophages.

        (b) HIV uses both the CD4 cell receptor and the chemokine receptors CCR5 and CXCR4 to gain entry into the cell.

          (i)   Different strains of HIV-1 have affinities for different co-receptors: (a) Non-syncytia-forming variants of HIV (NSI) bind preferentially to cells with the CCR5 co-receptors—these are the macrophage tropic strains of HIV; and (b) Syncytia-inducing (SI) T-cell tropic strains of HIV (typically found in late infection) use the CXCR4 co-receptor.

      (2) Entry

        (a) Following viral fusion with a target cell membrane, the virus uncoats and releases the HIV genome (RNA) and enzymes into the host cell's cytoplasm.

      (3) Transcription

(a) Reverse transcriptase transcribes the viral RNA to viral DNA in the host cell's cytoplasm.
   (i) Two linear strands of DNA assemble into a double-helical conformation.
   (ii) Single-stranded RNA template is degraded by viral ribonuclease H.
   (iii) Some of the double-stranded DNA join together to form a circle, while other strands remain in linear form.
(b) HIV entry into nucleus: Linear viral DNA is integrated into the host cell's DNA (facilitated by integrase enzyme), while some linear and circular viral DNA may remain in the host cell's cytoplasm. The integrated viral DNA is called the provirus.

    (4) Cellular latency
   (a) When host T cells are in a quiescent state, they serve as a reservoir for HIV.
   (b) Period of nonproductive expression of the integrated proviral DNA

ii) Active productive infection
   (1) Assembly
      (a) The infected host T cell is activated by antigens, mitogens, or cytokines.
      (b) Proviral DNA is transcribed into mRNA, which is then transported out of the nucleus into the cytoplasm.
      (c) The mRNA codons are then translated, generating polyprotein precursors, destined to become components of the viral protein core and virion envelope.
      (d) Protease modifies (cleaves) the larger polyproteins into active protein subunits (e.g., p24, p6, p7, p17, gpl20, gp4l) needed for assembly of new virions.
   (2) Budding
      (a) A virion core comprised of HIV RNA, structural proteins, and enzymes migrates to the plasma membrane of the host T cell.
      (b) The virion core buds from the host T cell's membrane, pushes itself into the extracellular space, taking with it a part of the host's cell membrane, which it uses for its own envelope.
      (c) During budding, gpl20 and gp4l are incorporated into the outer lipid membrane of the virion along with some of the host T cell's protein, which facilitates virion infection of other host T cells.

c. Differences between HIV-1 and HIV-2
   i) Absence of *vpu* gene (virulence factor) in HIV-2
   ii) Presence of the virulence factor gene *vpx* in HIV-2 genome
   iii) Amino acid sequences differ in envelope glycoproteins for HIV-l and HIV-2.
   iv) HIV-2 appears to be less virulent and may have a longer period of clinical latency.

d. Origin of AIDS
   i) HIV-1 (groups M, N, O) is closely related to SIVcpz virus found in the *Pan troglodytes,* a species of Central African chimpanzees. HIV-2 is closely related to the SIVsm virus found in the sooty mangabeys (*Cercocebus atys*), whose geographic boundaries appear to extend from Gabon and Cameroon in West Africa to as far east as Tanzania.
   ii) The emergence of HIV-1 and HIV-2 is considered to be the result of transmission of primate lentiviruses to humans (zoonotic transmission). Such transmission is thought

to have occurred as the result of hunting and dressing of infected chimpanzees and sooty mangabeys.

3. Normal immunology (Medzhitov, 2007)
   a. Cells of the immune system
      i) Types of leukocytes (white blood cells)
         (1) Neutrophils: Major phagocytic cells in the blood. They represent approximately 60% of circulating leukocytes. Production is regulated by inflammatory cytokines: GCSF and GMCSF.
         (2) Eosinophils: Participate in allergic reactions. They represent 5% of circulating leukocytes.
         (3) Basophils: Involved in early inflammatory reactions. They represent approximately 1% of circulating leukocytes.
         (4) Monocytes and macrophages (differentiated monocytes): Functions include phagocytosis, antigen presentation, cytokine secretion, and killing certain target cells. Monocytes are found within the blood and represent 5% to 10% of blood leukocytes. Macrophages are large phagocytic cells found in the brain (microglial), skin (Langerhans), spleen, liver (Kupffer), lungs (alveolar), and lymphoid tissues that participate in local immune responses.
         (5) Lymphocytes: Major participants in specific immune reactions. They represent 5% to 10% of circulating leukocytes. Postnatal lymphocyte differentiation takes place in the bone marrow (B cells) and thymus (T cells).
         (a) Types of lymphocytes
             (i) B cells are antibody-producing cells, and are one type of antigen-presenting cells. They represent approximately 10% of lymphocytes in peripheral blood, and are the major lymphoid cell in lymphoid organs outside of the blood. Antibody recognizes foreign antigens and marks them for destruction or removal from the body.
             (ii) T cells represent 70% to 90% of all circulating lymphocytes. They are found in lesser amounts in lymphoid tissues. They can serve as either effector cells or regulatory elements of the immune system. They can be identified by different surface markers (e.g., CD4, CD8, CD3). T-helper/inducer cells carry the surface marker of CD4. They secrete cytokines, such as interleukin-2 (IL-2), which help orchestrate antigen-specific immune responses against foreign materials. There are at least two categories of CD4 T cells: CD4-TH1 cells secrete gamma-interferon, IL-2, and TNF-beta and facilitate cell-mediated immune responses via activation of monocytes/macrophages and cytotoxic T cells; CD4-TH2 cells facilitate humoral immune reactions via secretion of IL-4, 5, 6, and 10. TH1 and TH2 cytokines are antagonistic (e.g., TH2 cytokine IL-10 inhibits TH1 secretion of IL-2 and TH1 cytokine gamma-interferon inhibits proliferation of TH2 cells). Cytotoxic T cells (CTLs) carry the marker of CD8 and have the ability to kill tumor cells or cells infected with intracellular pathogens (some viruses and bacteria).

(iii) Natural killer (NK) cells are neither B- nor T-lymphocytes. They represent 5% to 15% of circulating lymphocytes and kill virus and tumor targets. NK cells do not require antigen-presenting cells (APCs) to function. They attack either directly or through antibody-dependent cellular cytotoxicity (ADCC).

b. Characteristics of the immune system responses

  i) Nonspecific immunity

    (1) Physical, mechanical, chemical, and microbial barriers: skin, mucous membranes, soluble factors, and natural flora

    (2) Phagocytosis

      (a) Particle uptake by cells of the granulocytic and mononuclear (monocyte/macrophage) phagocytic lineages

      (b) Protective mechanisms against invading bacteria

    (3) Inflammatory response

      (a) Increased blood flow to site of injury

      (b) Increased capillary permeability

      (c) Accumulation of phagocytic cells

      (d) Complement system consists of 10 plasma proteins that are systematically activated during inflammatory and immune responses.

  ii) Specific immunity

    (1) Humoral immunity (B-cell involvement)

      (a) B cells secrete antibodies (immunoglobulins).

      (b) Basic structure of antibodies: Fab region (recognizes antigenic determinants); Fc region (activates complement and binds to phagocytic or natural killer cells)

      (c) B cells proliferate in response to antigen and differentiate into plasma cells that secrete a specific antibody. Differentiation is facilitated by TH2 cytokines.

      (d) Antibodies coat foreign materials (e.g., bacteria), rendering them more susceptible to phagocytosis (opsonization), and complement activation.

      (e) Generation of memory cells: Memory cells are generated at time of first exposure to a foreign antigen. Upon subsequent exposure to that antigen, memory cells are activated and facilitate generation of an immune response that is quicker, stronger, and more long-lasting than that following primary exposure.

    (2) Cell-mediated immunity (T-cell involvement)

      (a) Lymphocytes (T cells) undergo differentiation in the thymus gland.

      (b) Mature T cells have surface proteins that determine their function. The major functions of the cell-mediated responses are as follows:

        • Cytotoxicity: direct killing of tumor cells or virally infected targets

        • Delayed hypersensitivity: lymphocytes release mediators that influence monocytes/macrophages to kill pathogens post-phagocytosis

        • Memory: allows for generation of a secondary immune response

        • Control: regulation of both humoral and cell-mediated immune responses

(3) NK cells
   (a) Special groups of lymphocytes
   (b) Recognize altered structures on the surface of virally infected or transformed cells in an antigen-independent manner
   (c) Kill target cells following direct binding to altered cell membrane
   (d) Kill antibody-coated targets through ADCC mechanism; binding to NK cells is at Fc receptor

4. The immune system response to HIV infection (Burger & Poles, 2003; Zetola & Pilcher, 2007)
   a. CD4 T cells: targets for infection by HIV
      i)   If the mode of HIV transmission is sexual, HIV enters via macrophages in semen or vaginal secretions. Virus shed from the macrophages is carried to T cells via dendritic cells.
      ii) Chemokine receptors CCR5 or CXCR4 are required for target cell infection; different strains of HIV-1 have affinity for different co-receptors.
         (1) Non-syncytia-inducing (NSI) variants of HIV bind to CCR5 co-receptor and are macrophage tropic.
         (2) Syncytia-inducing (SI) T-cell tropic strains of HIV bind to the CXCR4 co-receptor and are typically found in late infection.
      iii) CD4 T cells become cellular reservoirs of latent virus early in HIV infection.
      iv) Progressive decline in CD4 cell numbers occurs over course of disease by direct and indirect mechanisms.
         (1) Decline in CD4 cell numbers may reflect effects of HIV at mucosal surfaces, particularly the gut.
         (2) HIV infection produces disruptions in gut mucosal integrity and leads to "microbial translocation" of bacteria from gut into the systemic circulation. This is postulated to lead to systemic immune activation and T-cell depletion (Brenchley et al., 2006).
      v)   There is progressive loss in proliferation and cytokine secretion by CD4-TH1 cells that promote cell-mediated immune responses.
      vi) There is excessive activation of CD4-TH2 cells that promote generation of humoral immune responses and turn off cell-mediated immune responses.
   b. CD8 T-cytotoxic cells
      i)   Increase in number during acute infection
      ii) Activated CD8 T cells are cytotoxic to HIV-infected CD4 cells with surface expression of *env, gag,* or *pol* proteins. Also are cytotoxic to uninfected CD4 T cells with surface-bound HIV envelope proteins.
      iii) Decline in numbers at time of AIDS diagnosis
      iv) Increased expression of activation markers on cell surface that correlates with stage of illness
      v)   Diminished HIV-specific cytotoxic lymphocyte activity as disease progresses
   c. NK cells
      i)   NK cells produce perforins that insert into cell membrane and create channels in the membrane resulting in cell death.

      ii) NK cells can be cellular reservoirs for latent virus. NK cells have IgGFc receptors that bind antibody attached to HIV and facilitate viral entry into NK cells.

  d. B lymphocytes

      i) Expression of activation markers on cell surfaces

      ii) Elevated levels of HIV-specific immunoglobulins in circulation

      iii) B cells differentiate into plasma cells that produce antibodies against HIV viral proteins. The major target is the viral envelope, especially gp120.

      iv) Via ADCC, antibodies facilitate viral clearance by macrophages and NK cells.

      v) Reduced specific humoral immune response to immunization is associated with late stages of illness.

  e. Mononuclear phagocytes

      i) Targets for infection by HIV

      ii) Macrophages can be cellular reservoirs of latent virus; HIV may gain entry via CD4 receptor engagement or via IgG Fc receptors in the case of IgG-coated virus particles.

      iii) Decreased migration to inflammatory stimuli

      iv) Diminished phagocytosis and bacterial killing

  f. Granulocytes: No consistent alterations reported.

  g. Lymphoid organs: main anatomical sites of early infection and clinically latent infection

  h. Follicular dendritic cells: antigen-presenting cells that help establish antibody or cell-mediated immune responses to HIV

5. The natural history of HIV infection (Burger & Poles, 2003)

  a. Primary infection (time 0)

      i) The period immediately after HIV infection of the host

      ii) Characterized by high levels of viremia and immune system activation. The viral load, if measured, usually exceeds 100,000 copies/mL and often exceeds 1 million copies/mL.

      iii) CD4 cells and CD8 cells decrease initially, but the decrease is transient and soon followed by lymphocytosis (greater than normal levels of lymphocytes).

      iv) Clinical manifestations include acute retroviral syndrome.

        (1) Occurs in 30% to 50% of people with primary infection.

        (2) Occurs 3 to 6 weeks post primary infection and lasts approximately 2 to 4 weeks.

        (3) Although most symptomatic patients seek medical consultation, the diagnosis is often missed because symptoms are nonspecific.

        (4) Common symptoms include fever, arthralgias, myalgias, lymphadenopathy, pharyngitis, anorexia, and weight loss.

        (5) Serum antibodies develop and are detectable after 2 to 5 weeks (seroconversion).

  b. Chronic infection

      i) Characterized by a decrease in the level of viremia and the resolution of symptoms associated with acute retroviral syndrome (if present)

      ii) After a period of viral load fluctuation, a balance between viral replication and immune control results in a steady state (often called the set point). After reaching the set point, the natural history of HIV progresses in the following manner:

(1) Clinical latency: a period before the development of clinically apparent disease (typically 12 weeks to 8 years). The length of time of clinical latency is largely influenced by the set point. This period is characterized by the following:
   (a) Sequestration of HIV, primarily in lymphatic tissue with ongoing viral replication
   (b) Chronic immune system activation
   (c) Continued viral spread to uninfected tissues and cells
   (d) CD4 cell count > 500 cells/mm^3 with a gradual attrition of CD4 lymphocytes
(2) Symptomatic HIV disease: a period after primary infection (typically 8 to 10 years) in which signs and symptoms of diseases associated with HIV infection begin to emerge. This period is characterized by the following:
   (a) Viral replication with increasing amount of virus detected in circulation
   (b) Deterioration of lymphoid microenvironment
   (c) CD4 cell count between 200 and 500 cells/mm^3 with a continued attrition of CD4 lymphocytes
(3) Advanced HIV disease (AIDS): period after primary infection (typically 10 to 11 years) in which the T cell count is < 200 cells/mm^3 or there is an AIDS indicator condition as defined by the CDC. This period is characterized by the following:
   (a) Failure of the immune system mechanisms to control viral replication; thus, large amounts of virus are detected in the circulation
   (b) Profound immunodeficiency, with CD4 lymphocyte counts between 0 and 200 cells/mm^3
(4) Clinical progression of HIV disease is dependent upon many factors including genetics of the host, viral virulence, and response to antiviral regimens.
(5) A small proportion ($< 5\%$) of HIV-infected individuals remain asymptomatic, showing no sign of disease progression in the absence of treatment. A greater understanding of these long-term non-progressors may yield information on how to prevent or better treat HIV disease.

REFERENCES

Blankson, J. N. (2008). *Johns Hopkins HIV guide*. Retrieved February 5, 2008, from http://www.hopkins-hivguide.org/pathogen/viruses/htlv_i_ii.html

Brenchley, J. M., Price, D. A., Schacker, D. W., Asher, T. E., Silvestri, G., Rao, S., et al. (2006). Microbial translocation is a cause of systemic immune activation in chronic HIV infection. *Nature Medicine, 12*(12), 1365–1371.

Burger, S. B., & Poles, M. A. (2003). Natural history and pathogenesis of human immunodeficiency virus infection. *Seminars in Liver Disease, 23*(2), 115–124.

Butler, I. F., Pandrea, I., Marx, P. A., & Apetrei, C. (2007). HIV genetic diversity: Biologic and public health consequences. *Current HIV Research, 5*(1), 23–45.

Gomez, C., & Hope, T. J. (2005). The ins and outs of HIV replication. *Cellular Microbiology, 7*(5), 621–626.

Medzhitov, R. (2007). Recognition of microorganisms and activation of the immune response. *Nature, 449*(7164), 819–826.

Zetola, N. M., & Pilcher, C. D. (2007). Diagnosis and management of acute HIV infection. *Infectious Disease Clinics of North America, 21*(1), 19–48.

1.5 HIV TESTING

1. Purpose of testing: HIV testing is used for both screening and clinical diagnosis, to determine if a person has been infected with HIV-1 or HIV-2, and may include quantifying the amount of virus (viral load) in a specimen.
   a. Fewer than 25% of HIV-positive people in the United States may be unaware of their infection.
   b. Three essentials ("3 Cs"):
      i) Consent: To comply with human rights principles and to ensure sustained public health benefits, testing must be voluntary.
         (1) Does not have to be written; oral assent is appropriate
         (2) Opt out versus opt in
            (a) The opt-out approach is recommended as the most effective. With this approach, individuals must explicitly decline the HIV test if they do not want it.
            (b) With an opt-in approach, individuals must affirmatively agree, at least orally, that they accept the specified test.
      ii) Confidentiality
      iii) Counseling
         (1) Pretest counseling: mandated in some states
            (a) Addresses not only HIV and related risks, but also explains testing procedures, when results will be available, risks and benefits of testing, and risks associated with disclosure of positive HIV status.
            (b) Is accomplished one-on-one, in a group, or via printed or audiovisual material
         (2) Posttest counseling
            (a) For a positive result this involves:
               (i)   Discussion of care needs
               (ii) Partner notification—informing current and previous (sexual and needle-sharing) contacts that they may be infected and should be tested.
               (iii) Education on preventing transmission
               (iv) Disclosure planning—implications of disclosures and anticipating others' responses (e.g., violence, support)
               (v)   Special considerations for pregnant women
                     1. Risk of and measures for preventing mother-to-child transmission (MCT)
                     2. Benefit to newborn of early diagnosis
            (b) For a negative result this involves:
               (i)   Explanation of window period and its implications
               (ii) Risk appraisal and risk reduction plan
               (iii) Introduction to harm reduction resources
               (iv) Referral for further prevention counseling, if indicated
               (v)   Future testing if the person has continuing experience of potential exposure
               (vi) Emphasis that periodic HIV testing is not a risk reduction or prevention plan

2. Approaches to HIV testing
   a. Voluntary counseling and testing (VCT)
      i)   VCT generally refers to a client-initiated process. The person actively seeks counseling and/or testing.
      ii) Anonymous counseling and testing occurs when the test providers (i.e., clinicians and laboratories) do not have identifying information for the person being tested, although demographic and risk history information may be collected for surveillance.
   b. Provider-initiated HIV counseling and testing (PIHCT, PICT) in healthcare facilities as a standard part of medical care, using an opt-out approach, is recommended by the U.S. CDC, WHO, and UNAIDS (UNAIDS, 2004, 2007; WHO, 2003, 2007; CDC, 2004, 2006).
      i)   Opt-out approach to routine PICT facilitates diagnosis and access to services (UNAIDS, 2004).
           (1) Testing is more likely to be accepted.
           (2) Not offering testing in the context of primary care or routine medical care may deter person from asking for test.
      ii) Training, supervision, and close monitoring of PICT programs are essential to ensure there is no coercion and to prevent adverse outcomes of disclosure.
      iii) Mandatory PICT: When effective antiretroviral prophylaxis of perinatal transmission became available, the need to integrate counseling and testing in reproductive health settings became more urgent.
           (1) Woman has right to decline the test because the mandate applies to providers, not patients.
   c. Anonymous unlinked HIV testing
      i)   May be used for research and surveillance. Blood samples that have been taken for other purposes are saved and additionally tested for HIV after personal identifying information has been removed. The test has no direct use for the individual whose blood is being tested.
   d. Mandatory testing
      i)   Screening of blood that may be used for transfusion or for the manufacture of blood products is mandatory. This testing is not anonymous. Donors who are positive are informed of the result and counseled.
      ii) Screening of donors prior to all procedures involving transfer of bodily fluids or body parts, such as artificial insemination, corneal and other tissue grafts, and organ transplant is mandatory.
      iii) Some countries require pre-recruitment and periodic HIV testing of military personnel and some require pre-immigration testing.
           (1) Such testing should be accompanied by both of the following:
               (a) Counseling regardless of the test result
               (b) Referral to medical and psychosocial services when result is positive (UNAIDS, 2004).
           (2) In November 1987, against the advice of the U.S. Public Health Service (PHS), President Reagan announced mandatory testing of immigrants and federal prisoners.
   e. Blind testing in which individuals do not know they are being tested or are not informed of the result is unethical; some states have explicit statutes outlawing this practice.
3. When to test (CDC, 2006; Frieden et al., 2006; Rietmeijer & Thrun, 2006)

a. Diagnostic testing is indicated whenever a person shows signs or symptoms of illness that could be HIV-related, including active tuberculosis.

b. Risk-based, targeted VCT

   i) Since March 1986, the CDC has recommended voluntary testing for all Americans with risks (e.g., MSM, pregnant women).

c. Routine PICT is an important complement to VCT, not an alternative.

   i) Rather than relying on individuals to seek testing themselves, the healthcare provider offers the test, explains the reason, and offers to do it.

   ii) PICT does not override the informed right of the patient to decline the provider's recommendation.

d. Benefits of integrating HIV testing into routine medical care

   i) Infected individuals who are unaware of their infection status cannot access and benefit from available life-saving, disease-delaying treatments.

   ii) Studies have found that in some areas, up to 70% of transmissions involve people who did not know they were infected.

4. Testing frequency: The frequency of testing following a negative result depends on risk behaviors.

   a. Every 6 to 12 months for people engaging in high risk behaviors is recommended, although the optimal interval for different populations has not been studied (e.g., sex workers, drug injectors, sexually active adolescents).

   b. Women should be retested as early as possible in every new pregnancy, particularly those who engage in high-risk behaviors or live in high-prevalence areas. If the results are negative at the beginning of pregnancy, women should be retested later in pregnancy and throughout the breastfeeding period if they live in high-prevalence regions or engage in high-risk behaviors.

5. HIV tests

   a. HIV antibody tests quantify antibodies to specific HIV antigens. Antibodies are usually detectable < 1 month following exposure. Most commercial antibody tests can detect the most common variants of HIV-1, as well as HIV-2.

   b. ELISA/EIA (enzyme-linked immunosorbent assay/enzyme immunoassay) may be used to test specimens of blood, urine, or oral fluid (not saliva).

      i) Antibody testing of specimens other than blood may be a practical, noninvasive option.

         (1) Oral fluid (not saliva)

            (a) Plasma-like fluid is drawn from within the gums using a small pad.

            (b) Because saliva may dilute the sample, oral tests may be less sensitive.

         (2) Urine

   c. Western blot assay—detects antibody reactivity to a specific combination of HIV antigens (gp120/160 plus either p24 or gp41).

   d. Indirect immunofluorescence assay (IFA) measures HIV antibodies in plasma using exogenous fluoresceinated antibodies.

   e. Polymerase chain reaction (PCR) amplifies plasma HIV RNA to measurable levels.

6. Interpreting test results

   a. ELISA tests are highly sensitive and able to detect antibodies at least 99.5% of the time that they are present (i.e., outside the window period). However, high sensitivity is associated with reduced specificity.

b. A specimen that is nonreactive by ELISA/EIA will be reported as a negative result. There is no need for further testing to confirm the result unless there is reason to suspect that the specimen was taken during the window period.

c. A specimen with a positive ELISA/EIA result will be retested and if it is repeatedly reactive by ELISA/EIA, it will be tested with a more specific, confirmatory test (Western blot or IFA).

d. The Western blot (WB) assay is the most frequently used confirmatory test in the United States. Different confirmation protocols are followed in some settings in low- and middle-income countries (WHO, 2004).

e. Indeterminate results may indicate that the individual is in the window period and seroconversion is incomplete. When the result is indeterminate, an IFA may then be performed on the same specimen, or the WB may be repeated in 3 to 6 months.

f. PCR tests are used to measure viral load. Because there are differences among commercially available tests, confirmatory and follow-up levels should be measured by the same laboratory using the same technique.

7. Rapid testing

a. Rapid, single-use antibody tests can use oral fluid or blood (from vein or finger stick) and produce results in 20 minutes. Positive results undergo confirmatory testing.

b. Rapid PCR results can be available within hours.

8. Consumer-controlled testing

a. With a home sampling kit, blood from a finger prick is placed on a specially treated card and sent to a laboratory. Results, along with counseling, are delivered by phone a few days later. If the result is positive, the phone counseling will include emotional support and referrals. Pretest counseling is optional.

b. Home testing that would allow the person to interpret the results at the point of testing is not approved in the United States and is illegal in many countries.

REFERENCES

Centers for Disease Control and Prevention (CDC). (2004). Voluntary HIV testing as part of routine medical care. *Morbidity and Mortality Weekly Report, 53*(24), 523–526.

Centers for Disease Control and Prevention (CDC). (2006). Revised recommendations for HIV testing of adults, adolescents, and pregnant women in health-care settings. *Morbidity and Mortality Weekly Report, 55*(RR14), 1–17.

Frieden, T. R., Das-Douglas, M., Kellerman, S. K., & Henning, K. J. (2006). Applying public health principles to the HIV epidemic. *New England Journal of Medicine, 353*(22), 2397–2402.

Joint United Nations program on HIV/AIDS (UNAIDS). (2004, June). *Policy statement on HIV testing.* Geneva, Switzerland: Author.

Joint United Nations program on HIV/AIDS/World Health Organization. (UNAIDS/WHO). (2007). *Guidance on provider-initiated HIV testing and counseling in health facilities.* Geneva, Switzerland: Author.

Rietmeijer, C. A., & Thrun, M. W. (2006). Mainstreaming HIV testing [editorial]. *AIDS, 20*(12), 1667–1668.

World Health Organization (WHO). (2003). *The right to know: New approaches to HIV testing and counseling.* Geneva, Switzerland: Author.

World Health Organization (WHO). (2007). *Strengthening health services to fight HIV/AIDS: Guidance on provider-initiated HIV testing and counseling in health facilities.* Geneva, Switzerland: Author.

CHAPTER 2

Clinical Management of the HIV-Infected Adolescent and Adult

2.1 BASELINE ASSESSMENT

1. Overview
   a. Chief complaint: HIV infection—the nurse should assess the patient's knowledge about his or her HIV infection, including risk factors, possible date or timing of infection, and client understanding of treatment options. The nurse should also assess the educational needs of the client and plan educational interventions as appropriate.
   b. The patient's coping mechanisms should be assessed. For example, is the patient having difficulty accepting his or her HIV diagnosis? Does the patient have a significant other, a support system, or both, available, and can these systems be easily accessed?
   c. The nursing team should assess the patient's HIV treatment history and experience with treatments, such as medications, side effects, and comfort level with healthcare providers, and expectations regarding treatment. The patient's previous records should be obtained when possible. The nurse should assess if the patient has any urgent questions about treatment options and plans.
   d. The nurse should help the patient prepare to discuss the short-term and long-term treatment goals with his or her primary care provider by providing reassurance and privacy during the visit and helping the client to explore his or her own treatment and healthcare expectations.
2. Health history
   a. Medical history: A complete assessment of the past medical history of the person with HIV is necessary. In addition to the patient's HIV medical history, it is also important to include other healthcare maintenance needs. This assessment includes exploration of concomitant medical problems or complaints (Bickley, 2003). General primary care and health maintenance have become a standard part of HIV care due to the aging of the HIV positive population and the associated conditions with aging, long-term HIV survival, and episodic (non-HIV related) illnesses.
   b. STD history: Because HIV can be a sexually transmitted disease (STD), the patient's history of sexually transmitted infections (STIs) should be noted. The nurse should also assess if appropriate treatment and follow-up was obtained for the condition (CDC, 2002).
   c. Surgical history: The date and outcome of any surgical procedures should be noted. The history should also include any appropriate and related laboratory results and any adverse sequelae.

d. Medication history: The health history should include a complete list of current medications including doses and frequency. Note any over-the-counter medications and nutritional supplements. Any allergic reactions or adverse symptoms experienced from medication use should be recorded. Details regarding the type of reaction (e.g., hives, rash, shortness of breath) should be noted.

e. Immunizations: The nurse must ascertain if the patient can recall or has documentation of childhood illnesses and immunizations. The patient's history of completion of all adult immunizations (i.e., diphtheria/tetanus, pneumococcal pneumonia) should be noted. Any allergic or sensitivity reactions to vaccines should be identified. Because hepatitis and HIV coinfection are increasing in prevalence and can contribute to the overall morbidity, careful attention should be paid to obtaining an accurate history of the patient's hepatitis A, B, and C status and the need for vaccinations. Currently vaccination is available only for hepatitis A and B and should be provided to HIV positive persons if they do not display serum antibodies conferring immunity.

f. Family history: The nurse should obtain a complete family history if possible. Long-term treatment of HIV infection is associated with many comorbid conditions, and care should be taken to assess for cancer, diabetes, cardiac disease, rheumatoid disease, renal disease, and other metabolic or endocrine conditions. Additionally, a complete mental health and psychiatric history of the patient should be obtained. A complete health database is especially important, because people with HIV live longer lives. It is important to continue age-appropriate health maintenance activities, such as colon cancer screening and mammography as appropriate.

g. Social history
   i)   Sexual history: A thorough sexual history is important to assess for ongoing risk factors of STIs and reexposure to HIV that might confer resistance to current treatment. The nurse should ask if the patient is sexually active and if he or she is having sex with men, women, or both. The patient's understanding of safer sex should be ascertained to determine risk-reduction education needs and to prevent further HIV transmission. Does the patient participate in other high-risk activities, such as sharing needles, self-tattooing, barebacking, or sharing of razors? Is the patient in a monogamous relationship, or does he or she have multiple sexual partners?

   ii)   Needle and blood exposure: Although all donor blood is screened for HIV and hepatitis B and C, the patient's history of blood or blood-product transfusions should be documented (the dates and reasons for transfusion should be recorded). The nurse should assess the patient's knowledge and need for education on needle safety and for implementation of any harm-reduction activities, such as needle exchange.

   iii) Tobacco use: The patient's history of tobacco use should be discussed, and if the patient is currently smoking cigarettes, the nurse should assess the patient's desire to quit and advise the patient to stop smoking. If the patient wishes to stop smoking, appropriate interventions should be determined. Additional educational needs about the risk of smoking should also be explored. Continued cigarette smoking can herald disease progression, opportunistic infections (OIs), and cardiac disease. The nurse should explore all possible psychosocial interventions and medications available to decrease or eliminate tobacco use.

iv) Alcohol use: The patient's alcohol use should be assessed, and the nurse should ascertain whether there is a history of alcohol abuse. A useful tool for screening is the CAGE alcohol assessment (Bickley, 2003). The following four questions should be asked: (1) Do you ever feel you should *C*ut down on drinking? (2) Do you get *A*ngry at others' criticism of your drinking? (3) Do you feel *G*uilty about your drinking? (4) Do you ever need an *E*ye opener to get going? A positive response to two or more questions indicates a need for further assessment.

v) Drug use: The patient's use of mood-altering substances should be assessed in a clear, nonjudgmental manner. It may also be important for the nurse to emphasize that gathering this data is for medical purposes only and not associated with legal issues. The types of drugs or substances and length of use should be documented. The nurse should explore whether the patient's use of such drugs or substances has altered the ability to perform activities of daily living, interfered with his or her responsibilities, or increased risk-taking behaviors (i.e., unsafe sexual practices). The nurse should also explore and document attempts to stop drug use, including interventions used and reasons for relapse into using behaviors.

vi) Health insurance: The nurse should assess the patient's health insurance resources and coverage. The nurse can assess whether the patient needs assistance with referrals to social services or supplemental programs, such as the AIDS Drug Assistance Program (ADAP), Medicare, or Medicaid.

vii) Travel: The patient's travel history and plans should be explored to assess whether there are risks for exposure to any opportunistic infections or a need for vaccinations or prophylactic medications for communicable disease. The nurse should also explore whether the patient requires any health education related to travel, such as safe drinking water and hygiene precautions.

viii) Exercise and sleep: The patient's sleep pattern and habits should be assessed. If the patient is experiencing sleep disturbances, causes of the problem should be explored as well as appropriate interventions. The patient's exercise routine should also be discussed to ensure that there is an appropriate outlet for stress and an adequate amount of activity given age, gender, and general state of health.

ix) Pets: The nurse should determine whether there are any pets in the patient's environment and if the pets have received recommended vaccinations. The facilities for pet hygiene and the patient's need for education about animal health should be explored (e.g., wearing face mask for cat litter box care).

x) Occupational history: The patient's current and past occupations should be discussed to assess whether there are any occupation-related health problems (i.e., injuries, risks, or problems associated with exposure to occupational hazards). Use of protective equipment and gear should be reviewed.

xi) Nutrition history: The patient's eating habits should be assessed and resources to meet nutritional needs, adequate food storage, preparation facilities, and dietary restrictions, food allergies, or intolerances should be determined. The patient's nutritional concerns or educational needs should also be explored; an HIV-knowledgeable dietician would be an appropriate resource referral.

xii) Women's health: The patient's obstetrics and gynecological history should be discussed. Previous records should be obtained, when available, to review all pertinent women's health examinations, procedures, and laboratory tests. Additional information should be obtained regarding obstetrics history (e.g., gravida and para status) and any contraceptive needs and education.

3. Review of systems (ROS) is completed at entry to the healthcare system and at the initial evaluation (Bickley, 2003). Care should be taken to ensure for patient privacy and comfort with the interview. The ROS should include, but is not limited to, a review of the following:

- General appearance, energy level, fatigue, weight changes, and acute complaints
- Skin ulcerations or lesions, itching, healing problems, alopecia, nail changes, and dryness
- Head: injuries, headaches; ears: hearing problems, pain, discharge, vertigo; eyes: blurred vision, floaters, pain, acuity problems, history of eye surgery or other conditions, last eye exam; nose/sinuses: drainage, nosebleeds, stuffiness, pain, injury; throat/mouth: gum sensitivity, bleeding, oral lesions or pain, last dental exam, difficult or painful swallowing
- Respiratory system: shortness of breath, dyspnea at rest or on exertion, sputum (color), wheezing, history of lung infection or other disease, last chest X-ray; breast: lumps, pain, nipple discharge, last mammogram
- Cardiovascular system: elevated blood pressure, chest pain, palpitations, murmurs, orthopnea, pedal edema, calf tenderness, paroxysmal nocturnal dyspnea (PND)
- Gastrointestinal system: nausea, vomiting, diarrhea, constipation, melena, flatulence/bloating, hemorrhoids, rectal bleeding, abdominal pain, irregular bowel habits, mucus in stools, history of gastrointestinal disorders (gallbladder, hepatic, or pancreatic problems), diagnostic workups (sigmoidoscopy, occult blood testing, colonoscopy)
- Genitourinary system: dysuria, nocturia, burning, frequency, urgency, incontinence, hematuria, pain, urinary infections or stones, STIs, erectile dysfunction and enlarged prostate (males), inorgasma (women), sexual interest and practices (safe sex assessment); gynecologic system: menstrual cycle, contraception history and use, discharge, dysuria, gravida/para status, abortion history
- Musculoskeletal system: myalgias, arthralgias, joint swelling or redness, injury or history of fractures
- Neurological system: syncope, headaches, seizures, weakness, parasthesias, tremors
- Psychiatric and emotional system: depression, mania, insomnia, panic attacks, anxiety, mood changes/swings, history of mental illness
- Endocrine system: increased thirst, hunger, or urination, hot flashes, cold spells, skin changes, temperature sensitivity
- Hematopoietic: fatigue, shortness of breath, bruising or bleeding, transfusion history

4. Physical examination should be completed in entirety at baseline. Ensure privacy and comfort as complete disrobing of the patient for a full evaluation is required. The complete exam should include the following:

- General examination: Include weight, height, and vital signs.

- Skin examination: Look for evidence of seborrheic dermatitis, Kaposi's sarcoma, folliculitis fungal infections, psoriasis, and dermatological manifestations of hepatitis C, such as prurigo nodularis.
- Head, ears, eyes, nose, and throat examination (includes a complete assessment of the mouth and oral cavity): Fundoscopic examination is essential in patient with advanced HIV disease. It may be appropriate to refer to ophthalmologist for detailed examination. The oropharynx should be examined for evidence of oropharyngeal candidiasis.
- Lymphatic system: Generalized adenopathy may be present in acute HIV infection. Localized adenopathy or splenomegaly may be a sign of infection or malignancy.
- Respiratory/thoracic examination: Include breast exam.
- Cardiovascular examination: Include peripheral vascular assessment.
- Abdominal examination
- Musculoskeletal examination
- Neurological examination includes a general assessment of cognitive function. Emphasis should be placed on gait, motor, vibratory, and sensory examinations because these may be altered in patients with distal sensory polyneuropathy.
- Genitourinary examination male/female: Conduct rectal, prostate, and pelvic examinations at baseline and as indicated/recommended. Carefully examine the anogenital area for evidence of STDs, such as condyloma or herpes lesions.

5. Laboratory and diagnostic evaluation: The following laboratory tests should be obtained at the baseline assessment. Previous results should be obtained to assess for clinically significant changes.

- Immunology profile (CD4/CD8 absolute and percent cell counts); HIV viral load testing (HIV polymerase chain reaction or branched DNA); complete blood count (CBC); multichemistry panel (fasting), including lipids, triglycerides, cholesterol, and glucose; urinalysis with microscopic; pregnancy testing and Papanicolaou (Pap) smear, if indicated; venereal disease research laboratory (VDRL) or rapid plasma reagin (RPR); gonorrhea/chlamydia cultures, if clinically indicated
- Tuberculin skin testing (PPD) should be completed if the patient has not had a positive test in the past. If the patient has a history of a positive PPD, an assessment of isoniazid treatment and a baseline chest X-ray should be obtained.
- The following testing should be obtained if not previously done or if records are not available:

a. Hepatitis A antibody; hepatitis B surface antigen, surface antibody, and core antibody; hepatitis C antibody
b. Toxoplasmosis, cytomegalovirus, and varicella antibody testing
c. Glucose-6-phosphate dehydrogenase level (G6PD) to ensure there are no contraindications with medications, such as Septra, which may be used as prophylaxis or treatment for opportunistic infections

- Immunizations as indicated and recommended
- Resistance testing if indicated; consider if newly or recently infected patient

REFERENCES

Bickley, L. (2003). *Bates' guide to physical examination and history taking.* Philadelphia: Lippincott Williams & Wilkins.
Centers for Disease Control and Prevention (CDC). (2002). Sexually transmitted disease treatment guidelines 2002. *Morbidity and Mortality Weekly Report, 51*(RR-6), 36–52.

2.2 IMMUNIZATIONS

1. Vaccine administration and patient education about vaccine preventable diseases (VPDs) are important nursing activities in contemporary HIV/AIDS nursing.
2. Persons with profound immunodeficiency may have impaired humoral response and may not respond to vaccines with the usual adult doses. It may be necessary to require supplemental doses to demonstrate serological evidence of protection from disease (Salvato & Thompson, 1999).
3. Live vaccines are associated with active replication of the bacteria or virus and generally should not be administered to those with severe immune deficiency. MMR (measles-mumps-rubella) vaccine is the only live vaccine recommended for persons with HIV infection who do not have immunity.
4. Vaccine preventable diseases
   a. Measles, mumps, and rubella
      i)   Measles, mumps, and rubella are three separate viral conditions that generally result in an acute systemic viral illness. Today, because of the success of childhood vaccination, complications from disease are rare.
      ii)   The MMR vaccine is commonly administered in childhood. Immunity is considered lifelong and can be demonstrated by antibody testing. Adults born before 1957 are considered immune.
      iii) One dose is recommended for those born in 1957 or later, if that person has not been previously vaccinated (a second dose of MMR may be required). The vaccine is given as a 0.5 ml subcutaneous (SC) injection.
      iv)   The vaccine is relatively contraindicated in patients who are severely immune compromised (CD4 percentage < 14) or receiving high doses of Prednisone.
      v)   Fever and rash are the most common side effects associated with this vaccine. Arthralgia and joint symptoms are reported in 25% of women and are attributed to the rubella component. Pregnant women should not receive the vaccine. Persons with a history of anaphylaxis to neomycin should not receive the rubella vaccine.
   b. Haemophilus influenzae type B
      i)   Haemophilus influenzae (Hib) is a bacterium that can cause a whole host of diseases that include, but are not limited to, meningitis, sepsis, epiglottis, pneumonia, and osteomyelitis. Bacterial infections with Hib commonly occur in children under the age of 5 and rarely cause disease in adults.
      ii)   The role of Hib vaccine in the HIV-infected adult has not been clearly established and is not currently recommended as a routine vaccination. The Advisory Committee on Immunization Practices (ACIP), however, recommends that this vaccine be considered in adults with HIV infection (CDC, 1993).

iii) The following Hib vaccines are available: ProHIBiT, HibTITER, PedvaxHIB, ActHib, and OmniHIB. Unvaccinated adults should receive one dose of one type of vaccine mentioned here. The recommended dosage is 0.5 ml, given as an intramuscular (IM) injection.

iv) Vaccine is considered safe. Swelling, redness, and pain at the injection site are the most common problems.

c. Influenza

i) Influenza is a viral illness contracted by direct contact with or inhalation of droplets. There are three subtypes of the influenza virus: influenza A, influenza B, and influenza C. Influenza A commonly affects adults and can cause a severe viral illness. Influenza B and C rarely affect adults.

ii) Influenza vaccine should be offered to all HIV-infected adults annually between September and mid-November. It is most effective when given 2 months prior to the influenza season, which, in the United States, is December. In some cases, the vaccine can be administered up to 4 months after the influenza season. Nasal spray influenza vaccine should not be used in people living with HIV infection.

iii) Patients with severe immune deficiency (CD4 < 100) may have a poor antibody response to the vaccine, providing them with little or no protection. A second dose does not improve response (Kroon, van Dissel, de Jong, & Furth, 1994).

iv) There are two types of vaccines available: whole and split vaccines. Whole-virus vaccines are prepared by using chick embryos. HIV patients can receive whole or split vaccines. Dosage is 0.5 ml given by IM injection.

v) Rare allergic reactions can occur in patients allergic to eggs and who receive the whole-virus vaccine; thus, vaccination should be deferred in patients who have documented or self-identified allergic reaction to eggs. Split-virus vaccines are prepared using organic solvents or detergents, and reaction to one of these components is rare. These vaccines can be used by people with egg allergies.

vi) Local reactions at the injection site, such as erythema, pain, and induration, can occur following vaccine administration. Nonspecific symptoms, including fever, chills, and myalgias, are reported in less than 1% of vaccine recipients and usually occur in individuals with no previous exposure to viral antigens in the vaccine (CDC, 2002).

vii) Vaccines are prepared annually and are formulated based on epidemiological forecasts. Effectiveness of the vaccine is determined by how close the vaccine matches the circulating influenza strains. Therefore, the nurse should inform the recipient that influenza can occur despite vaccination. Because of the potential for a viral illness to occur despite vaccination, the nurse should provide the patient with instructions for self-care during a viral illness. This includes information regarding the importance of bed rest and hydration, especially when febrile. Gargling with and drinking warm fluids, such as teas, will soothe the sore throat that accompanies illness, and using aspirin or Tylenol, if not contraindicated, will help relieve fever and myalgias.

d. Pneumococcal pneumonia

i) Pneumococcal pneumonia is a disease caused by the *streptococcus pneumonia* bacteria and is a common cause of hospital admission and a major cause of mortality in HIV disease.

   ii)   Pneumococcal vaccine (Pneumovax 23, Pnu-Immune 23) is administered as a 0.5 ml IM or SC injection. HIV-infected patients should be vaccinated 5 years after their initial dose.

      (1) Protection from the vaccine does not occur until 2 to 3 weeks after injection. Inform the patient that illness can occur during this period. Teach the patient how to protect from infection through such techniques as good hand washing.

      (2) Inform the patient that vaccination does not confer immunity from pneumococcal disease. At best, the vaccine has a protective efficacy of approximately 60% (DHHS, 1998).

      (3) The vaccine is considered safe; however, the recipient may complain of some mild pain at the injection site.

e. Hepatitis

   i)   Hepatitis is inflammation of the liver. Vaccines exist only for hepatitis A and B.

   ii)   Hepatitis A vaccine

      (1) The two licensed vaccines are HAVRIX and VAQTA. The recommended HAVRIX adult dose is 1,440 EL.U per 0.5 ml. The adult dose of VAQTA is 50 units in 1.0 ml. The recommended schedule for vaccination is at 0 months and then 6–12 months. Both vaccines are given as IM injections. Hepatitis A is also licensed as Twinrix in combination with hepatitis B. When this vaccine is administered, the recommended schedule is 0, 1, and 6 months.

      (2) The vaccine prompts an antibody response in only about 75% of HIV-positive patients, compared with 95% of the general population (Kemper et al., 2003).

      (3) Injection site pain, erythema, or swelling is reported in 20% to 50% of recipients. These symptoms are generally mild and self-limited.

   iii)   Hepatitis B vaccine

      (1) There are two licensed vaccines, Recombivax HB and Engerix-B. Both vaccines can be used interchangeably. However, the nurse should be alerted that for the immune-compromised patient, the recommended Recombivax dose is 40 mcg in 1 ml and the Engerix-B dose is 40 mcg in 2 ml. The recommended schedule for vaccination is at 0, 1, and 6 months. Hepatitis B is also licensed as Twinrix in combination with hepatitis A. When this vaccine is administered, the recommended schedule is 0, 1, and 6 months.

      (2) The vaccine prompts an antibody response in only about 50% of HIV-positive patients. Additional doses may be necessary to achieve an adequate antibody response. The vaccine provides protection from hepatitis B for a period of approximately 10 years (Bonacini, 1992).

      (3) Gluteal injections of hepatitis B vaccine should be avoided because immunogenicity is decreased via this route (Dolan, 1997).

      (4) Postvaccination antibody testing should be performed 30 to 60 days after the last vaccine to determine appropriate response.

      (5) The vaccine is considered safe, but fever and myalgias have been reported. The only known effect is some discomfort at the injection site. Teach the patient that application of heat to the affected area may improve vaccine-associated discomfort.

f. Tetanus-diphtheria (Td)

   i)   Tetanus is a serious disease caused by endotoxin produced by the bacillus *Clostridium tetani* that can cause painful spasms of the muscles. Diphtheria is a contagious disease caused by the bacillus *Corynebacterium diphtheriae.*

   ii)   Childhood vaccination programs generally administer tetanus in combination with diphtheria (DT or Td) or diphtheria and pertussis (DTP or DTaP). HIV-infected adults who have never been vaccinated should receive the full childhood series of three injections of Td, at 0 months, the second dose 1 to 2 months later, followed by the third dosage at 6 to 12 months.

   iii)   Adults who have received the full childhood series may be protected for life; however, in some adults protective immunity may decline over time. As a result, a booster of Td is recommended every 10 years for adults.

   iv)   The recommended adult dosage is 0.5 ml given IM, preferably in the deltoid muscle.

   v)   Local reactions at the injection site may occur, such as pain, redness, or induration. Inform the patient that a nodule may be palpable at the injection site for several weeks. The nurse must question the recipient about previous immunization. Patients should not receive the vaccine more than every 10 years. Frequent administration can lead to an exaggerated local reaction called Arthus hypersensitivity reaction. This manifests as a painful swelling from the shoulder to the elbow 2 to 8 hours after injection.

g. Other vaccines

   i)   Travel to foreign and exotic areas has become an attractive option for some HIV-infected individuals, and thus vaccination for travel is important to maintain clients' health abroad.

   ii)   Inactivated vaccines (e.g., rabies, cholera, plague, anthrax, Japanese encephalitis vaccines) can be safely administered to the HIV-infected person when required.

   iii)   Live travel vaccines (e.g., vaccinia, typhoid, yellow fever, polio) are contraindicated for persons with HIV. Persons at risk for exposure to typhoid fever should be administered an inactivated parenteral typhoid vaccine. When a polio vaccine is required for travel, the inactivated polio vaccine (IPV) is recommended.

REFERENCES

Bonacini, M. (1992). Hepatobiliary complications in patients with human immunodeficiency virus infection. *American Journal of Medicine, 92*(4), 404–411.

Centers for Disease Control and Prevention (CDC). (1993). Recommendations of the Advisory Committee on Immunization Practices (ACIP): Use of vaccines and immune globulins in persons with altered immunocompetence. *Morbidity and Mortality Weekly Report, 42*(RR-04), 1–18.

Centers for Disease Control and Prevention (CDC). (2002). Influenza. In *Epidemiology and prevention of vaccine-preventable diseases, pink book* (7th ed.). Washington, DC: Author.

Dolan, S. A. (1997). Vaccines for hepatitis A and B. *Postgraduate Medicine, 102*(6), 74–80.

Kemper, C. A., Haubrich, R., Frank, I., Dubin, G., Buscarino, C., McCutchan, J. A., et al. (2003). Safety and immunogenicity of hepatitis A vaccine in human immunodeficiency virus-infected patients: A double-blind, randomized, placebo-controlled trial. *Journal of Infectious Diseases, 187*(8), 1327–1331.

Kroon, F. P., van Dissel, J. T., de Jong, J. C., & Furth, R. (1994). Antibody response to influenza, tetanus and pneumo-coccal vaccines in HIV-seropositive individuals in relation to the number of CD4 + lymphocytes. *AIDS, 8*(4), 469–476.

Salvato, P. D., & Thompson, C. D. (1999). Clinical, virologic, and immunologic features of influenza vaccination in HIV infection. *AIDS Reader, 9,* 624–629.

U.S. Department of Health and Human Services (DHHS). (1998). *Clinician's handbook of preventive services* (2nd ed.). Washington, DC: U.S. Government Printing Office.

2.3 TEACHING FOR HEALTH PROMOTION, WELLNESS, AND PREVENTION OF TRANSMISSION

1. Health encounters with HIV positive patients should focus on the following:
   a. Self-care
   b. Relationships
   c. Staying healthy
2. Self-care
   a. Self-care is a philosophy that promotes personal responsibility through empowerment. It emphasizes psychosocial and biological balances and acknowledges the individual as a multidimensional being.
   b. Self-care requires connecting in caring relationships (Leenerts, 2003)
      i) Relationships to self
      ii) Relationships to family (defined by individual from biological to family of choice) and community (Hall, 2003)
      iii) Relationships to healthcare providers and resources
      iv) Relationships to meaning in life (Hall, 2003)
   c. HIV/AIDS care must be holistic. Treatment that focuses only on the medical condition is shortsighted and will very likely fail. Patient interaction must focus on more than lab values and medical therapy.
   d. The focus of treatment is healing (the attempt to regain balance), because HIV/AIDS has no cure. Healing may need to occur on many levels for the patient.
      i) Physical self
         (1) Physical illness has spiritual, mental, and emotional elements.
         (2) Physical illness is often a message:
             (a) Look more deeply at our needs and feelings.
             (b) Take better care of ourselves.
             (c) Be more true to oneself in some way.
      ii) Mental self
         (1) Recognize that individuals' beliefs, values, and personal philosophy may impact the treatment plan.
         (2) Do they define themselves based on those things external to them (job, status, etc.)?
         (3) What part does religion/spirituality play in how and what they think about themselves?
      iii) Emotional self
         (1) Many patients retain past pain.
         (2) Acknowledge buried feelings and repressed emotions.

        (3) Repressed feelings = blocked energy = emotional and physical ailments (Gawain, 1997)

    iv) Spiritual self

        (1) Help the individual differentiate between religious heritage and spirituality.

        (2) Explore how HIV/AIDS impacts one religiously/spiritually.

  e. Development of a wellness (self-care) plan for any patient acknowledges that HIV/AIDS is more than a physical ailment and must include all aspects of self.

  f. Skovholt (2001) identified 12 areas that should be considered in self-care: emotions, finances, humor, love, nutrition, physicality, playfulness, prioritization, recreation, relaxation-stress reduction, solitude, spirituality/religion.

  g. An individual care plan should be developed with each patient and reevaluated at regular intervals. This self-care plan helps the patient to see which areas need more focus in order to maintain balance and health.

  h. Self-care must also be addressed in relationship to an individual's culture. Providing healthcare professionals with avenues to achieve culturally competent care is especially vital amid the current effort to eliminate healthcare disparities (Hamill & Dickey, 2005).

  i. Culturally sensitive care improves health outcomes, and behavior change cannot occur until the factors that influence behavior choices are addressed (Blake & Taylor, 2006).

  j. Nurses need to remain aware of the myriad of factors that influence behavior and choices; HIV may not be a primary concern in someone's life (Blake & Taylor, 2006).

3. Relationships

  a. Healthcare providers need to evaluate their own clinical behaviors related to discussing sensitive issues that surround prevention. Failure to do so would be to provide suboptimal care and contribute to the prolongation of the HIV epidemic (Bradley-Springer & Cook, 2006; Fishman & Anderson, 2003).

    i) The nurse must evaluate his/her personal beliefs and/or knowledge in regard to sexual intimacy, in an effort to provide the patient with an environment of acceptance and openness when discussing sexual practice or preference (Blake & Taylor, 2006).

    ii) It is important that nurses develop a level of comfort when assessing sexual behaviors with diverse populations, recognizing that it is sexual behavior and not sexual orientation or identity that puts a person at risk for contracting HIV and other sexually transmitted diseases (Fishman & Anderson, 2003).

    iii) Stigma only promotes the voicelessness and suffering associated with HIV/AIDS (Duffy, 2005).

  b. Establishing and sustaining intimate relationships is often difficult for the person infected with HIV.

  c. It is important to emphasize that loving relationships can occur without sexual intimacy.

  d. Open discussion about sexuality may help the nurse discover:

    i) Beliefs about sex and love

    ii) Cultural practices/beliefs that may put the patient at risk for reinfection or other STDs

        (1) Condom use (Buseh et al., 2006)

           (a) Condom use takes that spontaneity out of sex (King, 2004).

           (b) Condom use makes sex a planned or thought-out action (King, 2004).

        (2) "Down low" (Buseh et al., 2006)

          (3) Stigma surrounding homosexuality (Buseh et al., 2006)

          (4) Open, nonjudgmental evaluation of "condomless" sex, known as barebacking

          (5) Review of harm reduction techniques

     iii) Personal beliefs/practices that may put the person at risk for reinfection or other STDs

          (1) Lack of commitment to safer sex practices (Gullette & Lyons, 2006)

          (2) Perception of risk (Brown & Van Hook, 2006)

          (3) Substance use (Robinson & Rempel, 2006)

          (4) Failure to embrace the barrier /condom use message (Griffin et al., 2006).

          (5) Use of Internet chat rooms for sexual encounters (Fields et al., 2006)

          (6) Magical thinking—"It will never happen to me" (Plowden et al., 2005)

     iv) The importance of body image and how the dysmorphic changes that occur as a result of highly active antiretroviral therapy (HAART) may impact self-esteem. The following psychosocial effects of bodily morphologic changes have been identified (Norris & Dreher, 2004):

          (1) Decline in body image

          (2) Lower self-esteem

          (3) Difficulty in social and sexual relationships

          (4) Anxiety related to disclosure of HIV status

  e. Patients often need advice regarding "how" and "when" to tell sexual partners (Gaskins, 2006; Sullivan, 2005).

     i) The following relationship factors affect disclosure (Sullivan, 2005):

          (1) Level of involvement

          (2) Degree of intimacy

          (3) Depth of relationship

     ii) Anxiety may be so overwhelming that the patients may fear that they will never again have intimate relationships.

     iii) Secrecy regarding sexual preference propagates risky behavior (down low), due to fear of being stigmatized by community (Buseh et al., 2006).

     iv) Nurses can prepare patients to disclose their serostatus by

          (1) Providing current and factual information about HIV transmission, treatment, and progression

          (2) Offering emotional support

          (3) Offering insight on how to respond appropriately to the various responses that they may encounter (Gaskins, 2006)

4. Staying healthy

  a. Health promotion for individuals infected with HIV should include discussion regarding the following:

     i) Physical activity (Clingerman, 2003)

     ii) Nutrition

     iii) Adherence

  b. Physical activity

     i) Aerobic physical activity is considered safe for 20 minutes three times per week (Nixon et al., 2002).

          (1) Aerobic exercise may have other benefits for the HIV patient, such as maintaining healthy cardiovascular status, resistance to pulmonary opportunistic infections (OIs), and healthy flow of lymph through the body (Arey & Beal, 2002).

          (2) Patients must consistently adhere to an exercise regimen to receive the protective benefits (Arey & Beal, 2002).

  ii) Patients with current OIs are at increased risk for wasting and should be encouraged to reduce energy expenditures to minimize loss of lean body mass (Arey & Beal, 2002).

  iii) The nurse must help the patient achieve balance between physical activity and rest through individualized intervention.

c. Nutrition

  i) Nutrition status is a predictor of survival and plays a role in slowing disease progression. Malnutrition is related to adverse outcomes.

  ii) Eighty-eight percent (88%) of persons with AIDS are considered malnourished. Anorexia, malabsorption, infection, or lack of access to food may cause compromised nutrition.

  iii) Nutritional intervention is indicated at the time of HIV diagnosis.

          (1) Dietary changes are difficult for patients to make and require repeated teaching sessions.

          (2) Evaluation by a registered dietician is key in this process.

          (3) Evaluation and intervention must include assessment in the context of the patient's ethnic, social, and economic circumstances.

d. Adherence

  i) Remaining healthy requires adherence to the treatment regime, including nonpharmacological interventions, that has been established between the healthcare team and the patient.

  ii) The alliance between the patient and the nurse will play a major role in promoting adherence behavior (Ramirez & Côte, 2003). In order to form such an alliance, nurses should be

          (1) Open to patients who choose not to take medication

          (2) Familiar with complementary and alternative therapies and the impact of these treatments when used in conjunction with antiretroviral therapy (Gore-Felton et al., 2003; Anastasi & McMahon, 2003)

          (3) Aware of the complexity of the treatment regime and the potential stigma associated with taking medication (Abel & Painter, 2003)

          (4) Sensitive to complaints regarding how side effects of medications impact quality of life (Abel & Painter, 2003)

          (5) Proactive in side effect management and education (Savini et al., 2003)

          (6) Aware of the unique body chemistry of each individual patient

          (7) Aware of the learning style of the patient (Abel & Painter, 2003)

          (8) Caring in every communication that they have with their patient (Abel & Painter, 2003)

          (9) Conscious of the physical health and psychological well-being of the formal/informal caregivers (Prachakul & Grant, 2003)

iii) Substance abuse has been identified as a factor that contributes to low adherence.

iv) The morphologic changes to the body may influence patients to delay or discontinue antiretroviral therapy (Norris & Dreher, 2004).

v) Low literacy may limit understanding medical instructions and adhering to treatment (Kalichman et al., 2005).

REFERENCES

Abel, E., & Painter, L. (2003). Factors that influence adherence to HIV medications: Perceptions of women and health care providers. *Journal of the Association of Nurses in AIDS Care, 14*(4), 61–69.

Anastasi, J., & McMahon, D. (2003). Testing strategies to reduce diarrhea in persons with HIV using traditional Chinese medicine: Acupuncture and moxibustion. *Journal of the Association of Nurses in AIDS Care, 14*(3), 28–40.

Arey, B., & Beal, M. (2002). The role of exercise in the prevention and treatment of wasting in acquired immune deficiency syndrome. *Journal of the Association of Nurses in AIDS Care, 13*(1), 29–49.

Blake, B., & Taylor, G. (2006). A portrait of HIV infection among men in the United States. *Journal of the Association of Nurses in AIDS Care, 17*(6), 3–13.

Bradley-Springer, L., & Cook, P. (2006). Prevention with HIV-infected men: Recommendations for practice and research. *Journal of the Association of Nurses in AIDS Care, 17*(6), 14–27.

Brown, E., & Van Hook, M. (2006). Risk behavior, perceptions of HIV risk, and risk-reduction behavior among a small group of rural African American women who use drugs. *Journal of the Association of Nurses in AIDS Care, 17*(5), 42–50.

Buseh, A., Stevens, P., McManus, P., Addison, J., Morgan, S., Million-Underwood, S., et al. (2006). Challenges and opportunities for HIV prevention and care: Insights from focus groups of HIV-infected African American men. *Journal of the Association of Nurses in AIDS Care, 17*(4), 3–15.

Clingerman, E. (2003). Participation in physical activity by persons living with HIV disease. *Journal of the Association of Nurses in AIDS Care, 14*(5), 59–70.

Duffy, L. (2005). Suffering, shame, and silence: The stigma of HIV/AIDS. *Journal of the Association of the Nurses in AIDS Care, 16*(1), 13–20.

Fields, S., Wharton, M., Marrero, A., Little, A., Pannell, K., & Morgan, J. (2006). Internet chat rooms: Connecting with a new generation of young men of color at risk for HIV infection who have sex with other men. *Journal of the Association of Nurses in AIDS Care, 17*(6), 53–60.

Fishman, S., & Anderson, E. (2003). Perception of HIV and safer sexual behaviors among lesbians. *Journal of the Association of Nurses in AIDS Care, 14*(6), 48–55.

Gaskins, S. (2006). Disclosure decisions of rural African American men living with HIV disease. *Journal of the Association of Nurses in AIDS Care, 17*(6), 38–46.

Gawain, S. (1997). *The four levels of healing.* New York: MJF Books.

Gore-Felton, C., Vosvick, M., Power, R., Koopman, C., Ashton, E., Bachmann, M., et al. (2003). Alternative therapies: A common practice among men and women living with HIV. *Journal of the Association of Nurses in AIDS Care, 14*(3), 17–27.

Griffin, R., Snook, W., Hoff, G., Cai, J., & Russell, J. (2006). Failure to embrace the barrier condom message. *Journal of the Association of Nurses in AIDS Care, 17*(4), 24–29.

Gullette, D., & Lyons, M. (2006). Sensation seeking, self-esteem, and unprotected sex in college students. *Journal of the Association of Nurses in AIDS Care, 17*(5), 23–31.

Hall, V. (2003). Bearing witness to suffering in AIDS: The testing of a substantive theory. *Journal of the Association of Nurses in AIDS Care, 14*(4), 25–36.

Hamill, S., & Dickey, M. (2005). Cultural competence: What is needed in working with Native Americans with HIV/AIDS? *Journal of the Association of Nurses in AIDS Care, 16*(4), 64–69.

Kalichman, S., Cherry, J., & Cain, D. (2005). Nurse-delivered antiretroviral treatment adherence intervention for people living with low literacy skills and living with HIV/AIDS. *Journal of the Association of Nurses in AIDS Care, 16*(5), 3–15.

King, J. (2004). *On the down low: A journey into the lives of "straight" black men who sleep with men*. New York: Broadway Books.

Leenerts, M. (2003). From neglect to care: A theory to guide HIV-positive incarcerated women in self-care. *Journal of the Association of Nurses in AIDS Care, 14*(5), 25–38.

Nixon, S., O'Brien, K., Glazier, R. H., & Tynan, A. M. (2002). Aerobic exercise interventions for adults living with HIV/AIDS (Issue 3). In *The Cochrane Library.* Oxford, UK: Update Software.

Norris, A., & Dreher, M. H. (2004). Lipodystrophy syndrome: The morphologic and metabolic effects of antiretroviral therapy in HIV infection. *Journal of the Association of Nurses in AIDS Care 15*(6), 46–64.

Plowden, K., Fletcher, A., & Miller, J. (2005). Factors influencing HIV-risk behaviors among HIV-positive urban African Americans. *Journal of the Association of the Nurses in AIDS Care, 16*(1), 21–28.

Prachakul, W., & Grant, J. (2003). Informal caregivers of persons with HIV/AIDS: A review analysis. *Journal of the Association of Nurses in AIDS Care, 14*(3), 53–71.

Ramirez Garcia, P., & Côte, J. (2003). Factors affecting adherence to antiretroviral therapy in people living with HIV/AIDS. *Journal of the Association of Nurses in AIDS Care, 14*(4), 37–45.

Robinson, L., & Rempel, H. (2006). Methamphetamine use and symptom self-management. *Journal of Association of Nurses in AIDS Care, 17*(5), 7–14.

Savini, C., James, C., & DiGuglielmo, D. (2003). Survey of patient and clinical attitudes on adherence in a rural HIV clinic. *Journal of the Association of Nurses in AIDS Care, 14*(3), 73–75.

Skovholt, T. M. (2001). *The resilient practitioner: Burnout prevention and self-care strategies*. Boston: Allyn & Bacon.

Sullivan, K. (2005). Male self-disclosure of HIV-positive serostatus to sex partners: A review of the literature. *Journal of the Association of Nurses in AIDS Care, 16*(6), 33–47.

2.4 HEALTHCARE FOLLOW-UP

1. Frequency of follow-up visits and laboratory monitoring depends on the patient's overall health status and immune function (Bartlett & Gallant, 2007).
   a. Asymptomatic patients with viral load and CD4 counts that have remained stable can be seen every 3 to 6 months for routine follow-up care unless symptoms develop or episodic illness occurs.
   b. Individuals who have had a change in antiretroviral therapy, new clinical symptoms, breakthrough in a previously stable viral load, or a CD4 count trending downward to below 200 cells/mm^3 or a CD4 percentage below 14% will need follow-up on a monthly basis until their condition stabilizes.
2. Laboratory parameters evaluated during routine follow-up visits are used to assess immune function, response to antiretroviral treatment, disease progression, drug toxicities, and evidence of opportunistic infections, new infections, or both. Additional laboratory data are collected for routine healthcare maintenance according to the patient's age and risk profile. Frequency will increase in the presence of concerns regarding drug toxicity, viral breakthrough, adherence, or a change in the patient's status (Bartlett & Gallant, 2007).
   a. The CD4 and CD8 absolute count and percentage parameters determine immunologic integrity and are evaluated every 3 to 6 months. They are repeated more frequently (e.g., every 2 to 4 weeks) if results vary from previous trends, if there is a change in drug therapy, or if levels approach those recommended for initiating or changing treatment (Kirton, 2001a). CD4 counts < 50/mm^3 do not require more frequent monitoring except in the context of monitoring antiretroviral response. The absolute count can vary considerably, even on separate specimens obtained on the same day. The CD4 percentage is less variable than the absolute count and hence a more stable marker of immune integrity (Bartlett &

Gallant, 2007; Kirton, 2001a). It is important to teach patients that the percentage and absolute counts are used when evaluating their results.

b. The viral load (VL) quantifies viral particles in the serum and is used as a measure of antiretroviral effectiveness. Ultrasensitive tests can detect viral particles down to < 50 copies/ml. When ultrasensitive tests are not available, a test that detects viral particles to < 400 copies/ml is performed. VL can be measured using either branched chain DNA (bDNA) or HIV RNA PCR methodologies. Consistency of type of test should be maintained to avoid misinterpretation of level of viremia. Concurrent illness or recent immunization can temporarily increase VL, and results should be interpreted accordingly (Kirton, 2001a).

c. A complete blood count (CBC) with differential is performed along with the CD4 count. The CBC monitors for anemia, thrombocytopenia, and other blood dyscrasias.

d. Blood chemistry testing includes, but is not limited to, evaluation of the levels of serum creatinine, blood urea nitrogen, bicarbonate, sodium, chloride, and glucose. These measures, as well as others, evaluate renal, endocrine, and metabolic functions.

e. Monitor liver functions, especially aminotransferases for individuals on hepatotoxic drugs (some protease inhibitors and nonnucleoside reverse transcriptase inhibitors), infected with hepatotrophic viruses, on lipid lowering agents, and those with alcohol abuse.

f. Monitor lipid profiles, such as total cholesterol, triglycerides, high-density lipoproteins (HDL), and low-density lipoproteins (LDL), at least every 3 to 4 months, especially in patients on protease inhibitors and nonnucleoside reverse transcriptase inhibitors. These drugs can cause dangerous increases in lipid levels, leading to pancreatitis and early coronary artery disease (Bartlett & Gallant, 2007).

g. Tuberculin skin testing should be done annually on patients with previous negative results and who are at risk for tuberculosis. Positive results for HIV patients include any induration of 5mm or greater. False negatives may occur in patients with depressed CD4 counts (Bartlett & Gallant, 2007; Talotta, 2001b).

h. Annual Papanicolaou (Pap) test from a cervical sample is recommended for routine healthcare maintenance in HIV-infected women. The CDC recommends a Pap smear every 6 months the first year after diagnosis, then annually if results are normal (CDC, 2002). Some women may require more frequent screening (e.g., those with human papilloma virus [HPV], advanced degree of immune suppression, and risk factors for new acquisition of any sexually transmitted infection). Women with symptomatic HIV or CD4 count < 400 cells/mm^3 should be checked every 6 months. Atypical squamous cells of undetermined significance (ASCUS) or low-grade squamous intraepithelial lesion (LGSIL) results require repeat Pap every 4 to 6 months. Colposcopy is recommended for women with abnormal Paps, with treatment as appropriate. Repeat Pap every 3 to 4 months following treatment of preinvasive lesions (Talotta, 2001a).

i. There is increasing evidence to support performing anal Pap smears on men and women who have had evidence of genital HPV or history of anal intercourse (Bartlett & Gallant, 2007; CDC, 2002).

j. Sexually transmitted infection testing is recommended annually or more frequently, depending on risk behaviors (Bartlett & Gallant, 2007; Kirton, 2001c). This should include a

VDRL (Venereal Disease Research Laboratory)/RPR (rapid plasma reagin) test and gonorrhea and chlamydia screening.

k. Serology testing for *Toxoplasmosis gondii* should occur annually for previously negative patients whose CD4 count drops below 100 cells/mm^3 (Bartlett & Gallant, 2007; Winson, 2001).

l. Additional testing and screening depends on patient history and presentation. Ongoing attention should be paid to age-appropriate routine health maintenance and screening, such as mammography, completion of vaccination series and annual flu shots, flexible sigmoidoscopy or colonoscopy, and prostate specific antigen levels.

3. Return visits for HIV follow-up will be built on the previously established relationships within the clinic setting. A comprehensive approach will facilitate building trust between the patient and the healthcare provider.

a. Health history taking and physical exam at follow-up visits involves exploration of any new chief complaint and a focused review of systems. Differential diagnosis of chief complaint may be guided by immune function.

b. Behavioral history taking should explore medication adherence, current mood, domestic abuse risk, sexual risk behaviors, and tobacco, alcohol, and drug use. The clinician should pay particular attention to new over-the-counter medications, herbal remedies, vitamin and dietary supplements, and therapies prescribed outside of the clinic setting.

c. Social history taking includes current travel and living arrangements, availability and interest in support networks, employment, and eligibility for assistance.

d. Patient teaching should be built on previous visits and the patient's willingness to acquire new knowledge. Because HIV disease is now considered a chronic illness, health promotion remains the emphasis at each healthcare visit. Health promotion teaching for the HIV-infected patient mirrors that of the non-HIV-infected patient.

e. Regular diet and exercise should be emphasized to minimize long-term metabolic changes often seen with antiretroviral therapy.

f. Food safety information should be reviewed with patients regularly. Food-borne illnesses are preventable and a source of opportunistic infections (e.g., toxoplasmosis) for the immune-compromised patient (CDC, 2002; Winson, 2001).

g. Review patient knowledge and practice of safer sex regularly (Kirton, 2001b). Emphasize both minimization of the spread of HIV and the acquisition of new and resistant viral strains. Discussion of family planning should be included as part of general healthcare follow-up.

h. Recommend annual eye exams with an ophthalmologist. Use Amsler eye tests with patients who have CD4 counts < 100 cells/mm^3 and those with symptomatic vision changes.

i. Recommend twice yearly dental check-ups for cleaning. Encourage ongoing daily flossing and regular brushing to minimize gingivitis. Gum disease can lead to the acquisition of new infections.

j. Although no current guidelines exist, recommending adequate calcium with vitamin D intake along with weight-bearing exercise is prudent for osteopenia/osteoporosis prevention, particularly for patients at increased risk (smokers, those with history of corticosteroid use).

REFERENCES

Bartlett, J. G., & Gallant, J. E. (2007). *2007 medical management of HIV infection.* Baltimore: Johns Hopkins University, Division of Infectious Disease.

Centers for Disease Control and Prevention (CDC). (2002). *Recommendations and reports.* Retrieved May 17, 2002, from http://www.cdc.gov/mmwr/preview/mmwrhtml/rr5107a1.htm

Kirton, C. A. (2001a). Clinical application of immunological and virological markers. In C. A. Kirton, D. Talotta, & K. Zwolski (Eds.), *Handbook of HIV/AIDS nursing* (pp. 26–42). St. Louis, MO: Mosby.

Kirton, C. A. (2001b). Risk assessment, identification, and HIV counseling. In C. A. Kirton, D. Talotta, & K. Zwolski (Eds.), *Handbook of HIV/AIDS nursing* (pp. 51–64). St. Louis, MO: Mosby.

Kirton, C. A. (2001c). Sexually transmitted diseases. In C. A. Kirton, D. Talotta, & K. Zwolski (Eds.), *Handbook of HIV/AIDS nursing* (pp. 452–465). St. Louis, MO: Mosby.

Talotta, D. (2001a). Gynecological and cervical disorders and therapeutics. In C. A. Kirton, D. Talotta, & K. Zwolski (Eds.), *Handbook of HIV/AIDS nursing* (pp. 121–149). St. Louis, MO: Mosby.

Talotta, D. (2001b). Tuberculosis screenings, diagnosis and infection control. In C. A. Kirton, D. Talotta, & K. Zwolski (Eds.), *Handbook of HIV/AIDS nursing* (pp. 110–120). St. Louis, MO: Mosby.

Winson, G. (2001). HIV/AIDS nutritional management. In C. A. Kirton, D. Talotta, & K. Zwolski (Eds.), *Handbook of HIV/AIDS nursing* (pp. 344–360). St. Louis, MO: Mosby.

2.5 MANAGING ANTIRETROVIRAL THERAPY

1. The therapeutic use of antiretroviral (ARV) medications requires a thorough understanding of the classes of currently approved drugs, appropriate combinations of classes and specific medications, and side effect management issues. Medication monitoring and side effect management are important facets of general HIV/AIDS nursing. The prescribing advanced practice nurse must have an even more thorough understanding of these important medication concepts. This section introduces the currently approved medications and the process through which antiretrovirals may be managed. Remember that this chapter provides general, introductory information and that the management of antiretroviral combinations is a complex skill acquired through knowledge and practice. The reader is cautioned that a more thorough reading about medications and consultation with an HIV-experienced clinician, as a mentor and resource, are necessary to become an expert HIV/AIDS nurse.

    a. Drug interactions: Many HIV medications affect or are affected by the cytochrome P450 (CYP) isoenzyme system. CYP isoenzymes are a family of enzymes that mediate phase I biotransformation reactions, of which oxidation is the most important. Oral medications can be rapidly inactivated by intestinal or hepatic CYP enzymes before they enter the systemic circulation. This is known as the first pass effect. Some medications and foods can induce CYP 450 isoenzyme expression and increase the metabolism of medications, whereas other substances inhibit enzyme expression and reduce drug metabolism. If metabolized too quickly, serum drug levels of antiretrovirals may decrease below the concentration necessary to inhibit viral replication. Conversely, if the CYP 450 system is inhibited by ARVs, serum drug concentrations may increase to potentially toxic levels.

2. HIV drug classes

    a. Nucleoside reverse transcriptase inhibitors (NRTIs): NRTIs are prodrugs that are analogues of cellular nucleosides. Once they're phosphorylated into the active drug, they compete with naturally occurring nucleotides for binding to reverse transcriptase and subsequent incorporation into the growing DNA chain. Because these analogues lack the attachment site for the next nucleotide, the DNA chain is terminated, thus arresting the viral lifecycle (Fischl, 2003). The first anti-HIV medication to be approved, zidovudine (Retrovir, AZT), is an NRTI. Other NRTIs include abacavir (Ziagen, formerly known as 1592), didanosine (Videx, ddI), emtricitabine (Emtriva, FTC), lamivudine (Epivir, 3TC), and stavudine (Zerit, d4T). Tenofovir DF (Viread) is usually included in this class but is in fact a *nucleotide* reverse transcriptase inhibitor (NtRTI). Tenofovir shares the same mechanism of action as the NRTIs, but unlike NRTIs, already exists in the active triphosphate form (Hoesley & Skowron, 2003). Several bi- and tri-NRTI combination medications (Combivir, Trizivir, Epzicom, Truvada) are available to reduce pill burden and promote adherence. Hyperlactatemia and potentially fatal lactic acidosis have been associated with NRTIs. Other metabolic complications including fat redistribution, dyslipidemia, and insulin resistance secondary to NRTI-induced mitochondrial damage (Bartlett & Gallant, 2007).

b. Non-nucleoside reverse transcriptase inhibitors (NNRTIs): NNRTIs bind to reverse transcriptase and inactivate its catalytic site (Demeter & Reichman, 2003). Unlike NRTIs, these drugs do not require intracellular phosphorylation to become active and do not terminate DNA chains. There is no evidence for cross-resistance between the NRTIs and NNRTIs (Deeks & Volberding, 1999). Drugs in this class include nevirapine (Viramune), delavirdine (Rescriptor), and efavirenz (Sustiva). Rashes and elevated serum transaminase levels are common side effects. Resistance can develop quickly, thus it is essential that patients understand that once they begin an NNRTI, the remaining NNRTIs will not be a future choice. Only one major NNRTI mutation (K103N) is required to confer resistance to the entire class of currently approved medications. NNRTIs, as all anti-HIV medications, need to be used in combination with other ART classes; single or monotherapy is unethical and clinically ineffective.

c. Protease inhibitors (PIs): These medications bind to the catalytic site of HIV protease and inhibit cleavage of newly formed viral precursor proteins into viral structural proteins and enzymes (Gulick, 2003). Use of PIs in combination with other classes disrupts the HIV life cycle at two different sites, and has led to significant virological and clinical improvement for many infected people (Bartlett & Gallant, 2007). Approved drugs in this class include saquinavir (Invirase), indinavir mesylate (Crixivan), ritonavir (Norvir), nelfinavir mesylate (Viracept), fosamprenavir (Lexiva), atazanavir (Reyataz), and lopinavir/ritonavir (Kaletra). Nelfinavir is contraindicated for use by pregnant women due to the presence of ethyl methanesulfonate (EMS), a substance with known carcinogenic, mutagenic, and teratogenic properties. Additionally, nelfinavir should not be a component of initial HAART regimens for pediatric patients (Pfizer Inc., 2007). Tipranavir (Aptivus) and darunavir (Prezista) inhibit replication of HIV mutants that are resistant to more commonly used PIs. At press time, these medications are approved only for those patients who are resistant to earlier PIs. Liver transaminase elevations have been associated with PI use and should be monitored closely. Other class side effects include metabolic changes including lipoatrophy, lipoaccumulation dyslipidemia, and insulin resistance.

d. Entry inhibitors: The fusion inhibitor enfuvirtide (Fuzeon, T-20) and the attachment inhibitor maraviroc (Selzentry) are classified as entry inhibitors. These medications target two distinct steps through which HIV enters CD4 cells. The first step, attachment, involves binding of gp120 to the surface CD4 receptor. This binding induces a conformational change in gp120 that exposes a second binding site that in turn binds to a chemokine co-receptor. There are two chemokine co-receptors, CCR5 and CXCR4; the virus preferentially binds to one co-receptor and is designated as either R5-tropic or X4-tropic. Binding of gp120 to the chemokine receptor induces a conformational change that exposes gp40. The second step involves the insertion of gp40 into the cell membrane that allows fusion of the viral envelope and host cell membrane (Merck & Co., 2007).

i) Enfuvirtide (Fuzeon, T-20) is a fusion inhibitor that binds to the GP-41 protein and prevents the insertion and fusion of the viral envelope and CD4 cell membrane. Currently, this medication is dosed at twice-a-day subcutaneous injections. Injection site reactions (ISRs) are problematic and are often the reason people discontinue the medication. Early success of the gas-powered Biojector injection system was thought to lead to fewer ISRs; however, in October of 2007, the drugmaker discontinued the Biojector system citing increased risk of bleeding from the injection site and increased nerve pain that can persist for up to 6 months (Cichocki, 2007). Other side effects include hypersensitivity reaction, abdominal pain, generalized fatigue, and an increased rate of bacterial pneumonia (Roche Laboratories Inc., 2007).

ii) Maraviroc (Selzentry) is a CCR5 inhibitor that is approved for treatment-experienced persons who carry only R5 tropic virus and are resistant to multiple antiretroviral medications. There are three dosing recommendations dependent upon concomitant medications and their effect on the CYP 450 system. Hepatotoxicity that may be preceded by evidence of a systemic allergic reaction has been reported.

e. Integrase inhibitors: A recent addition to the HIV medication armamentarium is the class known as integrase inhibitors. There is currently one approved drug in this class, raltegravir (Isentress). Raltegravir inhibits the activity of HIV-1 integrase, an enzyme that mediates integration of the provirus into the host cell DNA. Raltegravir is indicated for use in combination with other ARV agents for treatment-experienced adult patients with evidence of resistance to multiple other HIV medications. In addition to the common side effects of all HIV medications (headache, nausea, diarrhea), raltegravir is associated with creatinine kinase elevations and should be used with caution in persons at increased risk of myopathy or rhabdomyolysis (Merck & Co., 2007). Resistance to this drug requires only a few mutations and can happen quite quickly.

3. Prescription guidelines

a. Goals of therapy: The U.S. Department of Health and Human Services (DHHS, 2008) guidelines for the use of antiretroviral medications for adults and adolescents define the goals of therapy as (1) reduce HIV-related morbidity and mortality, (2) improve quality of life, (3) restore and preserve immunologic function, and (4) maximally and durably suppress viral load. Additionally, tools are offered to help the client reach these goals. These tools include (1) selection of combination regimen, (2) preservation of future treatment options, (3) pretreatment drug resistance testing, (4) drug sequencing, and (5) improving adherence. Nurses play vital roles in helping to attain and maintain these treatment goals, including interventions aimed at improving and maintaining medication adherence, ensuring appropriate use of resistance testing, managing HIV and medication-related symptoms, and helping the client to improve overall health.

b. Risks and benefits of therapy: Prior to starting antiretroviral therapy, the clinician and the client should perform a thorough risk-benefit assessment. Potential risks that must be considered include adverse effects of the medication on quality of life, inconvenience of life-long medication use requiring high levels of adherence to prevent emergence of resistance mutations, limitation of future drug options due to resistance, and the risk of transmission of resistant strains of HIV. Benefits to therapy, especially early therapy, include early suppression of the virus, preservation of immune function, longer period of disease-free living, and a decrease in the risk of viral transmission. These risks and benefits must also be considered in relation to other factors that may influence the decision to start medication. These factors include current level of viral activity and immune dysfunction (measured by HIV viral load and CD4 counts, respectively), presence of any symptoms that indicate immune dysfunction (e.g., thrush, recurrent severe herpetic infections) or opportunistic infections (OI; e.g., pneumocystis carinii pneumonia, or PCP), and the client's willingness or readiness to begin and maintain treatment.

c. Readiness to start treatment: One of the most important assessments prior to initiating therapy is determining the willingness and readiness of the client to begin treatment. Readiness should be established prior to writing the first prescription. Part of this assessment includes determining the client's usual lifestyle, daily schedule, and desires for treatment regimen (i.e., ease of dosing vs. strength of regimen). The medication regimen should have the highest potential for viral suppression and must also be acceptable to the client. Long-term strict adherence is required to maintain durable viral suppression.

d. Initiating therapy in asymptomatic disease: HIV clinicians differ in opinion regarding the optimal time for initiating HAART, and clinical trial data to settle the question are incomplete. In the meantime, clinicians are advised to consult published guidelines regarding the initiation of HAART. The DHHS recommendations can be accessed at http://www.aidsinfo.nih.gov/guidelines/. The goal of treatment is to achieve sustained suppression of plasma HIV RNA, a sustained increase in CD4 cells, and a favorable clinical outcome (i.e., delayed HIV progression). Most commonly, a combination of two NRTIs and a PI or NNRTI is recommended; in a PI-containing regimen, the use of ritonavir as a pharmacokinetic booster is recommended (U.S. Department of Health and Human Services, 2008). When initiating therapy, all drugs should be started simultaneously at full dose, the exception being the dose escalation regimens recommended for ritonavir (only when used as full-dose, which is rarely done) and nevirapine.

e. Initiating therapy in advanced disease: It is recommended that all persons with advanced HIV disease receive treatment with antiretroviral agents regardless of viral load (U.S. Department of Health and Human Services, 2008). Advanced HIV disease is defined as current or past history of condition meeting the 1993 CDC definition of AIDS. Additionally, HIV-infected persons without a diagnosis of AIDS but with symptomatic evidence of immune dysfunction (e.g., thrush, fever, wasting) should also be treated. When initiating HAART during an acute illness or opportunistic infection, the healthcare provider must consider all factors affecting ability to take a regimen prior to initiating therapy. These factors include, but are not limited to, drug toxicity, potential interaction with other OI therapies or medications, ability to adhere to treatment regimens, and laboratory abnormalities. HAART treatment should continue during the occurrence of an OI or malignancy unless drug toxicity, intolerance, or interactions are of concern (U.S. Department of Health and Human Services, 2008). Again, a maximally suppressive regimen, which is acceptable to the client, should be used. Care must be taken when prescribing HAART for the person with AIDS who is on multiple medications. Close assessment for potential interactions with other medications must be undertaken, and dangerous combinations of medications should be avoided.

f. Interruption of therapy: Therapy might be interrupted because of side effects of the medication, treatment fatigue, or, under certain circumstances, as a structured or supervised treatment interruption (STI). STIs have been studied in persons who have developed multiple medication resistance patterns (salvage therapy) in an effort to allow for the reemergence of HIV that is susceptible to ARV therapy. It has also been used to "auto-inoculate" infected hosts with their carried strains in an effort to stimulate immune function. Additionally, STIs have been used to decrease length of exposure to antiretrovirals. Data from the SMART study (El-Sadr et al., 2006) indicate that an interruption of more than 4 months leads to increased risk for progression of HIV, development of opportunistic infection, and greater potential for hepatotoxicity, renal toxicity, and cardiovascular toxicity. At this time, there are few data on the effects of STIs that are shorter than 4 months. If a patient elects to stop HAART, it is currently recommended to discontinue all antiretroviral agents simultaneously rather than continuing one or two agents. If short-term interruption is anticipated in the case of elective surgery, the pharmacokinetic properties and food requirements of specific drugs should be considered. This consideration is especially important in the case of drug regimens in which HIV medications have different half-lives. Detailed recommendations for specific scenarios are described in the ARV treatment guidelines (DHHS, 2008).

g. Changing therapy: There are many factors to assess when considering changing antiretroviral therapy. These factors include recent viral load levels and changes in those levels measured on two separate occasions, CD4 percentage and absolute count and any recent changes, history and physical findings, remaining treatment options, and potential for resistance already existing in the client. Additionally, similar to initiation of therapy, a thorough assessment of treatment readiness should be undertaken. This assessment is especially essential because any adherence problems that may have led to loss of viral suppression must be addressed. It is also important to determine if this change in therapy is secondary to side effects of the medications or drug failure. Side effects requiring therapy change in the presence of viral suppression allow for substitution of one drug in the treatment regimen. However, when drug failure has occurred, the clinician must rely on a thorough history of previously used medications, adherence issues, and other medications used by the client to determine recommendations for the next regimen, which will usually involve a significant change in medications and classes from those previously used.

h. The use of testing for antiretroviral resistance: Resistance testing has quickly become an invaluable tool in guiding antiretroviral therapy. There are currently two methods for testing: genotypic and phenotypic assays. Genotype assays measure drug resistance by sequencing the RT and protease genes to identify drug resistance mutations. This test is usually cheaper and quicker than phenotype testing, but interpretation of results requires an expert clinician. Phenotype assays measure the ability of the virus to grow in differing concentrations of antiretroviral drugs. Recombinant assays are available and can yield results in 2 to 3 weeks, but they still are generally more expensive than genotypic tests. Resistance assays should be performed when the person is taking ARV medications, and results need to be interpreted with the client's complete HIV medication history in mind. Currently, it is recommended to proceed with genotypic resistance testing when the client is experiencing acute HIV infection, especially if the decision is made to begin therapy. Drug resistance testing using the genotypic assay is also recommended for people with chronic HIV infection prior to initiation of therapy. When the person experiences virologic failure in the presence of HAART, genotypic and sometimes phenotypic testing is also recommended. Virologic failure can be defined as a confirmed HIV RNA level > 400 copies/mL after 24 weeks, > 50 copies/mL after 48 weeks, or a repeated HIV RNA level > 400 copies/mL after prior suppression of viremia to < 400 copies/mL. Also, testing is recommended when the client experiences suboptimal suppression of viral load after initiation of antiretroviral therapy. When a patient has had numerous drug class exposures, and is likely resistant to multiple HIV medications, the phenotypic test is invaluable in guiding selection of the best salvage regimen. Resistance testing should be completed while the client is taking his/her medication, or no later than 4 weeks after stopping HIV regimens. Finally, because amplification of the virus is unreliable at low values, resistance testing is not advised for people with plasma viral load levels less than 1000 copies/mL (U.S. Department of Health and Human Services, 2008).

i. Treating acute infection: Acute infection is defined as the postexposure time period during which the host mounts an immune response. This period usually occurs 2 to 6 weeks after the initial exposure and is often accompanied by a flulike illness, but may be asymptomatic. Patients will test seronegative during this time as antibody titers are insufficient to produce a positive ELISA; however, they will test positive for HIV RNA. Viral load is high during the acute infection period, and then declines as the host immune response begins to control viral replication. Viral load typically plateaus at a level known as the set point, which is prognostically significant. Theoretically, treatment during acute HIV infection could decrease the severity of acute disease, alter the initial viral set point, reduce the rate of viral mutation, and preserve immune function (DHHS, 2008). Whether treatment of acute HIV infections results in long-term virologic, immunologic, or clinical benefits is unknown. Treatment at this point is optional and dependent upon client readiness, ongoing symptoms, and potential for transmission.

j. Special considerations

i) The HIV-positive adolescent: Although adolescence is a period of growth and hormonal change, no evidence exists that these factors affect the use of HIV medications. Currently, it is recommended that antiretroviral dosing be based on the Tanner staging of puberty, rather than specific age. Adolescents in Tanner stage I–II should be dosed under pediatric guidelines, and those in late puberty (Tanner stage V) should be dosed using adult guidelines. Those adolescents in the midst of growth (Tanner III females and IV males) may use either guideline depending on physical characteristics, although they should be closely monitored for medication efficacy and toxicity.

Adherence can be a vexing problem for the HIV-infected adolescent. Reasons for adolescents' difficulty with adherence include (1) denial and fear of HIV infection, (2) misinformation, (3) distrust of the medical establishment, (4) fear and lack of belief in the effectiveness of medications, (5) low self-esteem, (6) unstructured and chaotic lifestyles, and (7) lack of familial and social support (U.S. Department of Health and Human Services, 2008). Treatment regimens must balance the goal of prescribing a maximally potent antiretroviral regimen with assessment of existing and potential social support systems to facilitate adherence.

ii) The HIV-infected pregnant woman: Generally, a pregnant woman with HIV should be offered the same treatment options as a nonpregnant woman with HIV. If clinical, immunological, and virological findings indicate that HAART should be initiated, there should be no delay due to pregnancy. However, an HIV-infected woman in the first trimester who is not already on therapy may wish to delay treatment until after the 10th or 12th week of gestation, assuming that the delay in treatment would not be harmful to the infected woman. Counseling for the infected pregnant woman should include information regarding the reduction of perinatal transmission through maternal antiretroviral therapy, as well as the administration of antiretrovirals during labor and delivery and to the infant after birth. Treatment of the infected pregnant woman should be monitored by an expert clinician who is familiar with changes in pregnancy that may require dosing alterations and correct medication administration to decrease the potential for perinatal transmission. Some ARVs may be harmful to mother or infant and should be used with extreme caution or avoided. The agents include (1) efavirenz, which is teratogenic, (2) combination of ddI and D4T due to reports of fatal and serious lactic acidosis with hepatic steatosis and/or pancreatitis, and (3) nevirapine, which has been associated with a 12-fold increased risk of hepatotoxicity in women whose CD4 cells counts are > 250 cells/mm^3. Clinicians caring for HIV-infected pregnant women are encouraged to report cases of prenatal exposure to ARV drugs to the Antiretroviral Pregnancy Registry (DHHS, 2008).

2. Adherence to prescribed regimens
   a. Overview of adherence to medication regimens in chronic disease: The concept of adherence was studied in other chronic illnesses before complex HIV therapies came into existence. Research examining adherence to medications for hypertension, asthma, diabetes, and congestive heart failure revealed adherence rates from 20% to 70%, with an average of approximately 50% (McDermott, Schmitt, & Wallner, 1997; Rand & Wise, 1994; Shaw, Anderson, Maloney, Jay, & Fagan, 1995). Typically, these studies defined adherence as correctly taking at least 80% of the prescribed doses. This level of adherence, though appropriate for other chronic illnesses, is clearly not at the 90–95% range required for continued HIV suppression (Paterson, Swindells, Mohr, et al., 2000). Studies of self-reported adherence to HIV medication regimens clearly reveal suboptimal self-medicating behavior. Data from the Adult AIDS Clinical Trials Group (AACTG) revealed low adherence in a representative national sample ($n = 75$). Ten centers throughout the United States administered the AACTG self-report adherence questionnaires to patients taking combination antiretroviral therapy, including at least one protease inhibitor (Chesney et al., 2000). Re-

sults indicated that 11% of patients reported missing at least one ART dose the day before the interview, and 17% (13) reported missing at least one dose during the prior 2 days. Of those reporting missed doses during the prior 2 days, 11 of 13 noted that their PI was the medication missed. In fact, these 13 nonadherent subjects skipped between 10% and 65% of their pills, with a median of 18% skipped. Clearly, people are having difficulty maintaining adherence to HAART, especially at the level necessary to maintain long-term viral suppression.

b. Client challenges to adherence: Factors associated with an individual's ability to adhere to a prescribed regimen are multifaceted and multidimensional. Included are client characteristics (e.g., psychosocial factors, substance use, sociodemographics), medication regimen factors (e.g., number of doses, complexity of regimen, medication side effects), client-provider relationship factors (e.g., client perception of provider communication, client's overall satisfaction with provider), disease factors (e.g., immunologic factors, symptomatology), and setting factors (clinical environment, confidentiality; Ickovics & Meisler, 1997). More than one factor might be exerting control on adherence at any given time. Additionally, these factors may hold differing levels of importance to any one individual (Crespo-Fierro, 1997). Any assumption on the part of a healthcare provider regarding a person's potential for adherence based on only one factor is myopic. It is important to remember that although overall factors suggesting problems with adherence may be determined, an assessment of the individual's unique potential for adherence is necessary.

c. The healthcare provider and adherence: It is important that healthcare providers do not make recommendations for treatment or to withhold treatment based on preconceived notions of what affects an individual's ability to adhere. This is especially true for clients who may have a history or may currently be using illicit drugs. An assessment of the individual nature of adherence for the drug-using client is necessary. Because adherence is multifaceted, a thorough evaluation of all life factors of the drug-using client should be considered in assessing readiness for HAART.

Another important aspect for the healthcare provider's consideration is the development of a trusting relationship with the client. This trusting relationship may be fostered through the provider's use of a harm reduction approach. The healthcare provider may also wish to explore other nonmedical model methods for assisting with adherence, such as the health belief model, transtheoretical model, or the theory of reasoned action (Glanz, Lewis, & Rimer, 2002).

d. Evidence-based strategies to enhance adherence: Although studies that examine strategies to improve adherence in HIV disease are ongoing, the U.S. Department of Health and Human Services (2008) does make recommendations based on the current literature regarding HIV medication adherence and adherence in other chronic illnesses. These recommendations include the following: (1) assessing client readiness to undertake ARV therapy; (2) providing education on medication dosing; (3) reviewing potential side effects; (4) anticipating and treating side effects; (5) utilizing educational aids including pictures, pillboxes, and calendars; (6) engaging family and friends; (7) to the extent possible, simplifying the regimen, dosing, and food requirements; (8) utilizing a multidisciplinary team approach; and (9) providing an accessible, trusting healthcare team. It is important to remember that it may take multiple encounters to negotiate a treatment plan that the client understands and finds acceptable. This process includes education regarding the goals of therapy and the importance of adherence. An adherence care plan should be developed, including concrete plans for specific regimens in relation to meals, daily activities, and side effects. Often reminder tools may be helpful, such as a daily written schedule that includes pictures of medications, pillboxes, alarm clocks, and pagers. Trials of medication schedules using jellybeans may also be helpful in identifying adherence issues to prevent the development of resistance if using real medications.

Nurses, physicians, pharmacists, case managers, peer educators, and other support personnel should all be considered when developing a team approach to adherence education and intervention. The adherence or treatment maintenance message should be provided by the entire healthcare team.

e. Theoretical models for behavior change

   i) The transtheoretical model: This model is so named because it incorporates elements from a number of psychotherapy and behavior change theories into its structure (Prochaska & Velecir, 1997). The major premise is that people progress through a series of stages when they attempt to change behavior. The first three stages (precontemplation, contemplation, and preparation) are stages in which the person is not yet ready to take the actual behavior change action, but may have begun preparations toward taking the action. Healthcare providers can intervene even when a person is not yet ready to undergo the actual behavior change by assisting in movement toward that healthier behavior. To ask persons to undergo a behavior change when they are not in the action phase of the model will result in failure. Related to HIV medications, an assessment of the stage of change might help prevent initiating HAART in a person who is not ready. If a person is not ready for HAART, nurses can develop interventions to assist the individual to move toward readiness for action. Interestingly, relapse, or a return to the unhealthy behavior, is addressed in this model as a part of the human change process. Thus, periods of nonadherence to HIV medications are expected as part of the human change process; a plan for return to adherent medication behavior is an important part of this model.

   ii) The harm reduction model: The harm reduction model was developed in Europe and the Netherlands to target injection drug use behavior. Harm reduction can be thought of as a philosophy of care rather than a true model. In this philosophy, health behaviors are thought of as beneficial, neutral, or harmful. The goal is to decrease the number of harmful behaviors and increase the number of beneficial behaviors. Inherent in this philosophy is the belief that although a person might not be able to completely remove all harmful behaviors, any reduction in these behaviors is beneficial. Thus, an injection drug user may be able to reduce potential harmful outcomes, such as HIV or hepatitis infection, by participating in a needle exchange program (Denning, Little, & Glickman, 2004). Application of the model to HIV-medication adherence does not mean that it is appropriate to encourage people to take medications when they are able or that taking medications some of the time is more beneficial than taking no medications. In fact, it is known that partial dosing encourages the development of drug-resistant viral mutations. However, the model might be applied to other medication-related factors. For example, if the client needs to take medication with a high-fat meal, but is able to do this only one time a day instead of two, the addition of a snack at the second dosing may improve absorption without requiring an entire meal. This model allows for the inability to follow instructions to the exact specifications.

iii) The Freirean approach: Developed in the 1970s by the Brazilian educator Paulo Freirean, this approach stresses the importance of considering racism, sexism, the exploitation of workers, and other forms of oppression in the development of curricula. Freirean suggests that any curriculum that does not consider these important variables supports the status quo or unequal distribution of power. He suggests that practical and expedient interests play a determining role in education (Heaney, 1995). Application of this approach to HIV-medication adherence would mean that power distribution in society affects individual power and the ability to be adherent to medications. Unequal societal distribution of power (i.e., oppression of some) affects an individual's ability to maintain drug adherence. It would be imperative then to consider these larger environmental and social factors when assessing an individual's potential for adherence.

iv) Other models: Other models may be helpful in understanding adherence issues and planning for adherence interventions. These include, but are not limited to, the health belief model, the theory of reasoned action, and the theory of planned behavior. Additionally, the model of adherence factors offered by Ickovics and Meisler (1997) is specific to HIV-medication-taking behavior and can be especially useful.

REFERENCES

Bartlett, J. G., & Gallant, J. E. (2007). *2007 medical management of HIV infection.* Baltimore: Johns Hopkins Medicine.

Cichocki, M. (2007, October 4). *Trimeris decides not to pursue needleless injection system for Fuzeon.* Retrieved October 28, 2007, from http://aids.about.com/b/a/257596.htm

Chesney, M. A., Ickovics, J. R., Chambers, D. B., Gifford, A. L., Neidig, J., Zwickl, B., et al. (2000). Self-reported adherence to antiretroviral medications among participants in HIV clinical trials: The AACTG adherence instruments. Patient Care Committee & Adherence Working Group of the Outcomes Committee of the Adult AIDS Clinical Trials Group (AACTG). *AIDS Care, 12*(3), 255–266.

Crespo-Fierro, M. (1997). Compliance/adherence and care management in HIV disease. *Journal of the Association of Nurses in AIDS Care, 8*(4), 43–54.

Deeks, S. G., & Volberding, P. A. (1999). Antiretroviral therapy for HIV disease. In P. T. Cohen, M. A. Sande, & P. A. Volberding (Eds.), *The AIDS knowledge base* (3rd ed., pp. 241–260). New York: Lippincott Williams & Wilkins.

Demeter, L. M., & Reichman, R. C. (2003). Delavirdine. In R. Dolin, H. Masur, & M. S. Saag (Eds.), *AIDS therapy* (2nd ed., pp. 122–133). New York: Churchill Livingstone.

Denning, J., Little, J., & Glickman, A. (2004). *Over the influence: The harm reduction guide for managing drugs and alcohol.* New York: Guilford Press.

El-Sadr, W. M., Lundgren, J. D., Neaton, J. D., Gordin, F., Abrams, D., Arduino, R. C., et al. (2006). CD4+ count-guided interruption of antiretroviral treatment. *New England Journal of Medicine, 355*(22), 2283–2296.

Fischl, M. A. (2003). Zidovudine. In R. Dolin, H. Masur, & M. S. Saag (Eds.), *AIDS therapy* (2nd ed., pp. 23–39). New York: Churchill Livingstone.

Glanz, K., Lewis, F. M., & Rimer, B. K. (2002). *Health behavior and health education: Theory, research and practice* (3rd ed.). San Francisco: Jossey-Bass.

Gulick, R. (2003). Indinavir. In R. Dolin, H. Masur, & M. S. Saag (Eds.), *AIDS therapy* (2nd ed., pp. 190–211). New York: Churchill Livingstone.

Heaney, T. (1995). Issues in Freirean pedagogy. *Thresholds in education.* Retrieved August 1, 2002, from http://nlu.nl.edu/ace/Resources/Documents/FreireIssues.html

Hoesley, C. J., & Skowron, G. (2003). Tenofovir disoproxil fumarate. In R. Dolin, H. Masur, & M. S. Saag (Eds.), *AIDS therapy* (2nd ed., pp. 245–252). New York: Churchill Livingstone.

Ickovics, J. R., & Meisler, A. W. (1997). Adherence in AIDS clinical trials: A framework for clinical research and clinical care. *Journal of Clinical Epidemiology, 50*(4), 385–391.

McDermott, M. M., Schmitt, B., & Wallner, E. (1997). Impact of medication nonadherence on coronary heart disease outcomes: A critical review. *Archives of Internal Medicine, 157*(17), 1921–1929.

Merck & Co., Inc. (2007, October). *Isentress package insert.* Whitehouse Station, NJ: Author.

Paterson, D. L., Swindells, S., Mohr, J., Brester, M., Vergis, E. N., Squier, C., et al. (2000). Adherence to protease inhibitor therapy and outcomes in patients with HIV infection. *Annals of Internal Medicine, 133*(1), 21–30.

Pfizer, Inc. (2007, September 10). *Dear Healthcare Professional* [letter]. New York: Author.

Prochaska, J. O., & Velicer, W. F. (1997). The transtheoretical model of health behavior change. *American Journal of Health Promotion, 12*(1), 38–48.

Rand, C. S., & Wise, R. A. (1994). Measuring adherence to asthma medication regimens. *American Journal of Respiratory and Critical Care Medicine, 149*(2, Pt. 2), 69–76, 77–78.

Roche Laboratories Inc. (2007, January). *Fuzeon package insert.* Nutley, NJ: Author.

Shaw, E., Anderson, J. G., Maloney, M., Jay, S. J., & Fagan, D. (1995). Factors associated with noncompliance of patients taking antihypertensive medications. *Hospital Pharmacy, 30*(3), 201–203, 206–207.

U.S. Department of Health and Human Services (DHHS). (2008). *Guidelines for the use of antiretroviral agents in HIV-infected adults and adolescents.* Washington, DC: Author.

CHAPTER 3

Symptomatic Conditions in Adolescents and Adults with Advancing Disease

3.1 HERPES ZOSTER

1. Etiology/epidemiology
   a. Varicella-zoster virus (VZV) is a member of the herpes family; humans are the only known reservoir for VZV.
   b. Intimate contact is associated with transmission; risk of developing zoster increases with age.
   c. Varicella infection is considered a childhood disease, and the majority of cases occur in children younger than age 15. The incidence of varicella has decreased with the use of vaccinations.
   d. An estimated 300,000 episodes of zoster occur annually, of which 95% are initial occurrences and 5% are recurrences (Atkinson, Hamborsky, McIntyre, & Wolfe, 2007).

2. Pathogenesis
   a. VZV infection results in two clinically distinct entities: primary infection with chicken pox or reactivation of latent infection known as herpes zoster (shingles).
      i) Primary VZV infection is thought to result from pulmonary inhalation of aerosolized viral particles.
      ii) Epithelial cells undergo degenerative changes characterized by ballooning, resulting in a characteristic vesicular rash that ruptures and releases infectious fluid.
      iii) VZV infection characteristically remains latent in the dorsal root ganglia or the ganglion semilunare after resolution of the primary infection.

3. Clinical presentation
   a. VZV is characterized by a painful, unilateral vesicular eruption with a dermatomal distribution; thoracic and lumbar dermatomes are most frequently involved. VZV can be disseminated with bilateral skin involvement.
   b. Onset of dermatomal pain precedes appearance of lesions by 48–72 hours; lesions form over 3–5 days and resolve in 10–15 days. Lesions may be very painful; acute pain (burning, stabbing) frequently occurs. Chronic pain syndrome (postherpetic neuralgia) can be a severe and disabling complication.
   c. VZV rarely results in disseminated disease; anorexia, fever, and cough may indicate dissemination, a potentially fatal complication. Retina or the central nervous system (CNS) may be involved, without concomitant skin involvement.

4. Diagnosis
   a. Immunofluorescent assay (IFA) or culture can detect virus antigens.

5. Prevention/treatment
   a. Varicella-naive persons (especially those who are older, debilitated, or pregnant) should avoid persons with chicken pox or herpes zoster. Administer zosterimmune globulin (VZIG) within 96 hours of exposure to persons with chicken pox or zoster.
   b. Acyclovir 800 mg by mouth 5x/day, Famciclovir 500 mg by mouth TID, or Valacyclovir 1 g by mouth TID all for 7–10 days (Sande, Eliopoulos, Moellering, & Gilbert, 2008)
      i)   Best response occurs if treatment is initiated within 72 hours of initial outbreak.
      ii) Parenteral therapy may be prescribed in severe disseminated skin infection, retinal involvement, or CNS disease. A maintenance dose may be required in AIDS patients with recurrent VZV.
   c. If famciclovir can be administered
      i)   Famciclovir is shown to decrease the incidence of postherpetic neuralgia in the elderly; clinical implications in persons with AIDS are unknown.
   d. Other treatment options may include valacyclovir, foscarnet, or ganciclovir.
   e. Varicella-zoster vaccines are contraindicated in people with weakened or compromised immune systems (Merck & Co., Inc., 2007).
6. Nursing implications
   a. Monitor laboratory values and other indices to monitor for adverse effects and response to therapy.
   b. Maintain strict isolation until all lesions are crusted; hospitalization may be necessary.
   c. Local lesion care is required because open lesions can develop superimposed bacterial infections.
   d. Teach pain management for both acute illness and postherpetic neuralgia.
   e. Provide patient education.
      i)   Teach local wound care.
      ii) Emphasize need for strict isolation.
      iii) Counsel varicella-naive visitors and staff not to enter the patient's isolation room.
      iv) Use separate cloth to clean affected areas to prevent autoinoculation and dissemination.

REFERENCES

Atkinson, W., Hamborsky, J., McIntyre, L., & Wolfe, S. (Eds.). (2007). *Epidemiology and prevention of vaccine-preventable diseases* (10th ed.). Washington, DC: Public Health Foundation.

Merck & Co., Inc. (2007). *Zostavax product label*. Retrieved January 11, 2008, from http://www.fda.gov/cber/label/zostavaxLB.pdf

Sande, M. A., Eliopoulos, G. M., Moellering, R. C., Jr., & Gilbert, D. N. (Eds.). (2008). *The Sanford guide to HIV/AIDS therapy 2008* (Rev. 16th ed.). Sperryville, VA: Antimicrobial Therapy.

3.2 IDIOPATHIC THROMBOCYTOPENIA PURPURA

1. Etiology/epidemiology
   a. Idiopathic thrombocytopenia purpura (ITP) occurs in as many as 40% of HIV-infected patients. Severe thrombocytopenia (platelet count $< 50,000/mm^3$) is seen in 5% of HIV-associated ITP.

    b. HIV-associated ITP is an early manifestation of HIV infection and occurs before the development of any AIDS-defining condition.

2. Pathogenesis
   a. Pathogenesis is unknown.
   b. Hypotheses include production of platelet-specific autoantibodies with early infection and direct HIV infection of megakaryocytes (Karpatkin, 2004).

3. Clinical presentation
   a. Patient is often asymptomatic, despite low platelet counts.
   b. Symptoms include ecchymosis, petechiae, purpura, abnormal menstrual bleeding, blood in urine or stool, epistaxis, and bleeding from the gums.
   c. Mild splenomegaly may be present.

4. Diagnosis
   a. Complete blood count reveals low platelets.
   b. Bone marrow biopsy may be normal or may show increased megakaryocytes.
   c. Coagulation profiles (PT/PTT) are normal.
   d. Platelet-associated antibodies may be detected (Karpartkin, 2004).

5. Prevention/treatment
   a. Effective prevention is not currently possible because the causes and risk factors are unknown.
   b. Treatment
      i) HAART increases platelet counts (Burbano et al., 2001; Carbonara et al., 2001).
      ii) Zidovudine stimulates thrombopoiesis (Aboulafia, Bundow, Waide, Bennet, & Kerr, 2000).
      iii) Steroid therapy (i.e., prednisone) may lead to short-lasting responses but may increase the risk of developing an opportunistic infection.
      iv) Anti-RhO-(d) IgG (WinRhO) has been shown to produce a response, but it is not usually sustained (Scaradavou et al., 1997).
      v) Splenectomy is indicated if the person does not respond to medication; however, the patient is at increased risk for fulminant infections.
      vi) High-dose gamma globulin injections produce a rapid rise in platelet counts, but the effect is generally temporary. Use is limited to acute episodes of life-threatening bleeding or before a surgical procedure or dental extraction in patients with low platelet counts ($< 30,000/mm^3$).
      vii) Danazol has been used as a second-line therapy.
      viii) Immunosuppressive agents (vincristine, vinblastine) can be used for refractory ITP.
      ix) Anecdotal use of rituximab has been reported (Ahmad, Ball, Height, & Rees, 2004).
      x) Platelet transfusions are reserved for patients whose platelet counts are $< 10,000/mm^3$ or in emergency cases.

6. Nursing implications
   a. Assess for changes related to bleeding: decreased or loss of consciousness, hematuria, blood in the stool, hemoptysis, and hematemesis.
   b. Provide soft toothbrushes or soft swabs for oral hygiene; avoid flossing, hard toothbrushes, or commercial mouthwashes.

   c. Instruct patient to avoid blowing or picking the nose, straining at bowel movements, douching, or using tampons. Patient should use electric razors to shave.

   d. Do not administer any injections intramuscularly. Do not insert rectal suppositories.

   e. Use paper tape and avoid strong adhesives that may traumatize the skin.

   f. Instruct patient to avoid medications that inhibit platelet production or function. Non-steroidal anti-inflammatory agents (NSAIDs) or aspirin-containing medications should be avoided.

   g. If patient is receiving immune globulin (Gamimune N), monitor vital signs during the infusion and observe for the following adverse reactions: fever; irritability; infusion reaction; headache; nausea; chest tightness; dyspnea; chest, back, or hip pain; aseptic meningitis syndrome; transient renal insufficiency; and anaphylaxis.

REFERENCES

Aboulafia, D. M., Bundow, D., Waide, S., Bennet, C., & Kerr, D. (2000). Initial observations on the efficacy of highly active antiretroviral therapy in the treatment of HIV-associated autoimmune thrombocytopenia. *American Journal of Medicine and Science, 320*(2), 117–123.

Ahmad, H. N., Ball, C., Height, S. E., & Rees, D. C. (2004). Rituximab in chronic, recurrent HIV-associated immune thrombocytopenic purpura. *British Journal of Hematology, 127*(5), 607–608.

Burbano, X., Miguez, M. J., Lecusay, R., Rodriguez, A., Ruiz, P., Morales, G., et al. (2001). Thrombocytopenia in HIV-infected drug users in the HAART era. *Platelets, 12*(8), 456–461.

Carbonara, S., Fiorentino, G., Serio, G., Maggi, P., Ingravallo, G., Monno, L., et al. (2001). Response of severe HIV-associated thrombocytopenia to highly active antiretroviral therapy including protease inhibitors. *Journal of Infection, 42*(4), 251–256.

Karpatkin, S. (2004). Autoimmune thrombocytopenias. *Autoimmunity, 37*(4), 363–368.

Scaradavou, A., Woo, B., Woloski, B. M. R., Cunningham-Rundles, S., Ettinger, L. J., Aledort, L. M., et al. (1997). Intravenous anti-D treatment of immune thrombocytopenic purpura: Experience in 272 patients. *Blood, 89*(8), 2689–2700.

3.3 ORAL HAIRY LEUKOPLAKIA

1. Etiology/epidemiology
   a. Definition: An oral infection associated with Epstein-Barr virus, which infects and replicates in epithelial cells and is characterized by frequent viral recombination (Walling, Ling, Gordadze, Montes-Walters, Flaitz, & Nichols, 2004)
   b. Prevalence: It occurs in both men and women; prevalence increases with immune deterioration, antiretroviral therapy failure, antifungal medication use, current recreational drug use, cigarette smoking, and male gender (Chattopadhyay, Caplan, Slade, Shugars, Tien, & Patton, 2005; Greenspan et al., 2004; Reznik, 2005/2006; Sroussi, Villines, Epstein, Alves, & Alves, 2007).

2. Pathogenesis
   a. A recombinant variant of an Epstein-Barr virus gene (ENBA-2) through modulation of ENBA-2 protein function is hypothesized to play a role in pathogenesis (Walling et al., 2004).

3. Clinical presentation

    a. White hairy or smooth areas on lateral, dorsal, or ventral surfaces of tongue; may extend to buccal mucosa

    b. Can occur concurrently with oropharyngeal candidiasis but cannot be scraped off like candidiasis

4. Diagnosis

    a. Presence of nonremovable, nonpainful, white, hairy or smooth tongue lesions

    b. Histopathological evidence of epithelial hyperplasia with little or no inflammation

    c. Evidence of Epstein-Barr virus DNA by polymerase chain reaction (PCR) with in situ hybridization (Mabruk et al., 2000)

    d. Difficulty chewing/swallowing, reduced/altered taste perception

    e. Rule out oropharyngeal candidiasis, squamous cell carcinoma, smoker's leukoplakia, epithelial dysplasia

5. Prevention/treatment

    a. Condition generally is asymptomatic and not treated.

    b. Antivirals (e.g., acyclovir, ganciclovir, foscarnet, cidofovir) and topical podophyllum resin (Bartlett & Gallant, 2007) provide temporary symptomatic relief; relapses are common.

    c. Antifungal therapy is given to minimize coinfection with oropharyngeal candidiasis.

    d. Meticulous oral hygiene and dental care are recommended.

6. Nursing implications

    a. Instruct patient to perform frequent oral assessments and oral care.

    b. If taking acyclovir, patient should drink adequate fluids to prevent dehydration and renal toxicity.

    c. If taste is altered, recommend eating seasoned, spicy, or pickled foods and avoid smoking before meals.

    d. If patient has difficulty chewing/swallowing, suggest eating soft or moist foods, drinking with a straw, and avoiding sticky foods.

REFERENCES

Bartlett, J. G., & Gallant, J. E. (2007). *Medical management of HIV infection*. Baltimore: Johns Hopkins Medicine Health Publishing Business Group.

Chattopadhyay, A., Caplan, D. J., Slade, G. D., Shugars, D. C., Tien, H-C., & Patton, L. L. (2005). Risk indicators for oral candidiasis and oral hairy leukoplakia in HIV infected adults. *Community Dentistry and Oral Epidemiology, 33*(1), 35–44.

Greenspan, D., Gange, S. J., Phelan, J. A., Navazeh, M., Alves, M. E. A. F., MacPhail, L. A., et al. (2004). Incidence of oral lesions in HIV-1-infected women: Reduction with HAART. *Journal of Dental Research, 83*(2), 145–150.

Mabruk, M. J., Antonio, M., Flint, S. R., Coleman, D. C., Toner, M., Kay, E., et al. (2000). A simple and rapid technique for the detection of Epstein-Barr virus DNA in HIV-associated oral hairy leukoplakia biopsies. *Journal of Oral Pathology Medicine, 29*(3), 118–122.

Reznik, D. A. (December 2005/January 2006). Oral manifestations of HIV disease. *Topics in HIV Medicine, 13*(5), 143–148.

Sroussi, H. Y., Villines, D., Epstein, J., Alves, M. C. F., & Alves, M. E. A. F. (2007). Oral lesions in HIV-positive dental patients—One more argument for tobacco smoking cessation. *Oral Diseases, 13*(3), 324–328.

Walling, D. M., Ling, P. D., Gordadze, A. V., Montes-Walters, M., Flaitz, C. M., & Nichols, C. M. (2004). Expression of Epstein-Barr virus replication latent genes in oral epithelium: Determinants of the pathogenesis of oral hairy leukoplakia. *Journal of Infectious Diseases, 190*(2), 396–399.

3.4 PERIPHERAL NEUROPATHY

1. Etiology/epidemiology
   a. There are a number of different HIV-related neuropathies, with varying etiologies (Pardo, McArthur, & Griffin, 2001; Verma et al., 2005).
   b. Peripheral neuropathy (PN) may be the result of direct HIV infection of nervous tissue; HIV infection of macrophages and lymphocytes, which results in immune dysregulation and cytokine elaboration; direct damage to mitochondria by antiretroviral drugs; or infection with cytomegalovirus (CMV) or other opportunistic organisms (Kolson & Gonzalez-Scarano, 2001; Pardo, McArthur, & Griffin, 2001; Verma et al., 2005).
   c. PN is the most common neurologic complication of HIV infection (Keswani et al., 2002).
   d. PN involves damage to nerves outside the brain and spinal cord. Although generally not life threatening, it causes significant morbidity in persons with HIV infection (Verma et al., 2005).
   e. About 30% of all HIV-infected persons have symptomatic PN, and at least another 15–20% have evidence of subclinical PN (Schifitto et al., 2002).
   f. With HAART, incidence of HIV-associated PN has declined; however, the incidence of antiretroviral-associated PN has increased (Sacktor, 2002).
   g. Risk factors for PN include advanced stage HIV infection, low CD4 count, high plasma viral load, and comorbid conditions such as diabetes mellitus (Verma et al., 2005).
2. Pathogenesis
   a. Depending on the etiological agent, there are a number of different pathophysiological responses to nerve injury (Keswani et al., 2002).
   b. Damage may occur at the afferent fiber, motor neuron, and/or dorsal root ganglion (Verma et al., 2005).
   c. Damage to sensory neurons results in increased sensitivity to external stimuli (Verma et al., 2005).
3. Clinical presentation
   a. Patients typically present with sensory loss or pain in the extremities, weakness, or motor dysfunction (Pardo, McArthur, & Griffin, 2001; Verma et al., 2004).
   b. Presentation differs depending on the type of PN disorder.
      i) Distal symmetric polyneuropathy (DSP) is the most common HIV-associated PN. It occurs in mid to late HIV infection and presents as pain, tingling, or burning, usually in the lower extremities (Simpson, 2002; Verma, 2001; Wulff, Wang, & Simpson, 2000).
      ii) Inflammatory demyelinating polyneuropathy (IDP) typically occurs as an early manifestation of HIV infection. It presents as motor weakness, with only minimal sensory loss (Simpson, 2002; Verma, 2001; Wulff, Wang, & Simpson, 2000).
      iii) Mononeuritis multiplex (MM) is a rare complication of late-stage HIV infection. It presents as multifocal asymmetric motor or sensory alterations, or both (Simpson, 2002; Verma, 2001; Wulff, Wang, & Simpson, 2000).

iv) Progressive polyradiculopathy (PP) most commonly occurs in the advanced stages of HIV infection. It commonly presents with pain in the sacrogenital area that rapidly progresses to motor loss and urinary and bladder incontinence (Simpson, 2002; Verma, 2001; Wulff, Wang, & Simpson, 2000).

v) Autonomic neuropathy is most likely to present in the later stages of HIV infection and is characterized by symptoms of sympathetic (e.g., palpitations, tachycardia) and parasympathetic (e.g., syncope, diarrhea) dysfunction (Simpson, 2002; Verma, 2001; Wulff, Wang, & Simpson, 2000).

4. Diagnosis
   a. Differential diagnosis of specific PN disorder is critical in choosing the appropriate treatment (Ferrari et al., 2006).
   b. Diagnostic work-ups involve a comprehensive history, neurological exam, blood studies, cerebrospinal fluid determinations, nerve conduction tests, and electromyelography (Ferrari et al., 2006).

5. Prevention/treatment
   a. Goal is to manage symptoms of PN as there is no known approach to reverse nerve damage. Treatment should begin early to prevent further loss of neurons (Ferrari et al., 2006).
   b. Once the underlying cause of the PN is determined, appropriate therapy is to be initiated. This may involve withdrawal of neurotoxic medications, adjustment of antiretroviral regimens to decrease viral load, or treatment of opportunistic infections (Ferrari et al., 2006).
   c. The World Health Organization (WHO) analgesic ladder is used to guide pain management (WHO, 1996).
   d. Some complementary therapies, such as relaxation therapy or transcutaneous electrical nerve stimulation, may be helpful (Forst et al., 2004; Nicholas et al., 2007; Verma et al., 2005).

6. Nursing implications
   a. Educate patients to identify early signs of PN.
   b. Routinely perform neurological assessments.
   c. Recommend good foot care, comfortable shoes, and walking aids.
   d. Assess home for safety hazards.
   e. Recommend exercise or massage to improve circulation to the feet.
   f. Advise regarding pain management strategies (e.g., analgesics, foot cradles to reduce pressure of bedcovers on feet, relaxation techniques).
   g. Refer to community resources for supportive/restorative care (e.g., support groups, podiatry clinics, physical therapists).

REFERENCES

Ferrari, S., Vento, S., Monoco, S., Cavallaro, T., Cainelli, F., Rizzuto, N., et al. (2006). Human immunodeficiency virus-associated peripheral neuropathies. *Mayo Clinic Proceedings, 81*(2), 213–219.

Forst, T., Nguyen, M., Disselhoff, B., Pohlmann, T., & Pfutzner, A. (2004). Impact of low frequency electrical transcutaneous nerve stimulation on symptomatic diabetic neuropathy using the new Salutaris device. *Diabetes Nutrition and Metabolism, 17*(3), 163–168.

Keswani, S. C., Pardo, C. A., Cherry, C. L., Hoke, A., & McArthur, J. C. (2002). HIV-associated sensory neuropathies. *AIDS, 16*(16), 2105–2117.

Kolson, D. L., & Gonzalez-Scarano, F. (2001). HIV-associated neuropathies: Role of HIV-1, CMV, and other viruses. *Journal of the Peripheral Nervous System, 6*(1), 2–7.

Nicholas, P. K., Mauceri, L., Slate Ciampa, A., Corless, I. B., Raymond, N., Barry, D. J., et al. (2007). Distal sensory polyneuropathy in the context of HIV/AIDS. *Journal of the Association of Nurses in AIDS Care, 18*(4), 32–40.

Pardo, C. A., McArthur, J. C., & Griffin, J. W. (2001). HIV neuropathy: Insights in the pathology of HIV peripheral nerve disease. *Journal of the Peripheral Nervous System, 6*(1), 21–27.

Sacktor, N. (2002). The epidemiology of human immunodeficiency virus-associated neurological disease in the era of highly active antiretroviral therapy. *Journal of Neurovirology, 8*(Suppl. 2), 115–121.

Schifitto, G., McDermott, M. P., McArthur, J. C., Marder, K., Epstein, L., Kieburtz, K., et al. (2002). Incidence of and risk factors for HIV-associated distal sensory polyneuropathy. *Neurology, 58*(12), 1764–1768.

Simpson, D. M. (2002). Selected peripheral neuropathies associated with human immunodeficiency virus infection and antiretroviral therapy. *Journal of Neurovirology, 8*(Suppl. 2), 33–41.

Verma, A. (2001). Epidemiology and clinical features of HIV-1 associated neuropathies. *Journal of the Peripheral Nervous System, 6*(1), 8–13.

Verma, S., Estanislao, L., & Simpson, D. (2005). HIV-associated neuropathic pain: Epidemiology, pathophysiology and management. *CNS Drugs, 19*(4), 325–334.

Verma, S., Micsa, E., Estanislao, L., & Simpson, D. (2004). Neuromuscular complications of HIV. *Current Neurology and Neuroscience Reports, 4*(1), 62–67.

World Health Organization (WHO). (1996). *Cancer pain relief, with guide of opioid availability* (2nd ed.). Geneva, Switzerland: Author.

Wulff, E. A., Wang, A. K., & Simpson, D. M. (2000). HIV-associated peripheral neuropathy: Epidemiology, pathophysiology and treatment. *Drugs, 59*(6), 1251–1260.

3.5 BACTERIAL PNEUMONIA

1. Etiology/epidemiology
   a. The most common etiologic agent in HIV infections is *S. pneumoniae.* Other causative pathogens are *H. influenza, Mycoplasma pneumoniae, C. pneumoniae, S. aureus, Streptococcus pyogenes, N. meningitides, Moraxella catarrhalis,* and *Klebsiella pneumoniae.*
   b. Population-based studies suggest pneumococcal pneumonia occurs 200 times more frequently in patients with HIV disease than in age-matched populations (Musher, 2000).
   c. Recurrence is relatively common. Thirteen percent of cases recur within 6 months, and the reported mortality rate among HIV-infected persons with bacteremic pneumococcal pneumonia is 5% to 11% (CDC, 1999).
2. Pathogenesis
   a. Bacteria are transmitted by respiratory droplets spread by close person-to-person contact.
   b. Bacteria adhere to pharyngeal cells and subsequently colonize.
   c. Complications include otitis media, sinusitis, and bronchitis.
3. Clinical presentation
   a. Symptoms of acute respiratory infection often include several of the following: fever, productive cough, chills, dyspnea, pleuritic chest pain, orthopnea, fatigue, and malaise.
4. Diagnosis
   a. Baseline assessments
      i) Chest radiography is performed to substantiate diagnosis of pneumonia and as a baseline to assess response to treatment.
      ii) Sputum gram stain and culture for conventional bacteria should be considered.

iii) Complete blood cell and differential counts, serum creatinine, urea nitrogen, electrolytes, bilirubin, and liver enzyme values are determined.

iv) Blood cultures from at least two different sites are taken before treatment.

v) A test is conducted for *Mycobacterium tuberculosis* using an acid-fast bacilli stain and culture for selected patients, especially those with cough or other symptoms suggestive of tuberculosis (TB).

5. Prevention/treatment
   a. Immunization with 23-valent pneumococcal polysaccharide vaccine should be offered to all HIV-infected patients. Vaccination can occur on initial clinical contact, and revaccination should occur every 3 to 5 years thereafter.
   b. The risk of pneumococcal pneumonia is greatly reduced in vaccinated individuals with CD4 counts > 500 cells/mm^3.
   c. *Pneumocystis carinii* pneumonia (PCP) prophylaxis with trimethoprim-sulfamethoxazole (TMP-SMX) may decrease risk of infection (Musher, 2000).
   d. Cefotaxime or ceftriaxone are the antibiotics of choice; fluroquinolones (levofloxacin, moxifloxacin, or gatifloxacin) are also used (Benson et al., 2004). In patients who are allergic to beta-lactam antibiotics, vancomycin or a quinolone antibiotic may be used. If bacteremia is suspected, treat with IV antipseudomonal beta-lactam (e.g., imipenem) combined with an aminoglycoside (e.g., tobramycin; Musher, 2000).

6. Nursing implications
   a. Promote optimal gas exchange (e.g., incentive spirometry, oxygen therapy, chest percussion, drainage therapy).
   b. Promote hydration with fluids, 2.5 to 3 L/day, and provide nutritional support, such as vitamin and mineral supplements and increased kilocalories.
   c. Monitor laboratory results, such as hemoglobin and hematocrit, white blood cell count, bilirubin, lactate dehydrogenase, and indices for side effects or adverse effects, such as empyema and response to therapy.

REFERENCES

Benson, C. A., Kaplan, J. E., Masur, H., Pau, A., & Holmes, K. K. (2004). Treating opportunistic infections among HIV-infected adults and adolescents: Recommendations from CDC, the National Institutes of Health, and the Infectious Diseases Society of America. *Morbidity and Mortality Weekly Report, 53*(RR-15), 1–118.

Centers for Disease Control and Prevention (CDC). (1999). USPHS/IDSA guidelines for the prevention of opportunistic infections in persons infected with human immunodeficiency virus: U.S. Public Health Service (USPHS) and Infectious Diseases Society of America (IDSA). *Morbidity and Mortality Weekly Report, 48*(RR10), 1–59, 61–66.

Musher, D. (2000). *Streptococcus pneumonia*. In G. Mandell, J. Bennett, & R. Dolin (Eds.), *Principles and practice of infectious diseases* (5th ed., pp. 2128–2147). Philadelphia: Churchill-Livingstone.

3.6 MYCOBACTERIUM AVIUM COMPLEX (MAC)

1. Etiology/epidemiology
   a. MAC consists of two closely related species, *M. avium* and *M. intracellulare,* that are ubiquitous in the environment (food, water, soil).

b. *M. avium* is the etiologic agent in $> 95\%$ of patients with AIDS who develop disseminated MAC disease (DMAC; CDC, 2004).

c. MAC is not considered contagious. Transmission most likely occurs with ingestion of contaminated water or by inhaling aerosolized contaminated water (Crowe, Hoy & Mills, 2002).

d. In the absence of effective ART or MAC prophylaxis in HIV infected, severely immune compromised patients, the incidence of DMAC is 20–40% (CDC, 2004).

2. Pathogenesis

a. Infects gastrointestinal or respiratory tracts; asymptomatic colonization is probably an essential step in the disease. *M. avium*–infected macrophages evade host defense by inactivating normal intracellular killing mechanisms. HIV infected monocytes may enhance intracellular replication of *M. avium;* widespread replication results in metastatic seeding.

b. Disseminated MAC (DMAC) most often occurs when CD4 cell counts are < 50 cells/mm^3. Only 10% of MAC bacteremia occurred in patients with CD4 > 100 cells/mm^3 with 57% occurring in those with CD4 < 50 cells/mm^3 (Crowe, Hoy & Mills, 2002).

3. Clinical presentation

a. GI: chronic diarrhea, abdominal pain, chronic malabsorption, and extrabiliary obstructive disease

b. DMAC: characterized by constitutional symptoms, such as fatigue, fever, weight loss, night sweats, abdominal pain, diarrhea, lymphadenopathy, organomegaly, and anemia (Zwolski & Talotta, 2001)

4. Diagnosis

a. Diagnosis of DMAC is based upon clinical signs and symptoms and isolation of MAC from blood, bone marrow, or other normally sterile tissues or body fluids.

b. Supportive diagnostic information may be obtained from AFB smears and culture of stool or tissue biopsies. *Note:* Because *M. avium, M. intracellulare,* and *M. tuberculosis* are acid-fast bacilli, a positive AFB smear is treated as *M. tuberculosis* infection until definitive diagnosis can be made.

5. Prevention/treatment

a. Prevention: Begin prophylaxis when CD4 cell counts < 50 cells/mm^3 and there is no evidence of DMAC. Prophylaxis may be discontinued in patients who have responded to HAART with CD4 counts >100 cells/mm^3 for ≥ 3 months (USPHS/IDSA, 2002).

   i) Preferred regimens:
      (1) Clarithromycin 500 mg PO BID
      (2) Azithromycin 1,200 mg PO weekly

   ii) Alternative regimens include the following:
      (1) Rifabutin 300 mg PO q day
      (2) Azithromycin 1,200 mg/week PO plus rifabutin 300 mg PO q day

b. Treatment: In ARV-naïve patients, HAART should be initiated simultaneously or within 1 to 2 weeks of initiation of MAC treatment. An immune reconstitution inflammatory syndrome (IRIS) may occur in those with a rapid or marked increase in CD4 cell count. Anti-inflammatory therapy may be required to alleviate symptoms (CDC, 2004).

   i) Preferred regimens:

      (1) Clarithromycin 500 mg PO BID plus ethambutol 15 mg/kg/day PO with or without rifabutin 300 mg/day PO.

      (2) Azithromycin 500 to 600 mg PO q day plus ethambutol 15 mg/kg/day PO with or without rifabutin 300 mg/day PO.

  ii) Alternative regimens:

      (1) Fluoroquinolones or parenteral amikacin may be used instead of rifabutin.

  iii) Salvage regimens:

      (1) Require customization based upon susceptibility testing. At least two active drugs should be used.

  c. Maintenance/prevention of recurrence:

    i) Preferred regimen:

      (1) Clarithromycin 500 mg PO bid plus ethambutol 15 mg/kg PO q day with or without rifabutin 300 mg PO q day

    ii) Alternative regimen:

      (1) Azithromycin 500 mg PO q day plus ethambutol 15 mg/kg PO q day with or without rifabutin 300 mg PO q day (Bartlett & Gallant, 2007; USPHS/IDSA 2002; Zwolski & Talotta, 2001)

6. Nursing implications

  a. If rifabutin is used for treatment or prophylaxis, must first exclude TB diagnosis and remember to adjust dose as appropriately given the HAART regimen.

  b. Monitor laboratory results (CBC with differential) and other indices for side effects, adverse effects (including IRIS), toxicity, and response to therapy.

  c. Perform blood cultures 4 to 8 weeks after initiation of therapy (Zwolski & Talotta, 2001).

  d. Provide patient education and monitor for multiple drug interactions, especially rifabutin and rifampin.

REFERENCES

Bartlett, J. G., & Gallant, J. E. (2007). *Medical management of HIV infection.* Baltimore: Johns Hopkins University, Department of Infectious Diseases.

Centers for Disease Control and Prevention (CDC). (2004). Treating opportunistic infections among HIV-infected adults and adolescents. *Morbidity and Mortality Weekly Report, 53*(RR-15).

Crowe, S., Hoy, J., & Mills, J. (2002). *Management of the HIV-infected patient.* London: Martin Dunitz.

United States Public Health Service & Infectious Diseases Society of America (USPHS/IDSA). (2002, June 14). *Guidelines for the prevention of opportunistic infections in persons infected with human immunodeficiency virus.* Retrieved November 5, 2007, from http://aidsinfo.nih.gov/contentfiles/OIpreventionGL.pdf

Zwolski, K., & Talotta, D. (2001). Bacterial infections. In C. Kirton, D. Talotta, & K. Zwolski (Eds.), *Handbook of HIV/AIDS nursing* (pp. 229–253). St. Louis, MO: Mosby.

3.7 MYCOBACTERIUM TUBERCULOSIS

1. Etiology/epidemiology

  a. Latent tuberculosis infection (LTBI) is caused by *Mycobacterium tuberculosis* (MTB), an acid-fast bacillus.

    b. Tuberculosis disease (TB) results when the immune system of the infected person is unable to control the replication of the bacillus.

    c. It is estimated that 2 billion people in the world (between 9.5 to 14.7 million people in the United States) are infected with MTB. Worldwide, about one-third of the people living with HIV are co-infected with MTB.

    d. Risk of tuberculosis (MTB) activation in an HIV-positive person is 8% to 10% per year versus a 5% to 10% lifetime risk for HIV-negative persons.

    e. In 2006, the U.S. case rate for TB was 2.3 per 100,000 for U.S.-born persons and 22 per 100,000 for foreign-born persons; over 55% of all reported cases in the United States were in the foreign-born group (CDC, 2006).

2. Pathogenesis

    a. Droplet nuclei containing aerosolized MTB bacilli are produced when a person with active pulmonary or laryngeal TB talks, coughs, sneezes, or sings. These droplets can remain airborne for 48 hours.

    b. MTB is inhaled and the organisms penetrate the lung parenchyma, establishing primary infection. The bacilli are transported to hilar lymph nodes by macrophages. The macrophages may disseminate organisms in the blood or sequester them in granulomas.

    c. Cell-mediated immunity is activated to halt the infectious process and dissemination. A breakdown of cell-mediated immunity can result in development of active TB.

3. Clinical presentation

    a. Constitutional symptoms of TB include fever, chills, weight loss, fatigue, and night sweats.

    b. Symptoms of active pulmonary TB include productive cough, hemoptysis, shortness of breath, and pleuritic chest pain.

    c. Tuberculosis can be disseminated to any organ of the body including bone, kidneys, lymph nodes, pericardium, and meninges. Symptoms of extrapulmonary TB vary depending on site(s) of disease.

    d. Persons with HIV disease have higher rates of extrapulmonary TB than HIV-negative persons.

4. Diagnosis

    a. Latent TB infection (LTBI) is diagnosed when there is evidence of infection with MTB and no evidence of active disease. A person with LTBI will have a positive tuberculosis skin test (TST per Mantoux method) and/or a positive interferon-gamma (IFNy) release assay. A 5 mm or greater area of induration is considered a positive TST in any person with HIV. TST is subject to both application and reader error, and results are not specific for MTB. New IFNy assays are being developed to improve specificity and avoid cross-reactivity with BCG vaccine and environmental mycobacteria. However, these assays are not as sensitive as the TST (CDC, 2005a).

    b. TB disease is suspected based upon evidence of TB infection, presentation of symptoms, positive acid-fast bacillus (AFB) smears of sputum and/or other body fluids, and abnormal chest radiographs and/or other imaging. Because persons with HIV may be anergic, a positive TST may not be obtained. Furthermore, atypical radiographic/imaging presentations can be expected. Diagnosis is confirmed with positive cultures (sputa or other fluids and tissues) for MTB and/or resolution of signs and symptoms with appropriate treatment.

5. Prevention/treatment
    a. Latent TB infection (LTBI): TST and IFN*y* assays can detect TB infection within 2 to 10 weeks. All HIV-infected patients should have an annual assessment for TB exposure including TST or IFN*y* assay. If LTBI is suspected, the chance of developing subsequent active disease can be reduced by providing LTBI using one of the following regimens (ATS/CDC, 2000; CDC, 2003):
        i) Isoniazid 300 mg daily for 9 months
        ii) Isoniazid 900 mg twice weekly by Directly Observed Therapy (DOT) for 9 months
        iii) Rifampin 600 mg daily for 4 months (if NOT on HAART)
        iv) Rifabutin (dosage varies depending on HAART regimen) daily for 4 months
    b. Tuberculosis disease: Treatment regimens and duration of treatment for TB vary depending upon the susceptibility profile of the MTB, the extent of the disease (pulmonary, extrapulmonary), the stage of HIV disease (CD4 count), and the specific HAART regimen in use (if any). In general, treatment of TB begins with at least 4 drugs taken once daily. Whenever possible, medication should be provided via directly observed therapy (DOT), which has been shown to improve outcomes (ATS/CDC, 2003). After 2 months of treatment of a susceptible MTB infection, the number of drugs is usually reduced and the regimen may be changed to 2 or 3 days a week. Note that any reduced frequency regimen MUST be provided by DOT and that when the CD4 count is < 100 cells/mm^3, drug administration should never be less than 3 days a week. Consult the most recent CDC guidelines for recommendations of acceptable regimens (http://www.cdc.gov/tb). Timing for initiating treatment is complicated by the fact that TB is itself immune suppressive and that treating TB can result in an immune reconstitution inflammatory syndrome (IRIS) even in the absence of HAART. Adding HAART increases the risk of IRIS. In a recent study, 25% of patients with CD4 count < 100 cells/mm^3 who started HAART and TB treatment at the same time experienced IRIS requiring steroid therapy (Nahid, et al., 2007).
6. Nursing implications
    a. Until patient has produced three AFB smear negative sputums (8 to 24 hours apart and with at least one specimen taken in the morning), airborne transmission precautions should be utilized (CDC, 2005b).
    b. Unlike other diseases, due to the public health implications, the successful treatment of tuberculosis is the responsibility of the care provider rather than the patient (CDC, 2005c). Educate about importance of adherence and utilize directly observed therapy (DOT) and incentives and enablers, as appropriate, whenever possible.
    c. Teach about and monitor laboratory results (e.g., complete blood count with differential, liver function test) and other indices to monitor for side effects, adverse effects, IRIS, toxicity, and response to therapy; test vision for ethambutol-induced optic neuritis. Patients may require more frequent laboratory assessments if they are older or have preexisting liver disease. Patients should be counseled frequently regarding avoidance of alcohol during TB treatment.
    d. When patients are taking HAART, they should not receive rifampin (CDC, 2004). Rifabutin may be substituted, but dose must be adjusted for interactions with PIs and NNRTIs. If HAART regimen is once daily, give HAART and TB medications at the same time per DOT to make sure rifabutin dose is appropriate. If rifabutin is given without HAART, underdosing or overdosing can occur and may lead to resistance or toxicity.

e. The Health Insurance Portability and Accountability Act (HIPAA) recognizes the need for public health activities and should "not be a barrier to the reporting of suspected and verified TB cases by health care providers, including health care institutions" (CDC, 2005c). Written permission from the patient is not required.

REFERENCES

American Thoracic Society/Centers for Disease Control and Prevention. (2000). Targeted tuberculin testing and treatment of latent TB infection. *Mortality and Morbidity Weekly Report, 49*(RR-6), 1–51.

American Thoracic Society, Centers for Disease Control and Prevention, and Infectious Diseases Society of America. (2003). Treatment of tuberculosis. *Mortality and Morbidity Weekly Report, 52*(RR-11), 1–77.

Centers for Disease Control and Prevention (CDC). (2003). Update: Adverse event data and revised American Thoracic Society/CDC recommendations against the use of rifampin and pyrazinamide for treatment of latent tuberculosis infection. *Mortality and Morbidity Weekly Report, 52*(31), 735–739.

Centers for Disease Control and Prevention (CDC). (2004). Notice to readers: Updated guidelines for the use of rifamycins for the treatment of tuberculosis among HIV-infected patients taking protease inhibitors or non-nucleoside reverse transcriptase inhibitors. *Mortality and Morbidity Weekly Report, 53*(2), 37.

Centers for Disease Control and Prevention (CDC). (2005a). Guidelines for using the QuantiFERON-TB Gold Test for detecting *Mycobacterium tuberculosis* infection, United States. *Mortality and Morbidity Weekly Report, 54*(RR-15), 49–55.

Centers for Disease Control and Prevention (CDC). (2005b). Guidelines for preventing the transmission of *Mycobacterium tuberculosis* in health care settings. *Mortality and Morbidity Weekly Report, 54*(RR-17), 1–141.

Centers for Disease Control and Prevention (CDC). (2005c). Controlling tuberculosis in the United States: Recommendations from the American Thoracic Society, CDC, and the Infectious Diseases Society of America. *Mortality and Morbidity Weekly Report, 54*(RR-12), 1–81.

Centers for Disease Control and Prevention (CDC). (2006). *Reported tuberculosis in the United States.* Retrieved March 3, 2009, from http://www.cdc.gov/tb/surv/surv2006/pdf/FullReport.pdf

Nahid, P., Gonzalez, L. C., Rudoy, I., de Jong, B. C., Unger, A., Kawamura, L. M., et al. (2007). Treatment outcomes of patients with HIV and tuberculosis. *American Journal of Respiratory Critical Care Medicine, 175*(11), 1199–1206.

3.8 CANDIDIASIS

1. Etiology/epidemiology
   a. *Candida albicans* is the most common of the species of candida that cause disease. Other disease-causing species include C. *glabrata,* C. *krusei*, C. *parapsilosis,* and C. *tropicalis* (Saccente, 2003).
   b. *Candida albicans* is a ubiquitous human commensal that lives in the gastrointestinal tract, and is also found in the environment. It can cause disease when the host's defenses are weakened locally or systemically (Dignani et al., 2003).
   c. Patients who have a low CD4+ T-lymphocyte count are at greatest risk for fungal infections (Saccente, 2003).
   d. About one-third of HIV-infected patients have esophageal symptoms, and mucosal candidiasis is the most frequent cause (Saccente, 2003). Oropharyngitis caused by candida usually occurs when the CD4+ count is less than 100 cells/mm^3 (Bartlett & Gallant, 2007). It is uncertain whether or not vaginal candidiasis occurs more frequently among HIV-infected women than women without HIV infection (Saccente, 2003).

2. Pathogenesis
   a. Most disease is caused by organisms that are ubiquitous in both the gut and the environment.
   b. Patients with low CD4+ T-lymphocyte counts are at greater risk for fungal infections (Saccente, 2003).
   c. Chronic recurrence is common, and drug-resistant strains are emerging.
3. Clinical presentation
   a. Four types of oropharyngeal disease are recognized: pseudomembranous (thrush), erythematous (atrophic), hyperplastic (candidal leukoplakia), and angular chelitis (Saccente, 2003). Symptoms include burning pain, altered taste sensation, and dysphagia.
   b. Esophageal candidasis
      i)   Symptoms include, but are not limited to, diffuse retrosternal pain, dysphagia, and odynophagia without fever (Bartlett & Gallant, 2007).
      ii) Considered an AIDS-defining condition.
   c. Vulvovaginal candidiasis
      i)   Symptoms include mucosal burning and pruritis combined with a creamy yellow-white discharge. May not be a true HIV-related condition (Saccennte, 2003).
4. Diagnosis
   a. Oropharyngeal and vulvovaginal candidiasis
      i)   Diagnosis is made on characteristic appearance; recovery of organism is not required, though helpful in confirming a diagnosis. The exam usually reveals erythema and yellow-white discharge that may show yeast or pseudohyphae on 10% potassium hydroxide (KOH) prep or gram stain (Bartlett & Gallant, 2007). Direct visualization of the mucosa with fiberoptic endoscopy is the procedure of choice to diagnose esophageal candidiasis (Saccente, 2003).
5. Prevention/treatment
   a. Oropharyngeal candidiasis (initial infection) can be treated with clotrimazole oral troches 10 mg 5x/day until lesions resolve, usually within 7–14 days (Bartlett & Gallant, 2007). Other options include nystatin 500,000 units (4–6 mL) gargled 4–5x/day or 1 to 2 flavored pastilles 4–5x/day for 7–14 days or fluconazole 100 mg/day PO for 7–14 days (Bartlett & Gallant, 2007). These treatments are easy to administer and are low cost. For refractory cases, other options include itraconazole 200 mg/day oral suspension swished and swallowed on an empty stomach; amphotericin B oral suspension (not currently available commercially but can be prepared by pharmacist) and amphotericin B IV 0.3mg/kg/day (Bartlett & Gallant, 2007).
   b. Esophageal candidiasis can be treated with fluconazole, 200–400 mg IV or PO once, then 100–200 mg 1x/day for 3–4 weeks or itraconazole 200 mg/day PO (Pappas et al., 2004), or an echinocandin (caspofungin, micafungin, or adnidulafungin; The Medical Letter, 2008). Maintenance therapy, only with relapsing disease, should include fluconazole 100–200 mg/day PO (Bartlett & Gallant, 2007).
   c. Vulvovaginal candidiasis should be treated with topical therapy including intravaginal creams, ointments, tablets, ovules, or suppositories. Topical drugs include butoconazole, clotrimazole, miconazole, tioconazole, or terconazole (The Medical Letter, 2008). Systemic therapy includes oral fluconazole and itraconazole (The Medical Letter, 2008;

Bartlett & Gallant, 2007). Treatment is identical for women with or without HIV infection (Bartlett & Gallant, 2007).

6. Nursing implications
   a. Frequent oral hygiene measures should be implemented in patients with oral candidiasis.
   b. Women with vaginal candidiasis should avoid pantyhose and douching, and they should adhere to good hygiene.
   c. Nutritional assessment and intervention may be necessary for patients with oropharyngeal candidiasis.

REFERENCES

Bartlett, J. G., & Gallant, J .E. (2007). *Medical management of HIV infection*. Baltimore: Johns Hopkins Medicine.
Dignani, M. C., Solomkin, J. S., & Anaissie, E. J. (2003). Candida. In E. J. Anaissie, M. R. McGinnis, & M. A. Pfaller (Eds.), *Clinical mycology* (pp. 195–239). Philadelphia: Churchill Livingstone.
Pappas, P. G., Rex, J. H., Sobel, J. D., Filler, S. G., Dismukes, W. E., Walsh, T. J., et al. (2004). Guidelines for the treatment of candidiasis. *Clinical Infectious Diseases, 38*(2), 161–189.
Saccente, M. (2003). Fungal infections in the patient with human immunodefiency virus infection. In E. J. Anaissie, M. R. McGinnis, & M. A. Pfaller (Eds.), *Clinical Mycology* (pp. 383–393). Philadelphia: Churchill Livingstone.
Medical Letter. (2008, January). Antifungal drugs. *Treatment Guidelines, 6*(65), 1–8.

3.9 COCCIDIOIDOMYCOSIS

1. Etiology/epidemiology
   a. Etiologic agent is *C. immitis,* a dimorphic fungus probably related to the ascomycetes. It appears as either a mycelium at room temperature or a spherule at body temperature.
   b. Mycelia grow in the soil during rainy seasons; they become airborne in dry seasons via wind and mechanical soil disruption.
   c. AIDS-associated coccidioidal disease is generally confined to endemic areas (i.e., southwestern United States, northern Mexico, and portions of Central and South America).
2. Pathogenesis
   a. The organism enters the pulmonary tract via inhalation. In an immunocompromised host, infection disseminates to the skin, central nervous system (CNS), bones, and lymph nodes.
   b. Disease in HIV-infected populations is generally associated with a CD4 count < 250 cells/mm^3 and impaired T-cell function. It may reflect reactivation of previously acquired infection or recent exposure.
3. Clinical presentation
   a. Clinical presentation is usually nonspecific and can range from asymptomatic presentation to life-threatening pneumonia or CNS disease.
   b. Constitutional symptoms of malaise, fever, dyspnea, cough, and fatigue are often present.
   c. Pulmonary disease may be indistinguishable from other opportunistic infections. Chest radiographic findings include focal alveolar infiltrates, discrete nodules, hilar adenopathy, or cavitary lesions.
   d. CNS involvement is characterized by the following cerebrospinal fluid CSF findings: high cell counts, decreased glucose, and elevated protein.

   e. Other focal findings are related to sites of end-organ disease, such as the skin, CNS, lymph nodes, liver, spleen, kidneys, adrenal glands, and peritoneum.
4. Diagnosis
   a. Diagnosis can be difficult and secondary to nonspecific presentation, especially in nonendemic areas. Review previous living and travel history to prevent diagnostic delay.
   b. Definitive diagnosis established by either culturing organism or by demonstrating spherule presence via histopathologic stains from clinical specimens.
   c. Differential diagnoses include all other pulmonary opportunistic infections.
5. Prevention/treatment
   a. Routine screening with skin testing has shown no predictive value for disease development; prophylaxis is not currently recommended.
   b. Avoiding endemic areas and excavation or construction sites may reduce risk of infection.
   c. Amphotericin B remains the principal therapy for initial and recurrent disease, although precise dose remains unclear. Most investigators recommend 1 mg/kg/day IV for a cumulative total dosage of 500–700 mg before switching to azole maintenance therapy (Ampel, 2005).
   d. Evidence suggests that fluconazole 400 to 800 mg daily or itraconazole 400 to 600 mg daily are effective for mild disease (Ampel, 2005).
   e. After completion of acute therapy, HIV-infected people usually require lifelong maintenance therapy with either fluconazole or itraconazole. No current evidence-based recommendations exist for discontinuing secondary prophylaxis even if CD4 count rises above 100 cells/mm^3 (Aberg, 2006).
6. Nursing implications
   a. Monitor for adverse effects and response to therapy.
      i) For patients treated with amphotericin B consider the following:
         (1) Concurrent hydration is required to minimize renal toxicity; liposomal form may be used for patients with significant amphotericin B–induced nephrotoxicity.
         (2) Shivering or rigors can be controlled with narcotics.
         (3) Monitoring includes the following—twice weekly: serum magnesium and potassium levels; weekly: complete blood and platelet count; every other day: serum creatinine and BUN while dosage is increased, then at least twice weekly.
      ii) For patients treated with fluconazole, monitor serum creatinine, BUN, and liver function tests as indicated.
      iii) For patients treated with itraconazole, monitor liver function tests and serum potassium as indicated; itraconazole levels may be monitored.
   b. Provide education about importance of maintenance therapy.
      i) Azoles are often associated with nausea. Itraconazole capsules must be taken with food to ensure adequate absorption.
      ii) Drug interactions can occur. Concomitant use of rifampin and rifabutin significantly increases itraconazole clearance and increases levels of rifabutin. Use of these agents as prophylaxis or treatment for mycobacterial infections must be avoided.
      iii) Relapse may occur despite maintenance therapy, and patient should report any symptom of recurrence.

REFERENCES

Aberg, J. A. (2006). Coccidioidomycosis and HIV. In L. Peiperl, S. Coffey, O. Bacon, & P. Volberding (Eds.), *HIV In-Site Knowledge Base* [online textbook]. Retrieved January 21, 2009, from http://hivinsite.ucsf.edu/InSite?page=kb-00&doc=kb-05-02-04

Ampel, N. M. (2005). Coccidioidomycosis in persons infected with HIV type 1. *Clinical Infectious Diseases, 41*(8), 1174–1178.

3.10 CRYPTOCOCCOSIS

1. Etiology/epidemiology
   a. Etiologic agent is *Cryptococcus neoformans,* a yeast characterized by distinctive polysaccharide encapsulations that can be divided into serotypic groups A, B, C, and D.
   b. Organism is ubiquitous in nature and distributed worldwide. Serotypes A and D are found in pigeon droppings and soil; serotype C has been isolated from fruit and fruit juices.
   c. Recurrent disease is thought to involve reactivation of initial infection.
   d. The incidence of cryptococcosis is 0.4 to 1.3 cases per 100,000 in the general population. In persons with AIDS, the annual incidence is 2 to 7 cases per 1,000 (Centers for Disease Control and Prevention, 2005) and is associated with both advanced HIV disease (CD4 counts < 100 cells/mm^3) and recrudescence of latent infection
2. Pathogenesis
   a. Aerosolized organisms enter pulmonary tract via inhalation. The most common extrapulmonary site of the disease is the central nervous system (CNS), but it can also involve skin, bone, and the genitourinary tract.
   b. *C. neoformans* produces tissue destruction secondary to yeast multiplication and tissue displacement. The infection elicits a variable inflammatory response, and well-formed granulomas are generally not seen.
      i) Characteristic lesions are cystic clusters of fungi with minimal inflammatory response (cyptococcoma, cyptococcocal granuloma).
      ii) CNS lesions tend to spread diffusely through the brain to involve basal ganglia, cortical gray matter, and meninges.
3. Clinical presentation
   a. Cryptococcosis among HIV+ patients most commonly occurs as a subacute meningitis or meningoencephalitis with fever, malaise, headache, and classic meningeal symptoms and signs (e.g., neck stiffness or photophobia). Some patients present with encephalopathic symptoms (e.g., lethargy, altered mentation, personality changes, and memory loss).
   b. Approximately half of patients with disseminated disease have evidence of pulmonary rather than meningeal involvement. Symptoms and signs of pulmonary infection include cough or dyspnea and pleuritic chest pain.
   c. Symptoms involving the CNS have an insidious or acute onset that can chronically wax or wane with asymptomatic intervals. CNS-specific symptoms include headaches, stiff neck, focal deficits, and seizures. Nonspecific symptoms of CNS infection include nausea, dizziness, irritability, somnolence, clumsiness, confusion or obtundation, and diarrhea.

    d. Other numerous sites of end-organ disease have been reported, including skin, bone, renal, oral mucosa, and GU tract.

4. Diagnosis
    a. Cryptococcal antigen is usually detected in the CSF at high titer in patients with meningitis or meningoencephalitis. A fungal blood culture can also be used and is helpful if disseminated disease is suspected in the absence of meningitis. Serologic testing for cryptococcal antigen (CRAG) is clinically useful for detecting organisms.
    b. Pulmonary cryptococcosis
       i) Radiographic findings often resemble a tumor with single or multiple circumscribed masses or nodules without hilar involvement. Other patterns include findings of lymphadenopathy or pleural effusions, most often with diffuse mixed interstitial infiltrates.
       ii) Bronchoscopic washings and brushings are usually diagnostic.
       iii) Sputum cultures can be negative with invasive disease; parenchymal and tissue samples are usually necessary for definitive diagnosis.
    c. CNS cryptococcosis
       i) Usually manifests as cerebrospinal fluid (CSF) abnormalities, including increased opening pressure ($<$ 200 mm H_2O), lowered glucose level, increased protein concentration, and leukocyte counts $>$ 20 cells/mm^3. Opening pressure (OP) $>$ 250 associated with lower survival rate.
       ii) Positive antigen titers and fungal cultures
       iii) CT scan or MRI findings may be normal or reveal diffuse atrophy, cerebral edema, hydrocephalus, or focal mass lesions.
       iv) Differential diagnosis is focused on ruling out other CNS space-occupying lesions, such as aspergillus, tuberculosis, toxoplasmosis, lymphoma, or other neoplasms.

5. Prevention/treatment
    a. Routine CRAG screening of HIV-infected people is not currently recommended because of limited sensitivity/specificity of the assay.
    b. Avoid sites that are likely to be contaminated with *C. neoformans;* tobacco-smoking cessation may reduce disease risk.
    c. Acute therapy (CDC, 2004) for the initial infection or recurrent infection includes the following:
       i) Amphotericin B (0.7–1.0 mg/kg IV daily) for minimum of 2 weeks, with or without 5-flucytosine (100 mg/kg orally QID, adjusted for any renal insufficiency development), followed by consolidation therapy of either fluconazole (400 mg orally daily for 8 to 10 weeks) or itraconazole (200 mg orally twice daily for 8 to 10 weeks).
       ii) In the absence of obstructive hydrocephalus, CNS disease may require serial lumbar punctures to release increased intracranial pressure. If lumbar puncture is insufficient to manage increased intracranial pressure, lumbar drain, ventriculostomy, or placement of a ventricular-peritoneal shunt may be performed.
    d. Maintenance suppressive therapy is fluconazole (200 mg orally daily). Alternative regimens are itraconazole (200 mg orally twice daily) or amphotericin B (1 mg/kg IV once or twice weekly). Secondary prophylaxis can be discontinued if CD4 count $>$ 100–200

cells/mm^3 for > 6 months and if initial acute therapy is completed and patient has no symptoms of cryptococcosis. Restart secondary prophylaxis if CD4 count falls below 100–200 cells/mm^3.

   e. Immune reconstitution inflammatory syndrome in cryptococcal meningitis has a presentation similar to relapsed meningitis and is associated with initial CSF titer > 1:1024 and is associated with antiretroviral initiation within 30 days of cryptococcccal meningitis diagnosis.

6. Nursing implications

   a. See Section 3.9, titled Coccidioidomycosis, for nursing implications relevant to treatment with amphotericin B, fluconazole, and itraconazole.

   b. For patients treated with 5-flucytosine, frequent monitoring of serum alanine aminotransferase (ALT), alkaline phosphatase, aspartate aminotransferase (AST), bilirubin, creatinine, and blood urea nitrogen is indicated.

   c. Ensure lumbar puncture opening pressure is recorded.

   d. Educate patient about prevention and importance of maintenance therapy (see Section 3.9 for specific interventions).

REFERENCES

Centers for Disease Control and Prevention (CDC). (2004). Treating opportunistic infections among HIV-infected adults and adolescents. *Morbidity and Mortality Weekly Report, 53*(RR15), 1–112.

Centers for Disease Control and Prevention (CDC). (2005). *Cryptococcus*. Retrieved February 5, 2009, from http://www.cdc.gov/nczved/dfbmd/disease_listing/cryptococcus_gi.html

3.11 HISTOPLASMOSIS

1. Etiology/epidemiology

   a. Etiologic agent is *Histoplasma capsulatum,* a fungus deposited in the soil via bird and bat droppings.

   b. *H. capsulatum* is endemic in the southern and midwestern United States from Alabama to southwest Texas and along the Ohio and Missouri river valleys. Hyperendemic areas include Indianapolis, Indiana, and Kansas City, Missouri. It is also found in eastern Mexico, the Caribbean, Central and South America, and parts of Southeast Asia.

   c. Infections in persons who live outside endemic areas are due to reactivation of previously acquired infection.

2. Pathogenesis

   a. Aerosolized spores enter the pulmonary tract via inhalation. Spores become activated and can spread via reticuloendothelial system to the liver, spleen, and lymph nodes. Infection is characterized by granuloma formation.

   b. Disseminated disease is associated with advanced HIV infection and median CD4 count of 50 cells/mm^3 at time of diagnosis.

3. Clinical presentation

   a. Constitutional symptoms are present in 95% of cases, and respiratory complaints are seen in 50–60% of cases; hepatosplenomegaly, lymphadenopathy, and septicemia are commonly present at time of diagnosis.

    b. Neurologic manifestations, such as meningitis, are reported in 18–20% of cases.

    c. Skin and mucosal ulcers may be present (Young & Goldman, 2006).

4. Diagnosis

    a. Diagnosis can be difficult secondary to nonspecific presentation, especially in nonendemic areas. Review previous living and travel history to prevent diagnostic delay.

    b. Detection of *Histoplasma* antigen in blood or urine is a sensitive method for rapid diagnosis of disseminated histoplasmosis, but insensitive for pulmonary infection. Antigen is detected in the urine of 95% and serum of 85% of patients with disseminated histoplasmosis and might be present in bronchoalveolar lavage fluid or CSF of patients with pulmonary or meningeal involvement (Young & Goldman, 2006). Fungal stain of blood smears or tissues also might yield a rapid diagnosis, but the sensitivity is < 50%. *H. capsulatum* can be isolated from blood, bone marrow, respiratory secretions, or localized lesions in > 85% of cases, but isolation can take 2–4 weeks (Young & Goldman, 2006). Serologic tests are positive in approximately two-thirds of cases but are rarely helpful in the acute diagnosis of histoplasmosis disease.

       i) Standard antibody serology test is not useful because it does not distinguish current from past infection.

       ii) Histoplasma specific antigen (HAG) can be assayed in both serum and urine specimens, although urine test is more sensitive. Most diagnoses of disseminated histoplasmosis are now made with this test because of its rapid turnaround time, compared with culture.

    c. Differential diagnoses include all other pulmonary opportunistic infections.

    d. Hematologic disturbances, primarily anemia, are frequently present.

    e. Diffuse or patchy infiltrates are the most common radiographic abnormality.

5. Prevention/treatment

    a. Routine skin testing is of little value in endemic areas because most people will test positive. Primary prophylaxis is not currently recommended.

    b. Avoiding endemic areas and excavation or construction sites may reduce risk of infection.

    c. Amphotericin B is the recommended acute therapy for severe initial or recurrent disease for 3–10 days or until clinically improved. Dosage is 0.7–1.0 mg/kg IV daily or liposmal amphotericin B 4mg/kg IV daily, followed by consolidational therapy with itraconazole 200 mg PO BID for 10–12 weeks. Itraconazole (200 mg PO TID for three days then BID) for 3 months can be used for treatment of mild disease (Young & Goldman, 2006).

    d. HIV-infected persons usually require lifelong maintenance therapy for suppression after completion of consolidation therapy. Maintenance therapy is usually itraconazole (200 mg PO QD).

6. Nursing implications: See "Nursing implications" in the Coccidioidomycosis section 3.9.

REFERENCES

Young, E. M., & Goldman, M. (2006). Histoplasmosis and HIV infection. In L. Peiperl, S. Coffey, O. Bacon, & P. Volberding (Eds.), *HIV InSite Knowledge Base* [online textbook]. Retrieved January 21, 2009, from http://hivinsite.ucsf.edu/InSite?page=kb-00&doc=kb-05-02-04

3.12 CRYPTOSPORIDIOSIS

1. Etiology/epidemiology
   a. Etiological agent is the sporozoa cryptosporidium.
   b. The global prevalence of cryptosporidiosis infection is 8%. The prevalence in the United States is estimated to be 4%. In developing countries, prevalence ranges from 12% to 48% of patients with AIDS and diarrhea (White, 2006).
2. Pathogenesis
   a. Cryptosporidium's oocyst releases four sporozoites upon excystation. The organism completes its entire life cycle within a single host. During the life cycle, four sporozoites are released and adhere to the surface of the intestinal mucosa. To enhance adherence, the organism releases a sporozoite-specific lectin adherence factor. Once attachment occurs, it is hypothesized that the epithelial mucosa cells release cytokines that activate phagocytes. The activated cells release histamine, serotonin, prostaglandins, leukotrienes, and platelet-activating factor. These soluble factors increase the intestinal secretion of water and chloride and also inhibit absorption. Epithelial cells are believed to be damaged by one of two ways: (a) direct result of parasite invasion, multiplication, or extrusion, or (b) T-cell-mediated inflammation produces villus atrophy and crypt hyperplasia (White, 2006).
   b. Either model produces distortion of the villus architecture and is accompanied by nutrient malabsorption and diarrhea.
3. Clinical presentation
   a. Debilitating, cholera-like diarrhea (up to 20 liters/day)
   b. Severe abdominal cramps
   c. Malaise
   d. Low-grade fever
   e. Weight loss
   f. Anorexia
   g. Cholangitis in persons with CD4 counts $\leq$ 50 cells/mm^3
4. Diagnosis
   a. History
      i)   Drinking water that is unfiltered and untreated
      ii) Involvement in farming practices such as lambing, calving, and muck-spreading
      iii) Engaging in sexual practices that lead to oral contact with feces of an infected individual
      iv) Being a patient in a healthcare setting with other infected patients or employees
      v)   Traveling to areas with untreated water
      vi) Living in densely populated urban areas
      vii) Owning an infected household pet (rare)
   b. HIV-infected persons with CD4 cell counts greater than 200 cells/mm^3 experience self-limiting disease, whereas those with counts less than 100 cells/mm^3 frequently experience chronic illness (Smith & Corcoran, 2004).
   c. Laboratory tests
      i)   Stool for ova and parasites
      ii) Stool studies using a modified acid-fast (Kinyoun) stain

      iii)   Differential diagnosis: diarrhea from other parasites; viral etiology: HIV, CMV; bacterial etiology: enteric pathogens, diarrhea from C. *difficile* toxin

      iv)   ELISA or antibody immunofluorescence assay for the presence of anti-cryptosporidial IgM, IgG, and IgA

5. Prevention/treatment

  a. Preventing transmission

      i)   Wash hands with soap and water after using the toilet, changing diapers, and before eating or preparing food.

      ii)   Avoid swimming in recreational water such as swimming pool, hot tubs, lakes, rivers, and so forth while experiencing diarrhea.

      iii)   Avoid fecal exposure during sex.

  b. General prevention

      i)   Wash hands after touching pets or animals.

      ii)   Avoid touching the stool of pets. Animals under the age of 6 months, strays, or animals with diarrhea pose the greatest risk.

      iii)   Wash hands after gardening even when wearing garden gloves.

      iv)   Avoid swallowing recreational water.

      v)   Avoid drinking untreated water from shallow wells, lakes, rivers, springs, ponds, and streams.

      vi)   Avoid drinking untreated water during community-wide outbreaks of disease caused by contaminated drinking water.

      vii)   Avoid using ice or drinking untreated water when traveling in countries where the water supply might be unsafe. If treated water is unavailable, boil water for at least 1 minute.

      viii)   A filter that has an absolute 1 micron or smaller pore size is useful for removing cysts. Filters that provide a "reverse osmosis" process protect against cryptosporidiosis. Reliable filters are labeled "Standard 53" and contain the words "cyst reduction" or "cyst removal."

      ix)   Wash and/or peel all raw vegetables and fruits before eating.

      x)   Avoid unpasteurized milk or dairy products.

      xi)   Use uncontaminated water to wash all food that is to be eaten raw.

      xii)   Avoid eating uncooked foods when traveling in countries with minimal water treatment and sanitation systems.

      xiii)   Safe bottled water is reverse-osmosis treated, distilled, or filtered through an absolute 1 micron or smaller filter.

  c. Treatment

      i)   Antiretroviral therapy improves immune status and will decrease or eliminate symptoms of cryptosporidiosis.

      ii)   Paromomycin has been shown to decrease the intensity of the infection and improve intestinal function. Relapse after paromomycin treatment is common.

      iii)   Nitazoxanide (Alinia) has demonstrated anti-cryptosporidial activity (Rossignol, 2006).

  d. Symptom management

      i)   Intravenous fluids or oral rehydration with electrolyte replacements may be necessary for voluminous, watery diarrhea. Oral rehydration can be accomplished with

  Gatorade, bouillon, or oral rehydration solutions that contain glucose, sodium bicarbonate, and potassium.
  ii)   Medications to slow GI motility: opiates, lomotil, sandostatin
  iii)   Antimicrobial agents may yield partial responses, such as reduced diarrhea or de-
         crease in the stool to oocyst number. These agents include spiramycin or dicalzuril.
6. Implications for nursing
    a. Patient education to avoid infection

REFERENCES

Rossignol, J. F. (2006). Nitazoxanide in the treatment of acquired immune deficiency syndrome-related cryptosporidiosis:
    Results of the United States compassionate use program in 365 patients. *Alimentary Pharmacology & Therapeutics,
    24*(5), 887–894.
Smith, H. V., & Corcoran, G. D. (2004). New drugs and treatment for cryptosporidiosis. *Current Opinions in Infectious
    Diseases, 17*(6), 557–564.
White, A. C. (2006). *Cryptosporidiosis.* Retrieved January 21, 2009, from http://emedicine.medscape.com/article/215490-
    overview

3.13 PNEUMOCYSTOSIS

1. Etiology/epidemiology
    a. The etiologic agent is the fungus *Pneumocystis jiroveci.*
    b. Incidence has decreased in industrialized countries as a result of augmentation of the im-
        mune system due to improved prophylaxis and HAART.
    c. Survey data suggest pneumocystosis (PCP) infection occurs in approximately 26% of pa-
        tients with AIDS without prophylaxis (Jones et al., 1999).
    d. Data indicate that it remains the most common AIDS-defining illness (Leoung, 2005).
    e. Risk of developing *Pneumocystis* pneumonia (PCP) has been correlated with a CD4 count
        of 200 cells/mm^3 or less (Leoung, 2005).
2. Pathogenesis
    a. Organism attaches to type 1 alveolar cells, replicates, and invades the epithelium of the
        lung.
    b. The immunocompromised host is unable to mount an alveolar macrophage response, re-
        sulting in pneumonia and interfering with the transport of fatty acid substrates, an essen-
        tial component of lung surfactant. Without surfactant, lung dispensability is diminished.
    c. Colonization with *Pneumocystis* is gaining greater attention, possibly due to detection fa-
        cilitated by the development of sensitive PCR techniques (Huang et al., 2006).
3. Clinical presentation
    a. Symptoms are insidious and slowly progress over the course of a few weeks; most com-
        mon symptoms are low-grade fever, nonproductive cough, and dyspnea.
    b. Fever, fatigue, and weight loss may precede respiratory symptoms (Kovacs, Gill, Mesh-
        nick, & Masur, 2001).
4. Diagnosis

a. The recovery of the organism from expectorated sputum is difficult. The diagnosis is often made on the presence of classic symptoms, chest radiograph (diffuse, bilateral infiltrates), and pulse oximetry (hypoxemia with activity).

b. Sputum induction via inhalation of a saline mist performed by specialists is an acceptable, noninvasive diagnostic alternative (Leoung, 2005).

c. *Pneumocystis jiroveci* may be identified in bronchoalveolar lavage or transbronchial biopsy but are not required for diagnosis.

d. Several PCR-based molecular assays for diagnosis and identifying trimethroprim-sulfamethoxazole drug resistance; specimens should be collected before initiation of treatment (Huang et al., 2006).

e. Laboratory data, such as arterial blood gases, should be monitored for hypoxemia because prognosis is related to oxygenation at time of presentation; alveolar-arterial oxygen gradient of > 29 mmHg is considered severe disease with a poor prognosis (Leoung, 2005).

5. Prevention/treatment

a. Primary prophylactic agents include trimethoprim-sulfamethoxazole (TMP-SMX, preferred therapy), dapsone, aerosolized pentamidine, dapsone/pyrimethamine, atovaquone, trimethoprim, and parenteral pentamidine. Pafuramidine maleate (DB289) is a promising investigational drug in clinical trials (ClinicalTrials, 2007).

b. Prophylaxis should be offered to any patient with a CD4 count less than or equal to 200 cells/mm^3 or less or a patient who has recovered from a previous episode of PCP. Prophylaxis may be discontinued if durable viral suppression is achieved with HAART and a stable CD4 count > 200 cells/mm^3 for > 3 months (Benson et al., 2004; Gottlieb, 1999; Mussini et al., 2000).

c. The preferred prophylactic regimen is Bactrim DS/day or 1 SS/day.

d. The treatment duration is 21 days (it may be extended with severe disease). Agents include TMP-SMX, pentamidine, trimetrexate with leucovorin rescue during length of infusion and 3 days beyond last dose, trimethroprim with dapsone, clindamycin with primaquine (especially if TMP-SMX treatment fails), atovaquone, and corticosteroids. The preferred treatment regimen is Bactrim 2 DS tablets TID.

e. Corticosteroids may be added during the first 72 hours of treatment in patients with an arterial oxygen pressure < 70 mmHg or an alveolar-arterial oxygen gradient > 35mmHg (Briel et al., 2006).

6. Nursing implications

a. Promote optimal gas exchange (e.g., incentive spirometry, oxygen therapy, chest percussion; Flaskerud & Ungvarski, 1999).

b. Do not place a coughing patient with PCP in a room with an immunocompromised patient until active tuberculosis (TB) is ruled out (Flaskerud & Ungvarski, 1999).

c. Monitor for side effects or adverse effects of medications, such as hypoglycemia, rash/photosensitivity, peripheral neuropathy, and liver function abnormalities; extreme caution should be used with desensitization to TMP-SMX; monitor for glucose-6-phosphate dehydrogenase deficiency to prevent hemolysis.

d. Monitor blood glucose during parenteral pentamidine treatment because hypoglycemia is an adverse effect (Flaskerud & Ungvarski, 1999).

REFERENCES

Benson, C. A., Kaplan, J. E., Masur, H., Pau, A., Holmes, K. K., CDC, National Institutes of Health, & Infectious Diseases Society of America. (2004). Treating opportunistic infections among HIV-infected adults and adolescents: Recommendations from CDC, the National Institutes of Health, and the HIV Medicine Association/Infectious Diseases Society of America. *MMWR Recommendations and Reports, 53*(RR15), 1–112.

Briel, M., Boscacci, R., Furrer, H., & Bucher, H. C. (2005). Adjunctive corticosteroids for *Pneumocystis jiroveci* pneumonia in patients with HIV infection: A meta-analysis of randomised controlled trials. *BMC Infectious Diseases, 98*(4), 287–290.

ClinicalTrials. (2007). *DB289 Versus TMP-SMX for the treatment of acute Pneumocystis jiroveci pneumonia (PCP)*. Retrieved January 21, 2009, from http://clinicaltrials.gov

Flaskerud, J. H., & Ungvarski, P. J. (1999). *HIV/AIDS: A guide to nursing care* (4th ed.). Philadelphia: W. B. Saunders.

Gottlieb, S. (1999). Some HIV patients can stop taking prophylaxis against infections. *British Medical Journal, 318*(7193), 1231.

Huang, L., Morris, A., Limper, A. H., & Beck, J. (2006). An official ATS workshop summary: Recent advances and future directions in *Pneumocystis* Pneumonia (PCP). *Proceedings of the American Thoracic Society, 3*(8), 655–664.

Jones, J. L., Handon, D. L., Dworkin, M. S., Alderton, D. L., Fleming, D. L., Kaplan, J. E., et al. (1999). Surveillance for AIDS-defining opportunistic illnesses, 1992–1997. *Morbidity and Mortality Weekly Report, 48*(SS-2), 1–22.

Kovacs, J. A., Gill, V. J., Meshnick, S., & Masur, H. (2001). New insights into transmission, diagnosis, and drug treatment of *Pneumocystic carinii* pneumonia. *Journal of the American Medical Association, 286*(19), 2450–2460.

Leoung, G.S. (2005). Pneumocystosis and HIV. In L. Peiperl, S. Coffey, O. Bacon, & P. Volberding (Eds.), *HIV InSite Knowledge Base* [online textbook]. Retrieved January 21, 2009, from http://hivinsite.ucsf.edu/InSite?page=kb-00&doc=kb-05-02-01

Mussini, C., Pezzotti, P., Govoni, A., Borghi, V., Antinori, A., d'Arminio Monforte, A., et al. (2000). Discontinuation of primary prophylaxis for *Pneumocystis carinii* pneumonia and toxoplasmic encephalitis in human immunodeficiency virus type I-infected patients. *Journal of Infectious Diseases, 181*(5), 1635–1642.

3.14 TOXOPLASMOSIS

1. Etiology/epidemiology
    a. *Toxoplasma gondii* is a coccidian feline parasite that uses mammals as its intermediate host and exists in three forms (Subauste, 2006):
        i) Oocysts, which are shed from the feline GI tract and released as sporozoites (inactive form) from dry feces
        ii) Tachyzoites (fast-growing, active form), which are found in mammalian tissue prior to mounting an immune response
        iii) Bradyzoites (slow-growing form), which continue to grow inside tissue cysts that form as part of the immune response
    b. Infection occurs via ingestion of oocysts in undercooked contaminated meats or feces-contaminated produce or via inhalation of sporozoites.
    c. Toxoplasmosis disease is rare in HIV-seronegative populations and is usually from latent cyst reactivation in HIV-positive populations. Most commonly seen in patients with CD4 count of < 200 cells/mm^3 with greatest risk at CD4 count < 50 cells/mm^3 (Subauste, 2006).
    d. The disease is found worldwide, with higher incidence of latent infection in Africa, Haiti, Europe, and Latin America.
2. Pathogenesis
    a. After primary exposure, *T. gondii* can invade and infect contiguous tissue by converting from bradyzoite to tachyzoite form. Cysts can be found in all tissue types.

      i) Most common sites are in brain, heart, and striated muscle.

      ii) There is evidence that cysts rupture and may cause recurrent asymptomatic infections.

3. Clinical presentation

  a. Disease is associated with advanced HIV disease, and clinical lab findings generally are too nonspecific to be of diagnostic value.

  b. Central nervous system disease is frequently multifocal, with a wide spectrum of clinical findings, including headache, fever, altered level of consciousness, mood changes, seizures, and strokelike symptoms.

  c. Retinochoroiditis, pneumonia, and evidence of other multifocal organ system involvement can be seen after dissemination of infection but are rare manifestations in this patient population.

      i) Pulmonary symptoms include fever, nonproductive cough, shortness of breath, or a combination of the three, that progresses more rapidly than *Pneumocystis jiroveci* pneumonia.

      ii) Ocular symptoms include decreased visual acuity and eye pain.

4. Diagnosis

  a. Definitive diagnosis of central nervous system disease is based on identification of the organism in tissue via biopsy, although this is rarely done.

      i) Empiric therapy based on typical head CT or MRI findings generally initiated without biopsy given high morbidity and mortality associated with brain biopsies. Serologic test (IgG) for *T. gondii* is also done to document latent infection because the disease is very unusual in AIDS patients with negative *T. gondii* serologic test results.

  b. CT scan or MRI of the brain will typically show multiple contrast-enhancing lesions, often with associated edema. CT is less sensitive than MRI but can show characteristic ring enhancing lesions.

  c. Differential diagnoses are central nervous system lymphoma, extra-pulmonary *M. tuberculosis,* fungal disease such as cryptococcosis, bacterial abscess, and rarely PML (Subauste, 2006).

5. Prevention/treatment

  a. All HIV-infected individuals should be tested for *T. gondii*-specific IgG antibodies as part of the baseline evaluation.

  b. Patients with findings on neuroimaging typical of toxoplasmic encephalitis should receive empiric toxoplasmosis therapy (Montoya & Remington, 2000).

      i) Pyrimethamine + leucovorin (to prevent pyrimethamine-associated bone marrow toxicity) + sulfadiazine or clindamycin is current standard of therapy and patients should be treated for at least 6 weeks or longer if disease is extensive or if response is incomplete.

      ii) Alternative regimens include the following: Pyrimethamine + leucovorin + either atovaquone or azithromycin.

  c. After completion of acute therapy, primary prophylaxis can be discontinued if CD4 count > 200 cells/mm^3 for at least 3 months. Secondary prophylaxis can be discontinued if CD4 count > 200 cells/mm^3 for > 6 months and if initial therapy has been completed and patient has no symptoms of toxoplasmosis. Restart primary prophylaxis if CD4 count falls below 100–200 cells/mm^3 and restart secondary prophylaxis if CD4 count falls below 200 cells/mm^3.

    d. Anticonvulsant therapy may be indicated for seizure prevention.
6. Nursing implications
    a. Teach patients to avoid contact with potentially contaminated sources.
       i) Use gloves when handling litter boxes or gardening.
       ii) Disinfect cat litter boxes when changing litter.
       iii) Eat only completely cooked or cured meats.
       iv) Wash hands and kitchen surfaces thoroughly after handling raw meat; avoid touching mucous membranes when handling raw meat.
       v) Wash all fruits and vegetables before eating.
    b. Monitor laboratory results and other indices for adverse drug effects and response to therapy.

REFERENCES

Montoya, J. G., & Remington, J. S. (2000). *Toxoplasma gondii*. In G. L. Mandell, J. E. Bennett, & R. Dolin (Eds.), *Principles and practice of infectious diseases* (pp. 2858–2888). Philadelphia: Churchill Livingstone.

Subauste, C.S. (2006). Toxoplasmosis and HIV. In L. Peiperl, S. Coffey, O. Bacon, & P. Volberding (Eds.), *HIV InSite Knowledge Base* [online textbook]. Retrieved January 21, 2009, from http://hivinsite.ucsf.edu/InSite?page=kb-00&doc=kb-05-04-03

3.15 CYTOMEGALOVIRUS (CMV)

1. Etiology/epidemiology
    a. CMV is a double-stranded DNA herpes virus that is found in semen, cervical secretions, saliva, urine, blood, and organs.
    b. Transmission modes include perinatal transmission, sexual contact, blood exchange, and transplantation of infected organs or tissues.
    c. In the United States, between 50% and 80% of adults are infected with CMV by 40 years of age (CDC, 2004).
2. Pathogenesis
    a. Can cause chorioretinitis, radiculopathy, encephalitis, colitis, esophagitis, and pneumonia (Drew & Lalezari, 2006).
3. Clinical presentation
    a. Seen with severe immunosuppression (CD4 count < 50 cells/mm^3).
    b. May be seen with the following: retinitis—decreased visual acuity, floaters, unilateral visual field loss, and scotoma; colitis—fever, weight loss, anorexia, abdominal pain, debilitating diarrhea, and malaise; radiculopathy—lower extremity weakness, spasticity, areflexia, and urinary retention; encephalitis—personality changes, poor concentration, headaches, and somnolence; esophagitis—odynophagia, fever, nausea (Drew & Lalezari, 2006).
4. Diagnosis
    a. CMV viremia can be detected by PCR, antigen assays, or blood culture and is generally detected in end-organ disease, but viremia also might be present in the absence of end-

organ disease. Retinal exam will reveal large, creamy to yellow-white granular areas with perivascular exudates and hemorrhages. CSF fluid analysis may be normal. Antigen testing of CMV DNA will be positive in affected tissues. Endoscopic examination generally reveals large, white-yellow plaques throughout the esophagus, and colon biopsy reveals ulceration and submucosal hemorrhages. Chest X-ray generally reveals diffuse infiltrates and histologic examination of sputum (Drew & Lalezari, 2006).

    b. Histologic diagnosis is the gold standard; tissue cultures may be positive but are not specific for active disease; urine culture may reveal viral shedding but is not indicative of active disease; CMV serology is necessary to determine active disease (Zwolski, 2001).

5. Prevention/treatment

    a. Avoid giving CMV-positive blood products to a CMV-negative patient; early detection can be determined by using a visual grid or routine ophthalmology exam to detect vision changes.

    b. The choice of initial therapy for CMV retinitis is dependent on the location and severity of the lesion(s), overall immune status, potential for drug interactions with concomitant medications, and ability to adhere to treatment. Oral valganciclovir, intravenous ganciclovir, intravenous ganciclovir followed by oral valganciclovir, intravenous foscarnet, intravenous cidofovir, and the ganciclovir intraocular implant coupled with valganciclovir are all effective treatments for CMV retinitis (CDC, 2004).

    c. For colitis or esophagitis, treatment is usually with intravenous ganciclovir or foscarnet (or with oral valganciclovir if symptoms are not severe enough to interfere with oral absorption) for 21–28 days.

    d. Oral ganciclovir 1 gm TID is not currently recommended for prophylaxis. Side effects outweigh any benefit derived by administration.

    e. Secondary prophylaxis can be discontinued if CD4 count > 100–150 cells/mm^3 for > 6 months, if there is a non-sight threatening lesion with adequate vision in the other eye, and patient has regular eye exams. Secondary prophylaxis should resume if CD4 count falls below 50 cells/mm^3.

6. Nursing implications

    a. Arrange for home care if intravenous medications are to be administered in the home. Teach self-administration of oral medications.

    b. Teach high-risk patients use of visual grid; offer visual aid devices if patient suffers visual loss.

    c. Monitor patient for response to therapy and adverse effects; monitor renal function, electrolytes, calcium, magnesium, and CBC with differential.

    d. With advanced immunosuppression, encourage serial ophthalmic exams.

REFERENCES

Centers for Disease Control and Prevention (CDC). (2004). Treating opportunistic infections among HIV-infected adults and adolescents. *Morbidity and Mortality Weekly Report, 53*(RR15), 1–112.

Drew, W. L., & Lalezari, J. P. (2006). Cytomegalovirus and HIV. In L. Peiperl, S. Coffey, O. Bacon, & P. Volberding (Eds.), *HIV InSite Knowledge Base* [online textbook]. Retrieved January 21, 2009, from http://hivinsite.ucsf.edu/InSite?page=kb-00&doc=kb-05-03-03

Zwolski, K. (2001). Viral infections. In C. Kirton, D. Talotta, & K. Zwolski (Eds.), *Handbook of HIV/AIDS nursing* (pp. 300–316). St. Louis, MO: Mosby.

3.16 HERPES SIMPLEX VIRUS (HSV)

1. Etiology/epidemiology
   a. There are two distinct viruses: HSV-1 and HSV-2.
   b. Initial infection is often during childhood; many infections are subclinical and undiagnosed.
   c. Many infections are acquired via sexual transmission. Genital HSV (most commonly HSV-2) is a chronic, lifelong infection. HSV-2 is one of the most common sexually transmitted viruses worldwide. About 80% to 100% of patients who are HIV-positive will become infected with one or more herpes viruses during the course of their HIV infection (Krzyzowska, Schollenberger, & Niemialtowski, 2000).
2. Pathogenesis
   a. Primary infection
      i)   Transmission occurs through direct contact, during which time the virus is inoculated onto mucosal surfaces or breaks in the skin. HSV shedding is increased in HIV-infected persons (CDC, 2006).
      ii) Virions travel from the site of inoculation along sensory nerves to the corresponding nerve root ganglion, where infections are permanently established.
      iii) Reactivation or recurrence can occur in response to a host of stimuli (e.g., stress, trauma, ultraviolet light).
3. Clinical presentation
   a. Manifestations of primary HSV infection include fever, adenopathy, malaise, and painful ulcerative lesions involving mucosal or cutaneous sites.
   b. Primary infection in HIV disease is rare; typically, subclinical HSV infection occurs prior to HIV infection.
      i)   Prodromal symptoms of paresthesias, itching, or tingling at the site of impending eruption may precede a recurrence or outbreak.
      ii) HSV lesions may present as small, localized ulcerations or can spread contiguously to cover large areas. Disease may also present as papules that rapidly evolve into painful, palpable fluid-filled vesicles.
      iii) Common sites of HSV lesions include orolabial, genital, and anorectal. Involvement of visceral organs can occur in HIV disease (e.g., esophagitis, encephalitis).
   c. Coinfection with HIV and HSV may lead to a prolonged and more severe clinical course than is seen in singly infected persons (CDC, 2006).
4. Diagnosis
   a. Direct virus culture taken from suspected lesions is the gold standard. Viral culture isolates should be typed to determine if HSV-1 or HSV-2 is the causative agent.
   b. Both type-specific and nontype-specific antibodies develop during the initial onset of infection and are present indefinitely, limiting their clinical utility (CDC, 2006).
5. Prevention/treatment
   a. Primary infection rates might be reduced by the use of latex condoms.
   b. Patients with primary infection should receive antiviral therapy, whereas patients with symptomatic, chronic HSV infections should be treated aggressively with antiviral chemotherapy.

  c. Antiviral agents used to prevent and treat HSV in HIV-infected persons
   i) Recommended regimens for daily suppressive therapy in persons infected with HIV (CDC, 2006, p. 19):
    (1) Acyclovir 400–800 mg orally twice or three times a day
    (2) Famciclovir 500 mg orally twice a day
    (3) Valacyclovir 500 mg orally twice a day
   ii) Recommended regimens for episodic infection in persons infected with HIV (CDC, 2006, p. 19):
    (1) Acyclovir 400 mg orally three times a day for 5–10 days
    (2) Famciclovir 500 mg orally twice a day for 5–10 days
    (3) Valacyclovir 1.0 gram orally twice a day for 5–10 days
   iii) Acyclovir, valacyclovir, and famciclovir are considered safe for use in immunocompromised persons in the doses recommended for treatment of genital HSV infection (CDC, 2006, p. 19).
   iv) For severe HSV disease, it may be necessary to initiate therapy with acyclovir 5–10 mg/kg body weight IV every 8 hours.
   v) Topical therapy with antiviral drugs offers minimal clinical benefit, and its use is discouraged.
  d. Although antiretroviral therapy reduces the severity and frequency of symptomatic genital herpes, shedding still occurs (CDC, 2006).
6. Nursing implications
  a. Local care of mucocutaneous lesions includes keeping lesions clean and dry, with gentle cleansing using mild soap and water.
  b. Pain can be severe and should be assessed; analgesia should be administered as needed.
  c. Stool softeners should be considered for patients with anorectal ulcers.
  d. Counseling should be given to prevent transmission of HSV infection. The goal of counseling is to help patients cope with the infection and to prevent sexual and perinatal transmission of HSV. Patient information services recommended by the CDC can be accessed by phone at 800-227-8922 or online at http://www.ashastd.org.

REFERENCES

Centers for Disease Control and Prevention (CDC). (2006). Sexually transmitted diseases treatment guidelines. *Morbidity and Mortality Weekly Report, 55*(RR-11), 1–94.
Krzyzowska, M., Schollenberger, A., & Niemialtowski, M. G. (2000). How human immunodeficiency viruses and herpesviruses affect apoptosis. *Acta Virologica, 44*(3), 203–210.

3.17 PROGRESSIVE MULTIFOCAL LEUKOENCEPHALOPATHY (PML)

1. Etiology/epidemiology
  a. PML is a demyelinating disease of cerebral white matter caused by the polyomavirus, JC virus (JCV). JCV is a neurotropic virus that chronically infects approximately 80% of all adults (Hou & Major, 2005; Koralnik, 2004). "JC" stands for the initials of the patient from whose brain this virus was first isolated (Padgett, Walker, ZuRhein, Eckroade, & Dessel, 1971).

      b. Approximately 4–8% of patients with advanced HIV disease will develop PML (Hou & Major, 2005; McGuire, 2003).

      c. PML occurs in patients with both HIV-1 and HIV-2 infection (Bienaime et al., 2006).

2. Pathogenesis

      a. JCV is thought to be transmitted by the respiratory route during childhood, although an oral-fecal route of transmission has also been proposed. The virus remains inactive for life in persons with a healthy immune system; acute JCV infection has not been described clinically (Hou & Major, 2005).

      b. Reactivation of the virus may occur in an immunocompromised host. Only patients with a high degree of immunosuppression (e.g., late-stage HIV disease/AIDS, lymphoproliferative diseases) or patients treated with highly immunosuppressive therapies (e.g., transplant recipients, patients with multiple sclerosis) are likely to develop PML.

      c. JCV causes selective demyelination in the CNS of immunocompromised hosts by lysis of oligodendrites and other CNS cell types (astrocytes and CNS progenitor cells; Hou & Major, 2005).

3. Clinical presentation

      a. PML is a subacute or chronic progressive illness characterized by focal neurologic findings and mental status or personality changes. A protracted, insidious clinical course is typical; fever, acutely altered consciousness, or other signs of acute encephalopathy are unusual.

      b. Manifestations depend on localization of lesions and may include weakness (found in most patients); decreased attention and memory; confusion; personality change; dementia; diplopia and other cranial nerve deficits; mono-, hemi-, or quadriplegia; ataxia; bradykinesia; rigidity; sensory deficits (face, arm numbness); headache; vertigo; seizures; coma; and alien hand syndrome (McGuire, 2003).

      c. PML may initially worsen in HAART-treated patients who show rapid improvements in CD4+ T lymphocyte counts and declines in viral loads (immune reconstitution syndrome). However, patients with immune reconstitution may still have more favorable outcomes, presumably due to restored immune function (Koralnik, 2004).

      d. Since the introduction of HAART, PML-related deaths appear to be decreasing, although there are conflicting findings on survival rates. The mortality rate for PML in the HAART era is 30–50% during the first 3 months post diagnosis (Hou & Major, 2005).

4. Diagnosis

      a. Magnetic resonance imaging (MRI) findings suggestive of PML include diffuse, white-matter, usually nonenhancing lesions without mass effect (Koralnik, 2004).

      b. JCV may be demonstrated by polymerase chain reaction (PCR) testing of cerebrospinal fluid (CSF; McGuire, 2003). Peripheral blood PCR for JCV has not been shown to be clinically useful, nor is routine CSF evaluation, which is usually normal (McGuire, 2003). Sensitivity and specificity may vary significantly by laboratory.

      c. Definitive diagnosis is by tissue acquired from stereotactic brain biopsy; occasionally, direct brain biopsy is required due to the anatomical location of a lesion.

      d. Brain biopsy is often refused by patients, however, and diagnosis may be based on radiologic and clinical findings, supported by confirmed presence of JCV in the CSF by PCR (McGuire, 2003).

   e. PML has been considered to be an AIDS-indicator illness since 1985 (CDC, 1985) and remains one of the 23 indicator illnesses included in the 1993 case definition for AIDS (CDC, 1992).

5. Prevention/treatment

   a. There is currently no known prophylaxis for PML, nor is there an accepted, recommended regimen for its specific treatment.

   b. A growing body of evidence suggests that HAART has significantly altered the typical course of PML in HIV-infected patients (Hou & Major, 2005; Koralnik, 2004; McGuire, 2003). Patients who had previously been naïve to antiretroviral therapy may do best when starting HAART at the time of PML diagnosis (Koralnik, 2004; Yoon, 2006). Patients with CD4 count >100 cells/mm^3 at time of PML diagnosis also experience a survival benefit (Drake et al., 2007).

   c. Several treatment strategies have been evaluated by clinical trial (including cytosine arabinoside, cidofovir, topotecan, interferons, and interleukins; Hou & Major, 2005). None of these treatments has been unequivocally successful, however, and further research to find an effective and safe treatment for PML is needed.

6. Nursing implications

   a. PML should be considered among possible diagnoses whenever a person with AIDS presents with unexplained neurological complaints or findings.

   b. In the early years of the HIV epidemic, a diagnosis of PML was uniformly fatal, usually within 2–4 months. In the HAART era, nurses may now have some hope to offer patients and their loved ones where before none existed.

   c. Effective treatment regimes specifically against PML, however, remain elusive. Randomized, controlled clinical trials continue to be required for definitive answers about therapy. Nurses can support and refer patients diagnosed with PML to appropriate research centers.

   d. In the meantime, concomitant HAART seems prudent, even though clinical trial evidence for the concurrent use of other efficacious agents is currently lacking.

   e. For patients whose PML remains progressive, appropriate counseling and planning for palliative and end-of-life care should be offered. Residential treatment in a long-term care facility or hospice care may be required if home care is not a viable option.

REFERENCES

Bienaime, A., Colson, P., Moreau, J., Zandotti, C., Pellissier, J.-F., & Brouqui, P. (2006). Progressive multifocal leukoencephalopathy in HIV-2-infected patient. *AIDS, 20*(9), 1342–1343.

Centers for Disease Control and Prevention (CDC). (1985). International notes update: Acquired immunodeficiency syndrome—Europe. *Morbidity and Mortality Weekly Report, 34*(11), 147–150, 155–156. Retrieved October 20, 2007, from http://www.cdc.gov/mmwr/preview/mmwrhtml/00000506.htm

Centers for Disease Control and Prevention (CDC). (1992). 1993 revised classification system for HIV infection and expanded surveillance case definition for AIDS among adolescents and adults. *Morbidity & Mortality Weekly Report, 41*(RR-17), 1–19. Retrieved October 20, 2007, from http://www.cdc.gov/mmwr/preview/mmwrhtml/00018871.htm

Drake, A. K., Loy, C. T., Brew, B. J., Chen, T. C. C., Petoumenos, K., Li, P. C. K., et al. (2007). Human immunodeficiency virus-associated progressive multifocal leucoencephalopathy: Epidemiology and predictive factors for prolonged survival. *European Journal of Neurology, 14*(4), 418–423.

Hou, J., & Major, E. (2005). Management of infections by the human polyomavirus JC: Past, present and future. *Expert Review of Antiinfective Therapy, 3*(4), 629–640.

Koralnik, I. J. (2004). New insights into progressive multifocal leukoencephalopathy. *Current Opinion in Neurology, 17*(3), 365–370.

Letendre, S., Ances, B., Gibson, S., & Ellis, R. J. (2007). Neurologic complications of HIV disease and their treatment. *Topics in HIV Medicine, 15*(2), 32–39.

McGuire, D. (2003). Neurologic manifestations of HIV. In L. Peiperl, S. Coffey, O. Bacon, & P. Volberding, (Eds.), *HIV InSite Knowledge Base* [online textbook]. Retrieved October 20, 2007, from http://hivinsite.ucsf.edu/InSite?page=kb-00&doc=kb-04-01-02

Padgett, B. L., Walker, D. L., ZuRhein, G. M., Eckroade, R. J., & Dessel, B. H. (1971). Cultivation of papova-like virus from human brain with progressive multifocal leukoencephalopathy. *Lancet, 1*(7712), 1257–1260.

Yoon, C. J. (2006). Progressive multifocal leukoencephalopathy in the era of highly active antiretroviral therapy. *AIDS Reader, 16*(6), 304–306, 309.

3.18 CERVICAL NEOPLASIA

1. Etiology/epidemiology
   a. The human papillomavirus (HPV) has been implicated as the cause of cervical cancer and some types of anal cancer.
   b. In HIV-infected women, cervical dysplasia (precursor to cervical cancer) is more likely to progress and do so more quickly and at a younger age than in noninfected women.
   c. HIV-infected women are also more likely to experience higher HPV viral loads (Lillo et al., 2005) and infection with multiple and high-risk strains of HPV.
   d. In one study, after 3 years of follow-up, 90% of HIV-infected women with CD4+ T lymphocyte counts < 200 cells/mm^3 were infected with HPV, compared with 55% of uninfected women (Ahdieh et al., 2001).
2. Pathogenesis
   a. There are an estimated 15 oncogenic HPV subtypes, and types 16, 18, 31, and 45 cause 80% of HPV-associated cancers (Abercrombie, 2006). Unlike the low-risk subtypes, the oncogenic subtypes integrate into the host cell DNA.
   b. HPV encodes for two regulatory proteins, E6 and E7, which inhibit cellular proteins that confer susceptibility to apoptosis. The net result is unsuppressed cell growth following DNA damage (Garcia, 2007).
   c. Cervical intraepithelial neoplasia (CIN) III is considered the true precursor to cervical cancer (Palefsky, 2006).
   d. Lesions are found in squamous epithelial cells at the squamocolumnar junction of the cervix and are considered invasive when extension begins into the basement membrane, stroma, and then endometrium.
3. Clinical presentation
   a. Early stages of disease are asymptomatic.
   b. Postcoital bleeding, metorrhagia, and foul-smelling vaginal discharge are common symptoms.
   c. Later symptoms are abdominal, pelvic, back, or leg pain; weight loss; anemia from vaginal bleeding; and lower extremity edema.
   d. Advanced symptoms, including hematuria and rectal bleeding, may be seen with extension of the tumor into the bladder and rectum.

4. Diagnosis
   a. Papanicolau (Pap) smear is the initial screening tool for abnormal cells and/or lesions. This should be initially performed twice at 6-month intervals in the first year of HIV diagnosis, and then once yearly if negative.
   b. HPV testing is used to determine the frequency of screening.
   c. Colposcopy with biopsy is the primary diagnostic tool and is warranted with positive Pap smear results (atypical squamous cells of undetermined significance, ASCUS) in all HIV-infected women.
      i) Biopsies are contraindicated in pregnancy.
      ii) Loop electrical excision procedure (LEEP) and conization/cone biopsy are used for both diagnostic and treatment purposes.
      iii) Frequency of colposcopic screening varies based on the grade of dysplasia.
5. Prevention/treatment
   a. HIV may exert a synergistic effect on HPV (Danso et al., 2006); therefore all grades of cervical dysplasia must be treated to prevent cervical cancer.
   b. The use of HAART has not consistently demonstrated a decrease in the incidence of cervical dysplasia/cancer (Bower et al., 2006).
   c. Hysterectomy is recommended for cervical carcinoma and beyond. Vulvar and anal cancer will still need to be treated.
   d. Radiation therapy
   e. Systemic chemotherapy using cisplatin, fluorouracil, hydroxyurea, methotrexate, bleomycin, doxorubicin
   f. Topical chemotherapy is an option with 5-FU.
   g. Modalities can be used alone or in combination.
   h. HPV therapeutic vaccines may be an option in the future (Palefsky, 2006).
6. Nursing implications
   a. Instruct on safer sex practices, because of increased risk of disease transmission with bleeding.
   b. Assess for signs and symptoms of psychological distress related to sexual trauma and/or gynecological exams.
   c. Instruct patient on prescribed treatment protocol.
   d. Use telephone reminders and/or mailings to increase adherence with treatment appointments.

REFERENCES

Abercrombie, P. (2006). Clinical management of lower genital tract neoplasia among women with HIV. In L. Peiperl, S. Coffey, O. Bacon, & P. Volberding (Eds.), *HIV InSite Knowledge Base* [online textbook]. Retrieved January 22, 2009, from http://hivinsite.ucsf.edu/InSite?page=kb-00&doc=kb-05-04-03

Ahdieh, L., Klein, R. S., Burk, R., Cu-Uvin, S., Schuman, P., Duerr, A., et al. (2001). Prevalence, incidence, and type-specific persistence of human papillomavirus in human immunodeficiency virus (HIV)-positive and HIV-negative women. *Journal of Infectious Diseases, 184*(6), 682–690.

Bower, M., Palmieri, C., & Dhillon, T. (2006). AIDS-related malignancies: Changing epidemiology and the impact of highly active antiretroviral therapy. *Current Opinion in Infectious Diseases, 19*(1), 14–19.

Danso, D., Lyons, F., & Bradbeer, C. (2006). Cervical screening and management of cervical intraepithelial neoplasia in HIV-positive women. *International Journal of STD & AIDS, 17*(9), 579–586.

Garcia, A. (2007). *Cervical cancer*. Retrieved January 22, 2009, from http://www.emedicine.com/MED/topic324.htm

Lillo, F. B., Lodini, S., Ferrari, S., Stayton, C., Taccagni, G., Galli, L., et al. (2005). Determination of human papillomavirus (HPV) load and type in high-grade cervical lesions surgically resected from HIV-infected women during follow-up of HPV infection. *Clinical Infectious Diseases, 40*(3), 451–457.

Palefsky, J. (2006). Human papillomavirus-related tumors in HIV. *Current Opinion in Oncology, 18*(5), 463–468.

3.19 KAPOSI'S SARCOMA (KS)

1. Etiology/epidemiology
   a. Human herpes virus 8/ Kaposi's sarcoma herpes virus (HHV8/KSHV) is the virus associated with Kaposi's sarcoma (KS).
   b. In HIV-infected persons, the transmission of HHV-8/KSV is primarily sexual, with the highest rates of transmission among men who have sex with men; it has also isolated in women whose sexual partners are bisexual. HHV-8/KSV has also been found in children, suggesting that other body fluids also carry the virus.
   c. KS was among the first diseases to be identified with AIDS in the late 1970s and early 1980s.
   d. After the introduction of HAART, there was a dramatic decline in the incidence of KS. The incidence ratio for KS before the era of HAART was 22,100 (1990–1995) and after it was 3,640 (1996–2002; Engels et al., 2006).
   e. HAART is associated with the development of immune reconstitution inflammatory syndrome (IRIS), which can lead to progression of KS (Connick et al., 2004).
2. Pathogenesis
   a. KS is the result of angiogenesis stemming from HHV-8/KSV infection of endothelial cells. The viral proteins are similar to various cytokines and are capable of triggering an inflammatory state (Di Lorenzo et al., 2007).
   b. HIV plays a direct role in the pathogenesis of KS. The tat protein enhances the oncogenic properties of HHV-8/KSV.
3. Clinical presentation
   a. Dermatologic: Lesions vary in presentation from macular papules to nodules; pink, purple or brown in color. Clusters of lesions can eventually lead to lymphedema, particularly in dependent regions.
   b. Internal organs: GI tract (most common), lungs, liver, and so forth with symptoms reflective of the organ involved.
4. Diagnosis
   a. Although dermatologic lesions are easily identified, biopsy is necessary to determine staging and tumor bulk, as well as course of treatment.
   b. With extracutaneous lesions, a differential diagnosis is necessary, because symptoms may be indicative of another disease entity.
5. Prevention/treatment
   a. Ganciclovir and foscarnet appear to have anti HHV-8/KSV properties.
   b. HAART affects HHV-8/KSV on various fronts: reduced HIV viral load, reduced levels of tat, improved immune response, and possible antiangiogenic activity (Di Lorenzo et al., 2007).
   c. Local treatments are useful when there are few lesions.

    i) Intralesional therapy is direct injection of chemotherapy (doxorubicin and rarely interferon alpha) into the lesions.

    ii) Topical treatment involves the use of aliretinoin gel

    iii) Cryotherapy

    iv) Laser treatments

    v) Photodynamic therapy

  d. Radiation therapy is used for lesions that are too large to be managed with local treatments.

  e. Systemic chemotherapy is warranted for extensive skin or oral lesions, lymphedema, symptomatic organ involvement, or IRIS-associated flares.

    i) Standard agents: doxorubicin, bleomycin, vinblastine, vincristine, and etoposide

    ii) Liposomal anthracyclines (doxorubicin and daunorubicin) allow the chemotherapy to more accurately target the highly vascular tumors (through increased permeability and longer plasma half-life) and result in a lessening of the side effects of the agents.

    iii) Taxanes: Paclitaxel has been used with favorable results when liposomal anthracyclines fail. Potential for drug–drug interactions due to its effects on the cytochrome P450 enzyme system.

  f. Immunotherapy with systemic interferon alpha is effective in combination with HAART and/or adequate immune function.

  g. Molecular agents seek to act on the pathways to oncogenesis triggered by HHV-8/KSV.

    i) Angiogenesis inhibitors: for example, thalidomide

    ii) Tyrosine kinase inhibitors: for example, Imatinib

    iii) Matrix metalloproteinase inhibitors: for example, Col-3 (chemically modified tetracycline)

6. Nursing implications

  a. Provide support for patient in dealing with body-image changes. Instruct on cosmetics that can camouflage lesions. Be aware that social isolation is a potential result.

  b. Instruct patient and significant other on safer sex practices (e.g., condoms).

  c. Instruct patient on potential side effects of various treatments and strategies for symptom management.

  d. Monitor patient for drug–drug interactions.

REFERENCES

Connick, E., Kane, M. A., White, I. E., Ryder, J., & Campbell, T. B. (2004). Immune reconstitution inflammatory syndrome associated with Kaposi's sarcoma during potent antiretroviral therapy. *Clinical Infectious Diseases, 39*(12), 1852–1854.

Di Lorenzo, G., Konstantinopoulos, P. A., Pantanowitz, L., Di Trolio, R., De Placido, S., & Dezube, B. J. (2007). Management of AIDS-related Kaposi's sarcoma. *The Lancet Oncology, 8*(2) 167–176.

Engels, E. A., Pfeiffer, R. M., Goedert, J. J., Virgo, P., McNeel, T. S., Scoppa, S. M., et al. (2006). Trends in cancer risk among people with AIDS in the United States 1980–2002. *AIDS, 20*(12), 1645–1654.

3.20 NON-HODGKIN'S LYMPHOMA (NHL)

1. Etiology/epidemiology

  a. Non-Hodgkin's lymphoma (NHL) is closely associated with declining CD4 counts, specifically at AIDS-defining levels, and with a history of other AIDS-defining illnesses. Age and no previous history of HAART are also related to development of systemic NHL (Palmieri et al., 2006).

   b. Epstein-Barr virus (EBV) has been linked with NHL.

   c. The use of HAART, in particular regimens that include NNRTIs and PIs, has been associated with a decline in the incidence of some types of NHL (Stebbing et al., 2004).

   d. NHL is more commonly diagnosed in men than women (Stebbing et al., 2004).

2. Pathogenesis

   a. Non-Hodgkin's lymphoma is a group of malignancies arising in lymphoid tissue that is of B-cell, T-cell, or NK-cell origin.

   b. EBV infection is postulated to induce clonal proliferation of immune cells. In the context of low CD4 counts, the proliferation is unregulated, increasing the probability of the accumulation of genetic defects that lead to malignant transformation (Ng & McGrath, 2002; Biggar et al., 2007).

3. Clinical presentation

   a. At presentation there may be nonspecific symptoms, such as enlarged lymph nodes, weight loss, fevers, and night sweats. Disease is usually widespread and at an advanced stage by this time.

   b. Incidence of central nervous system, bone marrow, gastrointestinal (GI), and liver involvement is high.

   c. Signs and symptoms will vary depending upon the location of the tumors.

      i) Alterations in mental status, seizures, or other cerebral changes with central nervous system involvement

      ii) Dyspnea with pulmonary involvement

      iii) Abdominal pain, constipation, diarrhea, or gastrointestinal bleeding with GI involvement

      iv) Elevated lactate dehydrogenase levels

      v) Diffuse effusion either in the pleura or as ascites with no visible tumor

4. Diagnosis

   a. CT scan of affected area (chest/abdomen/pelvis/brain) will reveal tumor(s) or sequelae (effusions) of those tumors in those areas.

   b. Gallium-67 nuclear medicine test may help identify areas of involvement.

   c. Positron emission tomography (PET) scan has a degree of sensitivity and specificity for lesions.

   d. Bone marrow biopsy and lumbar puncture are useful in disseminated disease.

5. Prevention/treatment

   a. There are currently no recommendations for primary prevention, although the use of HAART may delay onset and the use of acyclovir to control EBV is controversial.

   b. Depending on the location and size of the tumors, radiation and/or chemotherapy may be used.

   c. Chemotherapy agents include bleomycin, etoposide, vincristine, methotrexate, prednisolone/cyclophosphamide, and doxorubicin. Combination protocols include BEMOP, CA, CHOP, CDE, and EPOCH.

   d. Concomitant use of HAART allows for full dosing of chemotherapy protocols. Care must be taken in monitoring the regimens for synergistic effects leading to myelosuppression and other toxicities. The reduction of viral loads does improve overall immune function.

e. Rituximab is a monoclonal antibody that has an affinity for the CD20 antigen that is present with B-cell lymphomas. It is used in combination with chemotherapy with some improvement of response, but toxicity can be an issue (Palmieri et al., 2006).

f. Prophylactic CNS treatment is sometimes administered (Biggar et al., 2007; Palmieri et al., 2006).

g. Use of HAART in combination with chemotherapy can approximate response and survival rates similar to those without HIV disease (Lascaux et al., 2005).

6. Nursing implications

a. Provide education about the disease process, therapeutic regimens, side effects, and symptom management.

b. With CNS involvement, it is necessary to address the safety issues that can arise from motor and cognitive impairment.

c. Provide emotional support to the patient and caregivers regarding the loss of function and independence.

REFERENCES

Biggar, R. J., Chaturvedi, A. K., Goedert, J. J., & Engles, E. A. (2007). AIDS-related cancer and severity of immuno-suppression in persons with AIDS. *Journal of the National Cancer Institute, 99*(12), 962–972.

Lascaux, A. S., Hemery, F., Goujard, C., Lesprit, P., Delfraissy, J. F., Sobel, A., et al. (2005). Beneficial effect of highly active antiretroviral therapy on the prognosis of AIDS-related systemic non-Hodgkin's lymphoma. *AIDS Research in Human Retroviruses, 21*(3), 214–220.

Ng, V. L., & McGrath, M. S. (2002). Pathogenesis of HIV-associated lymphomas. In L. Peiperl, S. Coffey, O. Bacon, & P. Volberding (Eds.), *HIV InSite Knowledge Base* [online text]. Retrieved January 22, 2009, from http://hivinsite.ucsf.edu/InSite?page=kb-06-03-01

Palmieri, C., Treibel, T., Large, O., & Bower, M. (2006). AIDS-related non-Hodgkin's lymphoma in the first decade of highly active antiretroviral therapy. *QJM: An International Journal of Medicine, 99*(12), 811–826.

Stebbing, J., Gazzard, B., Mandalia, S., Teague, A., Waterston, A., Marvin, V., et al. (2004). Antiretroviral treatment regimens and immune parameters in the prevention of systemic AIDS-related non-Hodgkin's lymphoma. *Journal of Clinical Oncology, 22*(11), 2177–2183.

3.21 HIV-RELATED WASTING SYNDROME

1. Etiology/epidemiology

a. Definitions include the following:

i) The Centers for Disease Control and Prevention's (1987) pre-HAART-era definition of wasting syndrome is involuntary loss of $> 10\%$ body weight accompanied by chronic diarrhea, weakness, or fever for ≥ 30 days in the absence of a concurrent illness.

ii) Proposed HAART-era definition is "patient must meet one of the following criteria: 10% unintentional weight loss over 12 months; 7.5% unintentional weight loss over 6 months; 5% body cell mass (BCM) loss within 6 months; in men: BCM $< 35\%$ of total body weight (BW) and body mass index (BMI) < 27 kg/m^2; in women: BCM $<$ 23% of total BW and BMI < 27 kg/m^2; BMI < 20 kg/m^2" (Polsky, Kotler, & Steinhart, 2001, p. 413).

b. Etiologies include reduced food intake, malabsorption with or without diarrhea, and metabolic abnormalities (Dudgeon et al., 2006).

c. Prevalence ranges from 17% to 58% and is similar in HAART and HAART-naïve patients (Campa et al., 2005; Mangili, Murman, Zampini, & Wanke, 2006).

2. Pathogenesis

   a. Suppression of appetite due to elevated IL-1, TNF-alpha, delayed gastric emptying, oropharyngeal lesions, nausea and vomiting, taste alterations, diarrhea, fatigue, secondary infections, and psychosocial-economic factors (e.g., depression, altered cognition, drug use, food insecurity; Campa et al., 2005)

   b. Altered absorption resulting from medications, enteric pathogens, and changes in gastrointestinal tract structure and function

   c. Activation of abnormal metabolic pathways by IL-l, TNF-alpha, interferon-alpha, opportunistic infections, uncontrolled HIV, metabolic demands of HAART, testosterone deficiency, and growth hormone and factor resistance/deficiency (Dudgeon et al., 2006; Mangili, Murman, Zampini, & Wanke, 2006)

3. Clinical presentation

   a. Loss of body weight, skeletal muscle mass, and subcutaneous fat

   b. Reduced muscular strength and functional performance, associated with disease progression (Dudgeon et al., 2006)

   c. Fever, chronic diarrhea

4. Diagnosis

   a. Dietary/clinical history reveals weight loss, inadequate dietary intake, loss of functional status.

   b. Body composition measures—weight, lean body mass, body fat mass, and body mass index—are less than 95% standard.

   c. There is laboratory evidence of anemia, hypoalbuminemia, and hypogonadism.

5. Prevention/treatment

   a. Prevention includes ongoing nutritional assessment and counseling.

   b. Treatment includes managing symptoms, treating infections, administering hormone therapy (e.g., anabolic agents, recombinant growth hormone) and anti-cytokine therapies in selected individuals (Johns, Beddall, & Corrin, 2007), providing nutrition counseling and support (Ockenga et al., 2006), and incorporating progressive resistive and aerobic exercise (O'Brien, Nixon, Glazier, & Tynan, 2007; Shevitz et al., 2005).

6. Nursing implications

   a. Educate patient/family/significant other regarding the following:

      i) Eating foods high in protein and calories

      ii) Using vitamin/mineral and oral nutritional supplements as needed

      iii) Keeping appetite, weight, and symptom records

      iv) Maintaining appropriate exercise program to increase lean body mass

---

REFERENCES

Campa, A., Yang, Z., Lai, S., Xue, L., Phillips, J. C., Sales, S., et al. (2005). HIV-related wasting in HIV-infected drug users in the era of highly active antiretroviral therapy. *Clinical Infectious Diseases, 41*(8), 1179–1185.

Centers for Disease Control and Prevention (CDC). (1987). Revision of the CDC surveillance case definition for acquired immunodeficiency syndrome. *Morbidity and Mortality Weekly Report, 36*(Suppl. 1), 3–15.

Dudgeon, W. D., Phillips, K. D., Carson, J. A., Brewer, R. B., Durstine, J. L., & Hand, G. A. (2006). Counteracting muscle wasting in HIV-infected individuals. *HIV Medicine, 7*(5), 299–310.

Johns, K., Beddall, M. J., & Corrin, R. C. (2007). Anabolic steroids for the treatment of weight loss in HIV-infected individuals. *Cochrane Database of Systematic Reviews, 2,* 1–42.

Mangili, A., Murman, D. H., Zampini, A. M., & Wanke, C. A. (2006). Nutrition and HIV infection: Review of weight loss and wasting in the era of highly active antiretroviral therapy from the nutrition for healthy living cohort. *Clinical Infectious Diseases, 42*(15), 836–842.

O'Brien, K., Nixon, S., Glazier, R. H., & Tynan, A. M. (2007). Progressive resistive exercise interventions for adults living with HIV/AIDS. *Cochrane Database of Systematic Reviews, 2,* no pages.

Ockenga, J., Grimble, R., Jonkers-Schuitema, C., Macallan, D., Melchior, J-C., Sauerwein, H.P., et al. (2006). ESPEN guidelines on enteral nutrition: Wasting in HIV and other chronic infectious diseases. *Clinical Nutrition, 25*(2), 319–329.

Polsky, B., Kotler, D., & Steinhart, C. (2001). HIV-associated wasting in the HAART era: Guidelines for assessment, diagnosis, and treatment. *AIDS Patient Care and STDs, 15*(8), 411–423.

Shevitz, A. H., Wilson, I. B., McDermott, A. Y., Spiegelman, D., Skinner, S. C., Antonsson, K., et al. (2005). A comparison of the clinical and cost-effectiveness of 3 intervention strategies for AIDS wasting. *Journal of Acquired Immune Deficiency Syndromes, 38*(4), 399–406.

3.22 HIV-RELATED ENCEPHALOPATHY

1. Etiology/epidemiology
   a. HIV-related encephalopathy, also called AIDS dementia complex (ADC) or HIV-1-associated dementia (HAD) in adults, and HIV-1-associated progressive encephalopathy (PE) in children, results from HIV infection of cells in the central nervous system (Gonzalez-Scarano & Martin-Garcia, 2005; Schwartz & Major, 2006).
   b. In the pre-HAART era, HIV-related encephalopathy occurred in 20% to 30% of persons with advanced disease (Brew, 1999). With widespread use of HAART, fewer than 10% of adults exhibit HIV-related encephalopathy. A milder form of central nervous system (CNS) dysfunction, minor cognitive motor disorder (MCMD), is estimated to affect another 30% of HIV-infected persons (Gonzalez-Scarano & Martin-Garcia, 2005).
2. Pathogenesis
   a. HIV-related encephalopathy results from HIV infection of mononuclear phagocytes (microglial cells and perivascular macrophages) in the brain. It does not appear that astrocytes, oligodendrocytes, and neurons are infected with HIV (Gonzalez-Scarano & Martin-Garcia, 2005).
   b. Infected macrophages may fuse with microglial cells, leading to formation of multinucleated giant cells. The ensuing inflammatory response results in generation of neurotoxic substances, including cytokines and nitric oxide, which destroy neurons. Inflammatory factors may also change the permeability of the blood-brain barrier, facilitating the entry of HIV-infected peripheral blood monocytes into the brain (Gonzalez-Scarano & Martin-Garcia, 2005; Sperber & Shao, 2003).
   c. Also, HIV-1 viral proteins in the brain, such as gp 120, gp 41, tat, rev, and nef, may be directly neurotoxic to primary neurons through activation of N-methyl-D-aspartate (NMDA) receptors (Gonzalez-Scarano & Martin-Garcia, 2005; Lipton & Chen, 2004).
3. Clinical presentation
   a. Patients with HAD typically present with cognitive, motor, and behavioral symptoms. In the earliest stages, patients manifest attentional deficits, forgetfulness, and motor slowing.

In advanced stages, patients show personality changes, apathy, social withdrawal, more significant memory loss, and obvious motor dysfunction (Gonzalez-Scarano & Martin-Garcia, 2005; Sperber & Shao, 2003).

b. Although pediatric populations demonstrate similar neurological dysfunction, presentation of HIV-associated neuropathy is distinct from that of adults. Developmental delays typically are seen in infants, children, and adolescents infected with HIV-1 (Schwartz & Major, 2006).

4. Diagnosis

   a. Diagnosis of HIV-related encephalopathy is made after excluding other causes. There is no single clinical or laboratory diagnostic test.

   b. Diagnostic workup includes MRI, lumbar puncture, and neuropsychological testing (Ances & Ellis, 2007; Sperber & Shao, 2003).

      i) MRI scans reveal cortical atrophy and ventricular enlargement.

      ii) Cerebrospinal fluid (CSF) analyses often reveal the presence of HIV-1; however, some individuals on HAART may have undetectable CSF viral loads, despite brain infection.

      iii) Findings of neuropsychological testing are consistent with subcortical dementia (i.e., deficits on measures of attention, memory, information-processing speed, and motor speed). Useful screening tools include those measuring psychomotor speed, verbal and nonverbal learning, and sustained attention. The HIV Dementia Scale (HDS), although not as accurate as more comprehensive tests, is a quick and simple approach to evaluate suspected cases of HAD (Bottiggi et al., 2007; Power et al., 1995).

5. Prevention/treatment

   a. It remains unclear whether HAART is an effective prophylactic treatment for HIV-related encephalopathy, although cognitive impairment tends to be milder since the introduction of HAART (Ances & Ellis, 2007; Nath & Sacktor, 2006; Sperber & Shao, 2003).

   b. There is controversy as to whether HAART can effectively reverse neurological damage associated with HIV-related encephalopathy and restore cognitive function.

   c. Effective treatment of HAD with antiretroviral medications is limited by poor drug penetration of the blood-brain barrier, multidrug resistance protein-related efflux of drug from the brain, and emergence of drug-resistant virus in the brain (Ances & Ellis, 2007; Nath & Sacktor, 2006).

   d. Adjunctive therapies include antioxidants and NMDA antagonists, such as memantine (Ances & Ellis, 2007; Lipton & Chen, 2004; Nath & Sacktor, 2006; Pocernich et al., 2005).

6. Nursing implications (Vance & Burrage, 2006)

   a. Be alert for signs and symptoms of HIV-related encephalopathy to promote early detection/diagnosis.

   b. Promote activities to maintain cognitive function (e.g., good nutrition, restful sleep, physical activity, and social and mental stimulation).

   c. Assess for and manage factors that may have a detrimental effect on cognitive function (e.g., substance abuse, depression, and certain comorbidities and medications).

   d. Identify potential safety hazards in the home environment.

   e. Identify and reduce barriers to self-care, and encourage patients to perform as many activities of daily living as possible.

f. Serve as liaison between patients and other care providers (e.g., psychiatrists, psychologists, neurologists, social workers).

g. Assist with advance directives, home care, and assisted living referrals as cognitive function declines.

REFERENCES

Ances, B. M., & Ellis, R. J. (2007). Dementia and neurocognitive disorders due to HIV-1 infection. *Seminars in Neurology, 27*(1), 86–92.

Bottiggi, K. A., Chang, J. J., Schmitt, F. A., Avison, M. J., Mootoor, Y., Nath, A., et al. (2007). The HIV Dementia Scale: Predictive power in mild dementia and HAART. *Journal of the Neurological Sciences, 260*(1–2), 11–15.

Brew, B. J. (1999). AIDS dementia complex. *Neurologic Clinics, 17*(4), 861–881.

Gonzalez-Scarano, F., & Martin-Garcia, J. (2005). The neuropathogenesis of AIDS. *Nature Reviews Immunology, 5*(1), 69–81.

Lipton, S. A., & Chen, H.-SV. (2004). Paradigm shift in neuroprotective drug development: Clinically tolerated NMDA receptor inhibition by memantine. *Cell Death and Differentiation, 11*(1), 18–20.

Nath, A., & Sacktor, N. (2006). Influence of highly active antiretroviral therapy on persistence of HIV in the central nervous system. *Current Opinions in Neurology, 19*(4), 358–361.

Pocernich, C. B., Sultana, R., Mohmmad-Abdul, H., & Butterfield, D. A. (2005). HIV-dementia, Tat-induced oxidative stress, and antioxidant therapeutic considerations. *Brain Research Reviews, 50*(1), 14–26.

Power, C., Selnes, O. A., Grim, J. A., & McArthur, J. C. (1995). HIV Dementia Scale: A rapid screening test. *Journal of the Acquired Immune Deficiency Syndrome, 8*(3), 273–278.

Schwartz, L., & Major, E. O. (2006). Neural progenitors and HIV-1-associated central nervous system disease in adults and children. *Current HIV Research, 4*(3), 319–327.

Sperber, K., & Shao, L. (2003). Neurologic consequences of HIV infection in the era of HAART. *AIDS Patient Care and STDs, 17*(10), 509–518.

Vance, D. E., & Burrage, J. W. (2006). Promoting successful cognitive aging in adults with HIV: Strategies for intervention. *Journal of Gerontological Nursing, November, 32*(11), 34–41.

3.23 FAT REDISTRIBUTION SYNDROME

1. Etiology/epidemiology
   a. Definition: HIV-related changes in body fat distribution, also referred to as lipodystrophy syndrome, and often occurs in conjunction with insulin resistance and dyslipidemia
   b. Etiology: multifactorial, including protease inhibitors (PIs), nucleoside reverse transcriptase inhibitors (NRTIs), immune reconstitution, cytokine activation, abnormal immune or autoimmune responses, and hormonal disturbances (Morse & Kovacs, 2006)
   c. Prevalence: observed in approximately 20–80% of patients after 1–2 years of highly active antiretroviral therapy (HAART; Morse & Kovacs, 2006)
2. Pathogenesis
   a. Lipoatrophy is associated with NRTI-induced mitochondrial DNA depletion (Lee, Hanes, & Johnson, 2003).
   b. Fat accumulation may be associated with PI-based HAART, but also occurs in absence of PI use (Barrett & Gallant, 2007).
   c. Risk factors: older age, male, Caucasian, family history, overweight/obesity, high-fat/high-calorie diet, lack of exercise, extent of immune depletion/reconstitution, type/duration of HAART therapy

3. Clinical presentation
   a. Peripheral fat wasting (lipoatrophy): loss of subcutaneous fat in legs, arms, face, abdomen, and/or buttocks (Morse & Kovacs, 2006; Wohl et al., 2006)
   b. Central obesity: accumulation of fat in waist and intraabdominal/visceral cavity; dorsocervical fat accumulation ("buffalo hump"); breast enlargement
4. Diagnosis
   a. Clinical exam; self-report
   b. Anthropometric measures, such as waist-to-hip ratio, is ≥ 0.95 in men and ≥ 0.9 in women with fat accumulation.
   c. Single-slice CT or MRI at L4 shows intraabdominal fat deposits.
   d. Dual-energy X-ray absorptiometry (DXA) and bioelectrical impedance analysis (BIA) assess body fat amount, but not distribution.
5. Prevention/treatment
   a. Switch from thymidine analogue NRTI (e.g., stavudine) to NRTI-sparing regimen (Wohl et al., 2006).
   b. Other potential treatments include thiazolidinediones, metformin, testosterone, growth hormone, antioxidants, and mitochondrial co-factors, but data are inconclusive.
   c. Liposuction may be used for visceral fat removal; facial reconstruction to replace facial fat loss (Negredo et al., 2006).
6. Nursing implications
   a. Patients may refuse or discontinue HAART due to disfiguring body habitus changes.
   b. Assess impact of fat redistribution on patient's treatment decisions, compliance, and psychological and social well-being.
   c. Encourage lifestyle changes, such as low-fat/low-calorie diet, resistive and aerobic exercise.

REFERENCES

Bartlett, J. G., & Gallant, J. E. (2007). *Medical management of HIV infection*. Baltimore: Johns Hopkins Medicine Health Publishing Business Group.

Lee, H., Hanes, J., & Johnson, K. A. (2003). Toxicity of nucleoside analogues used to treat AIDS and the selectivity of the mitochondrial DNA polymerase. *Biochemistry, 42*(50), 14711–14719.

Morse, C. G., & Kovacs, J. A. (2006). Metabolic and skeletal complications of HIV infection: The price of success. *JAMA, 296*(7), 844–854.

Negredo, E., Higueras, C., Adell, X., Martinez, J. C., Martinez, E., Puig, J., et al. (2006). Reconstructive treatment for antiretroviral-associated facial lipoatrophy: A prospective study comparing autologous fat and synthetic substances. *AIDS Patient Care & STDs, 20*(12), 829–837.

Wohl, D. A., McComsey, G., Tebas, P., Brown, T. T., Glesby, M. J., Reeds, D., et al. (2006). Current concepts in the diagnosis and management of metabolic complications of HIV infection and its therapy. *Clinical Infectious Diseases, 43*(5), 645–653.

3.24 IMPAIRED GLUCOSE TOLERANCE (IGT)

1. Etiology/epidemiology
   a. Insulin resistance, hyperglycemia, and diabetes mellitus have an increased prevalence in patients with HIV. Diabetes mellitus is seen in approximately 7.0 percent of HIV-infected adults with lipoatrophy or fat accumulation (Hadigan et al., 2001).

b. New-onset diabetes mellitus occurs in 6–10% of patients taking HAART (Calmy, Hirschel, Cooper, & Carr, 2007). Insulin resistance and impaired glucose tolerance (IGT) are more common, with estimates of up to 60% of patients treated with protease inhibitors (PIs) having impaired fasting glucose (100–125 mg/dL; Rao, Disraeli & McGregor, 2004) or abnormal oral glucose tolerance test results (Walli et al., 1998). IGT is a metabolic stage intermediary between normal glucose homeostasis and diabetes, and is a risk factor for diabetes and cardiovascular disease.

c. The exact pathogenic mechanisms are not known. Glucose intolerance in HIV disease may relate to adverse effects of medications (PIs and non-nucleoside reverse transcriptase inhibitors [NNRTIs]) and metabolic dysfunction secondary to HIV disease itself (Galli, Ridolfo, & Gervasoni, 2001). Coinfections with hepatitis C (HCV) may also increase risk for glucose intolerance (Duong et al., 2001).

2. Pathogenesis

a. PIs are associated with both increased endogenous glucose production and resistance to multiple effects of insulin (van der Valk et al., 2001). Saquinavir, ritonavir, and indinavir all increase basal glucose transport but decrease insulin-stimulated glucose transport (Germinario et al., 2000).

b. Glucose intolerance is associated with lipodystrophy, but whether it is caused by or is the cause of lipodystrophy is unclear.

3. Clinical presentation

a. Patients with glucose intolerance are generally asymptomatic.

b. Some patients may present with symptoms of frank diabetes (i.e., polyuria, polydipsia, and polyphagia).

c. Morphological changes (i.e., central adiposity, increased waist-to-hip ratio, peripheral fat wasting) may be present and should heighten clinical suspicion.

4. Diagnosis

a. Fasting plasma glucose (FPG) is the preferred test. The American Diabetes Association (ADA) defines normal fasting plasma glucose as < 100 mg/dl (5.6 mmol/l); and a normal glucose tolerance test as a 2-h postload glucose < 140 mg/dl (7.8 mmol/l; Nathan et al., 2007). ADA further defines impaired fasting glucose as fasting plasma glucose of 100–125 mg/dl (5.6–6.9 mmol/l) and impaired glucose tolerance as a 2-h postload glucose of 140–199 mg/dl (7.8–11.0 mmol/l). A fasting plasma glucose of or above 126 mg/dl (7.0 mmol/l), or a 2-h postload glucose of or above 200 mg/dl (11.1 mmol/l) makes a provisional diagnosis of diabetes.

b. Increased fasting insulin levels may be seen but are not recommended as a diagnostic test.

c. Fasting glucose levels may be normal, requiring a 2-h oral glucose tolerance test. A 2-h postprandial glucose from 140 to < 200 (7.75 to < 11.1 mmol/L) is considered diagnostic of IGT.

5. Prevention/treatment

a. The goal is maintenance of normal glycemic control.

b. Lifestyle modifications, such as dietary moderation, exercise, weight loss, smoking cessation, and limitation of alcohol use, are effective in achieving normal glycemic control.

c. Metformin (500 mg twice daily) may improve glucose tolerance (Hadigan et al., 2001), but, although rare, its use has been associated with lactic acidemia. Thiazolidinediones also improve insulin sensitivity; rosiglitazone, but not pioglitazone, aggravates dyslipidemia (Calmy et al., 2007).

   d. Antiretroviral switching may improve the glycemic profile.

6. Nursing implications

   a. Nurses should remain aware of the increased prevalence of diabetes mellitus in HIV-infected patients. Assessment of symptoms of diabetes should be a routine part of the nursing assessment.

   b. If appropriate, counsel patients to maintain ideal body weight; encourage exercise, including strength training.

   c. Dietary counseling promoting low-glycemic-index foods may be helpful for patients with known glucose intolerance.

REFERENCES

Calmy, A., Hirschel, B., Cooper, D. A., & Carr, A. (2007). Clinical update: adverse effects of antiretroviral therapy, *Lancet, 370*(9581), 7–14.

Duong, M., Petit, J. M., Piroth, L., Grappin, M., Buisson, M., Chavanet, P., et al. (2001). Association between insulin resistance and hepatitis C virus chronic infection in HIV-hepatitis C virus-coinfected patients undergoing antiretroviral therapy. *Journal of Acquired Immune Deficiency Syndromes, 27*(3), 245–250.

Galli, M., Ridolfo, A. L., & Gervasoni, C. (2001). Cardiovascular disease risk factors in HIV-infected patients in the HAART era. *Annals of the New York Academy of Science, 946,* 200–203.

Germinario, R. J., Colby-Germinario, S. P., Cammalleri, C., & Wainberg M. (2000). The effects of a variety of protease inhibitors on insulin binding insulin-mediated sugar transport and cell toxicity in insulin target and non-target cell cultures. *Antiviral Therapy, 5*(Suppl. 5), 7.

Hadigan, C., Meigs, J. B., Corcoran, C., Rietschel, P., Piecuch, S., Basgoz, N., et al. (2001). Metabolic abnormalities and cardiovascular disease risk factors in adults with human immunodeficiency virus infection and lipodystrophy. *Clinical Infectious Diseases, 32*(1), 130–139.

Nathan, D. M., Davidson, M. B., DeFronzo, R. A., Heine, R. J., Henry, R. R., Pratley, R., et al. (2007). Impaired fasting glucose and impaired glucose tolerance. *Diabetes Care, 30*(3), 753–759.

Rao, S. S., Disraeli, P., & McGregor, T. (2004). Impaired glucose tolerance and impaired fasting glucose. *American Family Physician, 69*(8), 1961–1968, 1971–1972.

van der Valk, M., Bisschop, P. H., Romijn, J. A., Ackermans, M. T., Lange, J. M., Endert, E., et al. (2001). Lipodystrophy in HIV-1-positive patients is associated with insulin resistance in multiple metabolic pathways. *AIDS, 15*(16), 2093–2100.

Walli, R., Herfort, O., Michl, G. M., Demant, T., Jager, H., Dieterle, C., et al. (1998). Treatment with protease inhibitors associated with peripheral insulin resistance and impaired oral glucose tolerance in HIV-1 infected patients. *AIDS, 12*(15), 167–173.

3.25 DYSLIPIDEMIA

1. Etiology/epidemiology

   a. Dyslipidemia includes hyperlipidemia, hypercholesterolemia, and hypertriglyceridemia.

   b. The reported prevalence of HIV-related dyslipidemia is very high, with lipid abnormalities affecting the majority of individuals with HIV infection. Specific alterations include low total and high-density lipoprotein (HDL) cholesterol and elevated triglycerides levels.

   c. Etiology is unknown though often associated with fat redistribution and glucose intolerance.

2. Pathogenesis
   a. HAART has been implicated. Protease inhibitors (PIs) have been shown to stimulate triglyceride production (Lenhard, Croom, Weiel, & Winegar, 2000). Nucleoside reverse transcriptase inhibitors (NRTIs) have also been implicated because of their toxic effects on mitochondria (Brinkman, Smeitink, Romijn, & Reiss, 1999). Participants on regimens containing drugs from both the PI and NNRTI classes had the highest prevalence of dyslipidemia, suggestive of a possible additive effect of combinations of drugs from these drug classes (Friis-Møller et al., 2003).
   b. Dyslipidemia may be a secondary consequence of chronic suppression of HIV replication rather than a primary effect of HAART (Kotler, 1998).

3. Clinical presentation
   a. Lipid abnormalities are likely to be asymptomatic, except in the case of acute atherosclerotic infarction.

4. Diagnosis
   a. A fasting lipid profile, which includes total cholesterol, low-density lipoproteins (LDL), high-density lipoproteins (HDL), and triglycerides, should be obtained. Patients should receive baseline testing prior to starting any type of antiretroviral therapy. Subsequent lipid profiles should be performed every 3 to 6 months.
   b. Assess cardiovascular risk factors (i.e., hypertension, glucose intolerance, smoking).

5. Prevention/treatment
   a. Preventive efforts include encouraging appropriate caloric intake and physical activity. Refer overweight persons to a dietitian.
   b. Diet and exercise therapy using combined aerobic and resistance training have demonstrated benefit in reducing subcutaneous body fat, total cholesterol, and triglyceride concentrations (Jones, Doran, Leatt, Maher, & Pirmohamed, 2001).
   c. The potential benefit of switching antiretroviral medications to correct lipid abnormalities remains unclear; however, a systematic review found that switching may be beneficial (McGoldrick & Leen, 2007).
   d. Comorbidities such as alcohol abuse need to be identified due to the increased risk of pancreatitis in patients with lipid abnormalities, especially hypertriglyceridemia.
   e. For hypercholesterolemia, pravastatin or atorvastatin are most often used because their biotransformation is not affected by HAART (Calmy, Hirschel, Cooper, & Carr, 2007; McGoldrick, & Leen, 2007).
   f. Fish oil may have benefits for normalizing dyslipidemia in persons with HIV (Norman et al., 2007).

6. Nursing implications
   a. Assess family history for cardiovascular risk. Assess lifestyle risks (diet, physical activity, smoking). Provide patient education regarding risk factor modification.
   b. Encourage aerobic exercise and strength training as appropriate. Recommend dietary modifications consistent with the guidelines of the National Cholesterol Education Program and the Adult Treatment Panel-III (available at http://www.nhlbi.nih.gov/guidelines/cholesterol/atp3upd04.htm).

REFERENCES

Brinkman, K., Smeitink, J. A., Romijn, J. A., & Reiss, P. (1999). Mitochondrial toxicity induced by nucleoside-analogue reverse-transcriptase inhibitors is a key factor in the pathogenesis of antiretroviral-therapy-related lipodystrophy. *Lancet, 354*(9184), 1112–1115.

Calmy, A., Hirschel, B., Cooper, D. A., & Carr, A. (2007). Clinical update: Adverse effects of antiretroviral therapy. *Lancet, 370*(9581), 7–14.

Friis-Møller, N., Weber, R., Reiss, P., Thiébaut, R., Kirk, O., d'Arminio Monforte, A., et al. (2003). Cardiovascular disease risk factors in HIV patients—association with antiretroviral therapy: Results from the DAD study. *AIDS, 17*(8), 1179–1193.

Jones, S. P., Doran, D. A., Leatt, P. B., Maher, B., & Pirmohamed, M. (2001). Short-term exercise training improves body composition and hyperlipidaemia in HIV-positive individuals with lipodystrophy. *AIDS, 15*(15), 2049–2051.

Kotler, D. P. (1998). *Update on lipid abnormalities and cardiovascular complications in HIV infection.* Retrieved January 23, 2009, from http://www.medscape.com/viewprogram/295

Lenhard, J. M., Croom, D. K., Weiel, J. E., & Winegar, D. A. (2000). HIV protease inhibitors stimulate hepatic triglyceride synthesis. *Arteriosclerosis, Thrombosis, and Vascular Biology, 20*(12), 2625–2629.

McGoldrick, C., & Leen, C. L. S. (2007). The management of dyslipidaemias in antiretroviral-treated HIV infection: A systematic review. *HIV Medicine, 8*(6), 325–334.

Norman, L., Yip, B., Montaner, J., Arris, M., Frohlich, J., Bondy, G., et al. (2007). Use of metabolic drugs and fish oil in HIV-positive patients with metabolic complications and associations with dyslipidaemia and treatment targets. *HIV Medicine, 8*(6), 346–356.

3.26 ANEMIA

1. Etiology/epidemiology
   a. Anemia is characterized by abnormalities in the hematological system. It has multiple causes, including decreased erythropoiesis, ineffective erythropoiesis, or increased red blood cell destruction. Hematological complications such as anemia occur in up to 85% of AIDS patients (Sande, Eliopoulos, Moellering, & Gilbert, 2006).
   b. Anemia is the most common HIV hematological complication. The severity of anemia is an independent predictor of decreased survival (Sande et al., 2006).
   c. Anemia is the most common cytopenia seen in people with HIV. Independent of CD4 count and viral load, anemia has been shown to correlate with increased mortality (Fangman & Scadden, 2005).
2. Pathogenesis
   a. The pathogenesis of anemia in HIV is complex and may result from opportunistic infections, nutritional deficiencies, AIDS associated malignancies, medications, or HIV-induced alteration in hemitopoiesis (Fangman & Scadden, 2005).
   b. Bone marrow damage due to certain cancers, opportunistic infections, or myelosuppressive agents, such as zidovudine, ganciclovir, valganciclovir, foscarnet, flucytosine, sulfonamides, lamivudine, ribavirin, and vinblastine, can cause decreased erythropoiesis. Zidovudine and stavudine produce megaloblastic anemia. Indinavir and ribavirin are associated with hemolytic anemia (Sande et al., 2006). Additionally, macrocytosis has been increasingly observed in the HIV-infected population and is an early indicator of bone marrow toxicity (Khawcharoenporn, Shikuma, Williams, & Chow, 2007).
   c. Chronic disease has long been associated with anemia, which is characterized by decreased production of erythropoietin, erythropoietin resistance, abnormalities of iron me-

tabolism, decreased erythrocyte life span, and an increase in inflammatory cytokines which may interfere with erythropoietin production (Bartlett, 2007).

    d. Chronic blood loss and inadequate iron intake may lead to iron deficiency anemia (Bartlett, 2007). Blood loss can occur due to neoplastic disease (Kaposi sarcoma in the GI tract) or GI lesions from other causes (Volberding, Levine, Dieterich, Mildvan, Mitsuyasu, & Saag, 2004).

    e. Persistent parvovirus B-19 infection, found in one-third of HIV-infected persons, can cause anemia (Sande et al., 2006).

3. Clinical presentation

    a. Symptoms include fatigue, shortness of breath, decrease in cognitive function, impairment of activities of daily living, exercise intolerance, amenorrhea, and pallor.

4. Diagnosis

    a. The World Health Organization defines anemia as a hemoglobin of less than 12.5 g/dL in an adult (Yorba, Huff, & Mullins, 2005). Baseline evaluation should include the CBC. When anemia is confirmed by a lower than normal red blood cell count, hemoglobin, or hematocrit, the mean corpuscular volume (MCV) should be examined to determine if the anemia is microcytic (MCV < 84) or macrocytic (MCV > 96; Conrad, 2005).

    b. Physical signs include weight loss, hepatosplenomegaly, guaiac positive stool, mild peripheral edema, and retinal hemorrhages (NIH, 2008).

5. Prevention/treatment

    a. Identify and treat underlying cause.

    b. Substitute or discontinue myelosuppressive agents. Do not reduce dose of antiretroviral agents.

    c. Epoetin alfa is the treatment of choice for mild or moderate anemia. The initial dosage is 40,000 units subcutaneously weekly (Sande et al., 2006).

    d. For severe anemia, treatment includes red blood cell transfusions, administration of electrolyte and colloid solutions, and supplemental oxygen.

    e. Over the past decade, epoetin alfa dosing strategies have evolved, resulting in less frequent administration, improved patient convenience, and the potential for improved treatment adherence. Clinical studies have demonstrated that correction of anemia with epoetin alfa has been associated with prolonged survival and improved functional capacity in HIV-infected persons. Accordingly, epoetin alfa continues to play a therapeutic role in the management of HIV-related anemia beyond the reduction in transfusion requirements (Henry, Volberding, & Leitz, 2004).

6. Nursing implications

    a. Monitor lab work that is suggestive of anemia: red blood cell count, hemoglobin, hematocrit, and reticulocyte count.

    b. Educate patients to recognize and report early signs of anemia, such as fatigue, shortness of breath, and amenorrhea.

    c. Provide dietary counseling and nutritional support as needed. Iron is best absorbed from meat, fish, and poultry. Orange juice doubles the absorption of iron from an entire meal, whereas tea or milk reduces absorption to less than one half.

    d. The energy and physical functioning scales of the Medical Outcomes Study HIV Health Survey (MOS-HIV), the most widely used quality of life instrument in HIV studies, are reliable and have discriminate validity in HIV-infected patients (Martin, Gilpin, Jabs, & Wu, 2001).

e. Successful treatment of anemia has been shown to reduce risk of death compared to patients with similar immunologic and virologic parameters who are not treated. Women, blacks, injection drug users, and people with advanced disease are disproportionately affected by anemia and should be screened (Fangman & Scadden, 2005).

f. Monitor patients who take zidovudine-containing combination medications (i.e., Trizivir, Combivir) for the development of anemia (Bartlett, 2007).

REFERENCES

Bartlett, J. (2007). *Adult HIV/AIDS treatment: 2007 pocket guide*. Baltimore: Johns Hopkins University.

Conrad, M. (2005). *Anemia*. Retrieved January 23, 2009, from http://www.emedicine.com/med/topic132.htm

Fangman, J., & Scadden, D. (2005). Anemia in HIV-infected adults: Epidemiology, pathogenesis, and clinical management. *Current Hematology Reports, 4*(2), 95–102.

Henry, D., Volberding, P., & Leitz, G. (2004). Epoetin alfa for treatment of anemia in HIV-infected patients: Past, present, and future. *Journal of Acquired Immunology, 37*(2), 1221–1227.

Khawcharoenporn, T., Shikuma, C., Williams, A., & Chow, D. (2007). Lamivudine-associated macrocytosis in HIV-infected patients. *International Journal of STD & AIDS, 18*(1), 39–40.

Martin, B., Gilpin, A., Jabs, D., & Wu, A. (2001). Reliability and validity, and responsiveness of general and disease-specific quality of life measures in a clinical trial for cytomegalovirus retinitis. *Journal of Clinical Epidemiology, 54*(4), 376–386.

National Institutes of Health (NIH). (2008). *AIDS info*. Retrieved January 23, 2009, from http://aidsinfo.nih.gov

Sande, M., Eliopoulos, G., Moellering, R., & Gilbert, D. (2006). *The Sanford guide to HIV/AIDS therapy* (15th ed). Sperryville, VA: Antimicrobial Therapy.

Volberding, P., Levine, A., Dieterich, D., Mildvan, D., Mitsuyasu, R., & Saag, M. (2004). Anemia in HIV infection: Clinical impact and evidence-based management strategies. *Clinical Infectious Diseases, 38*(10), 1454–1463.

Yorba, P., Huff, S., & Mullins, M. (2005). *Anemia: Blood and lymphatic system*. Retrieved January 6, 2008, from http://www.emedicinehealth.com/articles/4893-1.asp

3.27 LEUKOPENIA

1. Etiology/epidemiology
   a. Leukopenia is defined as a white blood count $< 3,000$ cells/mm^3.
   b. Etiology involves HIV infection of white blood cells, altered stem cell differentiation, and cytokine dysregulation (Koka & Reddy, 2004).
   c. Prevalence increases as disease progresses. Neutropenia is reported in 10% of persons with early asymptomatic infection and increases to 50% to 75% of persons with full-blown AIDS (Crosby, 2007).
2. Pathogenesis
   a. Although HIV can infect CD34+ progenitor cells in vitro, it is not clear if they are infected in vivo and contribute to altered hematopoiesis (Koka & Reddy, 2004).
   b. HIV infection may indirectly contribute to leukopenia by altering the stromal/progenitor cell microenvironment required for hematopoiesis (Koka & Reddy, 2004).
   c. Myelosuppression related to drugs, concomitant infections, malignancies, autoimmune processes, and hypersplenism (Volberding, Baker, & Levine, 2003)

3. Clinical presentation
   a. Respiratory tract symptoms, such as cough and sputum production
   b. Urinary tract infection symptoms: frequency, urgency, and burning
   c. Fever
4. Diagnosis
   a. CBC with differential shows decrease in WBCs, including absolute neutrophil count < 1000 (Moore, 2006).
   b. Bone marrow biopsies have shown abnormalities in granulocytic precursors and megakaryocytes (Crosby, 2007).
5. Prevention/treatment
   a. Prevention: through durable suppression of viral replication and judicious use of myelo-suppressive medications
   b. Treatment
      i)   Antiretroviral therapy to suppress viral replication
      ii) Withdrawal of myelosuppressive therapies, if appropriate
      iii) Administration of hematopoietic growth factors, such as granulocyte colony-stimulating factor (G-CSF) and granulocyte-macrophage colony-stimulating factor (GM-CSF) are effective for reversing cytopenias, although it is not clear if they prolong survival (Crosby, 2007).
6. Nursing implications
   a. Education of patient, family, and significant other regarding the following:
      i) Strategies to reduce risk for infection (i.e., hand washing, food and water safety, avoidance of contact with infected persons)
      ii) Early detection of infections (i.e., regular monitoring of temperature, prompt reporting of any new signs or symptoms)

REFERENCES

Crosby, C. D. (2007). Hematologic disorders associated with human immunodeficiency virus and AIDS. *Journal of Infusion Nursing, 30*(1), 22–32.

Koka, P. S., & Reddy, S. T. (2004). Cytopenias in HIV infection: Mechanisms and alleviation of hematopoietic inhibition. *Current HIV Research, 2*(3), 278–282.

Moore, R. D. (2006). Neutropenia. *Johns Hopkins HIV Guide*. Retrieved September 7, 2007, from http://www.hopkinshivguide.org

Volberding, P. A., Baker, K. R., & Levine, A. M. (2003). Human immunodeficiency virus hematology. *Hematology, 2003*(1), 294–313.

3.28 THROMBOCYTOPENIA

1. Etiology/epidemiology
   a. In all risk groups, the prevalence is between 5% and 15% (Mannucci & Gringeri, 2000; Sullivan, Hanson, Chu, Jones, & Ciesielski, 1997).
   b. Medications associated with thrombycytopenia include hydroxyurea, zidovudine, ganciclovir, trimethoprim-sulfamethoxazole, acetylsalicylic acid (ASA), non-steroidal anti-inflammatories (NSAIDs), and chemotherapeutic agents.

    c. Infiltrative diseases of the bone marrow include MAC, fungal infections (*Coccidioides, Cryptococcus, Histoplasmosis*), and neoplasms (non-Hodgkin's lymphoma, KS).

    d. Other causes include chronic alcohol use, liver disease, HIV-associated idiopathic thrombocytopenic purpura, and recreational drug use (especially heroin).

    e. HIV-infected women with platelet counts of fewer than 50,000 per cubic millimeter had a five-fold increased risk of dying from any cause. Thrombocytopenia has also been associated with a three-fold increased risk of dying due to AIDS (Pearce et al., 2004).

2. Pathogenesis

    a. Generally a complication of an opportunistic infection, opportunistic neoplasm, side effect of a medication, or ITP

3. Clinical presentation

    a. Bleeding tendencies, including epistaxis, bleeding from gums, petechiae, blood in urine or stool, hemoptysis, and vaginal or rectal bleeding

    b. The potential risk for bleeding is related to the platelet count.

       i) Platelet count $< 100,00/mm^3$ is clinically significant and warrants monitoring.

       ii) Platelet count $< 50,000/mm^3$ indicates mild injury and may result in bleeding.

       iii) Platelet count $< 20,000/mm^3$ indicates serious risk for a major bleeding episode that may occur spontaneously.

       iv) Platelet count $< 10,000/mm^3$ indicates risk for life-threatening bleeding. Platelet transfusion is indicated.

4. Diagnosis

    a. May occur in association with certain factors, such as recreational drug use, especially heroin use

    b. Reduced platelet count as determined by CBC

    c. Selenium levels below 145 mcg/l are associated with thrombocytopenia.

    d. Platelet-associated antibodies may be detected with HIV-associated ITP.

5. Prevention/treatment

    a. Identify and manage the underlying cause.

6. Nursing implications

    a. Prevent bleeding secondary to trauma: Use electric razors and soft-bristled toothbrushes or toothettes, and avoid flossing teeth.

    b. When platelets are less than 50,000 cells/mm^3, avoid intramuscular injections, rectal temperatures or suppositories, and indwelling catheters.

    c. If venipuncture is performed, apply pressure to the site for at least 5 min.

    d. Teach patient not to take over-the-counter medications that contain aspirin or NSAIDs.

    e. Avoid penetrative anal or vaginal intercourse, vaginal or rectal suppositories, vaginal douching, and rectal enemas or thermometers.

    f. Report any signs of mental status changes, acute pain, nosebleeds, or blood in the urine, stool, or sputum.

    g. Teach patient to blow nose gently.

    h. Teach patient not to strain with bowel movements; stool softeners may be initiated.

    i. Teach female patients to avoid tampons and to keep count of the number of pads used during menstruation.

REFERENCES

Mannucci, P. M., & Gringeri, A. (2000). HIV-related thrombocytopenia. *Annals of Italian Medicine, 15*(1), 20–27.

Pearce, C. L., Mack, W. J., Levine, A. M., Gravnik, J., Cohen, M. H., Machtinger, E. L., et al. (2004). Thrombocytopenia is a strong predictor of all-cause and AIDS-specific mortality in women with HIV: The women's interagency HIV study. 46th Annual Meeting of the American Society of Hematology, San Diego, California.

Sullivan, P. S., Hanson, D. I., Chu, S. Y., Jones, J. L., & Ciesielski, C. A. (1997). Surveillance for thrombocytopenia in persons infected with HIV: Results from the Multistate Adult and Adolescent Spectrum of Disease Project. *Journal of Acquired Immunodeficiency Syndrome and Human Retrovirology, 14*(4), 374–379.

3.29 CARDIOMYOPATHY

1. Etiology/epidemiology
   a. The principal HIV-associated cardiomyopathy is dilated cardiomyopathy.
   b. The estimated annual incidence of dilated cardiomyopathy in the pre-HAART era was 15.9 per 1,000 asymptomatic patients (Barbaro, 2003); limited evidence suggests the incidence has declined in the HAART era (Rahklin, Hsue, & Cheitlin, 2005).
   c. Increasing immunodeficiency is closely related to the development of cardiomyopathy (Barbarini & Barbaro, 2003).
   d. Although it would appear that the use of HAART would reduce the incidence of cardiac complications by controlling HIV replication and delaying the onset of immune deficiency (Moroni & Antinori, 2003), the effects of the drugs themselves may contribute to the development of cardiomyopathy and other cardiac conditions (Breuckmann et al., 2005; Srivastava et al., 2004).
2. Pathogenesis
   a. It is not clear how HIV affects myocardial cells, because they do not express CD4 receptors. It is thought that HIV-infected monocytes in proximity to cardiac cells produce cytokines (e.g., TNF α and interleukins), which induce apoptosis of those cells and/or can affect the contractility of the cardiac muscle (Moroni & Antinori, 2003).
   b. Opportunistic infections with an affinity for cardiac muscle such as *Toxoplasma gondii, Cryptococcus neoformans,* herpes simplex virus type 2, Mycobacterium tuberculosis and avium intracellulare, coxsackie virus B3, cytomegalovirus and Epstein-Barr virus can also contribute to the pathogenesis (Barbarini & Barbaro, 2003; Barbaro, 2003).
   c. Nutritional deficiencies of trace elements such as selenium, vitamin B12, and carintine have been associated with cardiomyopathy.
   d. Cardiomyopathy has been associated with alterations in endocrine function (endocrinopathies), such as growth hormone and thyroid hormone deficiencies, adrenal insufficiency, and hyperinsulinemia.
3. Clinical presentation
   a. Patients are largely asymptomatic in the early stages of disease.
   b. When the ejection fraction falls below 30% and/or the left ventricular diastolic pressure rises above 60 mm, symptoms become apparent.
   c. The symptoms are similar to those found in non-HIV-related left- (pulmonary congestion) and right-sided (systemic venous congestion) heart failure.

      i) Left-sided heart failure symptoms include exertional dyspnea, orthopnea, and paroxysmal nocturnal dyspnea.

      ii) Right-sided heart failure symptoms include hepatic and abdominal distention, and peripheral edema.

4. Diagnosis

  a. Patient history will reveal a gradual increase in exercise intolerance and onset of congestive symptoms. This may include reports of chest pain and syncope or clinical embolic events.

  b. Electrocardiogram shows left ventricular dilation, with poor R-wave progression and higher voltage in V6 than in V5.

  c. Echocardiogram shows

      i) Left ventricular hypokinesis (an ejection fraction of $< 45\%$)

      ii) Left ventricular dilation (left ventricular end diastolic volume index > 80 ml per square measure)

  d. Chest X-rays typically show cardiomegaly.

  e. Serum levels of B-type natriuretic peptide (BNP), produced by ventricular myocytes, are elevated in volume overload states.

5. Prevention/treatment

  a. The use of routine echocardiograms as a screening tool has not been justified.

  b. The prognosis relies on the severity of the heart failure. A poor prognosis is associated with an ejection fraction less than 20%.

  c. Treatment is focused on symptom management (i.e., use of diuretics and salt-reduced diet to reduce edema and hypertension) and control of contributing factors.

  d. Angiotensin-converting enzyme (ACE) inhibitors are used to decrease intravascular volume. Digitalis and cardiac glycosides are used to improve the contractility of the heart. Beta-blocking agents (beginning with small doses and titrating upward to effective doses) improve ventricular function. Although beta blockers can slow the progression in stable heart failure, their use is not recommended for patients with unstable disease, volume overload, or heart block.

6. Nursing implications

  a. Monitor patient for early symptoms indicative of heart failure.

  b. In diagnosed patients, monitor for progression/stabilization of symptoms.

  c. Educate patient about causes of worsening symptoms and strategies for symptom management.

  d. Instruct on pacing and prioritization of activities when symptoms are severe.

  e. Teach the patient energy conservation techniques, such as delegation of chores, work organization, and small, frequent meals.

  f. Evaluate patient's response to prescribed regimen.

REFERENCES

Barbarini, G., & Barbaro, G. (2003). Incidence of the involvement of the cardiovascular system in HIV infection. *AIDS: Official Journal of the International AIDS Society, 17*(Suppl. 1), S46–S50.

Barbaro, G. (2003). Pathogenesis of HIV associated heart disease. *AIDS: Official Journal of the International AIDS Society, 17*(Suppl. 1), S12–S20.

Breuckmann, F., Neumann, T., Kondratieva, J., Ross, B., Nassenstein, K., Barkhausen, J., et al. (2005). Dilated cardiomyopathy in two adult human immunodeficiency positive (HIV+) patients possibly related to highly active antiretroviral therapy (HAART). *European Journal of Medical Research, 10*(9), 395–399.

Moroni, M., & Antinori, S. (2003). HIV and direct damage of organs: Disease spectrum before and during the highly active antiretroviral therapy era. *AIDS: Official Journal of the International AIDS Society, 17*(Suppl. 1), S51–S64.

Rakhlin, N., Hsue, P., & Cheitlin, M. D. (2005). Cardiac manifestations of HIV. In L. Peiperl, S. Coffey, O. Bacon, & P. Volberding (Eds.), *HIV InSite Knowledge Base* [online textbook]. Retrieved January 25, 2009, from http://hivinsite.ucsf.edu/InSite?page=kb-04-01-06

Srivastava, M., Verghese, C., & Sepkowitz, D. (2004). Acute reversible heart failure with highly active antiretroviral therapy. *American Journal of Therapeutics, 11*(4) 323–325.

3.30 PSORIASIS

1. Etiology/epidemiology
   a. Psoriasis is a chronic inflammatory condition characterized by a rapid turnover of the epidermal layer of the skin, an increase in the number of epidermal cells, and the subsequent formation of scales and well-marginated erythematous plaques.
   b. The etiology is unclear but may involve activity of cytotoxic/suppressor T cells in response to infected or dysfunctional Langerhans cells.
   c. Psoriasis may be exacerbated by stress, sunburn, streptococcal pharyngeal infections, medications, and localized trauma.
   d. Psoriasis is sometimes associated with arthritis.
   e. Prevalence of psoriasis in the HIV-infected population is similar to the prevalence in the general population, which is about 1–3% (Maurer & Berger, 1998).
2. Pathogenesis
   a. Psoriasis involves inflammation coupled with alteration of the skin cell cycle leading to chronic scaling of the skin.
   b. It is postulated that elevated gamma interferon levels secondary to HIV-induced expansion of the memory CD8 population is involved in the pathogenesis. Gamma interferon induces keratinocytes to express HLA-DR, which promotes the accumulation of white blood cells into psoriatic plaques (Fife, Waller, Jeffes, & Koo, 2007).
3. Clinical presentation
   a. Patients may present with chronic, scaly plaques on elbows, knees, lumbosacral areas, axillae, and groin.
   b. Diffuse dermatitis with thickening may be present; nail dystrophy also may be seen but is not present in many patients.
   c. Involvement is bilateral, rarely symmetrical.
4. Diagnosis
   a. The diagnosis of psoriasis is often made based on clinical presentation, the distribution and appearance of the lesions, and the response to therapy.
   b. It is important to exclude secondary infection by culture and stains.
   c. The only way to definitively diagnose the disease is by taking a biopsy of the lesion.
5. Prevention/treatment

    a. Treatment is variable, depending on the stage of disease and the site, extent, and degree of disability.

    b. Topical corticosteroids are commonly prescribed for application directly to the lesions.

    c. Small plaques may be treated with intradermal injections of triamcinolone acetonide aqueous suspension.

    d. Other treatments that may be applied are tars, salicylic acid, Denorex, Anthralin, ultraviolet B (UVB) light therapy, psoralens plus ultraviolet A (PUVA), retinoids, and immunosuppressives (e.g., methotrexate; Maurer & Berger, 1998).

    e. Systemic therapy may be used. AZT use may lead to improvement (Merrigan, Bartlett, & Bolognesi, 1999). HAART should be encouraged if appropriate; efficacy of HAART for psoriasis is unstudied (Maurer & Berger, 1998).

6. Nursing implications

    a. Teach patient not to scratch or rub lesions.

    b. Assist patient to implement self-care measures, such as avoidance of sun exposure and maintenance of adequate hydration and nutrition. Patient should avoid bathing more than once daily and avoid use of excessive soap and vigorous scrubbing. Stress and alcohol can trigger exacerbation of psoriasis, so stress management techniques and avoidance or decrease in alcohol consumption should be discussed with patient (Handel, 2001).

    c. Counsel patient about medications that could exacerbate the condition (i.e., systemic corticosteroids, lithium, chloroquine, beta blockers, and nonsteroidal antiinflammatory agents [NSAIDs]).

    d. Instruct patient on proper use of medications.

REFERENCES

Fife, D. J., Waller, J. M., Jeffes, E. W., & Koo, J. Y. M. (2007). Unraveling the paradoxes of HIV-associated psoriasis: A review of T-cell subsets and cytokine profiles. *Dermatology Online Journal.* Retrieved January 25, 2009, from http://dermatology.cdlib.org/132/reviews/HIV/fife.html

Handel, J. (2001). Dermatological care of clients with HIV/AIDS. In C. A. Kirton, D. Talotta, & K. Zwolski (Eds.), *Handbook of HIV/AIDS nursing* (pp. 323–325). St. Louis, MO: Mosby.

Maurer, T. A., & Berger, T. G. (1998). *Dermatologic manifestations of HIV.* Retrieved January 25, 2009, from http://hivinsite.ucsf.edu/InSite?page=kb-04-01

Merrigan, T., Bartlett, J. G., & Bolognesi, D. (Eds.). (1999). *Textbook of AIDS medicine.* Philadelphia: Lippincott Williams & Wilkins.

3.31 OSTEOPENIA, OSTEOPOROSIS, AVASCULAR NECROSIS

1. Etiology/epidemiology

    a. Osteopenia: bone thinning; osteoporosis: severe loss of bone mass with disruption of skeletal microarchitecture; avascular necrosis (AVN): bone necrosis secondary to circulatory insufficiency (Bongiovanni & Tincati, 2006)

    b. Etiology: incompletely understood. Evidence suggests that cytokine dysregulation contributes to bone demineralization. The contributions of HAART and HIV in activating bone-depleting cytokine pathways are unclear (Bongiovanni & Tincanti, 2006), although treatment with protease inhibitors has been shown to decrease bone mineral density (BMD).

   c. Prevalence: osteopenia: up to 67% of HIV-infected persons show reduced BMD; 15% have osteoporosis (Brown & Qaqish, 2006). HAART increases risk of reduced BMD by 2.5 fold (Brown & Qaqish, 2006). AVN: 4.4% (Miller et al., 2001).

2. Pathogenesis
   a. Osteopenia and osteoporosis: Both HAART and viral components, such as gp120 and Vpr, have been associated with overproduction of RANKL. RANKL, a cytokine secreted by T cells and osteoblasts, activates signal transduction pathways in osteoclasts that promote their differentiation and survival (Konishi et al., 2005; Wei et al., 2005). However, another study found evidence that HAART normalizes bone mineralization (Mondy et al., 2003). Tumor necrosis factor (TNF) has been shown to upregulate RANKL and thus may contribute to osteoclastogenesis (Wei et al., 2005).
   b. AVN: unknown; may involve deposition of lipids in subchondral bone vasculature with subsequent occlusion and ischemia, effects of ARV, chronic inflammation associated with persistent viral infection, and use of corticosteroids (Morse et al., 2007)

3. Clinical presentation
   a. Osteopenia and osteoporosis are clinically silent disorders.
   b. AVN most commonly involves the hip. Disabling pain may be insidious or sudden in onset and involves decreased range of motion.

4. Diagnosis
   a. Osteopenia and osteoporosis are diagnosed through bone density evaluations.
   b. AVN is best evaluated by magnetic resonance imaging (MRI).

5. Prevention/treatment
   a. Osteopenia and osteoporosis: smoking cessation, normalization of lipid profile, weight-bearing exercise, and adequate intake of calcium and vitamin D; biphosphonate therapy for osteoporosis. Limited clinical trial data suggest efficacy of alendronate for increasing hip and spine BMD (Guaraldi et al., 2004; Mondy et al., 2005; Negredo et al., 2005).
   b. AVN: activity modification, analgesic therapy, and prostethic replacement

---

REFERENCES

Bongiovanni, M., & Tincati, C. (2006). Bone diseases associated with human immunodeficiency virus infection: Pathogenesis, risk factors and clinical management. *Current Molecular Medicine, 6*(4), 395–400.

Brown, T. T., & Qaqish, R. B. (2006). Antiretroviral therapy and the prevalence of osteopenia and osteoporosis: A meta-analytic review. *AIDS, 20*(17), 2165–2174.

Guaraldi, G., Orlando, G., Madeddu. G., Vescini, F., Ventura, P., Campostrini, S., et al. (2004). Alendronate reduces bone resorption in HIV-associated osteopenia/osteoporosis. *HIV Clinical Trials, 5*(5), 269–277.

Konishi, M., Takahashi, K., Yoshimoto, E., Uno, K., Kasahara, K., & Mikasa, K. (2005). Association between osteopenia/osteoporosis and the serum RANKL in HIV-infected patients. *AIDS, 19*(11), 1240–1241.

Miller, K. D., Masur, H., Jones, E. C., Joe, G. O., Rick, M. E., Kelly, G. G., et al. (2002). High prevalence of osteonecrosis of the femoral head in HIV-infected adults. *Annals of Internal Medicine, 137*(1), 17–25.

Mondy, K., Powderly, W., Claxton, S. A., Yarasheski, K. H., Royal, M., Stoneman, J. S., et al. (2005). Alendronate, vitamin D, and calcium for the treatment of osteopenia/osteoporosis associated with HIV infection. *Journal of the Acquired Immune Deficiency Syndromes, 38*(4), 426–431.

Mondy, K., Yarasheski, K., Powderly, W. G., Whyte, M., Claxton, S., De Marco, D., et al. (2003). Longitudinal evolution of bone mineral density and bone markers in human immunodeficiency virus-infected individuals. *Clinical Infectious Diseases, 36*(4), 482–490.

Morse, C. G., Mican, J. M., Jones, E. C., Joe, G. O., Rick, M. E., Formentini, E., et al. (2007). The incidence and natural history of osteonecrosis in HIV-infected adults. *Clinical Infectious Diseases, 44*(5), 739–748.

Negredo, E., Martínez-López, E., Paredes, R., Rosales, J., Pérez-Alvarez, N., Holgado, S., et al. (2005). Reversal of HIV-1-associated osteoporosis with once-weekly alendronate. *AIDS, 19*(3), 343–345.

Wei, S., Kitaura, H., Zhou, P., Ross, F. P., & Teitelbaum, S. L. (2005). IL-1 mediates TNF-induced osteoclastogenesis. *Journal of Clinical Investigation, 115*(2), 282–290.

3.32 NEPHROPATHY

1. Etiology/epidemiology
   a. HIV-associated nephropathy (HIVAN) can directly result from HIV infection, or from secondary infections or adverse effects of medical therapies (Choi & Rodriguez, 2008).
   b. It is the most common cause of chronic renal disease in HIV-infected patients (Monahan, Tanji, & Klotman, 2001; Sothinathan, Briggs, & Eustace, 2001). In the United States there were more than 4,200 new cases of end-stage renal disease (ESRD) attributed to HIV between 2000 and 2004 (USRDS, 2004).
   c. The majority of HIVAN cases in the United States occur in African Americans; it is the leading cause of ESRD in African Americans (USRDS, 2004).
   d. Renal damage caused by antiretroviral agents can result in acute renal failure, tubular necrosis, kidney stones, or chronic renal disease.
      i)   Indinavir has been associated with adverse renal effects including nephrolithiasis, crystalluria, dysuria, papillary necrosis, and acute renal failure (Daugas et al., 2005).
      ii) Ritonavir at therapeutic doses of 800–1200 mg/day has been linked to reversible renal failure (Bochet et al., 1998; Chugh et al., 1997).
      iii) Tenofovir has been associated with renal tubular damage varying from acute tubular necrosis to possibly reversible tubular dysfunction, such as Fanconi syndrome (Barrios et al., 2004; Izzedine et al., 2005; Peyriere et al., 2004; Rifkin & Perazella, 2004; Zimmermann et al., 2006.)

2. Pathogenesis
   a. Pathogenesis likely involves HIV infection of renal tubular and epithelial cells (Choi & Rodriguez, 2008). Murine model data suggest that HIV gene expression in renal glomerular and epithelial cells underlies HIVAN histological changes (Bruggeman et al., 1997). Recent studies suggest that podocyte-specific expression of viral genes may be sufficient for the development of HIV-associated nephropathy (Zhong et al., 2005; Zuo et al., 2006), but it is also likely that HIV infection of lymphoid tissue also plays a role in the pathogenesis of HIVAN.

3. Clinical presentation
   a. HIVAN is often asymptomatic and undetected until proteinuria is found on a screening urinalysis.
   b. Symptomatic patients present with rapidly progressing azotemia and progressive renal failure (Betjes et al., 2001; Brook & Miller, 2001; Cosgrove, Abu-Alfa, & Perazella, 2002; Kirchner, 2002; Rajvanshi & Gupta, 2001).

4. Diagnosis
   a. Renal biopsy is necessary for a definitive diagnosis of HIVAN (Atta et al., 2006). Histopathological findings include focal segmental glomerulosclerosis with glomerular collapse, acute tubular necrosis, and mild interstitial inflammation.
   b. Other components of a diagnostic workup include ultrasonography, serology, and urinalysis (Betjes et al., 2001; Kimmel, 2000; Kirchner, 2002; Rajvanshi & Gupta, 2001).
      i) Ultrasound will show kidney enlargement.
      ii) Serological studies will reveal rapidly developing azotemia.
      iii) Urinalysis will reveal proteinuria.
5. Prevention/treatment
   a. The Infectious Diseases Society of America has published guidelines for the management of HIV-related chronic kidney disease, including HIVAN (Gupta et al., 2005).
   b. HAART has been shown to be effective in managing HIVAN (Atta et al., 2006; Betjes et al., 2001; Brook & Miller, 2001; Cosgrove et al., 2002; Kirchner, 2002).
   c. Decreased progression to ESRD can be achieved with cyclosporins, glucocorticoids, and angiotensin-converting enzyme (ACE) inhibitors (Choi & Rodriguez, 2008; Cosgrove et al., 2002; Kirchner, 2002).
6. Nursing implications
   a. Educate patient to avoid nephrotoxic agents and to maintain adequate hydration; reinforce self-care strategies to control hypertension (Sothinathan et al., 2001).
   b. Assess nutritional status (i.e., weight, body mass index, serum proteins, usual dietary intake) and risk for developing malnutrition before initiating a low-protein diet to slow renal disease progression.
   c. Educate patient with risk factors for kidney disease, such as diabetes, hypertension, hepatitis co-infection, or family history of kidney disease, for the need to be annually screened for decreased glomerular filtration rate and proteinuria (Gupta et al., 2005).

REFERENCES

Atta, M. G., Choi, M. J., Longenecker, J. C., Haymart, M., Wu, J., Nagajothi, N., et al. (2005). Nephrotic range proteinuria and CD4 count as noninvasive indicators of HIV-associated nephropathy. *American Journal of Medicine, 118*(11), 1288.

Atta, M. G., Gallant, J. E., Rahman, M. H., Nagajothi, N., Racusen, L. C., Scheel, P. J., et al. (2006). Antiretroviral therapy in the treatment of HIV-associated nephropathy. *Nephrology Dialysis Transplantation, 21*(10), 2809–2813.

Barrios, A., García-Benayas, T., González-Lahoz, J., & Soriano, V. (2004). Tenofovir-related nephrotoxicity in HIV-infected patients. *AIDS, 18*(6), 960–963.

Betjes, M. G., Weening, J., & Krediet, R. T. (2001). Diagnosis and treatment of HIV-associated nephropathy. *Netherlands Journal of Medicine, 59*(3), 111–117.

Bochet, M. V., Jacquiaud, C., Valantin, M. A., Katlama, C., & Deray, G. (1998). Renal insufficiency induced by ritonavir in HIV-infected patients. *American Journal of Medicine, 105*(5), 457.

Brook, M. G., & Miller, R. F. (2001). HIV associated nephropathy: A treatable condition. *Sexually Transmitted Infections, 77*(2), 97–100.

Bruggeman, L. A., Dikman, S., Meng, C., Quaggin, S. E., Coffman, T. M., & Klotman, P. E. (1997). Nephropathy in human immunodeficiency virus-1 transgenic mice is due to renal transgene expression. *Journal of Clinical Investigation, 100*(1), 84–92.

Choi, A. I., & Rodriguez, R. A. (2008). Renal manifestations of HIV. In L. Peiperl, S. Coffey, O. Bacon, & P. Volberding (Eds.), *HIV InSite Knowledge Base* [online textbook]. Retrieved January 25, 2009, from http://hivinsite.ucsf.edu/InSite?page=kb-04-01-10

Cosgrove, C. J., Abu-Alfa, A. K., & Perazella, M. A. (2002). Observations on HIV-associated renal disease in the era of highly active antiretroviral therapy. *American Journal of the Medical Sciences, 323*(2), 102–106.

Chugh, S., Bird, R., & Alexander, E. A. (1997). Ritonavir and renal failure. *New England Journal of Medicine, 336*(2), 138.

Daugas, E., Rougier, J. P., & Hill, G. (2005). HAART-related nephropathies in HIV-infected patients. *Kidney International, 67*(2), 393–403.

Gupta, S. K., Eustace, J. A., Winston, J. A., Boydstun, I. I., Ahuja, T. S., Rodriguez, R. A., et al. (2005). Guidelines for the management of chronic kidney disease in HIV-infected patients: Recommendations of the HIV Medicine Association of the Infectious Diseases Society of America. *Clinical Infectious Diseases, 40*(11), 1559–1585.

Izzedine, H., Hulot, J. S., Vittecoq, D., Gallant, J. E., Staszewski, S., Launay-Vacher, V., et al. (2005). Long-term renal safety of tenofovir disoproxil fumarate in antiretroviral-naive HIV-1–infected patients: Data from a double-blind randomized active-controlled multicentre study. *Nephrology Dialysis Transplantation, 20*(4), 743–746.

Kimmel, P. L. (2000). The nephropathies of HIV infection: Pathogenesis and treatment. *Current Opinion in Nephrology and Hypertension, 9*(2), 117–122.

Kirchner, J. T. (2002). Resolution of renal failure after initiation of HAART: 3 cases and a discussion of the literature. *The AIDS Reader, 12*(3), 103–105, 110–112.

Monahan, M., Tanji, N., & Klotman, P. E. (2001). HIV-associated nephropathy: An urban epidemic. *Seminars in Nephrology, 21*(4), 394–402.

Peyrière, H., Reynes, J., Rouanet, I., Daniel, N., de Boever, C. M., Mauboussin, J. M., et al. (2004). Renal tubular dysfunction associated with tenofovir therapy: Report of 7 cases. *Journal of the Acquired Immunodeficiency Syndrome, 35*(3), 269–273.

Rajvanshi, P., & Gupta, B. (2001). Human immunodeficiency virus-associated nephropathy. *Journal of the Association of Physicians of India, 49,* 813–818.

Rifkin, B. S., & Perazella, M. A. (2004). Tenofovir-associated nephrotoxicity: Fanconi syndrome and renal failure. *American Journal of Medicine, 117*(4), 282–284.

Sothinathan, R., Briggs, W. A., & Eustace, J. A. (2001). Treatment of HIV-associated nephropathy. *AIDS Patient Care and STDs, 15*(7), 363–371.

United States Renal Data System (USRDS). (2004). *USRDS 2004 annual data report: Atlas of end-stage renal disease in the United States.* Bethesda, MD: National Institutes of Health, National Institute of Diabetes and Digestive and Kidney Diseases.

Zhong, J., Zuo, Y., Ma, J., Fogo, A. B., Jolicoeur, P., Ichikawa, I., et al. (2005). Expression of HIV-1 genes in podocytes alone can lead to the full spectrum of HIV-1-associated nephropathy. *Kidney International, 68*(3), 1048–1060.

Zimmermann, A. E., Pizzoferrato, T., Bedford, J., Morris, A., Hoffman, R., & Braden, G. (2006). Tenofovir-associated acute and chronic kidney disease: A case of multiple drug interactions. *Clinical Infectious Diseases, 42*(2), 283–290.

Zuo, Y., Matsusaka, T., Zhong, J., Ma, J., Ma, L. J., Hanna, Z., et al. (2006). HIV-1 genes vpr and nef synergistically damage podocytes, leading to glomerulosclerosis. *Journal of the American Society of Nephrology, 17*(10), 2832–2843.

3.33 LACTIC ACIDOSIS

1. Etiology/epidemiology
   a. Hyperlactatemia is believed to be caused by mitochondrial dysfunction induced by nucleoside reverse transcriptase inhibitors (NRTIs; Monier & Wilcox, 2004).
   b. Lactic acidosis is a severe form of hyperlactatemia.
   c. Prevalence of hyperlactatemia in NRTI-treated persons is estimated to range from 10% to 20%; incidence of lactic acidosis is 4 to 5 per 1,000 patient years of NRTI therapy (Moyle, 2002; Cossarizza & Moyle, 2004). Risk factors associated with lactic acidosis include

pregnancy, female sex, inherited mitochondrial disorder, older age, obesity, and liver disease or steatosis (Khater et al., 2004).

d. Lactic acidosis is a rare complication of NRTIs, with an incidence estimated to be 0.4% per treatment year (Cossarizza & Moyle, 2004).

2. Pathogenesis
   a. NRTIs are thought to inhibit mitochondrial DNA polymerase-γ, which disrupts synthesis of mitochondrial enzymes and inhibits ATP formation. This leads to impaired fatty acid oxidation with subsequent anaerobic metabolism and lactate accumulation (Carr, 2003).

3. Clinical presentation
   a. Persons with mild or moderate hyperlactatemia may be asymptomatic or have mild GI symptoms (i.e., nausea, abdominal distension, pain). Laboratory findings include increased serum lactate and transaminase levels (McComsey & Lederman, 2002).
   b. Lactic acidosis is characterized by fatigue, dyspnea, nausea and vomiting, abdominal distention and pain, weight loss, myalgias, and hepatomegaly. Laboratory findings include elevated serum transaminase levels, and liver biopsy shows steatosis, inflammation, and necrosis (Carr, 2003).

4. Diagnosis
   a. Lactic acidosis is characterized by an arterial pH $<$ 7.30 and venous lactate levels $>$ 2.0 mmol/L (Monier & Wilcox, 2004).

5. Prevention/treatment
   a. Anecdotal data suggest that thiamine and riboflavin may prevent recurrence of hyperlactatemia in persons who must be maintained on NRTI therapy (McComsey & Lederman, 2002).
   b. Monitor lactate levels in NRTI-treated persons who present with suspicious signs or symptoms (i.e., fatigue, nausea and vomiting, increased anion gap, low plasma bicarbonate levels).
   c. Discontinue NRTIs in persons with lactatemia $>$ 10.0 mmol/L or symptomatic lactatemia $>$ 5.0 mmol/L (Carr, 2003).

6. Nursing implications
   a. Educate patient/family/significant other regarding early detection of hyperlactatemia.
   b. Recognize patients who are at higher risk for developing lactic acidosis (i.e., pregnant women, those with presence of other mitochondrial toxicity-mediated disorders, such as lipoatrophy and peripheral neuropathy).

REFERENCES

Carr, A. (2003). Lactic acidemia in infection with human immunodeficiency virus. *Clinical Infectious Diseases, 36*(Suppl. 2), S96-S100.

Cossarizza, A., & Moyle, G. (2004). Antiretroviral nucleoside and nucleotide analogues and mitochondria. *AIDS, 18*(2), 137–151.

Khater, F. J., Youssef, S., Iskandar, S. B., Myers, J. W., & Moorman, J. P. (2004). Lactic acidosis during nucleoside antiretroviral HIV therapy. *Southern Medical Journal, 97*(2), 208.

McComsey, G. A., & Lederman, M. M. (2002). High doses of riboflavin and thiamine may help in secondary prevention of hyperlactatemia. *AIDS Reader, 12*(5), 222–224.

Monier, P. L., & Wilcox, R. (2004). Metabolic complications associated with the use of highly active antiretroviral therapy in HIV-1-infected adults. *American Journal of Medical Science, 328*(1), 48–56.

Moyle, G. (2002). Hyperlactatemia and lactic acidosis: Should routine screening be considered? *AIDS Reader, 12*(8), 344–348.

3.34 HEPATITIS A

1. Etiology/epidemiology
   a. Hepatitis A virus (HAV) is an RNA virus classified as a picornavirus.
   b. Rates of hepatitis A infection in the United States have declined sharply due to changes in immunization practice. Overall U.S. incidence was 1.5/100,000 in 2005 (CDC, 2007).
   c. Blood-borne outbreaks of hepatitis A related to administration of contaminated blood products have sharply decreased due to improved screening of donors and changes in viral inactivation procedures used for processing factor VIII and factor IX.
   d. Predominant route of transmission is oral–fecal.
      i)   Contaminated water and food are vehicles for transmission.
      ii) HAV is sexually transmitted via oral–anal contact.
      iii) Person-to-person contact can occur through contamination of hands with feces.
   e. Average incubation period is 28 days (range 15–50 days).
   f. The following persons are at increased risk for hepatitis A infection (CDC, 2006):
      i)   Travelers to areas where hepatitis A is endemic
      ii) Men who have sex with men
      iii) Injection and noninjection drug users
      iv) Persons working with nonhuman primates (primates born in the wild)
      v)   Persons who work with HAV in a research laboratory setting
2. Pathogenesis (CDC, 2006)
   a. HAV is ingested or injected, replicates in the liver, is excreted in bile, and is shed in the stool.
   b. HAV is usually a mild, self-limiting infection and does not progress to chronic liver disease or hepatocellular carcinoma (CDC, 2007).
   c. HAV load is higher and prolonged in HIV-infected patients compared with HAV mono-infected persons (Ida et al., 2002).
3. Clinical presentation (CDC, 2006)
   a. Signs and symptoms of acute infection can include malaise, anorexia, fever, jaundice, nausea, and abdominal discomfort.
   b. The likelihood of symptomatic infection increases with age. Seventy percent of HAV infections are asymptomatic in children < 6 years old.
4. Diagnosis
   a. HAV infection is diagnosed by serologic evidence of IgM anti-HAV, which is present 5–10 days before onset of symptoms. IgG anti-HAV confers protective immunity to subsequent infections (CDC, 2006).
5. Prevention/treatment
   a. HAV vaccine should be administered to persons who are at increased risk for exposure (CDC, 2007).

b. HIV-infected persons coinfected with any hepatotrophic virus should be vaccinated with HAV vaccine.

c. HAV vaccine is immunogenic for persons with HIV infection. However, when CD4 counts are low (< 300 cells/mm^3), persons with HIV infection are less likely to acquire protective levels of hepatitis A antibodies. Protective antibody levels are achieved in 61–87% of HIV infected adults (CDC, 2006).

d. Immune globulin may be administered for short-term protection against hepatitis A, both pre- and post-exposure. Immune globulin must be administered within 2 weeks after exposure for maximum protection.

e. Symptomatic treatment is also administered when HAV-infected person becomes ill.

6. Nursing implications

a. Standard precautions must be used in the care of all patients. In addition, use transmission-based contact precautions for all HAV-infected persons who are diapered or incontinent of stool (Seigel et al., 2007).

b. Perform HAV risk assessment for all HIV-positive patients.

c. Conduct patient, family, and staff teaching regarding meticulous hand hygiene to prevent spread of infection.

d. Immune globulin can interfere with measles, mumps, rubella, and varicella vaccines.

e. Teach patient that the infectious state of hepatitis A in HIV/HAV coinfection may last as long as a year (Ida et al., 2002).

REFERENCES

Centers for Disease Control and Prevention (CDC). (2006). Prevention of hepatitis A through active or passive immunization: Recommendations of the Advisory Committee on Immunization Practices (ACIP). *Morbidity and Mortality Weekly Report, 55*(RR-7), 1–18.

Centers for Disease Control and Prevention, National Center for HIV/AIDS, Viral Hepatitis, STD, and TB prevention (CDC). (2007). Surveillance for acute viral hepatitis—United States, 2005. *Morbidity and Mortality Weekly Report, 56*(SS03), 1–24.

Ida, S., Tachikawa, N., Nakajima, A., Kaikodu, M., Yano, M., Kikuchi, Y., et al. (2002). Influence of human immunodeficiency virus type I infection on acute hepatitis A virus infection. *Clinical Infectious Disease, 34*(3), 379–385.

Siegel, J. D., Rhinehart, E., Jackson, M., Chiarello, L., & the Health Care Infection Control Practices Advisory Committee. (2007). 2007 guideline for isolation precautions preventing transmission of infectious agents in health care settings 2007. *American Journal of Infection Control, 35*(10, Suppl. 2), S65–S164.

3.35 HEPATITIS B

1. Etiology/epidemiology

a. Hepatitis B virus (HBV) is a double-stranded DNA virus and is classified as a hepadnavirus.

b. Overall U.S. incidence of acute HBV infection was 1.8/100,000 in 2005 (CDC, 2007).

c. Chronic HBV infection occurs in 90% of infected infants, 30% of infected children < 5 years of age, and $< 5\%$ of infected persons > 5 years of age.

d. Chronic HBV infection is associated with an increased risk for chronic liver disease and hepatocellular carcinoma (CDC, 2007).

e. Route of transmission is bloodborne and sexual.

f. Average incubation period is 90 days (range: 60–150 days).

g. The following persons are at risk for HBV infection (CDC, 2006):

    i)   Men who have sex with men

    ii)   Persons with multiple sex partners

    iii)   Persons with an HBV-infected sex partner

    iv)   Injection drug users

    v)   Infants born to HBV-infected mothers

    vi)   Hemodialysis patients

    vii) Household contacts of chronically infected persons

    viii) Healthcare and public safety workers with exposure to blood

    ix)   Infants/children of immigrants from areas with high rates of HBV infection

2. Pathogenesis

a. HBV enters the liver via the bloodstream. The primary site of HBV replication is the liver.

b. Chronic hepatitis B can cause hepatic necroinflammation, liver cirrhosis, and hepatocellular carcinoma (Lok & McMahon, 2007).

c. Reinfection or reactivation of latent HBV infection can occur in immunosuppressed persons.

d. Primary HBV infections become chronic more frequently in immunosuppressed persons.

3. Clinical presentation

a. Signs and symptoms of acute infection can include malaise, anorexia, nausea, vomiting, abdominal pain, and jaundice.

b. The likelihood of symptomatic infection increases with increased age. Seventy percent of infections are asymptomatic in children < 6 years of age.

c. Chronic hepatitis with liver cirrhosis may present with symptoms of jaundice, dark urine, ascites, pruritis, nausea, vomiting, coagulation disorders, and gastrointestinal bleeding.

4. Diagnosis

a. HBV infection is diagnosed by serologic evidence of antigens. Hepatitis B surface antigen (HBsAg) can be detected in blood during acute or chronic hepatitis and indicates the person is infectious.

b. HBV antibodies are produced in response to HBV antigens. Presence of antibodies usually indicates recovery and immunity from infection. Protective antibody response is reported quantitatively as 10 or more milliinternational units per milliliter.

c. Total hepatitis B core antibody (anti-HBc) is the first antibody to appear and is a lifelong marker of past exposure *or* ongoing infection. A positive anti-HBc in the absence of positive HBsAg could indicate a false positive result or there could be undetectable levels of HBsAg in the blood and the person may be chronically infected.

d. Research indicates that core antibody (anti-HBc) alone occurs more frequently in HIV-infected patients (Gandhi et al., 2003). Therefore, hepatitis B testing for HIV-infected patients should include anti-HBc in addition to HBsAg and anti-HBs.

e. Hepatitis B e antigen (HBeAg) is a marker for ongoing viral replication and indicates a high level of infectivity (CDC, 2007).

f. Presence of HBV DNA is the most certain indicator of HBV infection.

5. Prevention/treatment
   a. Prevention of hepatitis B is achieved through immunization and avoiding high-risk behaviors, such as injection drug use, sex with multiple partners, and unprotected sex (Lok & McMahon, 2007).
   b. Treatment for acute hepatitis B is symptomatic (CDC, 2005).
   c. Liver biopsy should be considered for persons who are HIV/chronic hepatitis B coinfected.
   d. Persons with HIV/chronic hepatitis B coinfection who are not on HAART may be treated with pegIFN-α, adefovir, or entecavir.
   e. Persons with HIV/chronic hepatitis B coinfection who are on effective HAART may be treated with pegIFN-α, adefovir, or entecavir.
   f. Patients who are beginning drug therapy for HIV infection and chronic hepatitis B may be treated with lamivudine and tenofovir or emtricitabine and tenofovir.
   g. Lamivudine has high rates of resistance to HBV in coinfected persons. The combination use of tenofovir with lamivudine seems to reduce HBV resistance to lamivudine.
6. Nursing implications
   a. Standard precautions must be used in the care of all patients (Seigel et al., 2007).
   b. Patients with HBV infection should be screened for hepatitis A and C infections.
   c. Patients with HBV infection should receive HAV vaccine, if indicated.
   d. Educate patient and family regarding prevention of disease transmission.
      i) Condoms should be used to prevent spread of HBV and other sexually transmitted diseases.
      ii) Patients with HBV infection should not share drug needles, injection equipment, toothbrushes, or razors.
      iii) Tattoos and body piercing should be performed with sterile equipment, by an experienced operator who can practice standard precautions.
      iv) Patients with HBV infection must not donate blood, organs, or sperm.
   e. Considerations for the care of persons who are susceptible to hepatitis B infection (HBsAg negative and anti-HBc negative and anti-HBs negative; CDC, 2005):
      i) Hepatitis B vaccine is contraindicated when patient has history of hypersensitivity to yeast or to any vaccine component.
      ii) Humoral response to hepatitis B vaccine is reduced in persons who are immunosuppressed. Modified dosing may increase response rate.
      iii) Injection into the buttock is associated with a decrease in the immunogenicity of the vaccine. Always administer vaccine in deltoid or anterolateral thigh.
   f. Counsel patient to abstain from alcohol.
   g. Review medications and adverse side effects with patient.
   h. Elicit history of botanical complementary therapy. Certain botanicals are hepatotoxic, such as comfrey and kava (Odom & Finkbine, 2001).

REFERENCES

Centers for Disease Control and Prevention (CDC). (2005). A comprehensive immunization strategy to eliminate transmission of hepatitis B virus infection in the United States: Recommendations of the Advisory Committee on Immunization Practices (ACIP): Part 1: Immunization of infants, children, and adolescents. *Morbidity and Mortality Weekly Report, 54*(RR-16), 1–31.

Centers for Disease Control and Prevention, National Center for HIV/AIDS, Viral Hepatitis, STD, and TB Prevention. (CDC). (2006). *Viral hepatitis B interpretation of the hepatitis B panel.* Retrieved February 5, 2009, from http://www.acphd.org/AXBYCZ/ADMIN/PUBLICATIONS/interprethepatitislabresults.pdf

Centers for Disease Control and Prevention, National Center for HIV/AIDS, Viral Hepatitis, STD, and TB Prevention (CDC). (2007). *Viral hepatitis B fact sheet.* Retrieved February 5, 2009, from http://www.cdc.gov/hepatitis/index.htm

Ghandi, R. T., Wurcel, A., Hang, L., McGovern, B., Boczanowski, M., Gerwin, R., et al. (2003). Isolated antibody to hepatitis B core antigen in human immunodeficiency virus type 1-infected individuals. *Clinical Infectious Diseases, 36*(12), 1602–1605.

Lok, A. S., & McMahon, B. J. (2007). *American Association for the Study of Liver Diseases Practice Guidelines: Chronic hepatitis B.* Retrieved March 4, 2009, from http://www.cdc.gov/hepatitis/index.htm

Odom, J., & Finkbine, S. (2001). Overcoming hepatitis C. *Alternative Medicine, 42,* 40–48.

Siegel, J. D., Rhinehart, E., Jackson, M., & Chiarello, L., for the Health Care Infection Control Practices Advisory Committee. (2007). 2007 guideline for isolation precautions preventing transmission of infectious agents in health care settings. *American Journal of Infection Control, 35*(10, Suppl. 2), S65–S164.

3.36 HEPATITIS C

1. Etiology/epidemiology
   a. Hepatitis C virus (HCV) is a single-stranded RNA virus and is related to flavivirus. HCV is divided into genotypes 1–6, based on genetic heterogeneity, and these are further subdivided into more than 50 subtypes. The prevalence of HCV genotypes varies in different parts of the world. Genotype 1 is most common in the United States (CDC, 2007).
   b. Approximately 3.2 million persons in the United States were chronically infected with HCV in 2005 (CDC, 2007b).
   c. Overall U.S. incidence of acute hepatitis C is 0.2/100,000 (CDC, 2007b).
      i) The most common risk factor for HCV infection is injection drug use. Fifty percent (50%) of all acute HCV-infected persons reported injection drug use. Prevalence of HCV infection among injection drug users may be as high as 80–90% (Khalsa et al., 2005).
      ii) Twenty-three percent (23%) of those infected with HCV reported having sex with multiple partners.
      iii) Fourteen percent (14%) of those infected with HCV reported having surgery 6 weeks to 6 months prior to diagnosis.
      iv) Eight percent (8%) of persons infected with HCV reported occupational exposure to blood.
   d. Additional issues related to risk for contracting HCV (CDC, 2006):
      i) During the past 20 years, < 1% of persons with acute hepatitis C reported a history of being tattooed. CDC is currently conducting a large study to evaluate tattooing as a potential risk (CDC, 2006).
      ii) Hemophiliacs treated with blood products made prior to 1987 are at increased for HCV infection (Strader et al., 2004).
      iii) Blood recipients receiving blood products prior to 1992 are at increased risk for HCV infection (Strader et al., 2004).
   e. Duration of survival in HIV/HCV coinfected persons is significantly decreased compared to mono-infected HCV persons (Anderson et al., 2004).

f. Route of transmission is blood borne. Sexual transmission is possible but is a less efficient mode of transmission (CDC, 2007a).

g. Acute hepatitis usually develops within 10–14 weeks after infection (Chung, 2005).

2. Pathogenesis

a. HIV and HCV envelope proteins cause apoptosis in hepatocytes, most likely through a mitochondrial pathway (Balasubramanian et al., 2005).

b. HCV infection is a major risk factor for development of end-stage liver disease and hepatocellular carcinoma (Strader et al., 2004).

c. Persons with HIV/HCV coinfection have more rapid progression to liver cirrhosis (Torre et al., 2001).

3. Clinical presentation

a. Between 60% and 70% of persons who have acute HCV infection are asymptomatic. An additional 10–20% have nonspecific symptoms (CDC, 2007b).

b. Signs and symptoms of HCV infection are usually mild and nonspecific. Fatigue, anorexia, weight loss, and muscle aches may be present (CDC, 2007a).

c. If progression to liver cirrhosis occurs, symptoms can include jaundice, dark urine, ascites, pruritus, nausea, vomiting, coagulation disorders, and gastrointestinal bleeding.

4. Diagnosis

a. HCV infection is diagnosed by serologic evidence:

i) Serum alanine aminotransferase levels higher than 7 times the upper limit of normal, *and*

ii) IgM anti-HAV negative, *and*

iii) IgM anti-HBc negative or, if not performed, HbsAg negative *and* one of the following:

(1) Antibody to hepatitis C virus (anti-HCV) screening test positive, verified by an additional, more specific assay (e.g., recombinant immunoblot assay [RIBA] for anti-HCV or nucleic acid testing for HCV RNA)

(2) Anti-HCV screening test positive with a signal-to-cutoff ratio predictive of a true positive, as determined for the particular assay (e.g., > 3.8 for the enzyme immunoassays)

b. Six percent (6%) of HIV/HCV coinfected persons do not develop antibodies to HCV; therefore, HCV RNA levels should be tested when there is evidence of liver disease and the person is anti-HCV negative (Strader et al., 2004).

5. Prevention/treatment

a. There is no hepatitis C vaccine available (CDC, 2006).

b. Prevention of hepatitis C consists of identifying and counseling uninfected persons at risk (CDC, 2007a).

c. Combination therapy, using pegylated interferon and ribavirin, is currently the recommended drug therapy for HIV/HCV coinfection (CDC, 2007a). Duration of treatment is dependent upon the HCV genotype (Strader et al., 2004).

d. It is not recommended to withhold HAART from persons with HIV/HCV coinfection due to concerns regarding hepatotoxicity (Strader et al., 2004).

6. Nursing implications

a. Standard precautions should be used on all patients (Siegel et al., 2007).

b. Screen patients with HCV for HAV and HBV infection. Immunize if indicated.

   c. Educate patients regarding adverse effects of medication, and monitor patients frequently.
   d. Counsel patient to abstain from alcohol. Alcohol use increases risk for mortality in patients with HCV infection.
   e. Elicit history of botanical complementary therapy use. Certain botanicals are hepatotoxic (Odom & Finkbine, 2001).
   f. Monitor HIV/HCV coinfected persons for liver toxicity, drug interactions, and psychiatric complications (Khalsa et al., 2005).
   g. Educate patient and family regarding prevention of disease transmission.
      i)   Condoms should be used to prevent spread of HCV and other sexually transmitted diseases.
      ii) Patients should not share drug needles, injection equipment, toothbrushes, or razors.
      iii) Patients must not donate blood, tissue, organs, or sperm.
      iv) Keep open wounds covered.

REFERENCES

Anderson, K. B., Guest, J. L., & Rimland, D. (2004). Hepatitis C virus coinfection increases mortality in HIV-infected patients in the highly active antiretroviral therapy era: data from the HIV Atlanta VA cohort study. *Clinical Infectious Diseases, 39*(10), 1507–1513.

Balasubramanian, A., Koziel, M., Groopman, J. E., & Ganju, R. K. (2005). Molecular mechanism of hepatic injury in coinfection with hepatitis C virus and HIV. *Clinical Infectious Diseases, 41*(Suppl. 1), S32–S37.

Centers for Disease Control and Prevention, National Center for HIV/AIDS, Viral Hepatitis, STD, and TB Prevention (CDC). (2006). *CDC's position on tattooing and HCV infection.* Retrieved April 22, 2009, from http://www.cdc.gov/hepatitis/index.htm

Centers for Disease Control and Prevention, National Center for HIV/AIDS, Viral Hepatitis, STD, and TB Prevention (CDC). (2007b). Surveillance for acute viral hepatitis—United States, 2005. *Morbidity and Mortality Weekly Report, 56*(SS03), 1–24.

Chung, R. T. (2005). Acute hepatitis C virus infection. *Clinical Infectious Diseases, 41*(Suppl. 1), S14–S17.

HepCnet. (2003). *Viral hepatitis C: Frequently asked questions provided by the National Center for Infectious Diseases.* Retrieved February 5, 2009, from http://hepcnet.net/hepatitiscfaq.html

Khalsa, J. H., Kresina, T., Sherman, K., & Vocci, F. (2005). Medical management of HIV-hepatitis C virus coinfection in injection drug users. *Clinical Infectious Diseases, 41*(Suppl. 1), S1–S6.

Odom, J., & Finkbine, S. (2001). Overcoming hepatitis C. *Alternative Medicine, 42,* 40–48.

Siegel, J. D., Rhinehart, E., Jackson, M., Chiarello, L., Health Care Infection Control Practices Advisory Committee. (2007). 2007 guideline for isolation precautions preventing transmission of infectious agents in health care settings. *American Journal of Infection Control, 35*(10, Suppl. 2), S65–S164.

Strader, D. B., Wright, T., Thomas, D. L., & Seeff, L. B. (2004). *American Association for the Study of Liver Diseases practice guideline: Diagnosis, management, and treatment of hepatitis C.* Retrieved February 5, 2009, from http://www.cdc.gov/ncidod/diseases/hepatitis/c/faq.htm

Torre, D., Tambini, R., Cadario, F., Barbarini, G., Moroni, M., & Basilico, C. (2001). Evolution of coinfection with human immunodeficiency virus and hepatitis C virus in patients treated with highly active antiretroviral therapy. *Clinical Infectious Diseases, 33*(9), 1579–1584.

3.37 GIARDIA

1. Etiology/epidemiology
   a. Giardia lamblia is a protozoal infection of the small intestine. It is also known as G. intestinalis, G. duodenalis, and Lamblia intestinalis.

b. Giardia occurs worldwide, with the highest frequency in areas with poor sanitation or contaminated water supplies. It is the most common intestinal protozoal parasite in North America and Europe and the most frequent cause of nonbacterial diarrhea.

c. The routes of transmission are fecal-oral, oral-anal sexual contact, waterborne, and fecal contamination of water or food.

d. Risk factors include exposure to children who attend day care, travel to endemic areas, and ingestion of well water or unfiltered water while hiking or camping. A nonhuman mammal reservoir has been suggested but not confirmed (FDA, 2007; McPhee et al., 2007).

2. Pathogenesis

a. The exact mechanism of pathogenesis is unknown (FDA, 2007; Pennardt, 2008).

b. Ingestion of one or more cysts may cause disease (FDA, 2007). After cyst ingestion, trophozoites may be seen in duodenum and jejunum. Cysts may survive in the environment for weeks to months (McPhee et al., 2007).

3. Clinical presentation

a. Giardia may be asymptomatic (especially in children) or cause GI symptoms.

b. Most patients have acute onset of diarrhea within 7 days. Symptoms may be mild and begin gradually within 1 to 3 weeks.

c. Weight loss of greater than 10 pounds occurs in 50% of adult patients (Vinetz, 2007).

d. Stool may be watery, malodorous, greasy, and in copious amounts. Diarrhea may be accompanied by malaise, bloating, cramps, anorexia, flatus, fever, and vomiting. Stools are heme-negative and do not contain pus.

e. Upper GI symptoms, including acid indigestion, nausea, heartburn, and sulfurous belching, may be present.

f. Illness is usually self-limiting within 2 weeks. However, chronic diarrhea may emerge, with resultant malabsorption and weight loss.

g. There is no extraintestinal disease.

h. HIV-infected persons may have more severe symptoms, and the infection may be more difficult to treat in the immunocompromised patient.

   i) Lactose intolerance may accompany symptoms and continue for 6 months.

4. Diagnosis

a. Diagnosis is made by microscopic visualization of stool for cysts or trophozoites.

b. Ninety percent (90%) of cases will be diagnosed with collection of 3 specimens collected at 2-day intervals (McPhee et al., 2007).

c. Immunoassays for cysts or excretory products of the organism in stool are also available.

5. Prevention/treatment

a. To prevent outbreaks, community water supplies must be filtered.

b. Hikers or campers should filter potentially contaminated water using a pore size less than 1 micron or boil the water for 1 minute.

c. Appropriate disposal of diapers (e.g., daycare centers) and frequent hand washing, especially after contact with human or animal feces, are critical for prevention.

d. Avoid untreated water.

e. Avoid fecal contact during sex.

f. Treatment may reduce severity of symptoms and duration of illness.

    i) Single-dose tinidazole is FDA approved for those 3 years and older, with a 90% cure rate (pregnancy class C).

    ii) Metronidazole is not FDA-approved for treatment of giardia, but has been the clinical standard with vast worldwide use. Its efficacy is 80–95% with 5- to 7-day TID dosing. Resistance has been demonstrated. It is used in combination with quinacrine in refractory cases (both at full doses). It is a pregnancy class B drug and has been used when treatment could not be delayed.

    iii) Quinacrine is effective, but difficult to obtain because it is not produced in the United States.

    iv) Paromomycin, pregnancy class C, is considered the drug of choice in early pregnancy, and is considered safe in lactating mothers. Its efficacy rate is lower, at 60–70%.

    v) Nitazoxanide is approved in children over 1 year, and is also used in adults (Gardner & Hill, 2001; Pennardt, 2008; Vinetz, 2007).

6. Nursing implications

    a. Safer-sex strategies, as well as screening and treating potentially infected sexual contacts, may decrease transmission risk, as sexual partners may be a reservoir source of infection/reinfection (Vinetz, 2007).

    b. Enteric precautions should be instituted for incontinent patients.

    c. Educate patients about lactose intolerance and nutritional strategies for maintaining hydration and weight.

    d. Frequent hand washing should also be reinforced.

    e. Patients receiving metronidazole or tinidazole *must* be counseled about the potential for disulfiram-like reaction in the presence of alcohol. All alcohol must be avoided during treatment, and for 24 hours after treatment is completed. Patients who are not able or willing to avoid alcohol should not receive these medications.

    f. Giardia is a CDC and health department reportable illness.

REFERENCES

Gardner, T. B., & Hill, D. R. (2001). Treatment of giardiasis. *Clinical Microbiology Reviews, 14*(1), 114–128.

McPhee, S. J., Papadakis, M. A., & Tierney, L. M. (Eds.). (2007). Giardiasis. *Current medical diagnosis and treatment 2007* (46th ed., pp. 402–403). New York: Lange.

Pennardt, A. (2008). *Giardiasis*. Retrieved February 5, 2009, from http://emedicine.medscape.com/article/782818-overview

U.S. Food and Drug Administration (FDA). (1992, with periodic updates). *Giardia lamblia. Bad Bug Book: Foodborne Pathogenic Microorganisms and Natural Toxins Handbook*. Retrieved February 5, 2009, from http://www.cfsan.fda.gov/~mow/chap22.html

Vinetz, J. (2007). *Giardia lamblia*. Johns Hopkins POC-IT Center. Retrieved February 5, 2009, from http://prod.hopkins-abxguide.org/pathogens/parasites/giardia_lamblia.html?contentInstanceId=255991

3.38 SYPHILIS

1. Etiology/epidemiology

    a. Syphilis is a systemic infectious disease caused by the bacterium *Treponema pallidum*.

    b. Syphilis is primarily sexually transmitted.

    c. Rates of syphilis have been labile in the past 50 years, with highs and lows in approximately decade-long cycles.

       i)   In the United States, highest rates are among men who have sex with men (MSM), accounting for 65% of primary and secondary syphilis cases (Zetola, Engelman, Jensen, & Klausner, 2007).

    d. HIV acquisition is increased 2- to 4-fold and HIV transmission is increased 2- to 9-fold during primary syphilis.

       i)   STDs, such as syphilis, which present with ulcerative lesions, disrupt the integrity of mucosal and endothelial barriers, facilitating HIV acquisition.

       ii)   It is speculated that transient increases in HIV viral load in blood and semen, and decreases in the CD4 count, may contribute to enhanced HIV transmission (Zetola et al., 2007; Zetola & Klausner, 2007).

2. Pathogenesis

    a. *T. pallidum* is a spirochete that may infect any organ or tissue and cause clinical symptoms.

    b. Although the site of exposure and transmission is usually genital, extragenital transmission is possible (Jacobs, 2006).

    c. Transmission usually occurs during sexual contact, including oral sex (Ciesielski, Tabidze, & Brown, 2004).

    d. The bacterium enters the body via minute abrasions of the skin or mucosa.

    e. Syphilis reaches the lymph nodes within hours of transmission, and quickly becomes systemic.

    f. Congenital syphilis may result from maternal–fetal transmission after the tenth week of pregnancy.

3. Clinical presentation

    a. The presentation and treatment of syphilis depends on the stage at which the individual enters care and is diagnosed.

    b. Syphilis is staged as primary, secondary, and tertiary, with periods of latency between symptomatic episodes.

    c. Primary syphilis

       i)   Presents with a chancre, a painless, nonpurulent ulcer with an indurated border, on the skin or mucous membranes of the genitals, perianal area, mouth, or pharynx. The chancre is present 2–6 weeks after exposure, and resolves spontaneously.

       ii)   Multiple lesions may occur in HIV-infected persons.

       iii)   Regional non-tender lymphadenopathy may be present. The primary stage lasts from 3 to 90 days.

       iv)   Up to 75% of persons with HIV may experience symptoms of both primary and secondary syphilis concomitantly at diagnosis (Zetola et al., 2007).

    d. Secondary syphilis

       i)   Presents with superficial lesions of the skin and mucosa, occurring 4–10 weeks after infection.

       ii)   A generalized maculopapular skin rash on the trunk and limbs is common, with lesions on the soles and palms in 50–80% of persons (Zetola et al., 2007).

       iii)   Mucocutaneous lesions may be ulcers or patches.

     iv)　A skin rash of 5–10 mm red- or copper-colored macules is characteristic. General-
ized lymphadenopathy is common; systemic symptoms may occur.

     v)　Lesions may mimic other disorders (Jacobs, 2006; Zetola et al., 2007).

     vi)　Symptoms resolve spontaneously. However, 25% of untreated patients will have re-
currences (Zetola et al., 2007).

e. Latency

     i)　This is an asymptomatic period, with diagnosis made only by serological testing.

     ii)　Typically, latency occurs after secondary syphilis.

     iii)　This period is described as either early latent in patients who have acquired syphilis
in the past year, or late latent or latent syphilis of unknown duration (Workowski &
Berman, 2006).

     iv)　Patients with early latent syphilis are considered potentially infectious; patients in the
late latent stage are not.

     v)　Testing is recommended for all pregnant women to allow treatment to prevent verti-
cal transmission and future symptoms in the mother.

     vi)　The goal of treatment of the patient with latent syphilis is prevention of the compli-
cations of tertiary syphilis, which occur in approximately 25% of those with untreated infections (Workowski & Berman, 2006; Zetola et al., 2007).

f. Tertiary syphilis

     i)　Patient may present with central or peripheral nervous system disorders including
ophthalmic or otologic disease, cardiovascular complications, or infiltrative tumors,
known as gummas, of the skin, bones, liver or other organs. Organomegaly may occur in the presence of gummas.

     ii)　Patients with any of these symptoms should be evaluated for neurosyphilis (Jacobs,
2006; Zetola et al., 2007).

g. Neurosyphilis

     i)　A complex diagnosis, as presentation may vary from that of asymptomatic disease to
extreme disability.

     ii)　Neurologic manifestations may include personality change, dementia, sharp pain,
psychosis, stroke, seizures, tremors, sensory impairment, auditory abnormalities,
loss of sexual function, bowel or bladder dysfunction, tabes dorsalis with muscle
weakness, paresthesias, abnormal reflexes, loss of coordination, or gait disturbance
(Jacobs, 2006; Workowski & Berman, 2006; Zetola et al., 2007).

     iii)　Neurosyphilis may result from untreated disease or treatment failure, and may occur
at any stage of illness.

     iv)　HIV-related immunosuppression may increase the risk of neurosyphilis (Marra,
Maxwell, Tantalo, et al., 2004).

4. Diagnosis

a. Syphilis is presumptively diagnosed in the presence of two positive serological tests.

     i)　Either of the nontreponemal tests for antibodies, the rapid plasma reagin (RPR) or
the venereal disease research laboratory (VDRL) test, is initially used.

     ii)　These tests become positive approximately 4 to 6 weeks after infection, or 1 to 3
weeks after a primary lesion (Jacobs, 2006).

     iii)　A positive test is then confirmed using a treponemal test; either the fluorescent tre-
ponemal antibody absorbed (FTA-ABS), or the *T. pallidum* particle agglutination
(TP-PA).

iv) Treponemal tests remain positive in most patients, despite successful therapy. Treponemal tests are not markers of disease activity.

v) Use of a single nontreponemal test is not sufficient for diagnosis, due to a high rate of false-positive responses that may be related to other conditions.

vi) Non-treponemal titers correlate to disease activity, and are used to determine response to treatment.

vii) Microscopic evaluation for presence of *T. pallidum* in lesions, tissues, or lymph nodes may also be used for diagnosis.

viii) Newer techniques, including PCR, are increasingly available, and will be useful to address unclear diagnoses using current methods (Zetola & Klausner, 2007).

b. The CDC (Workowski & Berman, 2006) and many experts recommend that patients with signs or symptoms of neurologic, ophthalmic, and possibly otologic disease should be evaluated for neurosyphilis, regardless of stage of syphilis.

c. Patients with evidence of tertiary syphilis or those with treatment failure should also receive CSF evaluation.

d. HIV-infected patients should be evaluated for neurosyphilis in the setting of late latent or syphilis of unknown duration (Workowski & Berman, 2006; Zetola & Klausner, 2007). Marra, Maxwell, Smith, et al. (2004) found that HIV-coinfected patients were more likely to have neurosyphilis when CD4 counts were 350 or less (3-fold increase) or when RPR titers were greater than or equal to 1:32 (nearly 11-fold). They suggest that these lab values should prompt evaluation for neurosyphilis, even in asymptomatic patients.

e. Cerebrospinal fluid (CSF) evaluation for neurosyphilis may reveal positive CSF VDRL, increased total protein, and presence of WBCs (pleocytosis) of > 20 cells/microL (CDC guidelines use > 5 cells/microL). However, CSF findings may be normal in the presence of neurosyphilis. If the CSF WBC is normal, neurosyphilis is not present (Jacobs, 2006; Marra, Maxwell, Smith, et al., 2004a; Workowski & Berman, 2006; Zetola & Klausner, 2007).

f. The distinction of primary, secondary, tertiary, and latent syphilis are serologic, symptomatic, and temporal diagnoses, as described above. A careful sexual history, and history of previous syphilis exposure, diagnosis, and treatment, is imperative to correctly identify temporal and risk factors. Patients diagnosed with syphilis should also be tested for HIV.

5. Prevention/treatment

a. Adults with primary, secondary, or early latent syphilis are treated with benzathine penicillin G, 2.4 million units IM in a single dose. Patients with penicillin allergy have been widely treated with doxycycline (100 mg twice daily for 14 days) or tetracycline (500 mg four times daily for 14 days). Ceftriaxone has also been used, although dose and duration have not been established. CDC guidelines for HIV-infected persons follow those of HIV-negative adults. However, these alternative treatments have not been adequately studied in HIV-infected persons. These guidelines state that pregnant women should receive penicillin desensitization, followed by benzathine penicillin G treatment (Workowski & Berman, 2006).

b. Adults with late latent or latent syphilis of unknown duration are treated with benzathine penicillin G 2.4 million units IM. Three separate 2.4 million unit doses are given, at 1-week intervals, for a total of 7.2 million units. Duration of treatment with doxycycline or tetracycline should continue for 28 days in patients with penicillin allergy.

c. Adults with tertiary syphilis, without neurosyphilis, are treated with benzathine penicillin G 2.4 million units, in three doses, at 1-week intervals (total 7.2 million units). Duration of treatment with doxycycline or tetracycline should continue for 28 days in patients with penicillin allergy.

d. Adults with neurosyphilis or syphilitic eye disease are treated with aqueous crystalline penicillin G 18–24 million units daily, either by continuous IV infusion or 3–4 million units IV every 4 hours for 10–14 days. Alternately, patients considered "compliant" may be treated with procaine penicillin 2.4 million units daily with probenecid 500 mg orally four times daily, both for 10–14 days. Some specialists recommend additional benzathine penicillin G IM up to 3 weeks after completion of IV neurosyphilis treatment (Workowski & Berman, 2006).

e. Treatment is considered successful when there is a four-fold decrease in non-treponemal titers within 12 months in HIV-infected patients with early syphilis and up to 24 months for those with late syphilis. HIV-infected patients with syphilis should be evaluated clinically and serologically at months 3, 6, 9, 12, and 24. Titers decrease more slowly in HIV-infected patients with a prior history of syphilis (Workowski & Berman, 2006; Zetola & Klausner, 2007).

f. Patients treated for neurosyphilis should have CSF examination every 6 months until cell counts return to normal. Retreatment should be considered if initially elevated WBC levels have not decreased in 6 months, or if the CSF is not normal within 2 years (Workowski & Berman, 2006).

g. Patients with persistent signs or symptoms, a four-fold increase in nontreponemal titers, or failure to achieve a four-fold decrease in nontreponemal titers within 12–24 months are considered to have treatment failure or reinfection. These patients should be retreated and evaluation for neurosyphilis considered. Reinfection is likely if titers increase after appropriate treatment (Workowski & Berman, 2006; Zetola et al., 2007).

h. Clinicians must be aware of, and educate patients to report symptoms of, Jarisch-Herxheimer ("Herx") reaction, which may occur within the first 24 hours after any treatment for syphilis. It is an acute febrile syndrome, with symptoms including headache, chills, muscle aches, malaise, and worsening of lesions. Tachycardia, tachypnea, and hemodynamic instability may also occur. The reaction peaks within 6–8 hours, and resolves in 12–24 hours. Although the mechanism of this reaction in not known, it is thought to be caused by cellular death of bacteria, with release of endotoxins after initiation of antibiotic therapy. The level of cellular toxins escalates more quickly than the liver and kidneys are able to detoxify. It is most common in early syphilis. It occurs more frequently in HIV-infected patients. This reaction is treated with antipyretics or corticosteroids (Jacobs, 2006; Knudsen & Sotero de Menezes, 2007; Workowski & Berman, 2006).

i. Prevention

  i)   Focus should be on safer sex and risk reduction, specifically the use of condoms or barriers for all types of sexual activity including oral sex.

  ii) Prevention of congenital syphilis is based on identification and treatment of maternal syphilis. It is important to retest pregnant women late in pregnancy if they have had potential exposure to syphilis or HIV during pregnancy.

  iii) HIV transmission may be inhibited by treatment of syphilis, which facilitates HIV acquisition and transmission and is an important public health consideration.

iv) Partner notification and aggressive location and identification of syphilis-infected persons are important public health prevention strategies, given the 3-week incubation period between acquiring infection and becoming infectious (Zetola et al., 2007).

v) Annual syphilis testing is recommended for HIV-infected individuals, and more often for those at risk, for example, two to four times yearly among active MSM and other high-risk groups (Zetola & Klausner, 2007).

vi) Partners of those diagnosed with syphilis should be tested and treated accordingly. Those exposed within 90 days preceding the partner's diagnosis should be presumptively treated, even in the presence of a negative test. Partners exposed prior to 90 days of diagnosis are also treated presumptively if serologic testing is not available or follow-up is uncertain (Workowski & Berman, 2006).

6. Nursing implications
   a. Results of RPR and VDRL titers are equally valid, but should not be compared. Each individual should be followed using the same serologic testing method as that used during initial diagnosis.
   b. Patients with syphilis and visual symptoms should be referred to an ophthalmologist to evaluate for ocular syphilis (Zetola et al., 2007).
   c. Nurses should be aware that unexplained decreases in CD4 counts or increases in HIV viral loads may result from syphilis infection in HIV-infected individuals. These transient lab variations may indicate a need for syphilis testing (Zetola & Klausner, 2007).
   d. Syphilis is a CDC and health department reportable illness.
   e. Innovative identification and prevention strategies, such as Internet-based interventions, including chat room and e-mail contacts, may improve case finding, partner notification, and prevention efforts (Zetola & Klausner, 2007).

REFERENCES

Ciesielski, C., Tabidze, I., & Brown, C. (2004). Transmission of primary and secondary syphilis by oral sex—Chicago, Illinois, 1998–2002. *Morbidity and Mortality Weekly Report, 53*(41), 966–968.

Jacobs, R. A. (2006). Syphilis. In M. A. Papadakis & S. J. McPhee (Eds.), *2006 Current Consult Medicine* (pp. 884–885). New York: Lange Medical Books/McGraw-Hill.

Knudsen, R. P., & Sotero de Menezes, M. (2007). *Neurosyphilis.* Retrieved November 24, 2007, from http://www.emedicine.com/neuro/topic684.htm

Marra, C. M., Maxwell, C. L., Smith, S. L., Lukehart, S. A., Rompalo, A. M., Eaton, M., et al. (2004). Cerebrospinal fluid abnormalities in patients with syphilis: Association with clinical and laboratory features. *Journal of Infectious Diseases, 189*(3), 369–376.

Marra, C. M., Maxwell, C. L., Tantalo, L., Eaton, M., Rompalo, A. M., Raines, C., et al. (2004). Normalization of cerebrospinal fluid abnormalities after neurosyphilis therapy: Does HIV status matter? *Clinical Infectious Diseases, 38*(7), 1001–1006.

Workowski, K. A., & Berman, S. M. (2006). Sexually transmitted diseases treatment guidelines. *Morbidity and Mortality Weekly Report, 55*(RR-11), 1–94.

Zetola, N. M., Engelman, J., Jensen, T. P., & Klausner, J. D. (2007). Syphilis in the United States: An update for clinicians with an emphasis on HIV coinfection. *Mayo Clinic Proceedings, 82*(9), 1091–1102.

Zetola, N. M., & Klausner, J. D. (2007). Syphilis and HIV infection: An update. *Clinical Infectious Diseases, 449,* 1222–1228.

CHAPTER 4

Symptom Management of the HIV-Infected Adolescent and Adult

4.1 ANOREXIA AND WEIGHT LOSS

1. Etiology
   a. Definitions
      i)   Anorexia: loss of appetite resulting in decreased food intake
      ii)   Weight loss: involuntary loss of body weight, which (1) occurs in early HIV infection regardless of HAART, (2) is accompanied by loss of body fat and cell mass, and (3) is associated with disease progression and death (Mangili, Murman, Zampini, & Wanke, 2006; Tang, Jacobson, Spiegelman, Knox, & Wanke, 2005).
   b. Esophagitis, medications (e.g., Fuzeon, Sustiva), psychosocial-economic factors, secondary infections, diarrhea and malabsorption, hormonal deficiencies (e.g., testosterone), nutrient deficiencies, fatigue, high viral load, and proinflammatory cytokines (Bartlett & Gallant, 2007; Keithley, Swanson, & Nerad, 2001; van Lettow, van der Meer, West, van Crevel, & Semba, 2005).
2. Nursing assessment
   a. Subjective data
      i)   Medication review (including dietary/herbal supplements; Hendricks, Sansavero, Houser, Tang, & Wanke, 2007)
      ii)   Current or previous secondary infections
      iii) Nutrition-related symptoms (e.g., nausea, vomiting, diarrhea, fever, difficulty swallowing, taste and smell changes, fatigue)
      iv)   Dietary patterns (e.g., typical daily intake, food likes and dislikes, food intolerances, special diets, use of dietary supplements)
   b. Objective data
      i)   Measurement of height, weight, body mass index, body composition (e.g., skinfold thickness), and body shape (e.g., waist circumference; Gerrior & Neff, 2005)
      ii)   Assessment of functional status, mood, and cognition (Williams, Waters, & Parker, 1999)
      iii) Comprehensive examination of oral cavity for abnormalities affecting nutritional intake
      iv)   Assessment of skin, hair, eyes, nails, thyroid, and musculoskeletal system for clinical signs of vitamin and mineral deficiency (e.g., vitamins A and B, iron) and loss of fat and lean body mass; assessment for hepatomegaly, splenomegaly, and edema

    v)   Laboratory studies: dependent on symptoms—stool cultures, blood cultures, serum testosterone, thyroid profile, serum proteins, serum lipids, and serum micronutrient levels

3. Nursing diagnosis
    a. Altered nutrition: less than body requirements related to inadequate dietary intake, increased energy and nutrient needs, impaired digestion/absorption of nutrients, cognitive changes, and drug interactions as evidenced by nutrition-related symptoms, loss of weight and muscle and fat mass, clinical signs of nutrient deficiency, impaired functional status, and abnormal laboratory studies
    b. Related nursing diagnoses: impaired physical mobility, diarrhea, fatigue, altered mucous membranes, self-feeding deficit, impaired swallowing, and knowledge deficit (Carpenito, 2006)

4. Goals
    a. Maximize nutrient intake.
    b. Minimize nutrient losses.
    c. Replenish body cell mass.
    d. Maintain functional status and quality of life.

5. Interventions and health teaching
    a. Nonpharmacological interventions
        i)   Assess nutritional status at regular intervals, incorporating objective and subjective measures (Gerrior & Neff, 2005).
        ii)   Conduct nutrition counseling, including nutritional implications of HIV/AIDS, principles of good nutrition, vitamin/mineral and oral supplements (available as nutrient-dense candy bars, soups, juices, coffees), and nutrition resources.
        iii)   Explain food safety measures, including safe handling, storage, and preparation of food; careful cleaning of cooking utensils and cutting boards; avoiding raw or undercooked eggs, meats, or fish; drinking treated water and pasteurized milk.
        iv)   Explain nutrition interventions for anorexia/weight loss, such as (1) eat small snacks or meals every 2 to 3 hours; (2) eat high-protein, high-calorie foods and snacks (e.g., peanut butter, cheese, ice cream, nuts); (3) drink high-calorie beverages (e.g., milk shakes, juices, liquid supplements); (4) drink a small glass of wine or fruit juice before meals to improve appetite; (5) eat cold or lukewarm foods, which have a better flavor than do hot foods; (6) go for a walk or exercise lightly before meals to stimulate appetite; (7) reduce fatigue associated with cooking by using prepared foods, takeout, or home-delivered meals; and (8) eat favorite foods in pleasant, relaxed environment to improve appetite.
        v)   Use enteral nutrition when oral intake is inadequate and accompanied by weight loss. Polymeric formulas (intact/complex nutrients) are used if digestive/absorptive function is normal; elemental formulas indicated if malabsorption is a problem. Enteral formulas fortified with immunostimulatory nutrients (i.e., arginine, omega-3 fatty acids, glutamine, antioxidants) have few or mixed beneficial effects (Keithley & Swanson, 2001).
        vi)   Reserve parenteral nutrition for patients with severe gastrointestinal disease or dysfunction (e.g., pancreatitis, intractable vomiting, or diarrhea) because of the high risk for infection and gut atrophy.

vii) Recommend resistive and aerobic exercise as tolerated to increase lean body mass and improve functional status and energy levels (O'Brien, Nixon, Glazier, & Tynan, 2007; Shevitz et al., 2005).

viii) Recommend frequent oral care (after meals and before bedtime) and regular preventive dental care (every 6 months).

ix) Suggest daily records/checklists of appetite, weight, and symptoms (Holzemer, Hudson, Kirksey, Hamilton, & Bakken, 2001).

b. Pharmacological interventions

i) Appetite stimulants (e.g., megestrol acetate, dronabinol) may be used, but weight gain is mostly fat.

ii) Anabolic agents (e.g., recombinant growth hormone, testosterone, nandrolone, oxandrolone, oxymetholone) may result in small increases in body weight and lean body mass (Johns, Beddall, & Corrin, 2007; Mwamburi et al., 2004).

iii) Anti-catabolic agents, such as ghrelin, are under investigation (Akamizu & Kangawa, 2007).

c. Alternative/complementary therapies used for anti-anorexia and anti–weight-loss properties include various dietary supplements (e.g., antioxidants, carotenoids, phytoestrogens, DHEA, flavonoids), herbal therapies, megavitamin/mineral therapy, and juice and enzyme therapy. Presently, little or no evidence exists to support the safety or efficacy of these products.

6. Evaluation

a. Daily caloric intake should be 30–40 kcal/kg, and daily protein intake should be 1.2–2.0 g/kg (Gerrior & Neff, 2005)

b. Weight, body mass index, and fat and muscle mass should be within 5% of standard

c. Adequate symptom management

d. Improved functional status and sense of well-being

REFERENCES

Akamizu, T., & Kangawa, K. (2007). Emerging results of anticatabolic therapy with ghrelin. *Current Opinion in Clinical Nutrition & Metabolic Care, 10*(3), 278–283.

Bartlett, J. G., & Gallant, J. E. (2007). *Medical management of HIV infection.* Baltimore: Johns Hopkins Medicine Health Publishing Business Group.

Carpenito, L. J. (2006). *Nursing diagnosis: Application to clinical practice* (11th ed.). Philadelphia: Lippincott Williams & Wilkins.

Gerrior, J. L., & Neff, L. M. (2005). Nutrition assessment in HIV infection. *Nutrition in Clinical Care, 8*(1), 6–15.

Hendricks, K. M., Sansavero, M., Houser, R. F., Tang, A. M., & Wanke, C. A. (2007). Dietary supplement use and nutrient intake in HIV-infected persons. *AIDS Reader, 17*(4), 211–216, 223–227.

Holzemer, W. L., Hudson, A., Kirksey, K. M., Hamilton, M. J., & Bakken, S. (2001). The revised sign and symptom checklist for HIV (SSC-HIVrev). *Journal of the Association of Nurses in AIDS Care, 12*(5), 60–70.

Johns, K., Beddall, M. J., & Corrin, R. C. (2007). Anabolic steroids for the treatment of weight loss in HIV-infected individuals. *Cochrane Database for Systematic Reviews, 2,* 1–42.

Keithley, J. K., & Swanson, B. (2001). Oral nutritional supplements in human immunodeficiency virus disease: A review of the evidence. *Nutrition in Clinical Practice, 16*(2), 98–104.

Keithley, J. K., Swanson, B., & Nerad, J. (2001). HIV/AIDS. In M. Gottschlich (Ed.), *The science and practice of nutrition support: A case-based approach* (pp. 619–641). Dubuque, IA: Kendall/Hunt.

Mangili, A., Murman, D. H., Zampini, A. M., & Wanke, C. A. (2006). Nutrition and HIV infection: Review of weight loss and wasting in the era of highly active antiretroviral therapy from the nutrition for healthy living cohort. *Clinical Infectious Diseases, 42*(15), 836–842.

Mwamburi, D. M., Gerrior, J., Wilson, I. B., Chang, H., Scully, E., Saboori, S., et al. (2004). Comparing megestrol acetate therapy with oxandrolone therapy for HIV-related weight loss: Similar results in 2 months. *Clinical Infectious Diseases, 38*(15), 895–902.

O'Brien, K., Nixon, S., Glazier, R. H., & Tynan, A. M. (2007). Progressive resistive exercise interventions for adults living with HIV/AIDS. *Cochrane Database of Systematic Reviews, 2,* no pages.

Shevitz, A. H., Wilson, I. B., McDermott, A. Y., Spiegelman, D., Skinner, S. C., Antonsson, K., et al. (2005). A comparison of the clinical and cost-effectiveness of 3 intervention strategies for AIDS wasting. *Journal of Acquired Immune Deficiency Syndromes, 38*(4), 399–406.

Tang, A. M., Jacobson, D. L., Spiegelman, D., Knox, T. A., & Wanke, C. (2005). Increasing risk of 5% or greater unintentional weight loss in a cohort of HIV-infected patients, 1995 to 2003. *Journal of Acquired Immune Deficiency Syndromes, 40*(1), 70–76.

van Lettow, M., van der Meer, J. W. M., West, C. E., van Crevel, R., & Semba, R. D. (2005). Interleukin-6 and human immunodeficiency virus load, but not plasma leptin concentration, predict anorexia and wasting in adults with pulmonary tuberculosis in Malawi. *Journal of Clinical Endocrinology & Metabolism, 90*(8), 4771–4776.

Williams, B., Waters, D., & Parker, K. (1999). Evaluation and treatment of weight loss in adults with HIV disease. *American Family Physician, 60*(3), 843–854.

4.2 COGNITIVE IMPAIRMENT

1. Etiology
   a. Primary to the pathogenic processes of HIV
      i)   HIV infection of the central nervous system (CNS) can result in HIV-associated neurocognitive impairment (HNCI).
      ii) Neurocognitive impairment can range from subtle cognitive deficits to HIV-associated minor cognitive motor disorder (MCMD) to HIV-associated dementia (HAD, previously referred to as "AIDS dementia complex" or "HIV encephalopathy"; Hinkin et al., 2001; Letendre et al., 2006).
   b. Secondary to physical and psychological/emotional problems
      i)   Systemic infections
           (1) Bacterial infections: bacterial meningitis, sepsis, neurosyphilis
           (2) Fungal infections: cryptococcosis, aspergillosis
           (3) Viral infections: cytomegalovirus, herpes zoster virus, herpes simplex virus, human papovavirus, JC virus
           (4) Mycoplasmic infections: tuberculosis, toxoplasmosis
      ii) CNS cancers: non-Hodgkin's lymphoma, advanced Kaposi's sarcoma, and primary central nervous system lymphoma
      iii) Cerebrovascular disease and accident
      iv) Metabolic imbalances: fluid and electrolyte imbalances, nutritional deficits, effects of sleep deprivation, hypoxia
      v)   Psychological illnesses and stress-related illnesses
      vi) Medications: histamine blockers, sedatives, anxiolytics, narcotics, steroids, antivirals, anti-TB medications, antidepressants, alcohol, and recreational drugs
2. Nursing assessment
   a. Subjective data

    i)   Patient and family assessment of cognitive, behavioral, motor, and affective symptoms

    ii)   Early manifestations

       (1) Cognitive: forgetfulness and loss of concentration, slowed information processing, impaired attention, sequencing problems, and memory loss

       (2) Behavioral: withdrawal, irritability, apathy, and loss of interest in usual activities

       (3) Motor: slowing, ataxia, tremor, incoordination, weakness, hyperreflexia, and handwriting change

       (4) Affective: depression and hypomania

    iii) Late manifestations

       (1) Cognitive: severe memory loss, word-finding problems or speech arrest, dysarthria, severe attention and concentration problems, and poor judgment with lack of insight

       (2) Behavioral: increasing severity of behaviors listed above in "Early manifestations," plus disinhibition and impetuous actions

       (3) Motor: incontinence, paraplegia, tremor, clonus, and marked slowing

       (4) Affective: severe depression, organic psychosis, and mania

    iv) Pharmacological history to evaluate for medications that may cause confusion, disorientation, decreased concentration, or memory problems

  b. Objective data

    i)   Physical examination (especially of nervous system)

    ii)   Assessment of cognition, attention, and memory using the Mini-Mental Status Exam, HIV Dementia Scale, Trail Making A/B tests, Symbol-Digit tests, and Grooved Pegboard test (Bartlett & Gallant, 2007; Tartar et al., 2004)

    iii) Psychological tests, such as the Beck Depression Inventory, Holmes and Rahe Stress Scale, and State/Trait Anxiety Inventory or Depression Anxiety Stress Scale (DASS), to screen for anxiety, stress, and depression

    iv)   Lab work (may be included in the etiologic investigation): CBC with differential; chemistry panel; serum B12, folate, and albumin; metabolic workup; serum toxoplasmosis IgG titer; cryptococcal antigen; RPR/VDRL

    v)   Neuroimaging

       (1) MRI/CT may be normal in the presence of symptoms or may show cortical atrophy, ventricular enlargement, subcortical atrophy (caudate nucleus and basal ganglia), and diffuse white matter changes or abnormalities (Paul et al., 2002).

       (2) Cranial computerized tomography is conducted to look for tumors, lesions, or atrophy.

    vi) Lumbar puncture to examine the cerebral spinal fluid (CSF) for infectious diseases

3. Nursing diagnosis

  a. Neurocognitive impairment related to HIV infection of the CNS, other systemic and CNS infections, CNS cancers, psychological and stress-related illnesses, and medications

4. Goals

  a. Remove or treat the underlying cause of the cognitive impairment

  b. Improve cognitive function

  c. Maintain self-care activities, including medication adherence

    d. Maintain social functioning

    e. Maintain client safety

    f. Prevent disease progression

5. Interventions and health teaching

    a. Nonpharmacological interventions

      i)   Refer to psychoeducational groups (Nelson, 1997) that assist the client in learning ways to overcome cognitive changes, including memory loss.

      ii) Refer client for cognitive-behavioral interventions (CBIs) to improve mental health and immune functioning (Crepaz et al., 2008).

      iii) Provide memory aids, such as calendars, timers, and pill boxes to ensure medication adherence.

      iv) Conduct a safety assessment of the client's home.

      v)   Provide instruction to family/significant others in monitoring the client for safety issues and changes in cognitive function.

      vi) Assist with advanced directives, wills, trusts, assisted-living referrals, and other legal concerns before disease progresses.

      vii) Teach client how to prevent HIV-related diseases that cause neurocognitive impairment, such as coccidioidomycosis, cryptococcosis, CMV, histoplasmosis, mycobacterial disease, disseminated M. tuberculosis, and progressive multifocal leukoencephalopathy (Ungvarski & Trzcianowska, 2000).

    b. Pharmacological interventions

      i)   Antiretrovirals have reduced the frequency of HIV dementia, but there is little evidence that shows the efficacy of antiretrovirals for reversing established dementia (Letendre et al., 2006; McCutchan et al., 2007; Robertson et al., 2004).

      ii) It is unclear whether drugs with better CNS penetration are more effective for treating HIV dementia; however, the nucleoside reverse transcriptase inhibitors, zidovudine, stavudine, and abacavir; the non-nucleoside reverse transcriptase inhibitors, nevirapine and efavirenz; and the protease inhibitor, indinavir, appear to have the best CNS penetration and have shown encouraging results for HIV dementia in clinical trials (Rumbaugh & Nath, 2006).

      iii) Psychotropic drugs are used for behavior management.

         (1) Agitation and anxiety: clonazepam, lorazepam, and buspirone; short-term use of diazepam or lorazepam for 1 to 4 weeks can help manage anxiety caused by acute life stress.

         (2) Mood swings and mania: valproic acid, lithium carbonate, and carbamazepine, all of which require monitoring of blood levels; lithium may not be tolerated by later-stage HIV clients, particularly those who have abnormalities on neuropsychological or neuroimaging tests (Hinkin et al., 2001).

         (3) Depression: fluoxetine, paroxetine, sertraline, venlafaxine, and citalopram; tricyclic antidepressants (nortriptyline or desipramine) can also be considered for depressed patients who are experiencing pain from common maladies.

         (4) Psychoses: haloperidol, chlorpromazine, molindone (depending on severity of symptoms), and perphenazine; newer atypical neuroleptics (risperidone and olanzepine) are likely to have more favorable side effect profiles.

(5) Psychomotor slowing: methylphenidate and dextroamphetamine (watch for irritability, which can be profound)

c. Alternative/complementary therapies

  i)   Vitamin therapy: Vitamins E, B6, and B12 can be used (Flaskerud & Miller, 1999).

  ii)   Aromatherapy: Use of essential oils may have moderately beneficial effects on reducing agitated behavior in persons with dementia. Dosages of aromatherapy oils vary: 1–2 drops of oil can be added to a bowl of freshly boiled water or oil can be used along with massage. Oils used in studies include lavender and lemon balm oil (Diamond et al., 2003).

  iii) Chinese herbs: Efficacy and safety of Chinese herbs have not been established, but the herbs are widely used. Clients should consult with a Chinese herbalist because there are no herbs or herbal formulas specific to treating HIV or cognitive impairment. Herbal formulas are individualized to clients' specific symptoms, as diagnosed in traditional Chinese medicine (TCM). Examples include liver Qi stagnation, heart and spleen deficiency, or heat toxins (Ryan & Shattuck, 1994).

  iv) Western herbs: Efficacy and safety of Western herbs also have not been established, but they are still widely used (Liu et al., 2005). Gingko biloba is commonly used for memory problems and has little interaction with antiretrovirals but can increase bleeding. Anyone considering using herbs should consult with a licensed herbalist as well as with a pharmacist who is knowledgeable about drug–herb interactions.

  v)   Energy work/healing: Anecdotal reports suggest that Reiki, therapeutic touch, and Shen are useful in calming the mind in persons with cognitive impairment. There is no scientific evidence to support this or improvement of cognitive function (Sierpina et al., 2005).

6. Evaluation
   a. Patient will show improved cognitive function.
   b. Patient will be able to perform activities of daily living.
   c. Patient will be able to engage in social interaction, work, and school activities.

REFERENCES

Bartlett, J. G., & Gallant, J. E. (2007). *Medical management of HIV infection*. Baltimore: Johns Hopkins Medicine Health Publishing Business Group.

Crepaz, N., Passin, W. F., Herbst, J. H., Rama, S. M., Malow, R. M., Purcell, D. W., et al. (2008). Meta-analysis of cognitive-behavioral interventions on HIV-positive persons' mental health and immune functioning. *Health Psychology, 27*(1), 4–14.

Diamond, B., Johnson, S., Torsney, K., Morodan, J., Prokop, B., Davidek, D., et. al. (2003). Complementary and alternative medicines in the treatment of dementia: An evidence-based review. *Drugs & Aging, 20*(13), 981–998.

Flaskerud, J. H., & Miller, E. N. (1999). Psychosocial and neuropsychiatric function. In P. J. Ungvarski & J. H. Flaskerud (Eds.), *HIV/AIDS: A guide to primary care management* (4th ed.; pp. 255–291). Philadelphia: W. B. Saunders.

Hinkin, C. H., Castellon, S. A., Atkinson, J. H., & Goodkin, K. (2001). Neuropsychiatric aspects of HIV infection among older adults. *Journal of Clinical Epidemiology, 54*(Suppl. 1), S44–52.

Letendre, S. L., Woods, S. P., Ellis, R. J., Atkinson, J. H., Masliah, E., van den Brande, G., et al. (2006). Lithium improves HIV-associated neurocognitive impairment. *AIDS, 20*(14), 1885–1888.

Liu, J. P., Manheimer, E., & Yang, M. (2005). Herbal medicines for treating HIV infection and AIDS. *Cochrane Database of Systematic Reviews, 3*, CD003937.

McCutchan, J. A., Wu, J. W., Robertson, K., Koletar, S. L., Ellis, R. J., Cohn, S., et al. (2007). HIV suppression by HAART preserves cognitive function in advanced, immune-reconstituted AIDS patients. *AIDS, 21*(9), 1109–1117.

Nelson, M. K. (1997). Psychoeducational group work for persons with AIDS dementia complex. In M. B. Winiarski (Ed.), *HIV mental health for the 21st century* (pp. 137–156). New York: New York University Press.

Paul, R., Cohen, R., Navia, B., & Tashima, K. (2002). Relationships between cognition and structural neuroimaging findings in adults with human immunodeficiency virus type-1. *Neuroscience & Biobehavioral Reviews, 26*(3), 353–359.

Robertson, K. R., Robertson, W. T., Ford, S., Watson, D., Fiscus, S., Harp, A. G., et al. (2004). Highly active antiretroviral therapy improves neurocognitive functioning. *Journal of Acquired Immune Deficiency Syndromes, 36*(1), 562–566.

Rumbaugh, J. A., & Nath, A. (2006). Developments in HIV neuropathogenesis. *Current Pharmaceutical Design, 12*(9), 1023–1044.

Ryan, M. K., & Shattuck, A. D. (1994). *Treating AIDS with Chinese medicine.* Berkeley, CA: Pacific View Press.

Sierpina, V. S., Sierpina, M., Loera, J. A., & Grumbles, L. (2005). Complementary and integrative approaches to dementia. *Southern Medical Journal, 98*(6), 636–645.

Tartar, J. L., Sheehan, C. M., Nash, A. J., Starratt, C., Puga, A., & Widmayer, S. (2004). ERPs differ from neurometric tests in assessing HIV-associated cognitive deficit. *Neuroreport, 15*(10), 1675–1678.

Ungvarski, P. J., & Trzcianowska, H. (2000). Neurocognitive disorders seen in HIV disease. *Issues in Mental Health Nursing, 21*(1), 51–70.

4.3 COUGH

1. Etiology: associated with pulmonary conditions, sinusitis, aspiration, esophageal reflux, auditory canal irritation, noxious substances, exercise/activity, and cold air; can occur postbronchoscopy
2. Nursing assessment
   a. Subjective data
      i)   When did the cough begin?
      ii) Is the cough productive?
      iii) What is the character of the cough?
      iv) Is there a time of day when the cough is more bothersome?
      v)   Is there a relationship to position or posture?
      vi) What makes the cough better? What makes it worse?
      vii) Are there any accompanying signs or symptoms such as hemoptysis, shortness of breath, wheezing, chest tightness, heartburn, edema or orthopnea, sinus pain, headache, or postnasal drip?
      viii) What are the patient's medical, surgical, and medication histories, including oxygen use and intubation?
   b. Objective data: pulmonary exam, including rate, amplitude of respiration, rhythm, symmetry of breathing, use of accessory muscles, and breath sounds
3. Nursing diagnosis
   a. Ineffective airway clearance related to smoking or secondhand smoke, airway spasm, mucus/secretions, infection, or allergic airways
   b. Risk for impaired gas exchange
   c. Risk for impaired comfort
4. Goals
   a. Promote optimal respiratory function.

    b. Promote effective cough effort.

    c. Eliminate or treat the underlying cause of a chronic cough.

    d. Minimize the discomfort associated with chronic cough.

5. Interventions and health teaching

    a. Nonpharmacological interventions

      i)   Prevent stasis of secretions by encouraging deep breathing/incentive spirometry; ambulation/frequent position changes, if on bed rest; and postural drainage/percussion, if necessary.

      ii)   Encourage fluid intake of 2.5 to 3L/day to maintain hydration and thin secretions; decrease or eliminate dairy products.

      iii) Use suction to remove secretions if cough is ineffective.

      iv) Promote oral hygiene if cough is productive; instruct on proper disposal of tissues and hand washing.

      v)   Position to prevent aspiration and reflux (i.e., elevate head of bed or use wedge-shaped pillow for sleep).

      vi) Teach splinting techniques to minimize pain associated with coughing.

      vii) Offer throat-soothing remedies, such as tea with honey and lemon, cough drops, warm saline gargle, warm mist humidifiers if immunocompetent (follow manufacturer's guidelines for daily cleaning; Althoff, Williams, Molvig, & Schuster, 1997).

      viii) Avoid activities or noxious substances that precipitate cough (e.g., cigarette smoke; Kozier, Erb, Berman, & Burke, 2000).

      ix) Encourage rest periods and energy conservation; plan daily activities with rest periods included.

      x)   Evaluate patient's ability to identify effective cough remedies, report changes in frequency and severity of cough, and demonstrate effective cough technique (Kozier et al., 2000).

    b. Pharmacological interventions: Administer cough medications (antitussives, expectorants) on a scheduled basis rather than prn.

6. Alternative/complementary interventions: Eucalyptus aromatherapy may be useful (Althoff et al., 1997).

REFERENCES

Althoff, S., Williams, P. N., Molvig, D., & Schuster, L. (1997). *A guide to alternative medicine.* Lincolnwood, IL: Publications International.

Kozier, B., Erb, G., Berman, A. J., & Burke, K. (2000). *Fundamentals of nursing: Concepts, process, and practice* (6th ed.). Upper Saddle River, NJ: Prentice Hall.

4.4 DYSPNEA

1. Etiology

    a. Pulmonary infections: *Pneumocystis jiroveci* pneumonia (PCP), bacterial pneumonias, mycobacterium avium complex (MAC), *M. tuberculosis,* cytomegalovirus (CMV), *C. albicans,* and *Cryptosporidium* (Benson, Kaplan, Masur, Pau, & Holmes, 2004)

b. Pulmonary malignancies: Kaposi's sarcoma (KS) and lymphomas

c. Autoimmune diseases: lymphocytic interstitial pneumonitis and diffuse infiltrative lymphocytosis syndrome

d. Anemia

e. Pneumothorax and pleural effusion

f. Exercise intolerance

g. Normal aging process and dying process

2. Nursing assessment

  a. Subjective data

    i)   Obtain patient's report of breathing difficulty (e.g., presence of orthopnea).

    ii) Ascertain relevant history of the symptoms: onset, duration, frequency of episodes, aggravating or relieving factors, and associated symptoms.

    iii) Two types of patient-rating tools are available.

      (1) Graphic rating scale: Ask patient to quantify the magnitude of dyspnea experienced on a scale of 1 to 5 (1 = *no difficulty breathing,* 5 = *severe difficulty breathing*).

      (2) Visual analog scale: This is a horizontal or vertical line with word descriptors or anchors at either end. The patient places a mark on the line indicating the degree of dyspnea experienced.

    iv) Ascertain medical and surgical history, including oxygen use and history of intubation.

    v)   Elicit medication, herbal, and nutritional supplement usage.

    vi) Conduct a thorough social assessment: living conditions, support systems, and presence of significant others and pets.

    vii) Obtain patient's report of activities of daily living abilities.

  b. Objective data

    i)   General appearance and color

    ii) Pulmonary exam: rate, amplitude of respiration, rhythm, symmetry of breathing, use of accessory muscles, nasal flaring, breath sounds, and clubbing

    iii) Cardiovascular exam: blood pressure and pulse

    iv) Lab and diagnostic data: pulse oximetry, chest X-ray, arterial blood gases (ABGs), and sputum studies, if appropriate

3. Nursing diagnosis

  a. Activity intolerance related to imbalance between oxygen supply and demand

  b. Anxiety related to ineffective breathing pattern

  c. Disturbed sleep pattern related to difficulty breathing and positioning required for effective breathing

  d. Fear related to threat to state of well-being and potential death

  e. Ineffective breathing pattern related to hyperventilation, hypoventilation, pain, anxiety, fatigue, perceptual or cognitive impairment, obesity, body position, and respiratory muscle fatigue

  f. Risk for impaired gas exchange

  g. Risk for sleep deprivation

  h. Risk for impaired comfort

4. Goals
    a. Identify and eliminate, or at least control, the causative factors.
    b. Promote optimal respiratory functioning.
    c. Manage stress and anxiety.
    d. Develop strategies to manage dyspnea to provide maximum independence.
5. Interventions and health teaching
    a. Nonpharmacological interventions
        i) Reassess respiratory status at appropriate frequency, including before and after respiratory treatments.
        ii) Eliminate or modify underlying causes of dyspnea.
        iii) Administer oxygen therapy, if indicated; teach patient safety issues, such as flammable hazards.
        iv) Assess need for bronchial hygiene (e.g., aerosol treatments, postural drainage, percussion, suctioning).
        v) Encourage adequate fluid intake to maintain hydration and help thin secretions, unless contraindicated.
        vi) Promote optimal nutrition.
        vii) Position patient to maximize both comfort and ventilation (e.g., sitting upright with pillows under elbows, leaning on overbed table); encourage frequent position changes and ambulation.
        viii) Pace activities and treatments to level of tolerance; encourage energy conservation.
        ix) Assist with activities of daily living, especially those that require use of the upper extremities (e.g., feeding, shaving); keep frequently used items within reach.
        x) Instruct to prolong exhalation phase of breathing using pursed-lip and diaphragmatic breathing techniques and incentive spirometry.
        xi) Counsel to avoid exposure to irritants, such as cigarette smoke, flowers, and perfume.
        xii) Counsel regarding smoking cessation or timing of smoking to occur between activities of daily living and meals to pace with rest periods.
        xiii) Evaluate patient's ability to do the following:
            (1) Participate in self-care activities, such as energy conservation and pacing activities.
            (2) Correctly use metered dose inhalers or other medications.
            (3) Report changes in frequency or severity of dyspnea.
            (4) Identify contributing factors related to dyspnea.
    b. Pharmacological interventions
        i) Antibiotics, corticosteroids, and bronchodilators, as indicated (Briel, Bucher, Boscacci, & Furrer, 2006; Huang, Morris, Limper, & Beck, 2006)
        ii) Opioids for palliation
6. Alternative/complementary therapies: Demonstrate relaxation and panic-control strategies and stress management (e.g., creative visualization, guided imagery, meditation, biofeedback, yoga; Ferrell & Coyle, 2001).

REFERENCES

Benson, C. A., Kaplan, J. E., Masur, H., Pau, A., & Holmes, K. K. (2004). Treating opportunistic infections among HIV-infected adults and adolescents: Recommendations from CDC, the National Institutes of Health, and the Infectious Diseases Society of America. *Morbidity and Mortality Weekly Report, 53*(RR-15), 1–118.

Briel, M., Bucher, H. C., Boscacci, R., & Furrer, H. (2006). *Adjunctive corticosteroids for Pneumocystis jiroveci pneumia in patients with HIV-infection.* Retrieved August 2, 2007, from http://www.ncbi.nlm.nih.gov/pubmed/16856118

Ferrell, B. R., & Coyle, N. (2001). *Textbook of palliative nursing.* New York: Oxford University Press.

Huang, L., Morris, A., Limper, A. H., & Beck, J. (2006). An official ATS workshop summary: Recent advances and future directions in *Pneumocystis* pneumonia (PCP). *Proceedings of the American Thoracic Society, 3*(8), 655–664.

4.5 DYSPHAGIA AND ODYNOPHAGIA

1. Etiology
   a. Definitions
      i) Dysphagia is defined as difficulty swallowing; often described as sensation of food sticking in mouth, pharynx, or esophagus.
      ii) Odynophagia refers to painful swallowing, usually characterized as burning or constricting esophagus.
   b. Etiologies
      i) Dysphagia may be caused by candidiasis and, to a lesser extent, HSV, CMV, aphthous ulcers; oral, pharyngeal, or esophageal neuromuscular dysfunction; malignancies; decreased saliva production; fatigue.
      ii) Odynophagia may be caused by HSV, CMV, aphthous ulcers, and, to a lesser extent, candidiasis; tumors; and medications (e.g., zidovudine, atazanavir) associated with mucosal ulceration, inflammation, obstruction, gastroesophageal reflux disease (Bartlett & Gallant, 2007).
2. Nursing assessment
   a. Subjective data
      i) Review of medications (including ASA, NSAIDs, anticholinergics, calcium channel blockers); problematic foods (e.g., peanut butter, spicy foods, citrus, liquids); current and previous opportunistic infections; presence and characteristics of coughing, choking, regurgitation, aspiration, and epigastric/retrosternal pain
   b. Objective data
      i) Inspection of oropharyngeal cavity for infections, lesions, malignancies, saliva production, parotid/sublingual/submandibular gland enlargement, and adequacy of oral hygiene
      ii) Observation of swallowing of foods and liquids of varying textures and consistencies (Terrado, Russell, & Bowman, 2001)
      iii) Assessment of mental and cognitive status
      iv) Assessment of nutritional status parameters: weight, body mass index, and fat and muscle mass
   c. Laboratory studies: cultures/biopsies to identify pathogens
3. Nursing diagnosis
   a. Impaired swallowing related to infections, tumors, medications, foods, gastroesophageal reflux disease, fatigue, and dental problems as evidenced by difficult or painful swallow-

ing of food and fluids; coughing, choking, or aspirating when swallowing; and loss of weight and fat and muscle mass.

   b. Related nursing diagnoses include altered mucous membranes, altered nutrition (less than body requirements), risk for aspiration, fatigue, and knowledge deficit (Carpenito, 2006).

4. Goals

   a. Increase knowledge of easy-to-swallow foods and fluids.

   b. Improve protein and calorie intake.

   c. Reduce swallowing pain and discomfort.

   d. Maintain ability to take oral medications.

   e. Prevent aspiration.

5. Interventions and health teaching

   a. Nonpharmacological interventions

     i) Provide nutrition counseling: (1) eat blenderized or soft foods (e.g., pudding, soups, canned fruits, scrambled eggs); (2) add sauces or gravies to meats and vegetables; (3) dip foods (bagels, cookies) in liquids (tea, coffee); (4) make liquids thicker by adding gravy, mashed potatoes, oatmeal, or Thick-It; (5) eat cold or lukewarm foods; (6) avoid sticky foods (e.g., peanut butter, caramels, gummy bears) and milk, if problematic; (7) use a straw, tilt head back, or sit upright to facilitate swallowing (Keithley, Swanson, & Nerad, 2001).

     ii) Give oral care counseling: (1) frequent oral care (before and after meals and before bedtime with soft toothbrush and nonirritating, saline or soda-based mouthwash); (2) daily assessment of tongue, pharynx, palate, gingiva, and buccal mucosa for lesions; (3) regular dental checkups and cleanings (every 6 months).

     iii) Refer to swallowing specialist for evaluation and swallowing retraining if indicated.

   b. Pharmacological interventions

     i) Topical or systemic pain medications (topical analgesics, oral or subcutaneous morphine)

     ii) Antifungal/antiviral medications based on causative agents

   c. Alternative/complementary therapies

     i) Chamomile, which has anti-inflammatory and antispasmodic properties, has been used to treat dysphagia, but its effectiveness is equivocal (Rotblatt & Ziment, 2002).

     ii) Capsaicin is sometimes used to reduce mouth and throat pain, but topical use may increase throat pain and be of limited value (Rotblatt & Ziment, 2002).

6. Evaluation

   a. Daily food/fluid intake meets targeted calorie and protein goals.

   b. Adequate pain relief and comfort occurs when swallowing.

   c. Choking, coughing, regurgitation, and aspiration are absent during swallowing.

   d. Oral medications are taken without difficulty.

REFERENCES

Bartlett, J. G., & Gallant, J. E. (2007). *Medical management of HIV infection.* Baltimore: Johns Hopkins Medicine Health Publishing Business Group.

Carpenito, L. J. (2006). *Nursing diagnosis: Application to clinical practice* (19th ed.). Philadelphia: Lippincott Williams & Wilkins.

Keithley, J. K., Swanson, B., & Nerad, J. (2001). HIV/AIDS. In M. Gottschlich (Ed.), *The science and practice of nutrition support: A case-based approach* (pp. 619–641). Dubuque, IA: Kendall/Hunt.

Rotblatt, M., & Ziment, I. (2002). *Evidence-based herbal medicine*. Philadelphia: Hanley & Belfus.

Terrado, M., Russell, C., & Bowman, J. B. (2001). Dysphagia: An overview. *MEDSURG Nursing, 10*(5), 233–250.

4.6 ORAL LESIONS

1. Etiology
   a. Infectious causes include Epstein-Barr virus (oral hairy leukoplakia), *Candida albicans* (thrush), bacterial infections (periodontal disease and necrotizing ulcerative gingivitis), herpes simplex virus, varicella zoster virus, cytomegalovirus, and human papillomavirus.
   b. Neoplasms include Kaposi's sarcoma and non-Hodgkin's lymphoma.
   c. Possible autoimmune manifestations include aphthous ulcers.
   d. Oral melanotic lesions have been associated with antiretrovirals, antifungals, low CD4 counts, and MAC-induced destruction of the adrenal cortex (Blignaut et al., 2006).
   e. Treatment-related causes include chemotherapy and radiation-induced stomatitis, and HAART-induced xerostomia (Frezzini, Leao, & Porter, 2005).
   f. Behavioral factors include smoking and ethanol-induced stomatitis.
   g. Prevalence of oral lesions has declined since the introduction of HAART, although HAART has been associated with oral warts and salivary gland disorders (Parveen et al., 2007).
2. Nursing assessment
   a. History
      i)   Current medications
      ii) Past opportunistic infections and neoplasms
      iii) Usual oral hygiene practices
      iv) Tobacco, alcohol, and illicit drug use
   b. Physical exam
      i)   Inspect oropharyngeal cavity for evidence of infection, lesions, or malignancies; note foul breath.
      ii) Inspect teeth and gums for tooth mobility; receding gums with exposure of tooth roots; gingival erythema, which suggests linear gingival erythema, a type of gingivitis; and necrosis of soft tissue.
      iii) Palpate for parotid/sublingual/submandibular salivary gland enlargement.
      iv) Assess GI system because oral lesions may indicate pathology in other regions of the GI tract (i.e., aphthous ulcers in mouth may be associated with similar lesions in the GI tract; esophageal candidiasis may occur concomitantly with thrush; Bartlett & Gallant, 2007).
      v)   Assess nutritional status: weight, body mass index, muscle mass, and serum albumin.
3. Nursing diagnosis
   a. Impaired oral mucous membrane
   b. Altered nutrition: less than body requirements
   c. Impaired comfort
   d. Impaired swallowing
4. Goals

    a. Maintain adequate protein and calorie intake for metabolic needs.

    b. Reduce pain.

    c. Maintain ability to take oral medications.

    d. Promote knowledge of strategies to manage pain and ensure adequate nutrition.

5. Interventions and health teaching

    a. Nonpharmacologic

       i) See Section 4.5, p. 151.

       ii) Provide resources for nonverbal communication if speaking is too painful (e.g., paper and pencil, erasable board and marker).

       iii) Encourage patient to limit or eliminate tobacco and alcohol use.

    b. Pharmacologic

       i) Pharmacological management depends on the etiology (i.e., antibiotic, antiviral, or antifungal medications; thalidomide or steroids for aphthous ulcers).

       ii) Topical or systemic pain medications can be used.

    c. Alternative/complementary therapies

       i) Ethanol propolis extract has been shown to have antifungal properties equivalent to nystatin when added to cultured *C. albicans* strains collected from HIV-infected persons (Santos et al., 2005). Garlic paste has shown preliminary evidence of efficacy for treating oral candidiasis (Sabitha et al., 2005).

       ii) Azole-resistant oral candidal lesions in HIV-infected persons have responded to treatments with an oral rinse derived from tea tree oil (Jandourek, Vaishampayan, & Vazquez, 1998) and a commercially available cinnamon preparation (Quale, Landman, Zaman, Burney, & Sathe, 1996).

       iii) An oral rinse derived from deglycyrrhizinated licorice has been associated with healing of aphthous ulcers (Das, Das, Gulati, & Singh, 1989).

       iv) Stress reduction may augment mucosal immunity in the mouth and reduce oral morbidity (Hand, Phillips, Dudgeon, & Skelton, 2005).

6. Evaluation

    a. Food and fluid intake are adequate for metabolic needs.

    b. Patient describes pain management as satisfactory.

    c. Oral medications are taken without difficulty.

REFERENCES

Bartlett, J. G., & Gallant, J. E. (2007). *Medical management of HIV infection*. Baltimore: Johns Hopkins Medicine Health Publishing Business Group.

Blignaut, E., Latton, L. L., Nittayananta, W., Ramirez-Amador, V., Ranganathan, K., & Chattopadhyay, A. (2006). (A3) HIV phenotypes, oral lesions, and management of HIV-related disease. *Advances in Dental Research, 19*(1), 122–129.

Das, S. K., Das, V., Gulati, A. K., & Singh, V. P. (1989). Deglycyrrhizinated liquorice in aphthous ulcers. *Journal of the Association of Physicians of India, 37*(10), 647.

Frezzini, C., Leao, J. C., & Porter, S. (2005). Current trends of HIV disease of the mouth. *Journal of Oral Pathology & Medicine, 34*(9), 513–531.

Hand, G. A., Phillips, K. D., Dudgeon, W. D., & Skelton, W. D. (2005). Stress reduction as a means to enhance oral immunity in HIV-infected individuals. *Journal of the Association of Nurses in AIDS Care, 16*(5), 58–63.

Jandourek, A., Vaishampayan, J. K., & Vazquez, J. A. (1998). Efficacy of melaleuca oral solution for the treatment of fluconazole refractory oral candidiasis in AIDS patients. *AIDS, 12*(9), 1033–1037.

Parveen, Z., Acheampong, E., Pomerantz, R. J., Jacobson, J. M., Wigdahl, B., & Mukhtar, M. (2007). Effects of highly active antiretroviral therapy on HIV-1-associated oral complications. *Current HIV Research, 5*(3), 281–292.

Quale, J. M., Landman, D., Zaman, M. M., Burney, S., & Sathe, S. S. (1996). In vitro activity of *Cinnamomum zeylanicum* against azole resistant and sensitive *Candida* species and a pilot study of cinnamon for oral candidiasis. *American Journal of Chinese Medicine, 24*(2), 103–109.

Sabitha, P., Adhikari, P. M., Shenoy, S. M., Kamath, A., John, R., Prabhu, M. V., et al. (2005). Efficacy of garlic paste in oral candidiasis. *Tropical Doctor, 35*(2), 99–100.

Santos, V. R., Pimenta, F. J., Aguiar, M. C., do Carmo, M. A., Naves, M. D., & Mesquita, R. A. (2005). Oral candidiasis treatment with Brazilian ethanol propolis extract. *Phytotherapy Research, 19*(7), 652–654.

4.7 FATIGUE

1. Etiology
   a. Etiology is unknown, but it is likely multifactorial, involving both physiologic and psychological causes.
      i)   Physiological causes
           (1) Factors that have been shown to be related to fatigue include anemia (Groopman, 1998; Semba, Martin, Kempen, Thorne, & Wu, 2005); nutritional deficiencies, particularly magnesium deficiency (Skurnick et al., 1996); zidovudine-induced myopathy (Cupler et al., 1995; Sinnwell et al., 1995); and low testosterone (Groopman, 1998).
           (2) Fatigue may result from endocrinological dysregulation, including abnormalities in hypothalamic-pituitary-adrenal axis functioning (Clerici et al., 1997; Stolarczyk, Rubio, Smolyar, Young, & Poretsky, 1998) and disruption of circadian variability of thyroid-stimulating hormone (Rondanelli et al., 1997), and liver disease (Bartlett, 1996; Braitstein et al., 2005).
           (3) Fatigue has been associated with a number of current AIDS-related physical symptoms, current treatment for HIV-related medical disorders, antiretroviral medications, and pain (Arendt, 2006; Carrieri et al., 2007; Phillips et al., 2004; Voss et al., 2007).
      ii) Psychological causes
           (1) Depression has been associated with HIV-related fatigue (Barroso, 1999, 2001; Voss, Portillo, Holzemer, & Dodd, 2007); however, explicating the relationship between the two is difficult because fatigue can cause depression, and depression can cause fatigue.
           (2) Anxiety may be related to fatigue as well (Barroso, 2001; Wessely, Hotopf, & Sharpe, 1998).
           (3) HIV-infected patients have a high incidence of poor nighttime sleep, which could have psychological as well as physiological causes (Pence, Barroso, Leserman, Harmon, & Salahuddin, 2008).
           (4) Recent evidence points to relationships among more childhood trauma, more recent stressful events, more depressive symptoms, and greater fatigue intensity and fatigue-related impairment in daily functioning. Recent stressors were a

more powerful predictor of fatigue than childhood trauma (Leserman, Barroso, Pence, Salahuddin, & Harmon, 2008).

2. Nursing assessment
   a. Subjective data: The nurse must rely on subjective data because there are no objective clinical indicators.
      i) There are many fatigue tools available; however, most of them are not appropriate for measuring fatigue in HIV-infected individuals because they simply measure the presence/absence of fatigue or intensity of fatigue, or they were developed and tested on non-HIV-infected samples (Barroso & Lynn, 2002; Harmon, Barroso, Pence, Leserman, & Salahuddin, 2008). The HIV-Related Fatigue Scale was developed specifically for patients with HIV (Barroso & Lynn, 2002); it contains 56 items, which measure the following:
         (1) Fatigue intensity (8 items; Cronbach's alpha 0.93)
         (2) Impact of fatigue on daily functioning (22 items; Cronbach's alpha 0.98), including three subscales: impact of fatigue on activities of daily living (ADL; 12 items; Cronbach's alpha 0.96), impact of fatigue on socialization (6 items; Cronbach's alpha 0.93), and impact of fatigue on mental functioning (4 items; Cronbach's alpha 0.93)
         (3) Responsiveness of fatigue to circumstances
      ii) The nurse should also assess the following:
         (1) Adequacy of the patient's sleep pattern
         (2) Patient's use or abuse of recreational drugs
         (3) Patient's nutritional intake
   b. Objective data: are of limited usefulness in diagnosing fatigue.
      i) Laboratory assessment may include hemoglobin, hematocrit, liver function tests, and thyroid function tests. Most studies show no relationship between either CD4 count (Barroso, 2001; Barroso, Carlson, & Meynell, 2003) or viral load (Barroso, 2001; Barroso, Carlson, & Meynell, 2003) and fatigue. Very recent evidence points to no physiological variables being associated with HIV-related fatigue (Barroso, Pence, Salahuddin, Harmon, & Leserman, 2008).

3. Nursing diagnosis
   a. Fatigue
      i) If fatigue affects activities of daily living, the following diagnoses may apply:
         (1) Impaired physical mobility
         (2) Bathing/hygiene self-care deficit
         (3) Dressing/grooming self-care deficit
         (4) Toileting self-care deficit
      ii) If fatigue affects relationships with others, the following diagnoses may apply:
         (1) Impaired social interaction
         (2) Social isolation
         (3) Risk for loneliness
         (4) Altered role performance
         (5) Altered parenting
         (6) Altered family processes

          (7) Altered sexuality patterns

          (8) Risk for caregiver role strain

     iii) For psychological sequelae of fatigue, the following diagnoses may apply:

          (1) Spiritual distress

          (2) Ineffective individual coping

          (3) Self-esteem disturbance

          (4) Hopelessness

          (5) Anxiety

4. Goals

   a. Determine the cause of fatigue.

   b. Characterize fatigue: the intensity, the circumstances surrounding the fatigue experience, and the consequences.

   c. Maintain or regain optimal functioning ability.

   d. Assist the patient in locating resources to help cope with fatigue.

5. Interventions and health teaching

   a. Nonpharmacological interventions

     i) Assess for undiagnosed opportunistic infections.

     ii) Assess for and treat underlying depression.

     iii) Control other symptoms that could be causing the fatigue (e.g., diarrhea).

     iv) If fatigue is medication-related, weigh the benefits of the medication against its side effects.

     v) Encourage patients to track their individual patterns of fatigue, keeping a fatigue diary if necessary, so they can best plan their activities each day (e.g., perform most strenuous activities during the times of peak energy, stagger activities to avoid excessive fatigue).

     vi) Napping and reducing strenuous activities have been reported to be helpful (van Servellen, Sarna, & Jablonski, 1998).

     vii) Refer the patient to community-based agencies for assistance with housekeeping support. Evaluate the need for occupational therapy (energy conservation techniques) or physical therapy (reconditioning and strengthening exercises).

   b. Pharmacological interventions

     i) One study found that thyroid hormone replacement improved HIV-related fatigue, although participants showed no evidence of thyroid abnormality (Derry, 1996).

     ii) Other successful interventions include dextroamphetamine (Wagner & Rabkin, 2000), DHEA (Rabkin, Ferrando, Wagner, & Rabkin, 2000), and hyperbaric oxygen (Jordan, 1998; Reillo, 1993).

   c. Alternative/complementary therapies

     i) Limited data support the usefulness of relaxation training (Fukunishi et al., 1997).

   d. Evaluation

     i) The patient will report being able to complete the most pressing tasks through careful planning.

     ii) The patient will maintain independence in ADLs.

     iii) The patient will access community-based resources, as needed.

     iv) The patient will maintain an overall optimal level of functioning.

REFERENCES

Arendt, G. (2006). Affective disorders in patients with HIV infection: Impact of antiretroviral therapy. *CNS Drugs, 20*(6), 507–518.

Barroso, J. (1999). A review of fatigue in people with HIV infection. *Journal of the Association of Nurses in AIDS Care, 10*(5), 42–49.

Barroso, J. (2001). "Just worn out": A qualitative study of HIV-related fatigue. In S. G. Funk, E. M. Tornquist, J. Leeman, M. S. Miles, & J. S. Harrell (Eds.), *Key aspects of preventing and managing chronic illness* (pp. 183–194). New York: Springer.

Barroso, J., Carlson, J. R., & Meynell, J. (2003). Physiological and psychological markers associated with HIV-related fatigue. *Clinical Nursing Research, 12*(1), 49–68.

Barroso, J., & Lynn, M. R. (2002). Psychometric properties of the HIV-Related Fatigue Scale. *Journal of the Association of Nurses in AIDS Care, 13*(1), 66–75.

Barroso, J., Pence, B. W., Salahuddin, N., Harmon, J. L., & Leserman, J. (2008). Physiological correlates of HIV-related fatigue. *Clinical Nursing Research, 17*(1), 5–19.

Bartlett, J. G. (1996). *Medical management of HIV infection.* Glenview, IL: Physicians and Scientists Publishing.

Braitstein, P., Montessori, V., Chan, K., Montaner, J. S. G., Schechter, M. T., O'Shaughnessy, M. V., et al. (2005). Quality of life, depression, and fatigue among persons co-infected with HIV and hepatitis C: Outcomes from a population-based cohort. *AIDS Care, 17*(4), 505–515.

Carrieri, M. P., Villes, V., Raffi, F., Protopopescu, C., Preau, M., Salmon, D., et al. (2007). Self-reported side-effects of anti-retroviral treatment among IDUs: A 7-year longitudinal study (APROCO-COPILOTE COHORT ANRS CO-8). *International Journal of Drug Policy, 18*(4), 288–295.

Clerici, M., Trabattoni, D., Piconi, S., Fusi, M. L., Ruzzante, S., Clerici, C., et al. (1997). A possible role for the cortisol/anticortisols imbalance in the progression of human immunodeficiency virus. *Psychoneuroendocrinology, 22*(Suppl. 1), 27–31.

Cupler, E. J., Danon, M. J., Jay, C., Hench, K., Ropka, M., & Dalakas, M. C. (1995). Early features of zidovudine-associated myopathy: Histopathological findings and clinical correlations. *Acta Neuropathologica, 90*(1), 1–6.

Derry, D. M. (1996). Thyroid hormone therapy in patients infected with human immunodeficiency virus: A clinical approach to treatment. *Medical Hypotheses, 47*(3), 227–233.

Fukunishi, I., Hosaka, T., Matsumoto, T., Hayashi, M., Negishi, M., & Moriya, H. (1997). Liaison psychiatry and HIV infection (II): Application of relaxation in HIV-positive patients. *Psychiatry and Clinical Neurosciences, 51*(1), 5–8.

Groopman, J. E. (1998). Fatigue in cancer and HIV/AIDS. *Oncology, 12*(3), 335–341.

Harmon, J. L., Barroso, J., Pence, B. W., Leserman, J., & Salahuddin, N. (2008). Demographic and illness-related variables associated with HIV-related fatigue. *Journal of the Association of Nurses in AIDS Care, 19*(2), 90–97.

Jordan, W. C. (1998). The effectiveness of intermittent hyperbaric oxygen in relieving drug-induced HIV-associated neuropathy. *Journal of the National Medical Association, 90*(6), 355–358.

Leserman, J., Barroso, J., Pence, B. W., Salahuddin, N., & Harmon, J. L. (2008). Trauma, stressful life events, and depression predict HIV-related fatigue. *AIDS Care, 20*(10), 1258–1265.

Pence, B. W., Barroso, J., Leserman, J., Harmon, J. L., & Salahuddin, N. (2008). Measuring fatigue in people living with HIV/AIDS: Psychometric characteristics of the HIV-Related Fatigue Scale. *AIDS Care, 20*(7), 829–837.

Phillips, K. D., Sowell, R. L., Rojas, M., Tavakoli, A., Fulk, L. J., & Hand, G. A. (2004). Physiological and psychological correlates of fatigue in HIV disease. *Biological Research for Nursing, 6*(1), 59–74.

Rabkin, J. G., Ferrando, S. J., Wagner, G. J., & Rabkin, R. (2000). DHEA treatment for HIV + patients: Effects on mood, androgenic and anabolic parameters. *Psychoneuroendocrinology, 25*(1), 53–68.

Reillo, M. R. (1993). Hyperbaric oxygen therapy for the treatment of debilitating fatigue associated with HIV/AIDS. *Journal of the Association of Nurses in AIDS Care, 4*(3), 33–38.

Rondanelli, M., Solerte, S. B., Fioravanti, M., Scevola, D., Locatelli, M., Minoli, L., et al. (1997). Circadian secretory pattern of growth hormone, insulin-like growth factor type I, cortisol, adrenocorticotropic hormone, thyroid-stimulating hormone, and prolactin during HIV infection. *AIDS Research and Human Retroviruses, 13*(14), 1243–1249.

Semba, R. D., Martin, B. K., Kempen, J. H., Thorne, J. E., & Wu, A. W. (2005). The impact of anemia on energy and physical functioning in individuals with AIDS. *Archives of Internal Medicine, 165*(19), 2229–2236.

Sinnwell, T. M., Sivakumar, K., Soueidan, S., Jay, C., Frank, J. A., McLaughlin, A. C., et al. (1995). Metabolic abnormalities in skeletal muscle of patients receiving zidovudine therapy observed by ^{31}P in vivo magnetic resonance spectroscopy. *Journal of Clinical Investigation, 96*(1), 126–131.

Skurnick, J. H., Bogden, J. D., Baker, H., Kemp, F. W., Sheffet, A., Quattrone, G., et al. (1996). Micronutrient profiles in HIV-1-infected heterosexual adults. *Journal of Acquired Immune Deficiency Syndromes and Human Retrovirology, 12*(1), 75–83.

Stolarczyk, R., Rubio, S. I., Smolyar, D., Young, I. S., & Poretsky, L. (1998). Twenty-four-hour urinary free cortisol in patients with acquired immunodeficiency syndrome. *Metabolism, 47*(6), 690–694.

van Servellen, G., Sarna, L., & Jablonski, K. J. (1998). Women with HIV: Living with symptoms. *Western Journal of Nursing Research, 20*(4), 448–464.

Voss, J., Portillo, C. J., Holzemer, W. L., & Dodd, M. J. (2007). Symptom cluster of fatigue and depression in HIV/AIDS. *Journal of Prevention and Intervention in the Community, 33*(1–2), 19–34.

Voss, J. G., Sukati, N. A., Seboni, N. M., Makoae, L. N., Moleko, M., Human, S., et al. (2007). Symptom burden of fatigue in men and women living with HIV/AIDS in Southern Africa. *Journal of the Association of Nurses in AIDS Care, 18*(4), 22–31.

Wagner, G. J., & Rabkin, R. (2000). Effects of dextroamphetamine on depression and fatigue in men with HIV: A double-blind, placebo-controlled trial. *Journal of Clinical Psychiatry, 61*(6), 436–440.

Wessely, S., Hotopf, M., & Sharpe, M. (1998). *Chronic fatigue and its syndromes.* Oxford, UK: Oxford University Press.

4.8 FEVER

1. Etiology
   a. Fever is an abnormally high body temperature caused by host defense responses to infectious or noninfectious molecular mediators called pyrogens. The temperature rise is regulated by the hypothalamic thermal control center when the pyrogen causes the thermoregulatory set point range to be reset at a higher level.
   b. Fever should not be confused with hyperthermia, which involves dysfunction of thermoregulatory mechanisms leading to an unregulated rise in temperature.
   c. Fever refers to the entire complex of thermal and acute-phase consequences producing symptoms of malaise and fatigue that are often more distressful than the elevated temperature.
   d. Fever heralds many HIV-related OIs (respiratory and urinary tract, central nervous system, abscesses, gingivitis, gastroenteritis, drug reactions, lymphoma), and noninfectious processes.
   e. Noninfectious pyrogens include blood products, drugs, and substances recognized as "foreign" by macrophages and other immune cells.
   f. Cytokines are believed to be responsible for mediating febrile temperature elevations by increasing synthesis of hypothalamic prostaglandins of the E group (PGE) that readjust the hypothalamic thermostat to a higher set point range (Boulant, 2000; Cooper, 1995).
   g. The cause of many HIV-related fevers is never detected. A recent large cotrimoxazole clinical trial for HIV-related OIs, documented that only half of the fevers could be attributed to specific causes (Anglaret et al., 2002).
   h. Several drugs used in treatment of HIV disease—TMP-SMX, atovaquone, amphotericin B (chills or rigors are secondary to fever), didanosine (ddI), amoxicillin-clavulanic acid, dapsone, ceftazidine, and ganciclovir—are known to induce fever, making it difficult to determine if the response is due to the disease or the treatment (Johnson, Stallworth, & Neilands, 2003; Lee, 1995).

     i. Fever is by far the most common symptom of acute retroviral syndrome, occurring in up to 96% of patients (Macneal & Dinulos, 2006).

2. Nursing assessment
   a. Subjective: Review body systems—fatigue, vomiting, diarrhea, lethargy, rashes, cough, congestion, or increased irritability, temperature duration.
      i) Review complete drug history to rule out acute retroviral syndrome, check duration of treatment, sequence of drug changes, combinations, possible incompatibilities, and physical clues such as asymptomatic macules and papules, involving primarily the face and trunk (Macneal & Dinulos, 2006).
      ii) Review exposure to any infectious diseases, animals (cats, dogs, reptiles, farm animals, birds), or molds. Inquire about whether the patient drinks well or city water at home, lives in an older/newer home, has eaten at any restaurants lately, has been exposed to anyone from a foreign country, has been incarcerated, or lives in a halfway house.
      iii) Inquire about travel history, any recent travel outside of the state (which states) or outside of the country
      iv) Inquire about any recent immunizations.
      v) Inquire about any recent medications.
   b. Objective: Select a monitoring schedule consistent with patient's clinical condition.
      i) Assess frequently during febrile episodes. Routine methods and twice-daily intervals between temperature measurements may not be adequate for detecting febrile episodes in hospitalized patients with evidence of infection, tissue injury, or inflammation (Taliaferro, 1996).
      ii) Increase the frequency of measurements when patients are receiving potentially pyrogenic agents, such as blood or antigenic drugs. Body temperature should be monitored at least every 4 hours.
      iii) Assess whether fever threatens safety. Temperatures approaching 40.5° C suggest hyperthermia and impose risk of irreversible central nervous system damage.
      iv) Monitor febrile shivering. During fever, mild heat loss can elicit shivering and vasoconstriction, making the patient vulnerable to chilling. Low levels of shivering may not be visible but are sufficient to contribute to heat generation and oxygen consumption.
      v) Monitor hydration. Significant amounts of body water are lost by compensatory cooling mechanisms of sweating and hyperventilation during fever.
      vi) Monitor pharmacologic fever therapies. Note responses, side effects, and achievement of therapeutic goals. Body temperature elevations often mark progress when drugs are aimed at controlling underlying infection or pathology.
      vii) Evaluate thermal comfort. Replace clothing with dry, warm clothing after sweating to avoid chilling.

3. Nursing diagnosis
   a. Risk for altered body temperature is related to febrile responses to altered thermoregulatory set point (NANDA, 1996).
   b. Altered thermoregulatory set point (an alternative diagnosis) is more precise and calls for attention to the underlying dynamics.

    c. Risk for fatigue is related to circulating cytokines and exertion from shivering.

    d. Risk for fluid volume deficit is due to fever-related compensatory sweating and insensible loss from respiration.

    e. Risk for shivering, hypothermia, and temperature drift occurs during aggressive cooling (Holtzclaw, 1998b).

4. Goals

    a. To monitor the patient's response to the febrile symptoms and treatment

    b. To promote comfort and adequate hydration

    c. To prevent febrile shivering or aggressive chilling

5. Interventions and health teaching

    a. Nonpharmacological interventions

       i) Tepid sponge baths, cooling fans or blankets, ice packs, or alcohol baths are contraindicated because they promote shivering, energy expenditure, and patient discomfort; they may actually raise body temperature (Holtzclaw, 2002).

       ii) Prevent chills and shivering of febrile response at onset of temperature rise by insulating extremities with protective wraps, socks, and absorbent blankets. As chilling subsides, remove heavy covering cautiously to avoid drafts (Holtzclaw, 1998a; 1998b; 1999).

       iii) When fever breaks and sweating occurs, remove wet clothing under bed covers to avoid drafts and chilling.

       iv) Avoid giving cold liquids to a febrile patient because rapid ingestion can abruptly cool the body core at a time when the elevated set point is highly sensitive to cooling. The patient can slowly lick or suck frozen juice or flavored Popsicles, which allows gradual ingestion and helps to avoid chilling.

    b. Pharmacological interventions

       i) Antipyretic therapy should not be instituted routinely for every febrile episode but should be based on therapeutic goals, relative risk of temperature elevation, and discomfort of fever-related symptoms (Holtzclaw, 2002).

       ii) NSAIDs (e.g., aspirin, indomethacin) are effective in diminishing fever, but they have significant side effects and may suppress signs of ongoing infection (Styrt & Sugarman, 1990).

       iii) When not contraindicated, antipyretics can be administered regularly around the clock rather than prn to people with chronic or frequent fevers to improve patient comfort.

    c. Alternative/complementary therapies

       i) Herbal extracts have long been used to treat fever, but they may interact with prescribed medications.

       ii) White willow bark (*Salix alba*) is similar in origin and action to aspirin.

       iii) Kava kava (*Piper methysticum*) and valerian (*Valeriana officinalis*) can manage fever-induced psychological distress, but they have significant drug interactions and toxic effects.

       iv) Cooling baths or rotary fans to cool the body temperature can initiate shivering and warming responses that defeat the purpose of cooling.

v) Warm baths, with temperatures 1 to 2 degrees lower than the body temperature, will often sedate the febrile patient and prevent shivering without increasing core temperatures.

6. Evaluation

a. Evaluate patient's response to the febrile symptoms and their treatment. Surveillance should include threat of neural damage from fever.

b. During fever, temperature should remain below 40° C.

c. Evaluate thermal comfort.

d. Evaluate hydration status.

REFERENCES

Anglaret, X., Dakoury-Dogbo, N., Bonard, D., Toure, S., Combe, P., Ouassa, T., et al. (2002). Causes and empirical treatment of fever in HIV-infected adult outpatients, Abidjan, Côte d'Ivoire. *AIDS, 16*(6), 909–918.

Boulant, J. (2000). Role of the preoptic-anterior hypothalamus in thermoregulation and fever. *Clinical Infectious Diseases, 31*(Suppl. 5), 157–161.

Cooper, K. (1995). Beyond the loci of action of circulating pyrogens: Mediators and mechanisms. In K. Cooper (Ed.), *Fever and antipyresis* (pp. 60–89). New York: Cambridge University Press.

Holtzclaw, B. J. (1998a). *Final Report: Febrile symptom management in persons with AIDS*. Bethesda, MD: National Institute of Nursing Research, National Institutes of Health.

Holtzclaw, B. J. (1998b). Managing fever in HIV disease. *Journal of the Association of Nurses in AIDS Care, 9*(4), 97–101.

Holtzclaw, B. J. (1999). Temperature regulation: Fever treatment. In G. M. Bulechek (Ed.), *Nursing interventions: Effective nursing treatments* (3rd ed., pp. 356–366). Philadelphia: Saunders.

Holtzclaw, B. J. (2002). Use of thermoregulatory principles in patient care: Fever management. *Online Journal of Clinical Innovations, 5*(5), 1–23. Retrieved September 19, 2007, from https://www.cinahl.com/cgi-bin/ojcishowdoc23.cgi?vol05.htm

Johnson, M. O., Stallworth, T., & Neilands, T. B. (2003). The drugs or the disease? Causal attributions of symptoms held by HIV-positive adults on HAART. *AIDS & Behavior, 7*(2), 109–117.

Lee, B. (1995). Drug interactions and toxicities in patients with AIDS. In P. Cohen, M. Sande, & P. Volberding (Eds.), *The AIDS knowledge base* (4th ed., pp. 161–182). Philadelphia: Saunders.

Macneal, R. J., & Dinulos, J. G. H. (2006). Acute retroviral syndrome. *Dermatologic Clinics, 24*(4), 431–438.

North American Nursing Diagnosis Association (NANDA). (1996). *Nursing diagnosis: Definitions and classification 1997–1998*. Philadelphia: Author.

Styrt, B., & Sugarman, B. (1990). Antipyresis and fever. *Archives of Internal Medicine, 150*(8), 1589–1597.

Taliaferro, D. (1996). *Monitoring fever patterns and hydration in hospitalized persons living with AIDS*. Paper presented at the Southern Nursing Research Society 10th Annual Research Conference, Miami, FL.

4.9 SLEEP DISTURBANCES

1. Etiology

a. Sleep disorders contribute to decreased quality of life (Davis, 2004) and can arise from the following:

i) HIV-related physical symptoms, such as pain, fever, and fatigue

ii) Side effects from medications, such as efavirenz, which can cause insomnia (NIH, 2007), mood-altering drugs, and alcohol

  iii) Mental health issues, such as depression and anxiety

  iv) HIV infection of the brain and nervous system

  v) Opportunistic infections and neoplasms

  vi) Social and environmental factors, such as sleeping in a room with a number of other adults (Robbins, Phillips, Dudgeon, & Hand, 2004)

b. Sleep disorders have been defined by the Cleveland Clinic (http://www.clevelandclinic.org/health/health-info/docs/3700/3743.asp?index=12137) and include the following:

  i) Insomnia, which refers to the complaint of difficulty falling asleep, staying asleep, or poor sleep quality in persons who have adequate opportunity for sleep (Buysse et al., 2007)

  ii) Periodic limb movement disorder

  iii) Parasomnias

  iv) Sleep apnea

  v) Narcolepsy

2. Nursing assessment

a. Subjective

  i) Sleep problems may be unreported unless the provider screens for them. An interactive sleep quiz (http://www.nhlbi.nih.gov/cgi-bin/tfSleepQuiz.pl) can assess knowledge about quality sleep, and the Sleepiness Scale (http://www.sleepeducation.com/Print_SleepinessScale.aspx) can identify whether a more thorough sleep assessment may be in order.

  ii) With the client's permission, speaking with the bed partner can yield valuable information about the client's sleep pattern.

  iii) Sleep problems are usually aggravated during withdrawal from mood-altering drugs, such as heroin, cocaine, and alcohol. These underlying withdrawal issues should be addressed before arriving at a diagnosis of chronic sleep disturbance.

b. Objective

  i) Sleep diaries and 24-hour sleep patterns recall (Meltzer, Mindell, & Levandoski, 2007) can be used to record naps, sleep latency (i.e., minutes required to fall asleep after going to bed), number and duration of awakenings, total sleep, quality of sleep, feelings on awakening, and whether or not the night was typical.

  ii) Self-report instruments, such as the Pittsburgh Sleep Quality Index, are available through the Internet but may be difficult to administer and score in a clinical setting.

  iii) Actigraphy devices may be used to measure movement over a period of 3 to 5 consecutive days. If there is clear evidence of pathology, a comprehensive assessment in a sleep laboratory using polysomnography is warranted.

3. Nursing diagnosis: sleep quality disturbance

4. Goals

a. Identify etiology and duration of sleep pattern disturbance.

b. Increase quality and duration of sleep.

5. Intervention and health teaching

a. Nonpharmacological interventions: A number of sleep hygiene strategies have been summarized by the Mayo Clinic (http://www.mayoclinic.com/print/sleep/HQ01387/) and include the following:

i)   Go to bed and get up at about the same time every day, even on the weekends.

ii)   Don't eat or drink large amounts before bedtime.

iii)   Avoid nicotine, caffeine, and alcohol in the evening.

iv)   Exercise regularly.

v)   Make your bedroom cool, dark, quiet, and comfortable.

vi)   Sleep primarily at night.

vii)   Choose a comfortable mattress and pillow.

viii) Start a relaxing bedtime routine.

ix)   Go to bed when you're tired and turn out the lights.

x)   Use sleeping pills only as a last resort.

b. Pharmacological interventions: Many persons with HIV/AIDS have liver disorders that can complicate the biotransformation of sleeping pills. Therefore, nonpharmacological interventions should be fully explored before drugs are administered. The Mayo Clinic provides information about the different medications used to treat sleep disorders (http://www.mayoclinic.com/print/sleeping-pills/SL00010/).

i)   Over-the-counter medications (diphenhydramine, doxylamine).

ii)   Non-benzodiazepine hypnotic medications (zolpidem tartrate, zaleplon, eszopiclone) are the newest class of hypnotic medications.

iii)   Benzodiazepine hypnotic medications (triazolam, estazolam, temazepam) are the oldest class of hypnotics and can be habit-forming. Some HIV-infected persons with a history of street drug use may have abused these drugs and so may be afraid of relapse.

c. Melatonin, a pineal gland hormone, has gained widespread use as a sleep-promoting substance, but there are many unanswered questions about its effectiveness.

d. Relaxation training, such as progressive relaxation or yoga, can be helpful.

e. Biofeedback, especially EMG (electromyography) feedback, might be beneficial.

f. Acupuncture has been shown to be effective in managing insomnia in HIV-infected persons (Phillips & Skelton, 2001).

g. Treat depressive symptoms. Sleep disturbance and depressive symptoms are associated and affect medication adherence (Phillips et al., 2005).

6. Evaluation

a. Match sleep hygiene strategies to the unique needs of individual clients. To determine which strategies are effective, introduce no more than two different strategies at any one time. Different strategies should be used for at least 1 week before assessing their effectiveness, unless they are exacerbating the problem.

b. Assess use of sleeping pills and other over-the-counter or street remedies and determine if there are interactions with prescribed treatments.

c. Refer to sleep laboratory for comprehensive follow-up if health insurance plans support clients' reimbursement for sleep studies.

REFERENCES

Buysse, D., Thompson, W., Scott, J., Franzen, P., Germain, A., Hall, M., et al. (2007). Daytime symptoms in primary insomnia: A prospective analysis using ecological momentary assessment. *Sleep Medicine, 8*(3), 198–208.

Davis, S. (2004). Clinical sequelae affecting quality of life in the HIV-infected patient. *Journal of the Association of Nurses in AIDS Care, 15*(Suppl. 5), 28S–33S.

Meltzer, L., Mindell, J., & Levandoski, L. (2007). The 24-hour sleep patterns interview: A pilot study of validity and feasibility. *Behavioral Sleep Medicine, 5*(4), 297–310.

National Institutes of Health (NIH). (2007). *Efavirenz.* Retrieved November 3, 2007, from http://www.nlm.nih.gov/medlineplus/druginfo/meds/a699004.html

Phillips, K., Moneyham, L., Murdaugh, C., Boyd, M., Tavakoli, A., Jackson, K., et al. (2005). Sleep disturbance and depression as barriers to adherence. *Clinical Nursing Research, 14*(3), 273–293.

Phillips, D., & Skelton, W. (2001). Effects of individualized acupuncture on sleep quality in HIV disease. *Journal of the Association of Nurses in AIDS Care, 12*(1), 27–39.

Robbins, J., Phillips, K. I., Dudgeon, W., & Hand, G. (2004). Physiological and psychological correlates of sleep in HIV infection. *Clinical Nursing Research, 13*(1), 33–52.

4.10 IMPAIRED MOBILITY

1. Etiology
   a. Limitation of movement (Carpenito, 2006); inability to move one or more body parts or inability to move freely within one's environment (Bergquist, Neuberger, & Jamison, 2006)
   b. May be caused by primary and secondary etiologies and is frequently multifactorial (Linton, 2007)
      i)   Neurological involvement that causes motor impairment, neuropathy, or pain (Brew, 2002; Price, 2003)
      ii)   Metabolic complications that may result in weakness and altered action potential of muscles
      iii) Muscle wasting resulting in weakness and increased risk of falls and injury
      iv)   Musculoskeletal injury precipitating mild to severe pain (McGuire & So, 1999)
      v)   Opportunistic infections and neoplasms
      vi)   HIV-associated dementia (HAD; Brew, 2002)
      vii) Polyneuropathies: primary due to HIV infection; secondary from pharmacologic agents (Bartlett, 2005; Cherry et al., 2006; Cornblath & Hoke, 2006; Ferrari et al., 2006; Koppel & Akfirat, 2004)
      viii) Fatigue resulting in inability to exercise to maintain muscle strength
      ix)   Osteopenia/osteoporosis subsequent to the use of highly active anti-retroviral therapy (HAART; Martin et al., 2004; Pan et al., 2006)
      x)   Psychological/psychospiritual complications (e.g., depression, bereavement, fear)
2. Nursing assessment
   a. Subjective data
      i)   Impact on quality of life, relationships
      ii)   Ability to perform activities of daily living (ADL)
      iii) Onset, severity, and character of associated signs and symptoms
            (1) Weakness (unilateral vs. bilateral; upper vs. lower extremities)
            (2) Decreased endurance, increased fatigue
      iv)   Other associated neurological symptoms (e.g., incontinence, urinary retention, sensory changes)

v) New or different pattern of constitutional signs and symptoms reported by patient (e.g., fever, weight loss)

vi) Recent changes in medication regimen

vii) Nutritional intake

b. Objective data

i) Musculoskeletal assessment: Conduct gait assessment; evaluate upper and lower body for muscle mass, strength, and equality; assess joint and muscle pain; assess agility; assess joints for evidence of rheumatologic/HIV-related conditions (Kaye, 2002).

ii) Neurological assessment: Assess presence of pain or headache, dizziness, tremors, consciousness, orientation and balance; evaluate sensory testing of upper and lower extremities along with bilateral comparisons.

iii) Pain assessment: Assess for control of pain and management strategies.

iv) Environmental assessment (home, institutional, social): Use Home Assessment Profile (Chandler, Duncan, Weiner, & Studenski, 2001; see Engberg & McDowell, 1999, and Stephens & Olson, 2004, for additional home safety screening information; see Stone & Wyman, 1999, for environmental hazards in institutional setting); Tinetti's Performance Oriented Mobility Test; Karnofsky Performance Status Index; and Katz Index of Activities of Daily Living, Instrumental Activities of Daily Living (Linton, 2007).

v) Mental status assessment: Use Folstein Mini-Mental Status Exam, Short Portable Mental Status Questionnaire, and Cognitive Capacity Screening Exam (see Williams & Salisbury, 1999).

vi) Conduct medication assessment to determine medication related sequelae/complications.

vii) Use the same instrument/assessment process consistently to track progression throughout the clinical course.

3. Nursing diagnoses

a. Risk for injury

b. Risk for impaired skin integrity

c. Altered role performance

d. Altered sexuality patterns

e. Impaired home maintenance

f. Potential for self-care deficit

g. Self-esteem disturbance

4. Goals

a. Maintain or rehabilitate to the maximal mobility level.

b. Minimize potential for injury.

c. Enhance well-being.

5. Interventions and health teaching

a. Nonpharmacological (Bergquist, Neuberger, & Jamison, 2006)

i) Recommend maintenance of normal physical activity, including activities of daily living, to the extent possible.

    ii)   Recommend incorporation of increased physical activity as appropriate, including flexibility training, resistance or strength training, and endurance or aerobic training.

    iii) Recommend consultation with a physical therapist and a primary care provider in the development of an exercise program.

    iv)   Assist with adequate nutritional guidelines for age and stage of HIV, considering food–drug interactions and indications.

    v)   Instruct in pain control methods (see Nedeljkovic, 2002, for more information).

    vi) Discuss alternative and self-care strategies for pain control (Nicholas et al., 2007; Ownby & Dune, 2007).

    vii) Recommend use of appropriate assistive devices to correct any sensory deficits and enhance mobility.

    viii) Conduct psychosocial interventions, including use of therapeutic communication with the patient, the family, and significant others. Consider referral to pastoral or psychological counseling, if indicated.

    ix)   Assess and recommend environmental adaptations, beginning with safety and functional assessment; be aware of financial or behavioral constraints inhibiting change in this area. Provide appropriate care and community referrals.

  b. Pharmacological

    i)   Recommend use of nonpharmacologic interventions as appropriate prior to the use of pharmacologic agents.

    ii)   Instruct patient to take pain medications as needed.

    iii) Provide specific information for recommended medications.

  c. Alternative/complementary therapies

    i)   There is some evidence to support the efficacy of diet and nutrition therapy, acupuncture, hyperthermia, and oxygen therapy (Goldberg, 1997).

    ii)   Herbal therapies, such as astragalus, schisandra, and ginseng, may increase stamina and energy; St. John's wort can be used topically for muscle soreness; kava and valerian are used to promote skeletal muscle relaxation (LaValle, Krinsky, Hawkins, Pelton, & Willis, 2000).

6. Evaluation

  a. Evaluate physical environment for safety.

  b. Evaluate strength, flexibility, and endurance.

  c. Evaluate for complications of immobility.

REFERENCES

Bartlett, J. G. (2005). *The Johns Hopkins Hospital 2005–6 guide to medical care of patients with HIV infection* (12th ed). Philadelphia: Lippincott Williams & Wilkins.

Bergquist, S., Neuberger, G. B., & Jamison, M. (2006). Altered mobility and fatigue. In I. M. Lubkin & P. D. Larsen (Eds.), *Chronic illness: Impact and intervention* (5th ed., pp. 147–163). Sudbury, MA: Jones and Bartlett.

Brew, B. J. (2002). Neurological manifestations of HIV infection. In S. Crowe, J. Hoy & J. Mills (Eds.), *Management of the HIV-infected patients* (2nd ed., pp. 161–181). London: Martin Dunitz.

Carpenito, L. J. (2006). *Nursing diagnosis: Application to clinical practice* (8th ed.). Philadelphia: Lippincott Williams & Wilkins.

Chandler, J. M., Duncan, P. W., Weiner, D. K., & Studenski, S. A. (2001). Special feature: Assessment profile—A reliable and valid assessment tool. *Topics in Geriatric Rehabilitation, 16*(3), 77–88.

Cherry, C. L., Skolasky, R. L., Lal, L., Creighton, J., Hauer, P., Raman, S. P., et al. (2006). Antiretroviral use and other risks for HIV-associated neuropathies in an international cohort. *Neurology, 66*(6), 867–873.

Cornblath, D. R., & Hoke, A. (2006). Recent advances in HIV neuropathy. *Current Opinion in Neurology, 19*(5), 446–450.

Engberg, S. J., & McDowell, J. (1999). Comprehensive geriatric assessment. In J. T. Stone, J. F. Wyman, & S. A. Salisbury (Eds.), *Clinical gerontological nursing: A guide to advanced practice* (2nd ed., pp. 63–80). Philadelphia: W. B. Saunders.

Ferrari, S., Vento, S., Monaco, S., Cavallaro, T., Cainelli, F., Rizzuto, N., et al. (2006). Human immunodeficiency virus-associated peripheral neuropathies. *Mayo Clinic Proceedings, 81*(2), 213–219.

Goldberg, B. (1997). *Alternative medicine: The definitive guide*. Tiburon, CA: Future Medicine.

Kaye, B. (2002). Rheumatological manifestations of HIV infection. In S. Crowe, J. Hoy & J. Mills (Eds.), *Management of the HIV-infected patients* (2nd ed., pp. 227–244). London: Martin Dunitz.

Koppel, B. S., & Akfirat, G. L. (2004). Neurologic complications of HIV and AIDS. In G. P. Wormser (Ed.), *AIDS and other manifestations of HIV infection* (pp. 479–535). San Diego, CA: Elsevier Academic Press.

LaValle, J. B., Krinsky, D. L., Hawkins, E. B., Pelton, R., & Willis, N. A. (2000). *Natural therapeutics pocket guide*. Hudson, OH: Lexi-Comp.

Linton, A. D. (2007). Nursing care of patients with musculoskeletal alterations. In A. D. Linton & H. W. Lach (Eds.), *Matteson & McConnell's gerontological nursing concepts and practice* (pp. 288–312). St. Louis, MO: Saunders Elsevier.

Martin, K., Lawson-Ayayi, S., Miremont-Salamé, G., Blaizeau, M. J., Balestre, E., Lacoste, D., et al. (2004). Symptomatic bone disorders in HIV-infected patients: Incidence in the Aquitaine cohort (1999–2002). *HIV Medicine, 5*(6), 421–426.

McGuire, D., & So, Y. T. (1999). The nervous system in HIV and AIDS. In P. T. Cohen, M. A. Sande, & P. A. Volberding (Eds.), *The AIDS knowledge base* (3rd ed., pp. 445–462). Philadelphia: Lippincott Williams & Wilkins.

Nedeljkovic, S. S. (2002). *Pain management of HIV/AIDS patients*. Boston: Butterworth-Heinemann.

Nicholas, P. K., Kemppainen, J. K., Canaval, G. E., Corless, I. B., Sefcik, E. F., Nokes, K. M., et al. (2007). Symptom management and self-care for peripheral neuropathy in HIV/AIDS. *AIDS Care, 19*(2), 179–189.

Ownby, K. K., & Dune, L. S. (2007). The processes by which persons with HIV-related peripheral neuropathy manage their symptoms: A qualitative study. *Journal of Pain & Symptom Management, 34*(1), 48–59.

Pan, G., Yang, Z., Ballinger, S., & McDonald, J. M. (2006). Pathogenesis of osteopenia/osteoporosis induced by highly active anti-retroviral therapy for AIDS. *Annals of the New York Academy of Sciences, 1068*, 297–308.

Price, R. W. (2003). Neurologic disease. In R. Dolin, H. Masur, & M. S. Saag (Eds.), *AIDS Therapy* (2nd ed., pp. 737–775). Philadelphia: Churchill Livingstone.

Stephens, J. A., & Olson, S. J. (2004). *Check for safety: A home fall prevention checklist for older adults*. Retrieved September 25, 2007, from http://www.cdc.gov/ncipc/pub-res/toolkit/Check%20for%20SafetyCOLOR.pdf

Stone, J. T., & Wyman, J. F. (1999). Falls. In J. T. Stone, J. F. Wyman, & S. A. Salisbury (Eds.), *Clinical gerontological nursing: A guide to advanced practice* (2nd ed., pp. 341–367). Philadelphia: W. B. Saunders.

Williams, M. P., & Salisbury, S. A. (1999). Cognitive assessment. In J. T. Stone, J. F. Wyman, & S. A. Salisbury (Eds.), *Clinical gerontological nursing: A guide to advanced practice* (2nd ed., pp. 129–154). Philadelphia: W. B. Saunders.

4.11 NAUSEA AND VOMITING

1. Etiology
   a. Side effects of antiretrovirals and medications used to manage opportunistic infections (OI; Capili & Anastasi, 1998)
   b. Chemotherapy
   c. Radiation therapy
   d. HIV-related autonomic neuropathy (Konturek, Fischer, Van Der Voort, & Domschke, 1997)

e. OI-induced endocrine dysfunction, including cytomegalovirus, cryptococcus, toxoplasma, mycobacteria, and candida (Etzel, Brocavich, & Torre, 1992)
f. Lactic acidosis (Calza, Manfredi, & Chiodo, 2005)
g. Acute gastroenteritis secondary to food-borne illness (Longstreth, 2006)
h. Postoperative nausea and vomiting
i. Vestibular neuritis
j. Functional vomiting
k. Gastroparesis
l. Gastroesophageal reflux
m. Gastric outlet obstruction
n. Eosinophilic gastroenteritis
o. Chronic idiopathic intestinal pseudo-obstruction
p. Rumination syndrome

2. Nursing assessment
a. Subjective data
   i) Assess pattern of nausea and vomiting: onset, duration, precipitating factors, appearance, amount, and odor of vomitus.
   ii) Assess associated symptoms (abdominal pain, shortness of breath, dizziness, and dysphagia) and impact of nausea and vomiting on lifestyle.
   iii) Question about history of gastrointestinal diseases, family medical history, stage of illness, weight loss, nutritional intake, and travel history.
   iv) Review prescribed medications and over-the-counter medications used.
   v) Obtain past and current treatments the patient has been prescribed to manage the symptoms and home remedies tried to self-manage the symptoms.
b. Objective data
   i) Examine the patient for signs of fluid depletion such as decreased blood pressure, increased heart rate, decreased skin turgor, and decreased urine output.
   ii) Perform an oral assessment for thrush, oral lesions, and ulcerations.
   iii) Conduct an abdominal assessment: observe for distention, auscultate for bowel sounds, and palpate for masses.
   iv) Obtain laboratory evaluations: complete blood count, chemistry, serum electrolytes, renal function, thyroid panel, and liver function.
   v) Radiology evaluations should be ordered according to the symptom and physical examination results.

3. Nursing diagnosis
a. Fluid volume deficit related to loss of fluids from the gastrointestinal tract secondary to vomiting
b. Altered nutrition, less than body requirement, related to the inability to ingest adequate nutrients due to nausea and vomiting

4. Goals
a. Identify and minimize the causative factors.
b. Control nausea and vomiting with pharmacological and nonpharmacological interventions.

    c. Support nutritional needs when experiencing nausea and vomiting.

5. Interventions and health teaching
    a. Nonpharmacological interventions
        i)   Avoid exposing patient to stimuli likely to produce or worsen nausea, which can precipitate vomiting and fluid loss.
        ii)   Maintain a calm and quiet environment.
        iii) Avoid moving the patient suddenly.
        iv) Encourage the patient to take deep breaths when nauseated.
        v)   Keep room well ventilated and free of strong odors.
        vi) Assist patient in rinsing and cleaning his or her mouth after each episode of vomiting.
        vii) If oral intake is not tolerated, maintain hydration by administering IV fluids and replace lost electrolytes as needed.
        viii) When oral intake is resumed, give clear fluids, such as water or ginger ale, in small amounts. If tolerated, gradually add foods such as gelatin, tea, and clear broth.
        ix) Discuss dietary changes to reduce nausea and vomiting and meet nutritional needs, such as the following: drink beverages between meals, not with meals; eat small frequent meals throughout the day; avoid foods high in fat; eat bland, dry foods such as crackers, bagels, and pretzels; and avoid acidic foods like vinaigrette salad dressing and tomatoes, and gas-producing vegetables like broccoli, cauliflower, cucumbers, green peppers, brussels sprouts, and sauerkraut.
        x)   Refer patient to a nutritionist for meal planning.
    b. Pharmacological interventions
        i)   Give antiemetics as prescribed.
        ii)   Monitor effectiveness of antiemetics.
        iii) Teach the patient and the caregiver the name, dose, frequency of use, and side effects of prescribed antiemetics.
    c. Complementary and alternative medicine (CAM)
        i)   Acupressure in Pericardium 6 acu-point has been shown to reduce chemotherapy-associated nausea and vomiting (Molassiotis, Helin, Dabbour, & Hummerston, 2007).
        ii)   Progressive muscle relaxation has been shown to reduce nausea and vomiting associated with chemotherapy (Campos de Carvalho, Martins, & dos Santos, 2007).
        iii) Cannabis has been shown to reduce nausea in people with HIV (Woolridge et al., 2005).
        iv) Ginger has been shown to reduce nausea and vomiting related to post-operative surgery (Ernst & Pittley, 2000).

6. Evaluation
    a. Assess patient's symptoms to see if they have resolved or are minimized.
    b. Evaluate patient and caregiver understanding of the appropriate use of antiemetics (e.g., dosing, administration).
    c. Evaluate patient and caregiver understanding of the appropriate use of nonpharmacologic therapies to manage nausea and vomiting.

REFERENCES

Calza, L., Manfredi, R., & Chiodo, F. (2005). Hyperlactataemia and lactic acidosis in HIV-infected patients receiving antiretroviral therapy. *Clinical Nutrition, 24*(1), 5–15.

Capili, B., & Anastasi, J. K. (1998). A symptom review: Nausea and vomiting in HIV. *Journal of the Association of Nurses in AIDS Care, 9*(6), 24–33.

Campos de Carvalho, E., Martins, F., & dos Santos, C. B. (2007). A pilot study of a relaxation technique for management of nausea and vomiting in patients receiving cancer chemotherapy. *Cancer Nursing, 30*(2), 163–167.

Ernst, E., & Pittley, M. H. (2000). Efficacy of ginger for nausea and vomiting: A systematic review of randomized clinical trials. *British Journal of Anesthesia, 84*(3), 367–371.

Etzel, J. V., Brocavich, J. M., & Torre, M. (1992). Endocrine complications associated with human immunodeficiency virus infection. *Clinical Pharmacy, 11*(8), 705–713.

Konturek, J. W., Fischer, H., Van Der Voort, I. R., & Domschke, W. (1997). Disturbed gastric motor activity in patients with human immunodeficiency virus infection. *Scandinavian Journal of Gastroenterology, 32*(3), 221–225.

Longstreth, G. F. (2006). Approach to the adult patient with nausea and vomiting. *UpToDate.* Retrieved August 7, 2007, from http://www.uptodate.com/patients/content/topic.do?topicKey=~TQcQwKoLyILd1

Molassiotis, A., Helin, A. M., Dabbour, R., & Hummerston, S. (2007). The effects of P6 acupressure in the prophylaxis of chemotherapy-related nausea and vomiting in breast cancer patients. *Complementary Therapies in Medicine, 15*(1), 3–12.

Woolridge, E., Barton, S., Samuel, J., Dougherty, A., & Holdcroft, A. (2005). Cannabis use in HIV for pain and other medical symptoms. *Journal of Pain and Symptom Management, 29*(4), 358–367.

4.12 DIARRHEA

1. Etiology
   a. Side effects of medications, including antiretroviral and broad-spectrum antibiotics (Anastasi & Capili, 2001)
   b. Diet: ingestion of undercooked food or contaminated food or water
   c. Bacterial infections: salmonella, shigella, campylobacter, *Clostridium difficile* (*C. difficile*), and *Escherichia coli* (*E. coli*)
   d. Parasites: cryptospordia, microspordia, isospora, giardia, and amoeba
   e. Invasive diseases affecting the bowel: *Mycobacterium avium* complex (MAC), cytomegalovirus (CMV), lymphoma, Kaposi's sarcoma (KS), and colon cancer
   f. Other causes: alcohol abuse, idiopathic HIV enteropathy, inadequate digestive enzymes or bile salts, lactose intolerance, low serum albumin levels, nonspecific colitis
2. Nursing assessment
   a. Subjective data
      i) Obtain current and previous history of medications, GI diseases, stage of illness, weight loss, dietary intake, and travel history.
      ii) Question patient about the pattern of diarrhea: amount, frequency, appearance, duration, and associated symptoms. Ask about precipitating events, cramping, flatus, abdominal distension, tenesmus; impact on lifestyle, quality of life, and ability to care for self.
   b. Objective data
      i) Examine patient for signs of dehydration, such as dry skin, dry tongue, decreased skin turgor, decreased urinary output, decreased blood pressure, and increased heart rate.

     ii)   Perform an abdominal assessment: Palpate for masses, observe for distension, auscultate bowel sounds, and conduct rectal examination.

     iii)   Obtain laboratory analyses: complete blood count, chemistry, C-reactive protein, erythrocyte sedimentation rate, stool analyses for fecal leukocytes, ova and parasite (three samples should be sent); culture enteric pathogens, salmonella, shigella, and campylobacter; assay for *C. difficile* and acid fast bacilli (AFB).

3. Nursing diagnosis
   a. Diarrhea related to medications, infections, bowel diseases, and other causes
   b. Fluid volume deficit related to loss of fluids through gastrointestinal tract
   c. Altered nutrition: less than body requirements due to malabsorption

4. Goals
   a. Identify and treat underlying cause(s).
   b. Reduce diarrhea with nonpharmacological interventions, medications, and alterations in diet.
   c. Prevent complications of diarrhea.

5. Interventions and health teaching
   a. Nonpharmacological interventions
       i)   Maintain hydration by encouraging oral intake and administering IV fluids.
       ii)   Replace lost electrolytes with clear liquids (e.g., sports drinks, tea, chicken broth, ginger ale) and saline IV fluids with potassium supplementation as needed.
       iii)   Maintain skin integrity by promoting the use of warm sitz baths, perineal hygiene cleaners, and soft toilet tissue.
       iv)   Discuss dietary changes to alleviate diarrhea and meet caloric needs, such as small frequent meals that are calorie dense. Avoid foods that are high in fat. Lactose, caffeine, alcohol, and spicy foods can worsen diarrhea. Encourage intake of foods that bind, e.g., bananas, plain white rice, applesauce, farina, toasted white bread, plain crackers, plain macaroni noodles, oatmeal, mashed potatoes, yogurt (Anastasi, Capili, Kim & Heitkemper, 2006).
       v)   Replace lost nutrients (e.g., fat-soluble vitamins, magnesium, potassium, and calcium).
       vi)   Refer undernourished patients to a dietitian for initiation of oral nutritional supplements.
       vii) Educate patients on food safety: wash hands before touching food; discard expired foods; thoroughly cook meat and fish; keep hot foods hot and cold foods cold; thaw frozen foods in the refrigerator, rather than on the countertop; clean all kitchen work surfaces with soap and warm water; use plastic rather than wooden cutting boards.
       viii) Encourage patients to use latex barrier condoms for oral and anal sex.
       ix)   Teach patients to avoid swimming in lakes or bodies of fresh water because they are likely contaminated with cryptosporidium.
   b. Pharmacologic interventions
       i)   Antibiotics, if bacterial etiology
           (1) *C. difficile* (Zaleznik & LaMont, 2006)
              (a) Stop offending antibiotic causing *C. difficile*.
              (b) First line: metronidazole po 500 mg three times daily or 250 mg four times daily for 10 to 14 days.

        (c) Second line: vancomycin po 125 mg four times daily for 10 to 14 days.
- (2) Salmonella (CDC, 2004)
  - (a) Ciprofloxacin po 500–750 mg twice a day for 7–14 days.
  - (b) Note: Duration of treatment for patients with CD4$^+$ T cell count less than 200 cells/mm^3 and/or with bacteremia should at least be 4–6 weeks.
- (3) Shigella (CDC, 2004)
  - (a) First line: ciprofloxacin po 500 mg twice a day for 3–7 days (duration of treatment with bacteremia is 14 days).
  - (b) Second line: TMP-SMX po double strength 1 tab twice a day for 3–7 days.
  - (c) Alternative second line: azithromycin po 500 mg on day 1, then 250 mg daily for 4 days.
  - (d) Note: Duration of treatment with bacteremia is 14 days.
- (4) Campylobacter (CDC, 2004)
  - (a) Ciprofloxacin po 500 mg twice a day for 7 days or
  - (b) Azithromycin po 500 mg once daily for 7 days
  - (c) Note: for mild disease may consider withholding therapy unless symptoms persist for several days. Duration of treatment with bacteremia is 14 days.
- (5) *E. coli* (Wanke, 2007)
  - (a) Ciprofloxacin po 500 mg twice a day for 3 days (use for enterotoxigenic *E. coli*. For *E. coli* 0157:H7, avoid antibiotics).

ii) Antidiarrheal agents include opioid preparations (e.g., opium tincture, paregoric) and absorbents (e.g., attapulgite).

iii) Other agent: Mesalamine has been shown to reduce chronic diarrhea and nonspecific colitis in HIV (Rodriguez-Torres et al., 2006).

iv) Antispasmodic agents can be used to treat abdominal cramps.

v) Pancreatic digestive enzymes are used for malabsorption.

c. Complementary alternative medicine (CAM)

i) Acupuncture and moxibustion have been shown to reduce the stool frequency and improve the stool consistency of chronic diarrhea in HIV (Anastasi & McMahon, 2003).

ii) SP-303, a proanthocyanidin oligomer that has been isolated from the plant family *Euphorbiaceae,* may be helpful in reducing diarrhea in HIV (Holodniy et al., 1999).

iii) L-Glutamine supplementation has been shown to improve protease inhibitor–associated diarrhea (Huffman, 2003).

6. Evaluation

a. Patient will show a reduction in the frequency and improvement in the consistency of stool.

b. Patient will show normalization of fluid and electrolyte balance and regain lost weight.

c. Patient will improve level of functional status.

REFERENCES

Anastasi, J. K., & Capili, B. (2001). HIV-related diarrhea and outcome measures. *Journal of Association of Nurses in AIDS Care, 12*(Suppl.), 44–50.

Anastasi, J. K., Capili, B., Kim, G., & Heitkemper, M. (2006). A randomized, controlled trial using a nutrition intervention to manage chronic diarrhea in patients with HIV/AIDS. *Journal for the Association for Nurses in AIDS Care, 17*(2), 47–57.

Anastasi, J., & McMahon, D. (2003). Testing strategies to reduce diarrhea using traditional Chinese medicine: Acupuncture and moxibustion. *Journal for the Association for Nurses in AIDS Care, 14*(3), 28–40.

Centers for Disease Control and Prevention (CDC). (2004). Treating opportunistic infections among HIV-infected adults and adolescents: Recommendations from CDC, the National Institutes of Health, and the HIV Medicine Association/Infectious Diseases Society of America. *Morbidity and Mortality Weekly Report, 53*(RR15), 1–112.

Holodniy, M., Koch, J., Mistal, M., Schmidt, J. M., Khandwala, A., Pennington, J. E., et al. (1999). A double blind, randomized, placebo-controlled phase II study to assess the safety and efficacy of orally administered SP-303 for the symptomatic treatment of diarrhea in patients with AIDS. *American Journal of Gastroenterology, 94*(11), 3267–3273.

Huffman, F. G., & Walgreen, M. E. (2003). L-Glutamine supplementation improves nelfinavir-associated diarrhea in HIV-infected individuals. *HIV Clinical Trials, 4*(5), 324–329.

Rodriguez-Torres, M., Rodriguez-Orengo, J. F., Rios-Bedoya, C. F., Fernandez-Carbia, A., Salgado-Mercado, R., & Marxuach, A. M. (2006). Double-blind pilot study of mesalamine vs. placebo for treatment of chronic diarrhea and nonspecific colitis in immunocompetent HIV patients. *Digestive Diseases and Sciences, 51*(1), 161–167.

Wanke, C.A. (2007). Diarrheagenic *Escherichia coli*. *UpToDate*. Retrieved August 3, 2007, from http://www.uptodate.com/patients/content/topic.do?topicKey=~c0LDfpA.sxNxR0

Zaleznik, D. F., & LaMont, J. T. (2006). Treatment of antibiotic-associated diarrhea caused by *Clostridium difficile*. *UpToDate*. Retrieved August 3, 2007, from http://www.uptodate.com/home/content/topic.do?topicKey=gi_infec/2874

4.13 PAIN

1. Etiology
   a. Gastrointestinal
      i) Oropharynx/esophageal: fungal infections (e.g., candidiasis, histoplasmosis), aphthous ulcerations, intraoral KS, dental abscesses, necrotizing gingivitis, herpes simplex, CMV ulcers, streptococcal infection, gastric reflux disorders
      ii) Abdominal: CMV colitis/ileitis, intestinal infections (e.g., cryptosporidia, shigella, salmonella, campylobacter, MAC, giardia lamblia, isospora bellis, entameba histolytica, cryptococcus, *Clostridium difficile*), HIV enteropathy/colitis, lymphoma, KS, pelvic inflammatory disease, and cholecystitis related to gallstones; pancreatitis related to IV pentamadine, ddI, ddC, CMV, alcohol, and toxoplasmosis; and peritonitis, ectopic pregnancy, appendicitis, perforated ulcer, ileus, and uterine fibroids
      iii) Anorectal: perirectal abscess or fistula; herpes simplex ulcers; anorectal carcinoma; hemorrhoids; foreign object; and proctitis related to herpes, CMV, *C. trachomatus,* or *N. gonorrhea*
   b. Genito-urinary: herpes simplex virus, epididymitis, cystitis, bartholinitis, and renal calculi
   c. Neurological: headaches; CNS toxoplasmosis; meningitis related to *cryptococcus,* syphilis, histoplasmosis, and *M. tuberculosis;* aseptic meningitis; CNS nocardia; herpes encephalopathy; progressive multifocal leukoencephalopathy; sinus infections; migraine; stress/tension; neuropathy; spinal/epidural abscess; spinal MAC; and lymphoma
   d. Dermatological: herpes zoster, postherpetic neuralgia, bacterial abscess, and bulky cutaneous KS
   e. Musculoskeletal: arthropathy; HIV-related arthralgia, hepatitis C-related arthralgia, or both; psoriatic-related arthritis; avascular necrosis associated with smoking, steroids, trauma, antiretrovirals, dyslipidemia, megace, and pancreatitis; myopathy; and fractures secondary to osteopenia/osteoporosis, osteoarthritis, degenerative disc disease, radiculopathy

f. Cardiovascular: pericarditis related to toxoplasmosis, CMV, *mycobacteria,* nocardiosis, Kaposi's sarcoma, lymphoma, herpes simplex, or *cryptococcus;* endocarditis related to *staphylococcus aureus* or nonbacterial thrombosis; angina pectoris related to dyslipidemia; and peripheral vascular disease

g. Pulmonary: infections related to PCP, bacteria, *histoplasmosis, aspergillosis, mycobacterium tuberculosis;* costal chondritis; PIP; emboli; and post-thoracotomy pain syndrome

2. Nursing assessment
   a. Subjective
      i)   Onset and duration, location, character (e.g., burning, sharp, dull), intensity, exacerbating and relieving factors, response to current and past treatments, cultural responses, and meaning of pain to the patient
   b. Objective
      i)   Numerical scale: 0–10 scale (0 = *no pain,* 10 = *worst imaginable*)
      ii) Verbal scale (*none, small, mild, moderate, severe*)
      iii) Pediatric faces pain scale (useful when the verbal skills are inadequate)
      iv) Nonverbal pain rating scales

3. Nursing diagnosis
   a. Alteration in comfort

4. Goals
   a. Achieve optimal level of patient comfort and functioning with the fewest medication-related side effects
   b. Achieve optimal level of patient comfort via the least invasive route
   c. Prevent pain

5. Interventions and health teaching
   a. Nonpharmacological
      i)   The nurse individualizes each patient's pain regimen.
      ii)   Relaxation techniques, imagery, biofeedback, hypnosis, massage, vibration, reflexology, acupressure, gentle stretches, and meditation may be helpful as adjunctive therapy.
      iii) Thermal modalities should be used as tolerated.
      iv)   Some patients may benefit from prayer.
      v)   Rhythmic breathing may be beneficial.
      vi)   Ultrasound, physical therapy, and TENS may be helpful.
      vii) Radiation therapy can be used for cancer-related pain (bulky KS, bone metastasis).
      viii) Recommend smoking cessation: Smoking has been found to decrease serum opiate levels, increase analgesia needs, and decrease pain tolerance (Creekmore et al., 2004; Ackerman & Ahmad, 2007).
      ix)   Those patients on methadone maintenance will need additional analgesia for their pain. Close supervision is required to monitor for and intervene as needed for aberrant behavior patterns.
   b. Pharmacological: World Health Organization analgesic guidelines (WHO, 2006)
      i)   Step 1: Nonopiate with or without adjuvants
         (1) Acetaminophen has no effect on platelet function or gastric mucosa and provides no anti-inflammatory effect; avoid use with hepatic insufficiency.

  (2) Nonsteroidal anti-inflammatory agents (NSAIDs): switch to an NSAID from a different class if sufficient analgesia is not obtained with one NSAID.

    (a) Salsalate and tolmetin produce less inhibition of platelet aggregation than other NSAIDs except for COX-2 inhibitors.

    (b) COX-2 inhibitors should be avoided with ACE inhibitors or diuretics.

    (c) Avoid celecoxib with sulfonamide-derived medications.

    (d) Use for throbbing, aching pain.

  (3) Tramadol

    (a) Centrally acting nonopiate

    (b) Can be combined with NSAIDs.

    (c) Available alone or with acetaminophen; available in long-acting or quick disintegrating form

    (d) Avoid with SSRIs and MAOIs to prevent serotonin syndrome.

    (e) Avoid in persons with seizure history.

ii) Step 2: Mild opiates with or without nonopiates with or without adjuvants

  (1) Use caution when using opiates in persons with asthma, increased ICP, and hepatic failure; assess need for bowel regimen to avoid constipation.

  (2) Maximum dose of combination agents is limited to ceiling dose of the nonopiate (usually acetaminophen or aspirin) and all are short-acting (3–4 hours).

  (3) Meperidine and propoxyphene are not recommended due to poor efficacy and accumulation of toxic metabolites.

  (4) Hydrocodone

    (a) Ritonavir, nelfinavir, indinavir, or saquinavir may increase hydrocodone levels

    (b) Neurotoxicity has been reported—monitor for hearing loss

    (c) Available in combination with ibuprofen or acetaminophen

  (5) Codeine

    (a) Ritonavir or nelfinavir may increase metabolism of codeine

    (b) Avoid with indinavir, which may interfere with codeine metabolism leading to poor pain relief.

iii) Adjuvants

  (1) Add at any step of analgesic ladder.

  (2) NSAIDs will provide additive effects to opiates, increasing duration.

  (3) Corticosteroids

    (a) Use in treating aphthous ulcers and cerebral edema.

    (b) Use with caution in persons with cavitary infections, bullous lung disease, renal insufficiency, and thrombocytopenia; can worsen osteoporosis with prolonged use.

  (4) Antidepressants (e.g., amitriptyline, doxepin, desipramine) can boost efficacy of opiates.

  (5) Provide independent analgesia for neuropathy and postherpetic neuralgia.

  (6) Anticonvulsants (e.g., gabapentin, lamotrigine; pregabalin) can be helpful in neuropathic pain and postherpetic neuralgia but may cause peripheral edema and weight gain; avoid carbamazepine due to neutropenia and thrombocytopenia.

       (7) Antihistamines (e.g., hydroxyzine) provide additive analgesia, anxiolytic, and antiemetic effect.

       (8) Caffeine increases opiate effect.

       (9) Topicals (e.g., lidocaine patch, lidocaine gel, capsaicin ointment, mentholated creams, compounded formulations)

          (a) Remove lidocaine patch every 12 hours.

          (b) Capsaicin ointment must be used qid and can cause initial burning; wear gloves during application to avoid contact with mucous membranes.

iv)   Step 3: Strong opiates with or without adjuvants

       (1) Morphine sulfate (MS)

          (a) MS available in immediate release (4 hours) and continuous release (8–12 hours; 24 hours)

          (b) Do not crush or break the long-acting pill; encourage high fluid intake to activate release of continuous release drug. Continuous-release sprinkle form can be used for patients with dysphagia.

          (c) Continuous-release MS may not be released in malabsorptive states.

          (d) Equianalgesic dose: 10 mg/SC = 20–30 mg po.

          (e) MS may increase zidovudine levels; ritonavir or nelfinavir may increase MS metabolism requiring dose or interval adjustment.

       (2) Hydromorphone

          (a) Immediate release only (3–4 hours)

          (b) Equianalgesic dose: 2 mg IM/SC = 4 mg po

       (3) Oxymorphone

          (a) Immediate release (4–6 hours); continuous release (12 hours)

          (b) Administer on empty stomach, 1h ac or 2 h pc.

          (c) Co-ingestion with alcohol can lead to fatal overdose.

       (4) Dolophine

          (a) Length of action: 6–8 hours

          (b) Can accumulate with repetitive dosing.

          (c) Phenytoin, abacavir, efavirenz, lopinavir/ritonavir combination, and nevirapine: lower dolophine levels

       (5) Meperidine

          (a) Meperidine is not recommended for use > 3 days.

          (b) Length of action is 2–3 hours.

          (c) Oral form is not recommended.

          (d) Toxic metabolites accumulate at doses > 300mg/day, leading to tremors and seizures.

          (e) Meperidine 100 mg IM equals morphine 10 mg IM.

          (f) Avoid use with ritonavir.

       (6) Fentanyl

          (a) Continuous release transdermal patch for chronic pain

             (i)   Place patch on intact, nonirritated skin.

             (ii) Fever or external heat source will increase release from patch, so monitor for sedation and decreased duration of analgesia.

(iii) Avoid use with ritonavir.

(b) Immediate release forms: submucosal lollipop, effervescent buccal tablets; use for breakthrough pain, acute pain, or both; patient should not chew lollipop.

(7) Oxycodone

(a) Available in immediate release (3–4 hours) and continuous release (8–12 hours)

(b) Available with and without acetaminophen

(c) Ritonavir, nelfinavir, indinavir, or saquinavir may increase oxycodone levels.

c. Alternative/complementary therapies

i) Aromatherapy

ii) Therapeutic touch/Reiki

iii) Movement therapy: yoga, stretching, Feldenkrais, Trager, tai chi

iv) Magnets: avoid in pregnancy due to a lack of safety data in this population.

v) Acupuncture

vi) Homeopathy

vii) Nutritional supplements (Carnitor, alpha lipoic acid, vitamin B complex): for neuropathic pain

6. Evaluation

a. Evaluate the response to the plan continually; change the drug, interval, dose, route, or modality as needed; and treat side effects.

b. Evaluate for sequelae of undermanaged pain.

i) Physical effects: difficulty sleeping, poor appetite, decreased mobility, shallow breathing, and suppression of immune system

ii) Psychological effects: anxiety/fear, depression, reduced quality of life, difficulty concentrating and suicidal ideation

iii) Social effects: impaired relationships and increased stress on friends/caregivers

iv) Spiritual effects: human suffering and hopelessness

REFERENCES

Ackerman, W., & Ahmad, M. (2007). Effect of cigarette smoking on serum hydrocodone levels in chronic pain patients. *Journal of Arkansas Medical Society, 104*(1), 19–21.

Creekmore, F., Lugo, R., & Weiland, K. (2004). Postoperative opiate analgesic requirements of smokers and nonsmokers. *Annals of Pharmacotherapy, 38*(6), 949–953.

World Health Organization (WHO). (2006). *Cancer pain release, 19*(1). Retrieved November 3, 2007, from http://whocancerpain.bcg.wisc.edu/index?q=node/15

4.14 FEMALE SEXUAL DYSFUNCTION

1. Etiology

a. Organic causes include vascular disease; neurological disease; hormonal/endocrine disorders; musculogenic, pelvic, or perineal surgery; trauma to pelvis or spine; pelvic anomalies or disease.

    b. Psychological causes of sexual dysfunction may be related to underlying psychiatric disorders, such as anxiety disorder, major depression, or panic disorder. Related issues such as low self-esteem, negative feelings about body image and quality of relationship with partner, and sociocultural influences such as religious background or definition of sex role may also impact sexuality.

    c. Dysfunction may also be caused by the secondary effects of medications: antihypertensives, chemotherapeutics, anticholinergics, anticonvulsants, antidepressants, antipsychotics, narcotics, sedatives/anxiolytics, antiandrogens, antiestrogens, birth control pills.

2. Nursing assessment: Sexuality is a complex issue that often is ignored by healthcare professionals. Nurses must be open to discussing these important issues with patients.

    a. Subjective data: Starting with a general question, presented in a nonthreatening manner, gives the patient permission to ask further questions. Begin with a question such as, "Many women have concerns and questions about sex. What questions do you have?" A more direct approach is, "How has this illness affected your sex life?"

    b. Objective data

      i) Evaluation of sexual dysfunction includes a thorough physical examination, including a pelvic examination, psychological and psychosocial assessment, and laboratory or hormonal studies, as indicated. The purpose of the examination is detection of dysfunction or disease. The examination also provides an opportunity to educate the patient about normal anatomy and sexual function. The suggested hormonal profile includes follicle-stimulating hormone, luteinizing hormone, prolactin, total and free testosterone levels, sex hormone-binding globulin, and estradiol levels.

      ii) Tools such as the Female Sexual Function Index (FSFI) can facilitate this discussion (see http://www.FSFIquestionnaire.com). The FSFI is a brief, reliable, and valid self-report measure of female sexual function. The tool evaluates the following areas of sexual functioning: desire and subjective arousal, lubrication, orgasm, satisfaction, and pain/discomfort (Bayer, Zonagen, Inc., & Target Health, Inc., 2000).

    c. Nursing diagnosis: altered sexual pattern

    d. Goal: Improved sexual functioning

    e. Interventions and health teaching

      i) Nonpharmacological interventions (Phillips, 2000)

        (1) Provide education about normal anatomy, sexual function, and normal changes with aging, pregnancy, and menopause.

        (2) Enhance stimulation and eliminate routine by encouraging use of erotic materials, masturbation, communication during sexual activity, use of vibrators, and varying positions, times of day, or places for sexual activity. Suggest patient make a date for sexual activity.

        (3) Provide distraction techniques by encouraging erotic or nonerotic fantasy, pelvic muscle contraction and relaxation exercises with intercourse, and use of background music, videos, or television.

        (4) Encourage noncoital behaviors, such as sensual massage, sensate-focus exercises that involve use of sensual massage without involvement of sexual areas of the body, and oral or noncoital stimulation, with or without orgasm.

(5) Minimize dyspareunia by superficial methods, such as female astride for control of penetration and to minimize deep thrusting, topical lidocaine, warm baths before intercourse, biofeedback, and use of nonsteroidal antiinflammatory agents before intercourse.

(6) A clitoral therapy device, also known as Eros-CTD, device fits over the clitoris and increases blood flow by a gentle suction action (http://www.eros-therapy.com).

(7) A topical massage oil, marketed under the name of Zestra, showed promising results in a phase 3 study (completed in March 2007) for women with acquired mixed interest/desire/arousal/orgasm disorders (http://www.zestra.com).

ii) Pharmacological interventions: Aside from hormone replacement therapy, pharmacologic management of female sexual dysfunction is in the early experimental stages. Most of the medications have been used in the treatment of male erectile dysfunction and are still in experimental stages for use in women. Pharmacological interventions currently include the following:

(1) Estrogen replacement therapy can be used by menopausal women.

(2) Methyl testosterone can be used in combination with estrogen in menopausal women for symptoms of inhibited desire, dyspareunia, or lack of vaginal lubrication.

(3) Sildenafil is a selective type V phosphodiesterase inhibitor that promotes relaxation of clitoral and vaginal smooth muscle.

(4) L-arginine is an amino acid that mediates relaxation of vascular and nonvascular smooth muscle. It has not been used in clinical trials with women, but studies in men have yielded promising results.

(5) Prostaglandin E1 delivered intravaginally is currently under investigation for use in women. In phase 2 trials as a transdermal cream for the treatment of Female Sexual Arousal Disorder, it has shown benefits for arousal success rates and other subjective measures of sexual arousal, but needs further study (Kielbasa & Daniel, 2006).

(6) Phentolamine in oral form causes vascular smooth muscle relaxation. A pilot study in menopausal women showed enhanced vaginal blood flow and improved subjective arousal.

(7) Apomorphine facilitates erectile response in men and is being examined for use in women.

(8) Tibolone is a synthetic steroid with estrogenic, androgenic, and progestagenic properties. Binding to estrogen receptors in bone is associated with decreased bone turnover and improved bone density, whereas binding to receptors in the vagina is associated with improved vaginal dryness and reduced dyspareunia. Binding to endometrial progesterone receptors is associated with bleeding, thus it is recommended only for patients who are at least 1 year postmenopausal. Impact on androgen receptors in the brain that are involved in libido are unclear. Effect on lipids and hemostasis related to effects on androgen receptors in the liver is also unclear (Modelska & Cummings, 2002).

iii) Alternative/complementary therapies

(1) Empirical data regarding the use of alternative/complementary therapies is limited.

(2) Yohimbine bark (Yohimbehe cortex) has been used as an aphrodisiac. It is thought to act as an alpha-adrenergic blocker. Contraindications include existing liver and kidney disease as well as chronic inflammation of the sexual organs (Blumenthal, 1998, 2000).

(3) Ginkgo biloba leaf extract (Ginkgo folium) has been used to treat patients with antidepressant-induced sexual dysfunction, especially related to the use of selective serotonin reuptake inhibitors (SSRIs). Studies showed women were more responsive to the sexually enhancing effects than men. It has been reported to have a positive effect on all four phases of the sexual response cycle: desire, excitement, orgasm, and resolution. It is thought that Gingko biloba leaf extract works by inhibiting platelet activation factor (PAF), which affects prostaglandins and enhances erectile function. Some researchers believe it has some type of norepinephrine receptor–induced effects on the brain. Contraindications include a noted hypersensitivity to gingko preparations (Blumenthal, 1998, 2000).

(4) Damiana leaf and herb (*Turnera diffusa*) has been used as an aphrodisiac and for prophylaxis and treatment of sexual disturbances. Little is known about the mechanism of action, as well as any contraindications (Blumenthal, 1998).

(5) Muira puama (*Ptychopetali lignum*) is used for prevention of sexual disorders, as well as an aphrodisiac. The mechanism of action and contraindications are poorly understood (Blumenthal, 1998).

  f. Evaluation
    i) Patient will be able to discuss cause of sexual dysfunction.
    ii) Patient will discuss alternative, satisfying, and acceptable sexual practices for self and partner.

REFERENCES

Bayer, A. G., Zonagen, Inc., & Target Health, Inc. (2000). *Female Sexual Function Index (FSFI)*. Retrieved December 19, 2002, from http://www.FSFIquestionnaire.com

Blumenthal, M. (Ed.). (1998). *The complete German Commission E monographs: Therapeutic guide to herbal medicines*. Boston: American Botanical Council.

Blumenthal, M. (Ed.). (2000). *Herbal medicine: Expanded Commission E monographs*. Newton, MA: Integrative Medicine Communications.

Kielbasa, L. A., & Daniel, K. L. (2006). Topical Alprostadil treatment of female sexual arousal disorder. *The Annals of Pharmacotherapy, 40*(7), 1369–1376.

Modelska, K., & Cummings, S. (2002). Tibolone for postmenopausal women: Systematic review of randomized trials. *Journal of Clinical Endocrinology & Metabolism, 87*(1), 16–23.

Phillips, N. A. (2000). Female sexual dysfunction: Evaluation and treatment. *American Family Physician, 62*(1), 127–136, 141–142.

4.15 MALE SEXUAL DYSFUNCTION

1. Etiology
  a. Premature ejaculation: primarily psychogenic

b. Erectile dysfunction
   i) Organic causes include vascular disease, neurological disease, endocrine disorders, renal failure, liver disease, malignancies, pelvic or perineal surgeries, trauma to pelvis or spine, penile anomalies or disease, drug abuse, and cigarette smoking.
   ii) Secondary causes of sexual dysfunction may be related to underlying psychiatric disorders, such as anxiety disorder, major depression, or panic disorder.
   iii) Dysfunction may also be caused by secondary effects of medications: antihypertensives, antidepressants, antiarrhythmics, antihyperlipidemics, antipsychotics, anticonvulsants, antiandrogens, histamine H2 receptor antagonists, narcotics, nonsteroidal anti-inflammatories, antimanics, cytotoxic medications, and ketoconazoles.

2. Nursing assessment
   a. Subjective data: Starting with a general question, presented in a nonthreatening manner, gives the patient permission to ask further questions. Begin with a question such as, "Many men have concerns and questions about sex. What questions do you have?" A more direct approach is, "How has this illness affected your sex life?"
   b. Objective data: Evaluation of sexual dysfunction includes a thorough physical examination, psychological and psychosocial assessment, and laboratory or hormonal studies, as indicated. The purpose of the examination is detection of dysfunction or disease. The examination also provides an opportunity to educate the patient about normal anatomy and sexual function. Diagnostic studies for erectile dysfunction include blood pressure, fasting blood glucose, total low-density and high-density lipoprotein cholesterol and triglycerides, luteinizing hormone and prolactin (measure of bioavailable testosterone), and thyroid studies.
   c. Nursing diagnosis: altered sexual pattern
   d. Goal: improved sexual functioning
   e. Interventions and health teaching
      i) Nonpharmacological interventions
         (1) Premature ejaculation
            (a) Psychotherapy (Holmes, 2000)
            (b) Couples counseling to improve communication skills
            (c) Behaviorally oriented psychotherapy
         (2) Erectile dysfunction: Advise patient to curtail or eliminate smoking, alcohol, caffeine, and drug abuse.
      ii) Pharmacological/treatment interventions
         (1) Premature ejaculation: low doses of clomipramine, sertraline, or Paroxetine to increase ejaculatory latency (Epperly & Moore, 2000; Holmes, 2000).
         (2) Erectile dysfunction: A stepped approach to the treatment of erectile dysfunction allows the primary caregiver to intervene with patients in Steps 1 and 2, based on a general assessment, before pursuing a urologic referral needed for interventions in Steps 3 and 4 (Epperly & Moore, 2000).
            (a) Oral agents such as sildenafil, L-arginine (investigational), or testosterone if hypogondal (Korenman, 1998)
            (b) Vacuum or constriction devices
            (c) Urethral therapies
               (i) Intracavernosal injections of prostaglandin E, paperverine, or phentolamine

        (ii)   Intraurethral insertion of prostaglandin E

    (d) Penile surgery

        (i)   Penile prostheses

        (ii) Penile vascular surgery

iii) Alternative/complementary therapies

    (1) Empirical data regarding the use of alternative/complementary therapies are limited.

    (2) Yohimbine bark (Yohimbehe cortex) has been used as an aphrodisiac. It is thought to act as an alpha-adrenergic blocker. Contraindications include existing liver and kidney disease, as well as chronic inflammation of the sexual organs (Blumenthal, 1998, 2000).

    (3) Ginkgo biloba leaf extract (Ginkgo folium) has been used to treat patients with antidepressant-induced sexual dysfunction especially related to the use of SSRIs. Although it is reported that women are more responsive to the sex-enhancing effects than men, it has been used successfully with men. It has been reported to have a positive effect on all four phases of the sexual response cycle: desire, excitement, orgasm, and resolution. It is thought that Gingko biloba leaf extract works by inhibiting PAF, which affects prostaglandins and enhances erectile function. It may also have effects on norepinephrine receptors in the brain. Contraindications include a noted hypersensitivity to gingko preparations (Blumenthal, 1998, 2000).

    (4) Ginseng root (*Ginseng radix*) has been used to treat erectile dysfunction. The mechanism of action is not understood. Hypertension is a contraindication for the use of ginseng (Blumenthal, 1998).

    (5) Damiana leaf and herb (*Turnera diffusa*) has been used as an aphrodisiac and for prophylaxis and treatment of sexual disturbances. Little is understood about the mechanism of action, as well as any contraindications (Blumenthal, 1998).

    (6) Muira puama (*Ptychopetali lignum*) is used for prevention of sexual disorders, as well as an aphrodisiac. The mechanism of action and contraindications are poorly understood (Blumenthal, 1998).

f. Evaluation

    i)   Patient will be able to discuss cause of sexual dysfunction.

    ii) Patient will discuss alternative, satisfying, and acceptable sexual practices for self and partner.

REFERENCES

Blumenthal, M. (Ed.). (1998). *The complete German Commission E monographs: Therapeutic guide to herbal medicines.* Boston: American Botanical Council.

Blumenthal, M. (Ed.). (2000). *Herbal medicine: Expanded Commission E monographs.* Newton, MA: Integrative Medicine Communications.

Epperly, T. D., & Moore, K. E. (2000). Health issues in men: Part 1. Common genitourinary disorders. *American Family Physician, 61*(12), 3657–3664.

Holmes, S. (2000). Treatment of male sexual dysfunction. *British Medical Bulletin, 56*(3), 798–808.

Korenman, S. G. (1998). New insights into erectile dysfunction: A practical approach. *American Journal of Medicine, 105*(2), 135–144.

4.16 VISION LOSS/VISUAL IMPAIRMENT

1. Etiology
   a. Vision loss is characterized by a change in the amount or patterning of incoming visual stimuli accompanied by diminished, exaggerated, distorted, or impaired interpretation (NANDA, 1996).
      i) The physiology of vision loss is predicated on the eye structures that do not undergo biological renewal. Anterior structures such as the optical lenses are formed during embryological development and are never replaced. Posterior structures such as the retina are a form of neural tissue, with no mitotic activity (Junqueira & Carneiro, 2005). Once damaged, scar tissue forms.
   b. Visual impairment from an opportunistic infection may be due to primary or secondary involvement; it may evolve from the anterior or posterior portion of the eye or the ocular adnexa (Cunningham, 1999).
   c. Anterior involvement (i.e., the cornea, anterior chamber, and iris) originates from tumors, external eye infections, and HIV-related opportunistic infections (Ahmed, Ai, & Luckie, 1999; Cunningham, 1999; Markomichelakis et al., 2002).
   d. Posterior involvement (i.e., the retina, choroids, and optic nerve head) originates predominantly from HIV-associated retinopathy and HIV-related opportunistic infections (Ahmed et al., 1999; Cunningham, 1999).
   e. The adnexa (i.e., eyelids, conjunctiva, and lacrimal drainage system) are susceptible to herpes simplex virus (HSV) infection and Kaposi's sarcoma (KS).
   f. Pharmacological therapies may contribute to vision loss or impairment (Cunningham, 2000; Kempen et al., 2003).
      i) Highly active antiretroviral therapy (HAART) has reduced the rate of visual impairment and loss among patients with posterior involvement by cytomegalovirus (CMV) retinitis and retinitis-related retinal detachment (Thorne, Jabs, Kempen, Holbrook, Nichols, & Meinert, 2006).
      ii) Successful immune recovery with HAART therapy may increase the inflammatory process and increase the risk of immune recovery uveitis (IRU), with cataract development and cystoid macular edema (CME; Robinson, Reed, Csaky, Polis, & Whitcup, 2000; Thorne, 2003).
      iii) IRU can be treated with anti-inflammatory drugs, such as NSAIDS, similar to other forms of ocular inflammatory disease (Thorne, 2003). The routine use of corticosteroid therapy is being studied.
   g. Nutritional deficiencies (e.g., vitamin A, B-complex vitamins) may cause or exacerbate vision loss or impairment (Eperjesi & Beatty, 2006).
2. Nursing assessment
   a. Subjective data
      i) Impact of visual loss on mood, self-concept, relationships: visual quality of life assessment tool (VisQOL; Misajon et al., 2005)

ii) Reported symptoms: decreased visual acuity, floaters, light flashes, blurred vision, pain, dryness, redness, swelling, discharge

iii) Reported date of last ophthalmic/fundoscopic examination

iv) Ability to manage activities of daily living and changes in self-care behaviors

v) Availability of social support and supportive services

vi) Emotional responses to changes in visual acuity

vii) Increased falls or injuries

b. Objective data

   i) Unilateral or bilateral field loss; initially, involvement is usually unilateral but becomes bilateral if underlying pathology is left untreated

   ii) Decreased visual acuity on examination: eye chart test (Snellen, Allen, LH test, HOTV test, Amsler grid, or Teich Target; Dew & Riley, 1998; Tingley, 2007); ability to read printed materials (determine literacy level before diagnosing a loss of visual acuity)

   iii) Visual field testing: peripheral or central vision loss

   iv) Observed photosensitivity

3. Nursing diagnosis

   a. Altered role performance

   b. Impaired home maintenance management

   c. Sensory or perceptual alterations (visual)

   d. Potential for self-care deficit

   e. Risk for loneliness

   f. Risk for injury

4. Goals

   a. Prevent visual impairment or loss via early detection and treatment.

   b. Promote the patient's safety and autonomy.

   c. Support the patient's adaptation to visual impairment or loss.

5. Interventions and health teaching

   a. Nonpharmacological

      i) Provide symptomatic relief using appropriate pain control techniques (e.g., cool compresses, eye drops, avoidance of bright lights).

      ii) Educate the patient, family, and significant other.

         (1) Advise patient that a sudden change/decrease in visual acuity constitutes an ophthalmic emergency in an HIV-infected individual. The individual should seek immediate medical attention to prevent additional vision loss.

         (2) Advise patient to have regular fundoscopic exams from a competent practitioner, especially if CD4+ T lymphocyte count < 50 cells/mm^3.

         (3) Refer patient to services for individuals with visual impairment or blindness for assistance in modifying home environment to maintain safety and promote independence (e.g., orientation and mobility training, sighted guide technique, magnification devices, books on tape, adaptive telecommunications equipment; occupational therapists may provide additional assistance with adaptive devices/technologies and home modifications for visual impairment).

        (4) To avoid patient disorientation and injury, remind caregivers not to move furniture or rearrange patient's belongings without the patient's consent.

        (5) Allow for verbalization of feelings (from both HIV-positive person and significant others) regarding visual impairment or vision loss.

        (6) Facilitate necessary community referrals to maintain a safe and adequate environment (e.g., Meals on Wheels, nutritional counseling, home health, paratransit services, individual counseling/support groups, crisis intervention services).

   iii) Pharmacological

        (1) Administer or instruct patient or caregiver regarding administration of prescribed eye medications, schedules for medications, and side effects. Modify medication taking to promote independence and safety.

        (2) When receiving intravenous medications for vision-related problems (e.g., cidofovir), instruct patient or caregiver in correct technique for managing venous access devices (e.g., flushing, site/dressing changes).

        (3) For medication side effects impairing vision, clarify with the primary care provider if alternative treatments are possible.

6. Complementary and alternative medicine (CAM) and therapies
   a. Stress reduction techniques: Guided imagery, relaxation, and mindfulness-based stress reduction (MSBR) approaches may reduce fear, enhance feelings of control, improve immune function, and limit the side-effect experiences of antiretroviral HIV therapies (Johnson, 2007).
   b. Herbal therapies include anxiety-reducing herbs, such as valerian, ashwagandha, chamomile, and passion flower (Bascom, 2002). Bilberry and eyebright are used to increase visual acuity. Goldenseal eyewashes are helpful in treating eye infections (Fetrow & Avila, 1999).
   c. Dietary modification therapies, including the use of lutein and zeaxanthin, have been proposed as means of preventing age-related declines in macular health (Stringham & Hammond, 2005).
   d. Acupuncture therapy as a modality for treatment of chronic disease may result in improvements in physiological and psychological coping (Paterson & Britten, 2003).
7. Evaluation
   a. Safety of physical environment
   b. Adaptation to visual impairment
   c. Progression of visual loss

REFERENCES

Ahmed, I., Ai, E., & Luckie, A. (1999). Ophthalmic manifestations of HIV infection. In P. T. Cohen, M. A. Sande, & P. A. Volderding (Eds.), *The AIDS knowledge base* (3rd ed., pp. 543–557). Philadelphia: Lippincott Williams & Wilkins.

Bascom, A. (2002). *Incorporating herbal medicine into clinical practice.* Philadelphia: F. A. Davis.

Cunningham, E. T., Jr. (1999). Ocular complications of HIV infection. In M. A. Sande & P. A. Volberding (Eds.), *The medical management of AIDS* (6th ed., pp. 171–184). Philadelphia: W. B. Saunders.

Cunningham, E. T., Jr. (2000). Uveitis in HIV positive patients. *British Journal of Opthalmology, 84*(3), 233–237.

Dew, T., & Riley, T. A. (1998). Visual changes. In M. E. Ropka & A. B. Williams (Eds.), *HIV: Nursing and symptom management* (pp. 484–492). Sudbury, MA: Jones and Bartlett.

Eperjesi, F., & Beatty, S. (2006). *Nutrition and the eye: A practical approach.* Philadelphia: Butterworth Heinemann Elsevier.

Fetrow, C. W., & Avila, J. R. (1999). *Complementary and alternative medicines.* Philadelphia: Springhouse.

Johnson, M. O. (2007). *A mindfulness based approach to HIV treatment side effects.* National Center for Complementary and Alternative Medicine. ClinicalTrials.gov #NCT 00312936. Retrieved November 17, 2007, from http://clinicaltrials.gov/ct2/show?term=mindfulness+based+approach+to+hiv&rank=1

Junqueria, L. C., & Carneiro, J. (2005) *Basic histology* (11th ed.). New York: McGraw-Hill.

Kempen, J. H., Martin, B. K., Wu, A. W., Barron, B., Thorne, J. E., & Jabs, D. (2003). The effect of cytomegalovirus retinitis on the quality of life of patients with AIDS in the era of highly active antiretroviral therapy. *Ophthalmology, 110*(5), 987–995.

Markomichelakis, N. N., Canakis, C., Zafirakis, P., Marakis, T., Mallias, I., & Theodossiadis, G. (2002). Cytomegalovirus as a cause of anterior uveitis with sectoral iris atrophy. *Ophthalmology, 109*(5), 879–882.

Misajon, R., Hawthorne, G., Richardson, J., Barton, J., Peacock, S., Iezzi, A., et al. (2005). Vision and quality of life: The development of a utility measure. *Investigative Ophthalmology & Visual Science, 46*(11) 4007–4015.

North American Nursing Diagnosis Association (NANDA). (1996). *NANDA nursing diagnoses: Definitions and classification 1997–1998.* Philadelphia: Author.

Paterson, C., & Britten, N. (2003). Acupuncture for people with chronic illness: Combining qualitative and quantitative outcome assessment. *Journal of Alternative and Complementary Medicine, 9*(3), 671–681.

Robinson, M. R., Reed, G., Csaky, K. G., Polis, M. A., & Whitcup, S. M. (2000). Immune recovery uveitis in patients with cytomegalovirus retinitis taking highly active antiretroviral therapy. *American Journal of Ophthalmology, 130*(1), 49–56.

Stringham, J. M., & Hammond, B. R. (2005). Dietary lutein and zeaxanthin: Possible effects on visual function. *Nutrition Reviews, 63*(2), 59–64.

Thorne, J. E. (2003). *Cytomegalovirus (CMV) retinitis.* American Uveitis Society. Retrieved November 17, 2007, from http://www.uveitissociety.org/pages/diseases/cmvr.html

Thorne, J. E., Jabs, D. A., Kemper, J. K., Holbrook, J. T., Nichols, C., & Meinert, C. L. (2006). Causes of visual acuity loss among patients with AIDS and cytomegalovirus retinitis in the era of highly active antiretroviral therapy. *Ophthalmology, 113*(8), 1441–1445.

Tingley, D. H. (2007). Vision screening essentials: Screening today for eye disorders of the pediatric patient. *Pediatrics in Review, 28*(2), 54–61.

CHAPTER 5

Psychosocial Concerns of the HIV-Infected Adolescent and Adult and Their Significant Others

5.1 RESPONSE TO AN HIV DIAGNOSIS: INFECTED PERSON

1. Initial diagnosis
    a. Shock is a common initial reaction. Communication between the patient and primary care provider may be distorted by shock. Encourage patients to have someone accompany them during office visits (Nichols, 1983).
    b. Anger can be directed at the diagnosis, self, or others.
    c. Denial, disbelief, and emotional numbness may be significant enough that the patient will ignore the need for treatment or support. It is important to involve the patient in a supportive group, individual counseling, or in a nonthreatening, structured social activity (Nichols, 1983).
    d. The patient may experience guilt and be concerned with how lifestyle choices impacted his or her HIV status (Nichols, 1983).
    e. Blaming can be directed at self or others.
    f. The nurse must assess the degree of helplessness and hopelessness because these feelings can lead to suicidal ideation.
2. Transitional issues
    a. Relationships with loved ones and families that have been altered by an HIV diagnosis must be restructured (Nichols, 1985). This includes disclosure issues.
    b. The patient must face fear of death and fear of losing the ability to care for him- or herself before being able to move into acceptance (Nichols, 1983).
    c. The patient may experience the loss of a job, income, housing, or all of these (Nichols, 1985). Loss of role also occurs (Murphy & Perry, 1988).
3. Acceptance
    a. Active participation in health care: Patients who are actively engaged in their care are more likely to adhere to their treatment plan and medication regimen (Remien & Rabkin, 2001; Roberts, 2002). Stress how advances in health care can assist in improved quality of life. Antiretroviral therapy has changed the dynamics of the disease, transforming it from a terminal illness to a chronic illness.
    b. Reengagement in relationships: It is important for patients to love and be loved throughout the course of the disease (Folkman, Chesney, & Christopher-Richards, 1994).
    c. Sexual functioning and decision making: Dilley, Woods, and McFarland (1997) showed that advances in treatment did not reduce the level of concern about infection or perception of

risk of infection. Procreation will need to be discussed honestly between partners and negotiated.
  d. Evaluation of spiritual beliefs (see Section 5.4: Spirituality and Related Concepts)
  e. Return of strength and vitality through stability in clinical conditions forces individuals to face the issue of returning to the workforce. This is an effort to master the uncertainty of a chronic illness and restore order in the face of a continued life threat (Rait, 1991).

REFERENCES

Dilley, J. W., Woods, W. J., & McFarland, W. (1997). Are advances in treatment changing views about high-risk sex? *New England Journal of Medicine, 337*(7), 501–502.

Folkman, S., Chesney, M. A., & Christopher-Richards, A. (1994). Stress and coping in caregiving partners of men with AIDS. *Psychiatric Clinics of North America, 17*(1), 35–53.

Murphy, P., & Perry, K. (1988). Hidden grievers. *Death Studies, 12,* 451–462.

Nichols, S. E. (1983). Psychiatric aspects of AIDS. *Psychosomatics, 24*(12), 1083–1089.

Nichols, S. E. (1985). Psychosocial reactions of persons with the acquired immunodeficiency syndrome. *Annals of Internal Medicine, 103*(5), 765–767.

Remien, R. H., & Rabkin, J. G. (2001). Psychological aspects of living with HIV disease. *Western Journal of Medicine, 175*(5), 332–335.

Roberts, K. J. (2002). Physician-patient relationships, patient satisfaction, and antiretroviral medication adherence among HIV-infected adults attending a public health clinic. *AIDS Patient Care and STDs, 16*(1), 43–50.

Rait, D. S. (1991). The family context of AIDS. *Psychiatric Medicine, 9*(3), 423–439.

5.2 RESPONSE TO AN HIV DIAGNOSIS: FAMILY AND SIGNIFICANT OTHER

1. Description
   a. Given the range of family constellations represented by people with HIV infection, a broad definition of family must be used to include both family of origin and family of choice, whether related biologically, legally, or not related at all.
   b. HIV infection presents as a major life transition that is out of sequence with what is expected. Critical points in HIV disease for alterations in family functioning include diagnosis of HIV or AIDS, first hospitalization, first opportunistic infection, new symptoms, recurrences or relapses, and terminal stage of disease.
   c. Alteration in family function occurs when the family is unable to do the following:
      i)   Adapt constructively to crisis or stress
      ii) Communicate openly among family members
      iii) Perform activities associated with family function (e.g., socialization, personal security, acceptance, companionship, and provision of physical necessities, such as food, clothing, shelter, and health care)
      iv) Seek or accept help appropriately
2. Risk factors and etiology are similar to risk factors for family/caregiver burden.
3. Goals of care
   a. Recognize a family in crisis that needs intervention.
   b. Support the family's adaptation to living with a life-threatening illness of one of its members in a manner that seems appropriate for the particular family.

   c. Identify resources that will support the family and individual members of the family to manage the demands of the loved one's illness.
4. Assessment (Carpentino, 2000)
   a. Family composition
   b. Family strengths
   c. Family rules/discipline
   d. Financial status
   e. Participation in community activities
   f. Family process
   g. Family communication patterns
   h. Family's emotional/supportive pattern (those that are both constructive and destructive)
5. Interventions (Carpentino, 2000)
   a. Acknowledge causative and contributing factors (e.g., sudden illness, hospitalization).
   b. Acknowledge your feelings about the family and their situation.
   c. Provide ongoing information.
   d. Promote cohesiveness.
   e. Discuss the implications of caring for ill family members.

REFERENCES

Carpentino, J. (2000). *Nursing diagnosis: Application to clinical practice* (8th ed.). Philadelphia: Lippincott.

5.3 CAREGIVER BURDEN/STRAIN

1. Definition/description
   a. There is no consistent, agreed-upon definition of caregiver burden.
   b. The terms *burden* and *strain* have been used interchangeably in the literature to describe the impact of caregiving.
   c. The prevalence is unknown but expected to increase as more people are living with HIV and the trend is moving toward home care.
   d. Signs and symptoms that caregiver burden/strain is present include the following:
      i) Anxiety, fear, and depression: These feelings are common for partners and significant others and are increased in partners who are also HIV infected.
      ii) Disrupted relationships: The person with HIV may have been an important source of support for the partner or spouse, leaving the caregiver feeling unappreciated and discouraged (Turner, Pearlin, & Mullan, 1998).
      iii) Conflicts: Problems can occur with friends and family over caregiving issues as well as with the patient (Turner et al., 1998).
      iv) Grief: Feelings of grief occur throughout the process of illness progression, for both the caregiver and patient (Folkman, Chesney, & Christopher-Richards, 1994).
2. Etiology
   a. Illness characteristics include severe illness, sudden onset of illness, and manifestations of new symptoms.

    b. Caregiver variables
- i) Gender: Women tend to show higher levels of distress than do men.
- ii) Age: Depending on age, the caregiver may not have had previous caregiving experiences (Matheny, Mehr, & Brown, 1997).
- iii) Socioeconomic status and economic burdens: Financial issues can precipitate strain and abuse.
- iv) Other life stressors such as poor health of caregiver or other member of family: Thirty-five percent of families report having several family members (sibling, partner, or extended family member) infected with HIV (Fiore et al., 2001).
- v) Other variables (Ruppert, 1996):
  - (1) Relationship communication style
  - (2) Family developmental stage
  - (3) Social support (see Figure 5.3a for assessment of social support)

    c. The unrelenting nature of caring for a person with a debilitating condition

    d. The vast array and large number of service organizations and providers with whom the caregivers must interact

    e. Financial constraints

    f. Isolation from friends, family, and community

    g. Fear of contagion

    h. Multiple losses, such as possible death of a loved one, a lifestyle, and a future

Table 5.3a Assessment of Social Support

Name, Address, Phone Number	Relationship Relative, Friend, Neighbor, Work Associate	Emotional Closeness High, Medium, Low	Perceived Willingness to Help High, Medium, Low	Types of Support Possible Emotional, Informational, Instrumental	Perceived Ability to Help High, Medium, Low
Jane Doe 123 Friend St. 348-6769	Friend	High	High	Informational	Low

      i. Pervasive uncertainty about the meaning of the symptoms, the future of caregiving, and strategies to provide the best care

3. Goals of care

    a. Enhance quality of life for caregiver and recipient of care.

    b. Prevent illness, disability, and psychiatric and physical morbidity of the caregiver.

4. Assessment

    a. Risk factors and etiologies

    b. Caregivers' subjective perception of tasks they perform

        i) How easy or difficult is each task?

        ii) To what extent does caregiving cause strain with regard to work, finances, social life, and emotional and physical status?

        iii) Are there resultant depression, anxiety, and changes in caregiver's health status? Fatigue is common, because demands of caregiving can be relentless.

5. Interventions

    a. The nurse works in partnership with the person with HIV/AIDS and caregiver to provide appropriate care (Ramirez, Addington-Hall, & Richards, 1998).

        i) Validate importance of the caregiving role, including commitment to PWA and the knowledge base related to caregiving.

        ii) Discuss strategies the caregiver can use to interact with healthcare providers to secure high-quality care for the loved one.

    b. Teach universal precautions and basic nursing skills as necessary.

    c. Assist caregivers to find meaning in their caregiving experiences by asking, "What does caregiving mean to you?" and "What has caregiving been like for you?"

    d. Explore the caregiver's strengths and weaknesses.

    e. Discuss the goals of caregiving as perceived by the caregiver.

    f. Refer to community services (e.g., caregiver courses, counseling, support groups, respite care services, home care) as needed.

    g. Discuss feelings associated with the possibility of deciding to institutionalize the ill person or end caregiving role, and assist the caregiver in problem solving.

    h. Provide information about the disease process, the expected course of illness, diagnostic tests, medical treatments, and symptom management as appropriate with interpretation of new symptoms and manifestations of illness, particularly changes in PWA's mental status.

    i. Facilitate problem solving related to treatment decisions.

    j. Refer for case management services to assist in coordinating care.

    k. Discuss coping options. Encourage caregiver to take each day as it comes, let go of what is not important, put the future on hold, and cherish special moments and time spent with loved ones.

    l. Discuss importance of the caregiver taking care of self through health-promotion activities, especially if the caregiver is HIV positive.

        i) Stress-reduction techniques

        ii) Proper nutrition and adequate rest/sleep

        iii) Maintenance of activity and exercise patterns and taking time-out periods

        iv) Avoidance of substance use/abuse

m. Assist in mobilizing resources to help in caregiving activities. Role-play asking for help.
n. Discuss, in conjunction with the PWA, healthcare durable power of attorney and living will. Refer for legal assistance if necessary.
o. Discuss uncertainty related to caregiving, its sources and manifestations, and ways to manage or accept it.
p. Discuss how the caregiver can promote the PWA's sense of autonomy and independence.
q. Encourage the caregiver to discuss relationship difficulties with PWA.
r. Facilitate caregivers' ability to provide care when PWA is hospitalized.

REFERENCES

Fiore, T., Flanigan, T., Hogan, T., Cram, R., Schuman, P., Schoenbaum, E., et al. (2001). HIV infections in families of HIV-positive and at-risk HIV-negative women. *AIDS Care, 13*(2), 209–214.
Folkman, S., Chesney, M. A., & Christopher-Richards, A. (1994). Stress and coping in caregiving partners of men with AIDS. *Psychiatric Clinics of North America, 17*(1), 35–53.
Matheny, S. C., Mehr, L. M., & Brown, G. (1997). Caregivers and HIV infection: Services and issues. *Primary Care, 24*(3), 677–690.
Ramirez, A., Addington-Hall, J., & Richards, M. (1998). ABC of palliative care: The carers. *British Medical Journal, 316*(7126), 208–211.
Ruppert, R. A. (1996). Psychological aspects of lay caregiving. *Rehabilitation Nursing, 21*(6), 315–320.
Turner, H. A., Pearlin, L. I., & Mullan, J. T. (1998). Sources and determinants of social support for caregivers of persons with AIDS. *Journal of Health and Social Behavior, 39*(2), 137–151.

5.4 SPIRITUALITY AND RELATED CONCEPTS

1. Definitions
    a. Spirituality: the essence of our being, which shapes our life journey, permeates our living, and infuses our unfolding awareness of who and what we are, our purpose in being, and our inner resources (Burkhardt & Nagai Jacobson, 2000). Spirituality can be defined as a search for the sacred, which includes the concepts of God, divinity, transcendence, and ultimate reality, and is a process through which people seek to understand, hold onto, and, when necessary, transform whatever they hold sacred in their lives (Roehlkepartain et al., 2005).
    b. Spiritual development: the process of growing the intrinsic human capacity for self-transcendence, in which the self is embedded in something greater than the self, including the sacred. It is the developmental "engine" that propels the search for connectedness, meaning, purpose, and contribution. It is shaped both within and outside of religious traditions, beliefs, and practices (Roehlkepartain et al., 2005).
    c. Spiritual wellness: a lifestyle that views life as purposeful and pleasurable, that allows people to seek out life-sustaining and life-enriching options to be chosen freely at every opportunity, and allows them to sink themselves deeply into spiritual values or specific religious beliefs (Pilch, 1998).
    d. Spiritual distress: the disruption in the life principle that pervades a person's entire being and that integrates and transcends one's biological and psychosocial nature (NANDA, 1994). Spiritual distress can manifest itself as guilt, recriminations and self-blame, hyper-

religiosity, rejection of significant others, and expressions of despair (Wilson & Kneisl, 1992). Although not all individuals identify with a religion or particular belief in a deity, all of humanity is seeking meaning and
acceptance.

2. Etiology
   a. Sources of spirituality
      i)   Faith tradition of origin or new spiritual journey or practices
      ii) Community, family/ancestors, and culture
      iii) Love, hope, justice, and forgiveness
      iv) Distant healing/distant prayer (Dossey, 1996; Sicher, Targ, Moore, & Smith, 1998)
      v)   Peaceful resolve about end of life
   b. Issues affecting spiritual wellness
      i)   Anger, shame, guilt, or powerlessness
      ii)   Demoralization and depression
      iii) Uncertainty and distrust
      iv)   Betrayal or forgiveness of self or others
      v)   Loss of perceived future, body image, and relationships
      vi)   Suffering, anguish, apprehension, and isolation
      vii) Anticipating death or future losses, despair or hopelessness
      viii) Rejection by family or community (homophobia, intolerance, stigmatization of substance abusers)
      ix)   Prolonged anger and negativistic thinking, inability to accept predicament
3. Goal of care
4. Assessment
   a. Belief systems, desired spiritual practices
      i) Does the individual believe in a concept of sin (dhanb, thanb in Islam, and Awen in Hebrew; most religious traditions have varying names for sin and gradations of sin) or transgressions against the self, other, and/or community? Does the individual believe in redemption and reconciliation? If the individual believes in an afterlife, does s/he believe this will be afforded the individual; if not, why not?
5. Interventions
   a. Establish a caring, supportive presence.
   b. Include family, significant others, community, and beloved pets in care plans, as appropriate.
   c. Listen nonjudgmentally.
   d. Explore the meaning of illness and how it has affected the individual's self-concept, connections to others, and so on. As people are living longer with HAART, explore with individuals how their life goals have changed.
   e. Encourage writing that seeks to identify meaning. Writing interventions have been shown to improve adherence in a sample of HIV+ women (Westling, Garcia, & Mann, 2007).
   f. Educate self about unfamiliar religions (e.g., Wicca, Santeria, Islam), cultural practices, and belief systems (Cantrell, 2001).
   g. For individuals who utilize prayer, explore the kind of prayer that is meaningful and helpful. Be mindful of gender and personality differences in individual prayer lives. Assess

for cultural differences and different methods of prayer including psalms, chants, mantras, mindfulness, meditation, specialized prayer formats/formulas, and so forth (see Coleman et al., 2006, for gender prayer differences in the African American community).

h. Assess degree of hope or despair, anger or alienation.

i. Refer for psychotherapy if symptoms of depression, anxiety, hopelessness, unremitting anger, guilt, or shame persist.

j. Encourage self-forgiveness and celebrations of life.

k. Discuss with the individual the research on the benefits of forgiveness. Listen for grievance stories that impede emotional growth (Luskin, 2002).

l. If assisted suicide is requested (assisted suicide is illegal in most states), evaluate patient's reasoning, mental status, and plans. Assess for situations that can impair judgment, including severe depression (illicit drug use, which can induce depression/delirium), compromised mental status, and uncontrolled pain (the major tenet of assisted suicide is patient autonomy; Crock, 1998; Saunders, 2000, 2001).

m. Reframe self-esteem in light of changes in body image and relationships.

n. Provide links to pastoral counselors, community programs, vocational training, and volunteerism.

o. When guilt or shame is present, do the following:

　　i) Remind individuals that HIV is a medical problem, not a moral issue.

　　ii) Provide an outlet for verbalizing shame and shameful behaviors.

　　iii) Remind individual that sometimes bad things happen to good people (Kushner, 1981) and that HIV is not retribution for falling short of values or ideals.

　　iv) Refer to pastoral counselor, priest, confessor, imam, therapist, and so forth for pastoral counseling and/or psychotherapy if shame/guilt is unremitting.

p. Listen for signs of grief, present or unresolved, and demoralization.

q. In cases of impending death, assist patient with good-byes (wills, video legacies, letters, making peace with self, others, and God). Include cultural or personal preferences (e.g., Hindus may prefer dying on the floor close to earth, and Muslims may elect to die facing east toward Mecca; Galanti, 1997; Hall, 1998; Lyon, Townsend-Akpan, & Thompson, 2001).

r. For the grieving who have lost family, friends, colleagues, and loved ones, explore meaningful memorials such as an AIDS memorial quilt, memorial gardens/planting of trees, inscribing names of the deceased in books of remembrances (such as in Grace Cathedral, SF, or the Cathedral of St. John the Divine, NYC), volunteerism in HIV-related organizations, or donations in honor of loved ones to HIV/AIDS service organizations including ANAC, and so forth.

s. Instill hope and acceptance.

　　i) As appropriate, employ touch; even minimal contact implies acceptance.

　　ii) Discuss what the patient hopes for (e.g., a cure, more time, reconciliation, absence of pain).

　　iii) Assess for hopelessness, which is frequently a symptom of depression.

　　iv) Inquire about what brings individual comfort or joy (e.g., music, friends, family, nature, prayer, meditation, yoga or exercise, service to others).

v) Determine which spiritual practices or beliefs provide meaning to life, hope, and transcendence to the individual

t. Engage in prayer, meditation, or rituals with patient, as mutual comfort levels and appropriateness dictate. Employ sensitive humor if it is appropriate.

u. Facilitate patient's involvement in meaningful spiritual practices and outlets, such as worship, meditation, yoga, chakras, healing oils, aromatherapy, imagery, and therapeutic touch (Buckle, 2002; Foster, 1999).

v. Work for justice, locally and internationally, in accessing appropriate medical care, pain control, medications, and housing. Support organizations, whether by volunteerism or donations, that work for basic human rights across the globe.

REFERENCES

Buckle, J. (2002). Clinical aromatherapy and AIDS. *Journal of the Association of Nurses in AIDS Care, 13*(3), 81–99.

Burkhardt, M., & Nagai Jacobson, M. G. (2000). Spirituality and health. In B. Dossey, L. Keegan, & C. Guzzetta (Eds.), *Holistic nursing: A handbook for practice* (3rd ed., pp. 91–121). New York: Aspen.

Cantrell, G. (2001). *Wiccan beliefs and practices: With rituals for solitaries and covens.* St. Paul, MN: Llewellyn.

Coleman, C. L., Holzemer, W. L., Eller, L. S., Corless, I. B., Reynolds, N. R., Nokes, K. M., et al. (2006). Gender differences in use of prayer as a self-care strategy for managing symptoms in African Americans living with HIV/AIDS. *Journal of the Association of Nurses in AIDS Care, 17*(4), 16–23.

Crock, E. A. (1998). Breaking (through) the law—Coming out of the silence: Nursing, HIV/AIDS and euthanasia. *AIDS Care, 10*(Suppl. 2), 137–145.

Dossey, L. (1996). *Prayer is good medicine: How to reap the healing benefits of prayer.* San Francisco: HarperOne.

Foster, B. (1999). The mind-body connection: Yoga for HIV/AIDS. *Body Positive,* 32–36.

Galanti, G. A. (1997). *Caring for patients of different cultures: Case studies from different American hospitals* (2nd ed.). Philadelphia: University of Pennsylvania Press.

Hall, B. (1998). Patterns of spirituality in persons with advanced HIV disease. *Research in Nursing & Health, 21*(2), 143–153.

Kushner, H. (1981). *When bad things happen to good people.* New York: Schocken Books.

Luskin, F. (2002). *Forgive for good: A proven prescription for health and happiness.* New York: HarperSanFrancisco.

Lyon, M., Townsend-Akpan, C., & Thompson, A. (2001). Spirituality and end of life care for an adolescent with AIDS. *AIDS Patient Care and STDs, 15*(11), 555–560.

North American Nursing Diagnosis Association (NANDA). (1994). *Classification of nursing diagnosis: Proceedings of 10th Conference.* St. Louis, MO: Author.

Pilch, J. (1998). Wellness spirituality. *Health Values, 12*(3), 28–31.

Roehlkepartain, E. C., Benson, P. L., Ebstyne King, P., &Wagener, L. M. (2005). *The handbook of spiritual development in childhood and adolescence* (The SAGE Program on Applied Developmental Science). New York: Sage.

Saunders, J. (2000). AIDS nursing and physician-assisted suicide: Part I. *Journal of the Association of Nurses in AIDS Care, 11*(6), 45–53.

Saunders, J. (2001). AIDS nursing and physician-assisted suicide: Part 2. *Journal of the Association of Nurses in AIDS Care, 12*(1), 71–82.

Sicher, F., Targ, E., Moore, D., & Smith, H. (1998). A randomized double-blind study of the effects of distant healing in a population with advanced AIDS. *Western Journal of Medicine, 169*(6), 356–367.

Westling, E., Garcia, K., & Mann, T. (2007). Discovery of meaning and adherence to medications in HIV-related infected women. *Journal of Health Psychology, 12*(4), 627–635.

Wilson, H. S., & Kneisl, C. R. (1992). *Psychiatric nursing* (4th ed.). Reading, MA: Addison-Wesley.

5.5 DEPRESSION

1. Definitions/descriptions
   a. Major depressive disorder: a mood disorder characterized by symptoms that persist over a minimum of a 2-week period and reflect a change from previous functioning. These symptoms cannot be accounted for by bereavement, a general medical illness, medications, or alcohol/drug use. The presence of these symptoms results in significant impairment in social and occupational function. A person must have at least five of nine diagnostic symptoms, one of which must be a depressed mood or loss of interest or pleasure, also known as anhedonia. Other symptoms include feelings of worthlessness or excessive or inappropriate guilt, suicidal thoughts, sleep disturbance, appetite/weight changes, attention/concentration changes, energy level changes or fatigue, and psychomotor agitation or retardation (APA, 2000a).
   b. Other *DSM-IV-TR* mood disorders
      i)   Adjustment disorders: Patients with HIV are at higher risk because of numerous emotional responses to HIV, multiple stressors that impact one's ability to cope, and in some patients, the increased need for dependency and/or history of exposure to chronic stress (Holder-Perkins & Akman, 2006). Adjustment disorder with depressed mood or adjustment disorder with mixed anxiety and depressed mood may occur. Patients return to normal functioning after resolution of stressors; therefore, it is imperative to connect the client with resources to cope with these stressors. Medications may or may not be necessary for full recovery.
         (1) Adjustment disorder with depressed mood: development of symptoms of depressed mood, tearfulness, and/or feelings of hopelessness that occur in response to a stressor within 3 months of the stressor. Symptoms are clinically significant because they are evidenced by either marked distress in excess of what would be expected as a result of the stressor or causes significant impairment in social or occupational functioning (APA, 2000a).
         (2) Adjustment disorder with mixed anxiety and depressed mood: development of symptoms of depressed mood, tearfulness, and/or feelings of hopelessness as well as nervousness, worry, or jitteriness in response to a stressor within 3 months of the stressor. See above for discussion of stressors and clinical significance of symptoms (APA, 2000a).
   c. Dysthymic disorder: depressed mood lasting more than 2 years. Although this is a milder form of depression, it is accompanied by low self-esteem, sleep difficulties, poor concentration or difficulty making decisions, and feelings of hopelessness (APA, 2000a).
   d. Depressive disorder not otherwise specified: These are disorders with depressive features that don't meet criteria for other mood disorders. Examples include premenstrual dysphoric disorder, minor depressive disorder, or recurrent brief depressive disorder (APA, 2000a).
   e. Mood disorders secondary to medical conditions: This is more likely to occur as HIV progresses. Conditions to consider include opportunistic infections, CNS malignancies, neurosyphilis, HIV-related neuropathological changes, nutritional deficiencies (i.e., B12,

folate), hypogonadism, thyroid dysfunction, diabetes, inflammatory diseases, and anemia (Stolar, Catalano, Hakala, Bright, & Fernandez, 2005).

f. Substance-induced mood disorder: This can occur as a result of recreational drugs, anti-retrovirals, or medications used to treat other conditions. Stolar et al. (2005) note that trimethoprim-sulfamethoxazole, interferon-alpha, isoniazid, steroids, efavirenz, zidovu-dine, the PIs, vinblastine, and vincristine have been reported to cause depression. The following medications have been associated with depressive symptoms of tearfulness, decreased appetite, irritability, and insomnia: abacavir, didanosine, acyclovir, ganciclovir, and amphotericin B (Stolar et al., 2005).

g. Bereavement: This is not considered a major depressive episode, although symptoms are similar unless these symptoms persist more than 2 months. Normal grief generally lasts more than 6 months and is considered a self-limiting condition (Bonanno & Kaltman, 1999).

2. Prevalence and impact

a. HIV-infected persons have a two- to fourfold increase in depressive disorders (Morrison et al., 2002). Rates of depressive disorders range between 2% and 35% in HIV-infected individuals (Bing et al., 2001; Morrison et al., 2002; NYSDHAI, 2001; Rabkin, 1997; Work Group on HIV/AIDS, 2000). One prevalence study estimated that 39% of clinic patients had a mood or anxiety disorder, 21% had a substance abuse diagnosis, and 8% had both; of those with a mood/anxiety diagnosis, 76% had clinically relevant depression and 11% had posttraumatic stress disorder (Pence et al., 2006). Another study of non-substance-abusing participants reported depressive disorder rates of 19% for HIV seropositive women versus 5% in a matched HIV seronegative group (Morrison et al., 2002).

b. Depression increases with disease progression. Rates of major depressive disorder were 2–11% in asymptomatic HIV-infected and 4–18% in symptomatic HIV-infected persons globally (Morrison et al., 2002).

c. Comorbidity of HIV and depression is common. Depression occurs twice as frequently in HIV patients versus non-infected persons (Gomez & O'Dowd, 2006).

d. Compared with HIV-infected men, women with HIV infection have higher rates of depressive disorders, with prevalence rates ranging from 2% to 35% (Morrison et al., 2002).

3. Etiology

a. Major depression is a complex psychobiological condition that results from neuroanatomical and neurochemical changes. Multiple factors also impact its occurrence.

b. Genetic: First-degree relatives of persons with major depression have two to three times greater risk for depression. This is supported by data from twin and adoption studies (Sadock & Sadock, 2003).

c. Biological: The dysregulation of neurotransmitters, especially norepinephrine, serotonin, and dopamine, are thought to be involved in depression. Changes in the limbic system, basal ganglia, and hypothalamus are also believed to play a role (Sadock & Sadock, 2003).

d. Social and psychological factors: Depression may be triggered by adverse early life events, intrapsychic conflicts, or reactions to life events (i.e., stressors).

e. Medications that can cause depressive symptoms; analgesics/anti-inflammatory (indomethacin, opiates), anticonvulsants (phenobarbital), antihypertensives (methyldopa, reserpine), anti-infectives, antimicrobial, antineoplastics, anti-Parkinson agents (levodopa), antiretrovirals (efavirenz, zidovudine), hormones, immunosuppressives (corticosteroids), neuroleptics, sedatives/tranquilizers (abused), stimulants (abused), and other drugs (Valente, 2003).

 f. Chronic illnesses can increase the incidence of depression.

4. Goals of care

 a. Reduce symptoms of depression and improve functioning.

 b. Help patients learn a more effective coping style.

 c. Increase hope and optimism, which can lead to more active involvement in care.

 d. Establish a positive outlook, which research links with improved immune response.

 e. Increase adherence to HAART through effective treatment of depression (Basu, Chwastiak, & Bruce, 2005).

5. Assessment

 a. Mental status

  i) Appearance: Lack of self-care may be evident. Patient may exhibit poor eye contact, although culture may impact this and must be taken into consideration.

  ii) Mood and affect: Patient may acknowledge feeling depressed, sad, irritable, or having crying spells. Affect may appear blunted, sad, or depressed. (Note: It is important to distinguish between mood and affect. Mood is subjective, and we must question patient about this, whereas affect is an objective assessment made by the clinician.)

  iii) Cognition: Patient displays poor attention and concentration, which may impair learning ability and short-term memory.

  iv) Thought processes: Themes of guilt, self-deprecation, and worthlessness are common.

  v) Perception: Patient may have distorted perception, and may perceive everything as bad or his or her fault. Symptoms of psychosis, such as hallucinations and delusions, may present in persons with severe depression.

 b. Tools can be used to differentiate among depression, neurocognitive changes as a result of AIDS, dementia, prior neurologic assaults, and substance abuse (Herfkens, 2001), and other mental disorders.

  i) Cognitive assessment tools

   (1) Folstein Mini Mental State Examination (MMSE) is used as a quick cognitive screen for cortical signs.

   (2) The Johns Hopkins HIV Dementia Scale tests memory-registration, attention, psychomotor speed, memory recall, and constructional abilities in a short, easy-to-administer format (Power, Selnes, Grim, & McArthur, 1995).

   (3) High Sensitivity Cognitive Screen (HSCS) screens for the absence or presence of cognitive dysfunction (Levy, 2006).

 c. Depression assessment tools

  i) Hamilton Depression Rating Scale (HAM-D) is one of the oldest and most psychometrically sound rating scales (Andreasen & Black, 2001).

  ii) PRIME-MD screens for somatoform, depressive, anxiety, eating, and alcohol disorders. The PHQ is the self-administered version of this tool (Spitzer et al., 1999).

  iii) Center for Epidemiologic Studies Depression Scale (CES-D) is a short, 20-question Likert-type scale developed by L. Radloff at the National Institutes of Health (NIH). It is commonly used to assess depression in persons with HIV (Herfkens, 2001).

iv) Hospital Anxiety and Depression Scale (HADS) is a tool designed to screen for anxiety or depression in medically ill patients. Despite its name, it can be used in both inpatient and outpatient settings. It is useful to exclude those patients who are experiencing only somatic symptoms (APA, 2000b; Basu et al., 2005). Some evidence indicates that the PHQ has superior validity compared to the HADS (Löwe et al., 2004).

d. Suicide assessment

i) Directly question about the presence of suicidal ideation and the patient's plan. Then assess suicidality, which includes the patient's suicidal intent and lethality of plan (APA, 2003).

ii) It is important to explore past psychiatric history, with a focus on previous suicide attempts, and history of suicide by a family member or friend (Basu et al., 2005).

iii) Assess patient's perception of current level of social and financial support (Basu et al., 2005).

iv) Assess patient beliefs about his/her illness and support system (Basu et al., 2005).

v) Presence of any of the following psychological symptoms increases the risk of suicide: anxiety, hopelessness, command hallucinations, impulsiveness, and aggression (APA, 2003).

vi) Periods associated with increased risk of suicide in persons with HIV include the following:

(1) Immediately after HIV diagnosis

(2) Advanced HIV disease, especially if accompanied by significant health issues and side effects of treatment (Catalan, 2005)

vii) Potential for suicide rises when energy increases (early in the treatment of depression) or with decreased inhibition (during rage or when intoxicated; Risk Management Foundation, 1996).

viii) Presence of suicidal ideation in the context of an active plan requires immediate psychiatric intervention. There is a 15% risk of death by suicide in patients who have been previously hospitalized for depression (Andreasen & Black, 2001).

ix) Differentiate from rational suicide when terminally ill. Nurses must examine their own beliefs and philosophies regarding this issue (Fontana, 2002). The American Nurses Association (ANA) and ANAC provide guidelines in this area.

6. Interventions

a. Nonpharmacological

i) Depressed individuals experience varied emotions and emotional responses including unworthiness and guilt. Staff must be able to provide support to help decrease the patient's sense of loss and promote feelings of being accepted and cared for.

ii) Individual or group support, professional or peer facilitated, can decrease feelings of isolation. Encourage social and community activities to decrease behaviors that create environments that maintain negative self-views.

iii) Determine risk of self-harm and harm to others through direct and indirect means (neglect).

iv) Refer for psychotherapy. Cognitive behavioral therapy (CBT) and interpersonal therapy have been shown to decrease depressive symptoms (Basu et al., 2005).

    v)   Provide appropriate coping and social skills training: assess coping styles, support systems, and repertoire. Self-care strategies can be used when patients are unable to access or refuse to accept psychiatric care; however, the effectiveness of these strategies is variable (Eller et al., 2004).

    vi)   Provide grief counseling if appropriate.

    vii)   Monitor and educate the patient regarding purpose and side effects of medications and ways to manage them.

    viii)   Consider cultural variations in expression of depressed feelings.

        (1) Culturally appropriate affect ranges from open, demonstrative expression to stoicism.

        (2) The expression of depression is not a reliable indicator of the degree of feeling.

    ix)   Provide education and support to significant others.

        (1) Understand that nurturing the patient and encouraging independence are supportive behaviors.

        (2) Patients who have the support of friends and family tend to cope better with their illnesses.

        (3) Dealing with illness and concern about mortality of a loved one can cause sadness, anger, and ambivalence.

        (4) Support groups can decrease feelings of isolation and help in working out feelings and problem solving.

    x)   Encourage a balanced diet to offset depletion in essential elements and vitamins. Consider vitamin and mineral supplementation. Folic acid deficiency has been associated with a suboptimal response to selective serotonin reuptake inhibitors (Fava et al., 1997).

    xi)   Alternative modalities such as body work, therapeutic touch, and acupuncture may be beneficial.

    xii)   Exercise is effective in decreasing symptoms of depression (Basu et al., 2005).

    xiii)   Weekly massage decreases both depression and anxiety in a study of HIV-infected adolescents (Basu et al., 2005).

b. Pharmacologic

    i)   Selective serotonin reuptake inhibitors (SSRIs): fluoxetine, sertraline, paroxetine, citalopram, escitalopram

        (1) SSRIs are one of the first-line choices for the treatment of depression in HIV patients (Vergara-Rodriguez & Watts, 2008).

        (2) Most troubling side effect of SSRIs is sexual dysfunction, which can be managed with dose reductions, drug holidays, or switching to another drug in the same class. Other side effects include headache, irritability/agitation, nausea, difficulty sleeping, and dry mouth.

        (3) SSRIs should be used with caution in patients taking PIs and NNRTIs because these antiretroviral medications can inhibit cytochrome P450 (CYP450) isoenzymes and lead to serotonin syndrome (NYSDHAI, 2001). Ritonavir boosting can increase the CYP450 inhibition and further increase levels of SSRIs. SSRIs, especially fluoxetine and paroxetine, can increase GI symptoms when used concurrently with PIs (Vergara-Rodriguez & Watts, 2008).

(4) Sertraline, citalopram, and escitalopram are preferred because both fluoxetine and paroxetine can inhibit CYP450 2D6, which may increase the adverse effects of PIs. Escitalopram is least likely to have drug interactions with PIs or NNRTIs (Vergara-Rodriguez & Watts, 2008).

(5) Both SSRIs and efavirenz can worsen neuropsychiatric symptoms. These symptoms include headache, dizziness, insomnia or somnolence, anxiety/agitation, and akathesia (Vergara-Rodriguez & Watts, 2008).

ii) Mixed serotonin/norepinephrine reuptake inhibitors (SNRIs): venlafaxine, duloxetine

(1) Another first-line choice for the treatment of major depression in HIV patients (Vergara-Rodriguez & Watts, 2008)

(2) Relatively safe and well tolerated. Caution should be used in patients taking NNTRIs or PIs as their use may lead to increased level of antidepressant (NYSDHAI, 2001).

(3) May increase GI side effects and motility (Vergara-Rodriguez & Watts, 2008).

(4) Venlafaxine can be associated with treatment-emergent hypertension, so it's necessary to monitor vital signs.

iii) Mixed norepinephrine/dopamine reuptake inhibitors (NRI/DRIs)-buproprion

(1) Another first-line choice for the treatment of major depression in HIV patients (Vergara-Rodriguez & Watts, 2008)

(2) Used to improve energy and often used in combination with SSRIs (Vergara-Rodriguez & Watts, 2008).

(3) Does not increase risk of seizures, but seizure risk is increased with certain HIV-related organic brain disorders. Risk also increases with HIV-related CNS disease and infections (CNS lymphoma, HIV dementia, CNS toxoplasmosis, progressive multifocal leukoencephalopathy, fungal and tubercular meningitis/encephalitis; Vergara-Rodriguez & Watts, 2008).

iv) Atypical antidepressant: mirtazepine

(1) Preferred due to minimal drug interactions (Vergara-Rodriguez & Watts, 2008)

(2) Increases appetite and causes sedation, which is helpful with HIV wasting (Vergara-Rodriguez & Watts, 2008).

v) Psychostimulants (methyphenidate, dextroamphetamine)

(1) Rapid onset of action. Given to improve energy and apathy. Have positive effects on symptoms of depression, especially in advanced HIV disease (Vergara-Rodriguez & Watts, 2008).

(2) Psychostimulants may be contraindicated in individuals in recovery from substance abuse because they are highly addictive. Also contraindicated for patients who abuse amphetamines. Other antidepressants are safe to use in individuals with substance abuse issues.

(3) May increase risk of hallucinations, tics, tremors, and agitation (Vergara-Rodriguez & Watts, 2008). Use with caution in patients with seizure disorders.

vi) Tricyclic antidepressants (TCAs)

(1) Generally avoided due to issues of safety and tolerability.

(2) TCAs can be lethal in overdose. Assess suicidal ideation regularly.

    (3) Use with PIs or NNRTIs can lead to increased levels of antidepressant due to inhibition of CYP450 3A4 and 2D6 (Vergara-Rodriguez & Watts, 2008).

    (4) Side effects include drowsiness, dry mouth, blurred vision, and constipation.

vii) Other agents

    (1) Monafinil has been studied as adjunctive therapy for atypical depression and depression associated with fatigue (Vaishnavi et al., 2006).

    (2) Dehydroepiandrosterone (DHEA) has been studied as adjunctive therapy for depression in HIV associated with fatigue (Rabkin et al., 2006).

viii) Herbal supplements: Used in the treatment of depression and neurological symptoms, they may have unexpected interactions with antiretroviral medications. Cytochrome P450 enzymes metabolize many antiretroviral medications and dietary supplements may be P450 inducers or inhibitors. This interaction can result in subtherapeutic or toxic plasma concentrations of antiretroviral medications. St. John's wort (hypericum perforatum) should not be used with protease inhibitors (PIs) or non-nucleoside reverse transcriptase inhibitors (NNRTIs) because it may result in suboptimal antiretroviral drug concentrations (NYSDHAI, 2001). Other herbal supplements that are used in the treatment of depression that affect the P450 pathway include garlic, ginseng, ginkgo, melatonin, and skullcap (Delgoda & Westlake, 2004; Greenblatt et al., 2006; Haouzi et al., 2000; Ma et al., 2005).

REFERENCES

American Psychiatric Association (APA). (2000a). *Diagnostic and statistical manual of mental disorders* (4th ed., text revision). Washington, DC: Author.

American Psychiatric Association (APA). (2000b). *Handbook of psychiatric measures*. Washington, DC: Author.

American Psychiatric Association (APA). (2003). *Practice guideline for the assessment and treatment of patients with suicidal behavior*. Washington, DC: Author.

Andreasen, N. C., & Black, D. W. (2001). Mood disorders. *Introductory Textbook of Psychiatry* (3rd ed., pp. 260–314). Washington, DC: American Psychiatric Publishing.

Basu, S., Chwastiak, L. A., & Bruce, R. D. (2005). Clinical management of depression and anxiety in HIV-infected adults. *AIDS, 19*(18), 2057–2067.

Bing, E. G., Burnnam, M. A., Longshore, D., Fleishman, J. A., Sherbourne, C. D., London, A. S., et al. (2001). Psychiatric disorders and drug use among human immunodeficiency virus-infected adults in the United States. *Archives of General Psychiatry, 58*(8), 721–728.

Bonanno, G., & Kaltman, S. (1999). Toward an integrative perspective on bereavement. *Psychological Bulletin, 125*(6), 760–776.

Catalan, J. (2005). Suicidal behavior and HIV infection. In K. Citron, J. Brouillette, & A. Beckett (Eds.), *HIV and psychiatry: Training and resource manual* (2nd ed.; pp. 110–119). New York: Cambridge University Press.

Delgoda, R., & Westlake, A. C. (2004) Herbal interactions involving cytochrome p450 enzymes: A mini review. *Toxicological Reviews, 23*(4), 239–249.

Eller, L. S., Bunch, E. H., Wantlant, D. J., Portillo, C. J., Reynolds, N., Nokes, K. M., et al. (2004). Self-care strategies for depression in people living with HIV, XV International AIDS Conference, Bangkok, Thailand, Abstract # MoPeD3738.

Fava, M., Borus, J. S., Alpert, J. E., Nierenberg, A. A., Rosenbaum, J. F., & Bottiglieri, T. (1997). Folate, vitamin B12, and homocysteine in major depressive disorder. *American Journal of Psychiatry, 154*(3), 426–428.

Fontana, J. S. (2002). Rational suicide in the terminally ill. *Journal of Nursing Scholarship, 34*(2), 147–151.

Gomez, M. F., & O'Dowd, M. A. (2006). Psychiatric assessment. In F. Fernandez & P. Ruiz (Eds.), *Psychiatric aspects of HIV/AIDS* (pp. 39–47). Philadelphia: Lippincott Williams & Wilkins.

Greenblatt, D. J., Leigh-Pemberton, R. A., & von Moltke, L. L. (2006). In vitro interactions of water-soluble garlic components with human cytochromes p450. *Journal of Nutrition, 136*(Suppl. 3), 806S–809S.

Haouzi, D., Lekehal, M., Moreau, A., Moulis, C., Feldmann, G., Robin, M. A., et al. (2000). Cytochrome P450-generated reactive metabolites cause mitochondrial permeability transition, caspase activation, and apoptosis in rat hepatocytes. *Source Hepatology, 32*(2), 303–311.

Herfkens, K. M. (2001). Depression, neurocognitive disorders and HIV in prisons. *HEPPNews, 4*(1), 1–9. Retrieved March 11, 2009, from http://www.aegis.com/pubs/hepp/2001/HEPP2001-0101.html

Holder-Perkins, V., & Akman, J. S. (2006). Psychological reactions. In F. Fernandez & P. Ruiz (Eds.), *Psychiatric aspects of HIV/AIDS* (pp. 71–78). Philadelphia: Lippincott Williams & Wilkins.

Levy, J. K. (2006). Psychological and neurological testing. In F. Fernandez & P. Ruiz (Eds.), *Psychiatric aspects of HIV/AIDS* (pp. 48–62). Philadelphia: Lippincott Williams & Wilkins.

Löwe, B., Gräfe, K., Zipfel, S., Witte, S., Loerch, B., & Herzog, W. (2004). Diagnosing ICD-10 depressive episodes: Superior criterion validity of the Patient Health Questionnaire. *Psychotherapy and Psychosomatics, 73*(6), 386–390.

Ma, X., Idle, J. R., Krausz, K. W., & Gonzalez, F. J. (2005). Metabolism of melatonin by human cytochromes p450. *Drug Metabolism & Disposition, 33*(4), 489–494.

Morrison, M. F., Petitto, J. M., Have, T. T., Gettes, D. R., Chiappini, M. S., Weber, A. L., et al. (2002). Depressive and anxiety disorders I women with HIV infection. *American Journal of Psychiatry, 159*(5), 789–796.

New York State Department of Health AIDS Institute (NYSDHAI). (2001). *Mental health care for people with HIV infection: HIV clinical guidelines for the primary care practitioner*. New York: Author.

Pence B. W., Miller, W. C., Whetten, K., Eron, J. J., & Gaynes, B. N. (2006). Prevalence of DSM-IV-defined mood, anxiety, and substance use disorders in an HIV clinic in the Southeastern United States. *Journal of Acquired Immune Deficiency Syndrome, 42*(3), 298–306.

Power, C., Selnes, O. A., Grim J. A., & McArthur, J. C. (1995). HIV Dementia Scale: A rapid screening test. *Journal of Acquired Immune Deficiency Syndromes and Human Retrovirology, 8*(3), 273–278.

Rabkin, J. G., Ferrando, S. J., Jaconsberg, L. B., & Fishman, B. (1997). Prevalence of axis I disorders in an AIDS cohort: A cross-sectional, controlled study. *Comprehensive Psychiatry, 38*(3), 146–154.

Rabkin, J. G., McElhiney, M. C., Rabkin, R., McGrath, P. J., & Ferrando, S. J. (2006). Placebo-controlled trial of dehydroepiandrosterone (DHEA) for treatment of nonmajor depression in patients with HIV/AIDS. *American Journal of Psychiatry, 163*(1), 59–66.

Risk Management Foundation. (1996). *Guidelines for identification, assessment and treatment planning for suicidality*. Retrieved February 22, 2009, from http://www.rmf.harvard.edu/files/documents/suicideAs.pdf

Sadock, B. J., & Sadock, V. A. (2003). *Kaplan and Sadock's synopsis of psychiatry: Behavioral sciences/clinical psychiatry* (9th ed.). Philadelphia: Lippincott Williams & Wilkins.

Spitzer, R. L., Kroenke, K., Williams, J. B. W., & the Patient Health Questionnaire Primary Care Study Group. (1999). Validation and utility of a self-report version of the PRIME-MD. *JAMA, 282*(18), 1734–1744.

Stolar, A., Catalano, G., Hakala, S. M., Bright, R. P., & Fernandez, F. (2005). In K. Citron, J. Brouillette, & A. Beckett (Eds.), *HIV and psychiatry: Training and resource manual* (2nd ed., pp. 88–109). New York: Cambridge University Press.

Vaishnav, I. S., Gadde, K., Alamy, S., Zhang, W., Connor, K., & Davidson, J. R. (2006). Modafinil for atypical depression: effects of open-label and double-blind discontinuation treatment. *Journal of Clinical Psychopharmacology, 26*(4), 373–378.

Valente, S. M. (2003). Depression and HIV disease. *Journal of the Association of Nurses in AIDS Care, 14*(2), 41–51.

Vergara-Rodriguez, P., & Watts, J. (2008). Use of psychotropic medications in the HIV-positive patient: Part I. *Psychopharm Review, 43*(8), 59–66.

Work Group on HIV/AIDS. (2000). Practice guidelines for the treatment of patients with HIV/AIDS. *American Journal of Psychiatry, 157*(Suppl. 11), 1–62.

5.6 BIPOLAR DISORDER

1. Definitions/descriptions
   a. Bipolar disorder: a mood disorder characterized by symptoms consistent with both major depressive disorder and manic or hypomanic episodes.

  i)   Manic episode: a distinct period of abnormally and persistently elevated, expansive, or irritable mood that lasts for at least 1 week. This is accompanied by three or more of the following symptoms (four if the mood is irritable only): inflated self-esteem or grandiosity, decreased need for sleep, more talkative than usual or pressure to keep talking, flight of ideas or subjective experience that thoughts are racing, distractibility, increase in goal-directed activity or psychomotor agitation, and excessive involvement in pleasurable activities that have a high potential for painful consequences (e.g., engaging in unrestrained buying sprees, sexual indiscretions, foolish business investments). These symptoms cause significant impairment in occupational functioning, social activities, and relationships with others, and necessitate hospitalization for safety or if psychotic features are present. These symptoms are not due to the physiological effects of a substance or a general medical condition.

  ii) Hypomanic episode: similar, but requires only 4 days of an elevated, expansive, or irritable mood. It also is accompanied by symptoms described above and represents a change in functioning. The disturbance in mood and change in functioning are noted by others. Unlike manic episodes, hypomanic episodes don't cause marked impairment in social or occupational functioning, necessitate hospitalization, or include psychotic features. Like manic episodes, they cannot be the result of direct physiological effects of a substance or a general medical condition (APA, 2000a).

b. Substance-induced mania: The following agents play a role: drugs of abuse, especially amphetamines and cocaine, corticosteroids, NRTIs, NNRTIs, ganciclovir, and adrenergic agonists (Ruiz, 2006). Antidepressants can cause mania in persons diagnosed with major depressive disorder, but who actually have bipolar disorder.

c. Mania due to a general medical condition: The following conditions play a role: opportunistic infections of the CNS, neurosyphilis, CNS malignancies, cerebrovascular changes (Stolar, Catalano, Hakala, Bright, & Fernandez, 2005). Herpes and vitamin B12 deficiency may also be responsible (Ruiz, 2006).

d. HIV-associated mania: due to HIV infection of the brain or "multiple infections, metabolic, neoplastic, and pharmacologic insults to the brain" (Wyszynski et al., 2005, p. 189) that occur with HIV disease. Patients are less likely to have a family history. Patients experience more irritability, psychomotor slowing, and cognitive impairment, and have a more chronic course (Wyszynski et al., 2005).

2. Prevalence

a. National Comorbidity Study reports lifetime prevalence rate of bipolar disorder as 2.1%. Merikangas et al. (2007) also reported the rate for subthreshold bipolar disorder as 2.4%. They defined subthreshold bipolar disorder as "recurrent hypomania without a major depressive episode or with fewer symptoms than required for threshold hypomania" (Merikangas et al., 2007, p. 543). Combining these two rates increases the prevalence rate to 4.5%.

b. Judd and Akiskal (2003) reexamined the Epidemiological Catchment Area (ECA) database to determine the prevalence of bipolar disorder. They report the lifetime prevalence for bipolar spectrum disorders as 6.4%. This rate reflects the combined rates of manic episodes, hypomanic episodes, and subsyndromal manic/hypomanic symptoms (SSM). They defined persons with SSM as those who experienced two or more lifetime manic symptoms without meeting full criteria for a hypomanic or manic episode (Judd & Akiskal, 2003).

3. Etiology
   a. Etiology is complex, although it is thought to be the result of an interplay of changes in brain chemistry and structure. Genetics also play a role.
   b. Genetics: Individuals with a first-degree relative with bipolar disorder are at significantly higher risk than those without. Biological children of bipolar parents are at increased risk for bipolar disorder even if they are raised in an environment with nonaffected adoptive parents (Sadock & Sadock, 2003).
   c. Changes in brain chemistry: This is due to alterations in norephinephrine, serotonin, dopamine, glutamate, signaling pathways, and the "master clock."
   d. Changes in brain structure: Chemical and structural changes in the prefrontal cortex play a role in bipolar disorder, especially mania.

4. Goals of care
   a. Help reduce symptoms of depression or mania and improve functioning.
   b. Help patients learn a more effective coping style.
   c. Increase hope and optimism, which can lead to more active involvement in care.
   d. Establish a positive outlook, which research links with improved immune response.

5. Assessment
   a. Mental status exam
      i) Appearance: Patients may be very talkative and hyperactive, as well as either extremely happy or irritable.
      ii) Mood and affect: They may state that they feel the best they have ever felt in their life or that they are "on top of the world." Also, they may feel they are very "cranky" or irritable. Affect may be very bright, irritable, or labile.
      iii) Speech: Pressured speech may be present. It may be very difficult to interrupt or redirect.
      iv) Cognition: Memory and orientation are intact.
      v) Thoughts: Usually patients are easily distracted. Thoughts, as well as flow of thoughts, may be disorganized.
   b. Tools
      i) Structured Clinical Interview for DSM-IV Axis I Disorders (SCID) has a nonpatient version that can be used in outpatient medical settings and is easy to administer (APA, 2000b).
      ii) The Young Mania Rating Scale (YMRS) is used to assess severity of symptoms and can measure effects of treatment on symptoms (APA, 2000b). This scale is frequently used in research studies.
   c. Data gathering
      i) Gather information specific to presenting symptoms.
      ii) Obtain thorough medical, psychiatric, social, and family histories.
      iii) Assess for underlying medical conditions and substances (prescription, over-the-counter, illicit drugs, herbal supplements) that could cause or exacerbate mania.

iv)   Assess level of stress, including suicidality.

v)   Consider cultural variations in expression of mania.

6. Interventions focusing on mania

   a.   Nonpharmacologic

      i)   Psychoeducation (group or individual) to teach the patient about his/her illness and treatment options. Help him/her to learn to recognize signs and symptoms of mania to prevent relapse (National Institute of Mental Health [NIMH], 2007).

      ii)   Refer for psychotherapy. Cognitive behavioral therapy helps the patient to change negative thought patterns and inappropriate thoughts. Family therapy assists the patient and his/her family to decrease the stress in the family unit. This stress (a) may be caused by the patient experiencing symptoms associated with depression or mania or (b) may worsen symptoms for the patient. Interpersonal or social rhythm therapy helps the patient to improve relationships and establish a regular routine. Regular routines may help protect against mania (NIMH, 2007).

      iii)   Determine risk of self-harm and harm to others through direct and indirect means (neglect). See section on suicide in "Depression" for further information.

      iv)   Monitor and educate the patient regarding purpose and side effects of medications and ways to manage them.

      v)   Consider cultural variations in expression of mania.

      vi)   Provide education and support to significant others.

         (1)   Understand that nurturing the patient and encouraging independence can help support the patient.

         (2)   Patients who have the support of friends and family tend to cope better with their illnesses.

   b.   Pharmacologic

      i)   Valproate (valproic acid)

         (1)   Can be hepatotoxic, so monitor liver function tests regularly. Should be used in patients free of hepatic disease (Vergara-Rodriguez & Watts, 2008).

         (2)   Toxicity can develop, especially in advanced HIV disease. Signs/symptoms of toxicity include incoordination, ataxia, and tremor (Vergara-Rodriguez & Watts, 2008).

         (3)   Concurrent use with PIs can have mixed effects on valproate levels. PIs can inhibit CYP 450 2C9 (increase valproate levels) and induce urine glucuronyl transferase (decrease valproate levels) (Vergara-Rodriguez & Watts, 2008).

         (4)   Divalproex sodium, another available preparation of valproate, is better tolerated than valproic acid due to fewer gastrointestinal side effects, and it can be dosed less frequently.

      ii)   Lithium

         (1)   Used in patients free of renal dysfunction (Vergara-Rodriguez & Watts, 2008).

         (2)   Avoid in patients with advanced HIV disease due to tolerability issues and risk of toxicity (Stolar et al., 2005).

         (3)   Lithium has a narrow therapeutic index, and drug levels should be monitored to prevent toxicities (Vieta & Rosa, 2007).

(4) Use with caution in patients with HIV-related nephropathy because illness can cause decreased lithium clearance and possible lithium toxicity (APA, 2000a).

iii) Carbamazepine: Avoid with concurrent HAART. Can reduce levels of NNRTIs and PIs via CYP450 3A4 induction (Vergara-Rodriguez & Watts, 2008).

iv) Lamotrigine

   (1) Approved for maintenance treatment of bipolar disorder

   (2) Can be used with HAART but should be started at lower doses and titrated slowly to avoid development of rash or Stevens-Johnson syndrome (Vergara-Rodriguez & Watts, 2008)

   (3) Metabolized by UGT system so ritonavir and tipranavir may decrease levels of lamotrigine (Vergara-Rodriguez and Watts, 2008)

   (4) Has also been studied in the treatment of neuropathy (Wiffen & Rees, 2007)

REFERENCES

American Psychiatric Association (APA). (2000a). *Diagnostic and statistical manual of mental disorders* (4th ed., text rev.). Washington, DC: Author.

American Psychiatric Association (APA). (2000b). *Handbook of psychiatric measures*. Washington, DC: Author.

Judd, L. L., & Akiskal, H. S. (2003). The prevalence and disability of bipolar spectrum disorders in the U.S. population: Re-analysis of the ECA database taking into account subthreshold cases. *Journal of Affective Disorders, 73*(1–2), 123–131.

Merikangas, K. R., Akiskal, H. S., Angst, J., Greenberg, P. E., Hirschfeld, R. M. A., Petukhova, M., et al. (2007). Lifetime and 12-month prevalence of bipolar spectrum disorder in the National Comorbidity Survey replication. *Archives of General Psychiatry, 64*(5), 543–552.

National Institute of Mental Health (NIMH). (2007). *Bipolar disorder*. Bethesda, MD: National Institute of Mental Health, National Institutes of Health, and U.S. Department of Health and Human Services.

Ruiz, P. (2006). Mood disorders. In F. Fernandez & P. Ruiz (Eds.), *Psychiatric aspects of HIV/AIDS* (pp. 93–100). Philadelphia: Lippincott Williams & Wilkins.

Sadock, B. J., & Sadock, V. A. (2003). *Kaplan and Sadock's synopsis of psychiatry: Behavioral sciences/clinical psychiatry* (9th ed.). Philadelphia: Lippincott Williams & Wilkins.

Stolar, A., Catalano, G., Hakala, S. M., Bright, R. P., & Fernandez, F. (2005). Mood disorders and psychosis in HIV. In K. Citron, J. Brouillette & A. Beckett (Eds.), *HIV and psychiatry: Training and resource manual* (2nd ed., pp. 88–109). New York: Cambridge University Press.

Vergara-Rodriguez, P., & Watts, J. (2008). Use of psychotrophic medications in the HIV-positive patient: Part I. *Psychopharm Review, 43*(8), 59–66.

Vieta, E., & Rosa, A. R. (2007). Evolving trends in the long-term treatment of bipolar disorder. *World Journal of Biological Psychiatry, 8*(1), 4–11.

Wiffen, P. J., & Rees, J. (2007). Lamotrigine for acute and chronic pain. *Cochrane Database of Systematic Reviews, 2*, CD006044.

Wyszynski, A. A., Bruno, B., Ying, P., Chuang, L., Friedlander, M., & Rubenstein, B. (2005). The HIV-infected patient. In A. A. Wyszynski and B. Wyszynski (Eds.), *Manual of psychiatric care for the medically ill* (pp. 171–200). Washington, DC: American Psychiatric Publishing.

5.7 ANXIETY DISORDERS

1. Definitions

   a. Generalized anxiety disorder (GAD): a mood disorder in which a person experiences excessive anxiety and worry that is difficult to control. This is accompanied by three or more of the following symptoms: restlessness or feeling keyed up or on edge, easily fatigued, difficulty concentrating or mind going blank, irritability, muscle tension, or sleep disturbance. These symptoms cause clinically significant distress or impairment in functioning. Symptoms are not due to the direct effects of a medical condition or substance (APA, 2000).

b. Adjustment disorder with anxiety or adjustment disorder with mixed anxiety and depressed mood: See discussion in "Depression" for further information.

c. Panic disorder: a mood disorder in which a person experiences recurrent and unexpected panic attacks. A panic attack is a distinct period of intense fear or discomfort during which four or more of the following symptoms develop abruptly and reach a peak within 10 minutes: palpitations, pounding heart, or accelerated heart rate; sweating; trembling or shaking; sensations of shortness of breath or smothering; feeling of choking; chest pain or discomfort; nausea or abdominal distress; feeling dizzy, lightheaded, or faint; feelings of unreality or being detached from oneself; fear of losing control or going crazy, fear of dying, numbness, or tingling sensations; chills; hot flushes. At least one panic attack has been followed by at least 1 month of one or more of the following: persistent concern about having additional panic attacks; worry about the implications of having an attack or its consequences; or a significant change in behavior related to the attacks. Panic attacks are not due to the direct effects of a medical condition or substance (APA, 2000).

d. Posttraumatic stress disorder (PTSD): a response to significant life trauma from a variety of sources, including interpersonal violence, multiple AIDS-related losses, or notification of an HIV test. The traumatic event is persistently reexperienced in one or more of the following ways: recurrent and intrusive distressing recollection of the event; recurrent distressing dream of the event; acting or feeling as if the traumatic event were recurring; intense psychological distress when exposed to cues that symbolize or resemble an aspect of the event; or physiological reactivity when exposed to cues that symbolize or resemble an aspect of the traumatic event. Some additional symptoms include nightmares, intrusive thoughts and flashbacks, and poor self-care, including HIV management.

e. Anxiety disorder due to a general medical condition: The following disorders have anxiety as a component: fever, dehydration, opportunistic central nervous system (CNS) diseases, neurosyphilis, respiratory conditions, endocrinopathies, metabolic complications, cardiovascular disease, hyperventilation syndrome, neurocognitive disorders (HIV-associated dementia and minor cognitive motor disorder), and delirium.

f. Substance-induced anxiety disorder: Withdrawal or intoxication of substances is associated with anxiety. Anxiety associated with withdrawal is seen with nicotine, alcohol, sedative-hypnotics, heroin, and benzodiazepines. Intoxication with amphetamines (including methamphetamine, also known as crank, crystal, candy, ice, party, speed, Tina, or T), caffeine, cocaine (crack, freebase, rock, ski, smoke, snow), ecstasy (MDMA, E, X), gamma hydroxybutyrate (GHB), ketamine (K, Special K), and opiates is associated with anxiety.

2. Prevalence and impact

a. It is estimated that 2–40% of HIV-infected persons have an anxiety disorder (APA, 2002).

b. One prevalence study estimated that 39% of HIV-infected outpatients have a mood/anxiety disorder, and of these, 11% had posttraumatic stress disorder (Pence et al., 2006). Anxiety disorders can occur throughout the spectrum of HIV infection. HIV-related anxiety is common with milestones such as HIV testing; news of HIV-positive status; appearance of first symptoms; declining CD4 counts; increasing viral loads; onset of AIDS-defining illness; initiation of antiretroviral therapy (ART); onset of functional or cognitive disabilities, including multisystem medical conditions; negotiation of new sexual life; disclosure of HIV status; chronic pain; and end-of-life preparation.

3. Etiology
   a. Genetic or familial tendencies: Studies have shown that there is an increased rate of anxiety disorders in the first-degree relatives of individuals with anxiety disorders (Sadock & Sadock, 2003).
   b. Biological factors: It is thought that the limbic system mediates general anxiety, worry, and vigilance. The following neurochemicals appear to have a role in the regulation of anxiety: gamma-aminobutyric acid (GABA), serotonin, glutamate, and corticotrophin releasing factor. The amygdala and its many connections to other parts of the brain also play a role in anxiety (Stahl, 2008).
   c. Social and psychological factors: Cognitive-behavioral theory postulates that anxiety stems from an inaccurate assessment of perceived environmental dangers. Psychoanalytic theory proposes that anxiety results from unresolved unconscious conflicts. HIV-infected persons may have sexual orientation issues, a history of incarceration, or interpersonal violence that contributes to high levels of anxiety, both chronic and acute, or both. Poor social support and maladaptive coping strategies contribute to anxiety triggers.
   d. Effects of medications: Medications that can contribute to anxiety include acyclovir, zidovudine, efavirenz, indinavir, anabolic and corticosteroids, isoniazid, interferons, interleukin-2, and pentamidine. Psychotropic medications (e.g., selective serotonin reuptake inhibitors, venlafaxine, bupropion, psychostimulants, neuroleptics) can have the side effect of anxiety. Polypharmacy can also contribute to anxiety.
   e. Some psychiatric disorders have anxiety symptoms associated with them. These include adjustment disorders, depressive disorders, alcohol and other substance abuse, and bereavement.

4. Goals of care
   a. Reduce patient's level of discomfort.
   b. Help patient identify source of anxiety.
   c. Assist patient in developing alternative ways of coping.
   d. Decrease symptoms of anxiety and improve functioning.

5. Assessment
   a. Tools useful in evaluating anxiety
      i) The Structured Clinical Interview for *DSM-III-R* Non-Patient Version-HIV (SCID-NP-HIV) excludes HIV-related worries, but has a module for diagnosing HIV-specific adjustment disorders.
      ii) The Modified Hamilton Anxiety Rating Scale (some somatic anxiety symptoms are omitted) can also be useful.
   b. Data gathering

    i)   Gather information specific to presenting symptoms.

    ii)   Obtain a thorough past medical, psychiatric, social history (recent stressful events including homelessness, loss of loved one or job, incarceration, interpersonal violence), and family history.

    iii) Assess for underlying medical conditions and substances (prescription, over-the-counter, illicit drugs, herbal supplements) that could cause or exacerbate anxiety.

    iv)   Assess level of stress including suicidality.

    v)   Assess past history of interpersonal violence including sexual abuse.

    vi)   Consider cultural variations in expression of anxiety. Use language and interventions that are culturally appropriate and meaningful to the patient.

c. Physical signs associated with anxiety

    i)   Autonomic/somatic symptoms that can mimic medical conditions: shortness of breath and palpitations, chronic abdominal pain without pathology, gastrointestinal (GI) symptoms, and central and peripheral nervous systems. Sympathetic nervous system response includes increased heart rate, increased blood pressure, and dilated pupils.

    ii)   Other physical symptoms that can indicate anxiety: muscle tension, worried facial expression, tingling hands or feet, hand wringing, tremors or twitching, restlessness, GI disturbance, chest pain, palpitations, headache, shortness of breath, lightheadedness and dizziness, faintness, dry mouth, and increased motor activity.

d. Psychological symptoms associated with anxiety: worry, unexplained feeling of discomfort, difficulty with concentration, preoccupation with self, and complaints of chronic fatigue or lack of energy.

7. Interventions

a. Nonpharmacological

    i)   Supportive therapy

        (1) Express empathy.

        (2) Reassure patients about cause of physical symptoms of anxiety.

        (3) Identify patients' strengths and weaknesses.

        (4) Teach patients simple relaxation exercises, such as diaphragmatic breathing, progressive muscle relaxation, meditation, self-hypnosis, and imagery (APA, 2002; Blalock, Sharma & McDaniel, 2005; NYSDHAI, 2001).

    ii)   Electromyographic biofeedback, acupuncture, therapeutic touch

    iii) Weekly massage decreased both depression and anxiety in a study of HIV-infected adolescents (Basu, Chwastiak, & Bruce, 2005).

    iv)   Aerobic exercise

    v)   Coping strategies, such as goal setting, information seeking, skill mastery, help seeking, distraction (physical or mental), meditation, and prayer (Kemppainen et al., 2006)

    vi)   Cognitive-behavioral therapy, which deals with distorted patterns of thinking and maladaptive behaviors (Blalock, Sharma, & McDaniel, 2005). Exposure techniques can also be used by experienced therapists for panic disorder.

    vii) Psychoeducation can be done individually or in groups.

    viii) Peer support groups that are gender and culturally appropriate can provide basic information to reduce anxiety from knowledge deficit.

b. Pharmacologic

   i)   Selective serotonin reuptake inhibitors (SSRIs), such as fluoxetine, sertraline, paroxetine, citalopram, and escitalopram, are considered to be the first-line choice for the treatment of GAD, panic disorder, and PTSD. See discussion under "Depression."

   ii)   Mixed serotonin/norepinephrine reuptake inhibitors (SNRIs), such as venlafaxine, duloxetine, are also considered to be a first-line choice for the treatment of GAD, panic disorder, and PTSD. See discussion under "Depression."

   iii)   Buspirone: used for patients with persistent anxiety. Helpful for patients with anxiety and a history of substance abuse because there is no potential for abuse (APA, 2002; NYSDHAI, 2001). Need to start at low doses to avoid akathesia. Can see increased levels of nelfinavir, ritonavir, and efavirenz due to CYP 2D6 inhibition (Vergara-Rodriguez & Watts, 2008).

   iv)   Benzodiazepines: no longer a first-line treatment for anxiety disorders. Can be used as short-term adjunctive treatment (usually about 6 weeks) when first starting patients on SSRIs or SNRIs. Use with caution due to potential for physical and psychological dependence. Cytochrome P450 inhibition may lead to drug–drug interactions with PIs and NNTRIs. Midazolam and triazolam are contraindicated due to potential for oversedation. Lorazepam, temazepam, and oxazepam are preferred, especially for patients with liver dysfunction, as they are metabolized by the kidneys (Vergara-Rodriguez & Watts, 2008).

REFERENCES

American Psychiatric Association (APA). (2000). *Diagnostic and statistical manual of mental disorders* (4th ed., text revision). Washington, DC: Author.

American Psychiatric Association, Office on HIV Psychiatry (APA). (2002). *HIV and anxiety*. Retrieved February 13, 2009, from http://www.psych.org/Resources/OfficeofHIVPsychiatry/Resources/HIVMentalHealthTreatmentIssues_1/Anxiety.aspx

Basu, S., Chwastiak, L. A., & Bruce, R. D. (2005). Clinical management of depression and anxiety in HIV-infected adults. *AIDS, 19*(18), 2057–2067.

Blalock, A. C., Sharma, S. M., & McDaniel, J. S. (2005). Anxiety disorders and HIV disease. In K. Citron, J. Brouillette, & A. Beckett (Eds.), *HIV and psychiatry: Training and resource manual* (2nd ed., pp. 120–127). New York: Cambridge University Press.

Kemppainen, J. K., Eller, L. S., Bunch, E., Hamilton, M. J., Dole, P., Holzemer, W., et al. (2006). Strategies for self-management of HIV-related anxiety. *AIDS Care, 18*(6), 587–607.

New York State Department of Health AIDS Institute (NYSDHAI). (2001). *Mental health care for people with HIV infection: HIV clinical guidelines for the primary care practitioner*. New York: Author.

Pence, B. W., Miller, W. C., Whetten, K., Eron, J. J., & Gaynes, B. N. (2006). Prevalence of DSM-IV-defined mood, anxiety, and substance use disorders in an HIV clinic in the southeastern United States. *Journal of Acquired Immune Deficiency Syndrome, 42*(3), 298–306.

Sadock, B. J., & Sadock, V. A. (2003). *Kaplan and Sadock's synopsis of psychiatry: Behavioral sciences/clinical psychiatry* (9th ed.). Philadelphia: Lippincott Williams & Wilkins.

Stahl, S. M. (2008). *Stahl's essential psychopharmacology: Neuroscientific basis and practical applications* (3rd ed.). New York: Cambridge University Press.

Vergara-Rodriguez, P., & Watts, J. (2008). Use of psychotrophic medications in the HIV-positive patient: Part I. *Psychopharm Review, 43*(8), 59–66.

5.8 DELIRIUM

1. Definition
   a. Characterized by a disturbance of consciousness and change in cognition that develops over a short period of time and is caused by the direct physiologic consequences of a medical condition (APA, 2000a)
2. Prevalence
   a. Most common neuropsychiatric complication in hospitalized AIDS patients (NYSDHAI, 2001)
   b. Patients at high risk for developing delirium: those in advanced stages of immunosuppression; those with a history of opportunistic infections, substance use, or head/brain injury; those with previous episodes of delirium or dementia, or those with infection or malignancies of the central nervous system (CNS; NYSDHAI, 2001)
3. Etiology
   a. Single or multiple simultaneous etiologies may be present.
   b. Toxic causes are related to medications, alternative or complementary therapies, or drug or alcohol intoxication/withdrawal. Newly introduced medications should be high on the list of differential diagnoses.
   c. Metabolic causes include electrolyte disturbances, endocrine disorders, hypoxia, fever, and renal or liver insufficiency.
   d. Infectious causes include cryptococcal or toxoplasmosis or HIV disease itself.
   e. Vascular causes include congestive heart failure, cerebrovascular accidents, and anemia.
   f. Neurologic causes include encephalopathy, CNS malignancies and infections, seizures, and postictal state.
3. Goals of care
   a. Swiftly recognize and treat underlying cause(s).
   b. Apply appropriate therapies to reverse or control symptoms.
   c. Prevent injury to patient and others.
4. Assessment
   a. A sudden change in mental status warrants immediate nursing intervention with referral for emergency evaluation.
   b. Level of alertness may vary from agitation to lethargy, stupor, or coma.
   c. Patients are generally drowsy and may require repeated explanations from caregivers/examiners. Consider that a patient's ability to focus may be impaired, and modify instructions and education plans accordingly.
   d. Abrupt disturbances in sleep patterns or changes in level of activity should raise suspicions.
   e. Early signs and symptoms of delirium may be inaccurately attributed to anxiety.
   f. Clinical manifestations of delirium in patients with HIV may include the following:
      i)   Impairment of memory, orientation, prefrontal executive functions: difficulty with abstraction, difficulty with sequential thinking, impaired temporal memory, impaired judgment
      ii) Disturbances in thought and language with decreased verbal frequency

     iii)   Disturbances in perception: visual hallucinations and paranoid delusions

     iv)   Disturbances in psychomotor function: hypoactive, hyperactive, or mixed

     v)   Disturbances in the sleep-wake cycle with daytime lethargy, nighttime agitation

     vi)   Affective lability: rapid changes from one emotional state to another

     vii)   Neurologic abnormalities: tremors, myoclonus, asterixis, nystagmus, ataxia, cranial nerve palsies, and cerebellar signs (NYSDHAI, 2001)

  g. Interview caregiver and observe patient to assess functional status, medications, substance use, other new clinical signs and symptoms, and any history of delirium or precipitating event.

  h. Screening tools for delirium

     i)   Delirium Rating Scale Revised-98: Used clinically and in research studies, it has 3 diagnostic questions and 13 severity items; useful to monitor changes over time (APA, 2000b; Wyszynski, 2005).

     ii)   Confusion Assessment Method (CAM): bedside tool used by clinicians and researchers; has a version that substitutes nonverbal tasks for verbal responses in patients on ventilators (CAM-ICU; APA, 2000b; Wyszynski, 2005)

     iii)   Memorial Delirium Assessment Scale (MDAS): good for assessing patients with advanced disease (APA, 2000b; Kerrihard & Breitbart, 2004).

5. Interventions

  a. Nonpharmacological

     i)   Provide safe and consistent environment and increase supervision of patient as indicated.

     ii)   Institute appropriate treatment for causative condition, monitor patient's response, and report adverse effects of treatment.

     iii)   Communicate in clear, simple terms to avoid misperceptions.

     iv)   Educate patient, family, and significant other regarding care and diagnostic procedures, medications given and expected effects, and the need to orient the patient to person, time, place, and situation.

     v)   Ensure patient's activities of daily living are met.

     vi)   Attempt to organize care to ensure patient's nighttime sleep is undisturbed.

     vii)   Evaluate patient/caregiver resources for continuing care when hospitalization is no longer required.

     viii)   If patient does not sleep through the night, nighttime help or temporary placement may be necessary until the patient's sleep and activity needs are reestablished.

     ix)   Avoid restraints due to potential to cause injury and increase agitation (Wyszynski, 2005).

     x)   Implement relaxation techniques such as massage, music, and relaxation tapes to decrease agitation and enhance sleep (Wyszynski, 2005).

  b. Pharmacologic

     i)   Correct underlying conditions that have led to delirium.

     ii)   Short-term low doses of antipsychotics may be used to treat confusion or agitation (Lacasse, Perreault, & Williamson, 2006).

REFERENCES

American Psychiatric Association (APA). (2000a). *Diagnostic and statistical manual of mental disorders* (4th ed., text revision). Washington, DC: Author.

American Psychiatric Association (APA). (2000b). *Handbook of psychiatric measures*. Washington, DC: Author.

Kerrihard, T. N., & Breitbart, W. (2004). General issues in hospital HIV psychiatry. In K. Citron, J. Brouillette, & A. Beckett (Eds.), *HIV and psychiatry: Training and resource manual* (2nd ed., pp. 128–137). New York: Cambridge University Press.

Lacasse, H., Perreault, M. N., & Williamson, D. R. (2006). Systematic review of the treatment of hospital-associated delirium in medically or surgically ill patients. *The Annals of Pharmacotherapy, 40*(11), 1966–1973.

New York State Department of Health AIDS Institute (NYSDHAI). (2001). *Mental health care for people with HIV infection: HIV clinical guidelines for the primary care practitioner*. New York: Author.

Wyszynski, A. A. (2005). The delirious patient. In A. A. Wyszynski & B. Wyszynski (Eds.), *Manual of psychiatric care for the medically ill* (pp. 1–26). Washington, DC: American Psychiatric Publishing.

5.9 MENTAL ILLNESS AND SUBSTANCE USE

1. Definition
   a. Dual diagnosis refers to the concurrence of mental health disorders and substance abuse disorders (alcohol or drug dependence or abuse, or both).
   b. Dual diagnosis and dual/multiple disorders profiles may include the following:
      i) Severe/major mental illness and a substance disorder(s)
      ii) Substance disorder(s) and personality disorder(s)
      iii) Substance disorder(s), personality disorder(s), and substance-induced acute symptoms that may require psychiatric care (i.e., hallucinations, depression, and other symptoms resulting from substance abuse or withdrawal)
      iv) Substance abuse, mental illness, and organic syndromes in various combinations. Organic syndromes (e.g., HIV) may be a result of substance abuse, or they may be independent of substance abuse.
   c. Acronyms that define various dual disorders
      i) MICA(A): mentally ill, chemical abusers (and addicted)
      ii) MISA: mentally ill substance abuser
   d. Many studies of comorbidity show that people with alcohol and drug use disorders have high rates of personality disorder, bipolar depression, major depression, and, to a lesser extent, anxiety disorders. Whereas only a small number of substance users suffer from severe psychotic disorders, a sizable portion of people with severe psychotic disorders appear to have comorbid substance abuse disorders (Cournos & McKinnon, 1997).
2. Etiology and epidemiology
   a. The association between drug use and high-risk behaviors and mental illness
      i) The CDC reports that 17% of new AIDS cases in 2006 occurred among injection-drug users (CDC, 2006).
      ii) Studies of the sexual activity of the mentally ill have demonstrated that a significant portion of the mentally ill are engaging in sexual activity and those who do report recent sexual activity have engaged in multiple risk behaviors (Cournos & McKinnon, 1997).

iii) One prevalence study estimated that 39% of HIV clinic patients had a mood or anxiety disorder, 21% had a substance abuse diagnosis, and 8% had both (Pence et al., 2006).

iv) The prevalence of alcohol problems or alcohol use disorder in HIV-infected populations has been estimated to range from 22% to 60% of patients (Fiellin, 2004).

v) Men who have sex with men (MSM) who use methamphetamine are more likely to contract HIV through receptive anal intercourse than MSM who do not use the drug (Halkitis et al., 2005).

3. Goals of care
   a. Maintain the safety of the patient regardless of the setting.
   b. Decrease the symptoms associated with the specific mental illness.
   c. Decrease the negative effects of substance use for the patient and others (harm reduction).

4. Assessment
   a. Alcohol Use Disorders Identification Test (AUDIT; Babor et al., 1992)
   b. CAGE Screening Tool (Mayfield et al., 1974)
   c. CAGE-AID Screening Tool (Brown & Rounds, 1995)
   d. Drug Abuse Screening Test (DAST; Skinner, 1982)
   e. Fagerstrom Test for Nicotine Dependence (Fagerstrom et al., 1992)
   f. RAFFT Screening Tool (Riggs & Alario, 1989)

5. Interventions
   a. Nonpharmacologic
      i) Acupuncture
      ii) Day treatment programs
      iii) Inpatient treatment programs
      iv) Motivation interviewing (pros and cons)
      v) Needle exchange
      vi) 12-step programs (AA, CA, CMA, NA, etc.)
   b. Pharmacologic (Naegle & D'Avanzo, 2001)
      i) Alcohol abuse/dependency/withdrawal
         (1) Benzodiazepines can be used to ameliorate signs and symptoms of alcohol withdrawal.
         (2) Beta-blockers can modify some of the hyperactivity of the autonomic nervous system associated with alcohol withdrawal.
         (3) Carbamazepines, phenytoin, and naltrexone can be used in the treatment of seizures associated with alcohol withdrawal, but should be used with caution due to the potential drug–drug interactions with antiretroviral agents.
         (4) Disulfiram (Antabuse) is an alcohol-abuse deterrent. It works by blocking the biotransformation of alcohol, causing unpleasant side effects (e.g., vomiting, upset stomach) when even a small amount of alcohol is consumed. It should not be used with metronidazole or an alcohol-containing medicine. (Note: capsule and liquid formulation of antiretrovirals contain alcohol.)
         (5) Kudzu and other herbal remedies have demonstrated some effectiveness in reduction of alcohol intake (Lukas et al., 2005; Overstreet et al., 2003).
         (6) Vitamin therapy, including large doses of B vitamins, is currently being used investigationally in the treatment of alcohol and other drug addictions.

    ii) Opiate dependency/withdrawal

       (1) Buprenorphine is an opioid drug with partial agonist and antagonist activity used in the treatment of opioid addiction in patients with HIV infection (Fiellin, 2004; Khalsa et al., 2006).

       (2) Methadone is a synthetic opioid used medically in the treatment of narcotic addiction.

       (3) Levo-alpha-acetylmethadol (LAAM) is a synthetic opioid, similar in structure to methadone, that has a long duration of action due to its active metabolites.

    iii) Stimulant dependency withdrawal

       (1) Selective serotonin reuptake inhibitors (SSRIs) are currently being used investigationally in the treatment of methamphetamine addiction.

    iv) Tobacco dependency

       (1) Bupropion hydrochloride (wellbutrin) is an atypical antidepressant. It acts as norepinephrine reuptake inhibitor, dopamine reuptake inhibitor, and nicotinic antagonist. It is used as an antidepressant and as a smoking cessation aid.

       (2) Nicotine replacement therapy (NRT), in various forms of nicotine delivery methods, is used to replace nicotine obtained from smoking or other tobacco usage.

       (3) Varenicline tartrate is the first approved nicotinic receptor partial agonist used in the treatment of tobacco addiction.

REFERENCES

Babor, T. F., de la Fuente, J. R., Saunders, J., & Grant, M. (1992). *AUDIT: The Alcohol Use Disorders Test: Guidelines for use in primary health care*. Geneva, Switzerland: WHO.

Brown, R. L., & Rounds, L. A. (1995). Conjoint screening questionnaires for alcohol and drug abuse. *Wisconsin Medical Journal, 94*(3), 135–140.

Centers for Disease Control and Prevention (CDC). (2006). *HIV/AIDS Surveillance Report, 18*.

Cournos, F., & McKinnon, K. (1997). Substance use and HIV risk among people with severe mental illness. *NIDA Research Monograph, 172,* 110–129.

Fagerstrom, K. O., Heatherton, T. F., & Kozlowski, L. T. (1992). Nicotine addiction and its assessment. *Ear, Nose, and Throat Journal, 69*(11), 763–767.

Fiellin, D. A. (2004). Perspective: Substance use disorders in HIV-infected patients: Impact and New Treatment Strategies. *Topics in HIV Medicine, 12*(3), 77–82.

Halkitis, P. N., Shrem, M. T., & Martin, F. W. (2005). Sexual behavior patterns of methamphetamine-using gay and bisexual men. *Substance Use and Misuse, 40*(5), 703–719.

Khalsa, J., Vocci, F., Altice, F., Fiellin, D., & Miller, V. (2006). Buprenorphine and HIV primary care: New opportunities for integrated treatment. *Clinical Infectious Diseases, 43*(Suppl. 4), S169–S172.

Lukas, S. E., Penetar, D., Berko, J., Vicens, L., Palmer, C., Mallya, G., et al. (2005). An extract of the Chinese herbal root kudzu reduces alcohol drinking by heavy drinkers in a naturalistic setting. *Alcohol Clinical and Experimental Research, 29*(5), 756–762.

Mayfield, D., McLeod, G., & Hall, P. (1974). The CAGE questionnaire: Validation of a new alcoholism screening instrument. *American Journal of Psychiatry, 131*(10), 1121–1123.

Naegle, M. A., & D'Avanzo, C. E. (2001). *Addictions and substance abuse: Strategies for advanced practice nursing*. Upper Saddle River, NJ: Prentice Hall.

Overstreet, D. H., Keung, W.-M., Rezvani, A. H., Massi, M., & Lee, D. Y.-W. (2003). Herbal remedies for alcoholism: Promises and possible pitfalls. *Alcohol Clinical and Experimental Research, 27*(2), 177–185.

Pence, B. W., Miller, W. C., Whetten, K., Eron, J. J., & Gaynes, B. N. (2006). Prevalence of DSM-IV-defined mood, anxiety, and substance use disorders in an HIV clinic in the southeastern United States. *Journal of Acquired Immune Deficiency Syndrome, 42*(3), 298–306.

Riggs, S. R., & Alario, A. (1989). Adolescent substance use instructor's guide. In C. Dube, M. Goldstein, D. Lewis, E. Meyes, & W. Zwick (Eds.), *Project ADEPT curriculum for primary care physician training* (Vol. II, pp. 1–57). Providence, RI: Brown University.

Skinner, H. A. (1982). The Drug Abuse Screening Test. *Addictive Behavior, 7*(4), 363–371.

5.10 HIV-ASSOCIATED DEMENTIA COMPLEX

1. Definitions
   a. HIV-associated dementia (HAD): constellation of cognitive, motor, and behavioral dysfunctions frequently observed in persons with AIDS. HAD may occur at any stage of HIV, but is usually associated with later stages of disease, variable severity, and progressive nature (Hult, Chana, Masliah, & Everall, 2008).
   b. Minor cognitive motor disorder (MCMD): presence of cognitive or motor dysfunction. Milder than HAD as person is able to work and perform ADLs, except those that are most demanding (Wyszynski et al., 2005). Does impact ability to function in areas such as medication adherence and driving (McArthur, 2004).
   c. Subclinical cognitive motor impairment: minimal cognitive or motor dysfunction that doesn't impair work or ADLs. Gait and strength are normal (Wyszynski et al., 2005).
2. Prevalence and factors
   a. HAD is the most common of the neurological disorders resulting from HIV infection. The effect of HAART on the prevalence of HAD is not clear. One study found no decline from pre-HAART levels in the post-HAART era (Cysique, Maruff, & Brew, 2004), whereas another study found significant declines (Dilley et al., 2005).
   b. Some studies suggest that CD4 count is inversely related to the risk of developing HAD, whereas HIV viral load is directly related to the risk of developing HIV related CNS disease (Childs et al., 1999; d'Arminio Monforte et al., 2004).
   c. Mild motor and psychomotor decline is evident shortly after onset of HIV infection, even in the absence of specific CNS AIDS-defining illnesses or HIV dementia (Clifford, 2002).
   d. MCMD is associated with worse HIV disease prognosis (Gonzalez-Scarano & Martin-Garcia, 2005).
   e. Women may have greater risk of HIV-associated cognitive impairment (McArthur, 2004).
   f. May be associated with decreased quality of life, decreased survival, sense of decreased performance at work, and unemployment (Maggi, Rourke, & Halman, 2004).
   g. HAD may be incorrectly diagnosed as Alzheimer's disease (AD), but differs from AD in that it is more likely to present with behavioral changes and progresses more rapidly, but is rarely associated with aphasia (Meehan & Brush, 2001); the cortical brain damage associated with AD is slowly progressive and is first characterized by memory impairment, and eventually by disturbances in reasoning, planning, language, perception, and social behavior (Stopford et al., 2008).
3. Etiology
   a. HIV infects brain macrophages and microglia in the central nervous system (Gonzalez-Scarano & Martin-Garcia, 2005).

   b. HIV dementia is a subcortical disorder, whereas AD is a cortical disorder with three characteristics found only at autopsy: neurofibrillary tangles, neuritic plaques, and neuronal loss (Alzheimer, 1907; Brew et al., 2005).
4. Goals of care
   a. Reduce cognitive, behavioral, and/or psychomotor symptoms and improve functioning.
   b. Assist patients in developing mechanisms to cope with cognitive, behavioral, and/or psychomotor symptoms.
5. Assessment
   a. Tools used to screen for HIV-associated dementia complex
      i)   HIV Dementia Scale (HDS): tests memory-registration, attention, psychomotor speed, memory recall, and constructional abilities in a short, easy-to-administer format (Power et al., 1995).
      ii) International HIV Dementia Scale (IHDS): consists of three subtests that include timed alternating hand sequence test, timed finger-tapping, and recall of four items after 2 minutes. Ability to speak English not required, takes a few minutes to complete, and only instrument needed is a watch with a second hand. Useful in settings with few resources (Sacktor et al., 2005).
   b. Cognitive changes: mental slowing, decline in attention and concentration, difficulties with problem solving, abstraction, and using previously acquired knowledge (Wyszynski et al., 2005)
   c. Behavioral: personality changes, social withdrawal, apathy, and agitated psychosis (Wyszynski et al., 2005)
   d. Motor: unsteady gait, leg weakness, loss of coordination, tremor, eye movement abnormalities, and fine motor difficulties, such as impaired handwriting (Wyszynski et al., 2005).
6. Interventions
   a. Prevention
      i)   Current research indicates that HIV infection may be associated with an increased risk for vascular disease, diabetes, and heart disease.
      ii) There is evidence that HIV can sequester in the central nervous system and brain within a few days of initial infection (Ghorpade et al., 1998; Gonzalez-Scarano & Martin-Garcia, 2005).
      iii) Aging may place HIV-infected persons at greater risk for dementia and increase the need for primary and secondary prevention interventions. Promoting a healthy diet and exercise, as well as quitting smoking, are indicated; addressing risk factors related to diabetes, glucose elevations, and metabolic abnormalities may help prevent or slow disease progression.
   b. Nonpharmacologic
      i)   For patients
           (1) Avoid multitasking; do one thing at a time.
           (2) Utilize stress reduction and relaxation techniques.
           (3) Use memory aids.
           (4) Talk aloud as you complete a task.
           (5) Get enough rest to avoid fatigue.

(6) Plan activities ahead of time to avoid stress.

(7) Maintain a regular exercise routine.

(8) Ask for help when tasks become too difficult to do (Wyszynski et al., 2005).

ii) For caregivers

(1) Have a consistent routine.

(2) Orient person as needed.

(3) Keep items in the same place.

(4) Keep level of stimulation low.

(5) Avoid confrontation.

(6) Use redirection or distraction with inappropriate behavior.

(7) Stay calm (Wyszynski et al., 2005).

c. Pharmacologic

i) Antiretroviral therapy can delay or mitigate the symptoms of HAD (Hult et al., 2008).

ii) Consider treatment of associated depression, anxiety, and/or fatigue.

iii) Psychostimulants can improve fatigue and cognitive impairment (Wyszynski et al., 2005).

iv) In a small preliminary study, Lexipafant was shown to improve the memories of people with HIV-related cognitive dysfunction (Schifitto et al., 1999).

v) In two pilot studies, selegiline patches were associated with improved verbal memory and psychomotor speed test results (Sacktor et al., 2000).

REFERENCES

Alzheimer, A. (1907). Über eine eigenartige erkrankung der hirnrinde [About a peculiar disease of the cerebral cortex]. *Allgemeine Zeitschrift für Psychiatrie und psychisch-gerichtliche Medizin, 64,* 146–148. English translation in *Archives of Neurology* (1967), *21,* 109–110.

Brew, B. J., Pemberton, L., Blennow, K., Wallin, A., & Hagberg, L. (2005). CSF amyloid beta42 and tau levels correlate with AIDS dementia complex. *Neurology, 65*(9), 1490–1492.

Childs, E. A., Lyles, R. H., Selnes, O. A., Chen, B., Miller, E. N., Cohen, B. A., et al. (1999). Plasma viral load and CD4 lymphocytes predict HIV-associated dementia and sensory neuropathy. *Neurology, 52*(3), 607–613.

Clifford, D. B. (2002). AIDS dementia. *Medical Clinics of North America, 86*(3), 537–550.

Cysique, L. A., Maruff, P., & Brew, B. J. (2004). Prevalence and pattern of neuropsychological impairment in human immunodeficiency virus-infected/acquired immunodeficiency syndrome (AIDS) patients across pre- and post-highly active antiretroviral therapy eras: A combined study of two cohorts. *Journal of Neurovirology, 10*(6), 350–357.

d'Arminio Monforte, A., Cinque, P., Mocraft, A., Goebel, F.-D., Antunes, F., Katlama, C., et al. (2004). Changing incidence of central nervous system disease in the EuroSIDA cohort. *Annuals of Neurology, 55*(3), 320–328.

Dilley, J. W., Schwarcz, S., Loeb, L., Hsu, L., Nelson, K., & Scheer, S. (2005). The decline of incident cases of HIV-associated neurological disorders in San Francisco, 1991–2003. *AIDS, 19*(6), 634–635.

Ghorpade, A., Nukuna, A., Che, M., Haggerty, S., Persidsky, Y., Carter, E., et al. (1998). Human immunodeficiency virus neurotropism: An analysis of viral replication and cytopathicity for divergent strains in monocytes and microglia. *Journal of Virology, 72*(4), 3340–3350.

Gonzalez-Scarano, F., & Martin-Garcia, J. (2005). The neuropathogenesis of AIDS. *Nature Reviews Immunology, 5*(1), 69–81.

Hult, B., Chana, G., Masliah, E., & Everall, L. (2008). Neurobiology of HIV. *International Review of Psychiatry, 20*(1), 3–13.

Maggi, J. D., Rourke, S. B., & Halman, M. (2004). Cognitive disorders in people living with HIV disease. In K. Citron, J. Brouillette, & A. Beckett (Eds.), *HIV and psychiatry: Training and resource manual* (2nd ed., pp. 30–55). New York: Cambridge University Press.

McArthur, J. C. (2004). HIV dementia: An evolving disease. *Journal of Neuroimmunology, 157*(1–2), 3–10.

Meehan, R. A., & Brush, J. A. (2001). An overview of AIDS dementia complex. *American Journal of Alzheimer's Disease & Other Dementias, 16*(4), 225–229.

Power, C., Selnes, O. A., Grim, J. A., & McArthur, J. C. (1995). HIV dementia scale: A rapid screening test. *Journal of Acquired Immune Deficiency Syndromes and Human Retrovirology, 8*(3), 273–278.

Sacktor, N., Schifitto, G., McDermott, M. P., Marder, K., McArthur, J. C., & Kieburtz, K. (2000). Transdermal selegiline in HIV-associated cognitive impairment: Pilot, placebo-controlled study. *Neurology, 54*(1), 233–235.

Sacktor, N. C., Wong, M., Nakasujja, N., Skolasky, R. L., Selnes, O. A., Musisi, S., et al. (2005). The international HIV dementia scale: A new rapid screening test for HIV dementia. *AIDS, 19*(13), 1367–1374.

Schifitto, G., Sacktor, N., Marder, K., McDermott, M. P., McArthur, J. C., Kieburtz, K., et al. (1999). Randomized trial of the platelet-activating factor antagonist lexipafant in HIV–associated cognitive impairment. *Neurology, 53*(2), 391–396.

Stopford, C. L., Snowden, J. S., Thompson, J. C., & Neary, D. (2008). Variability in cognitive presentation of Alzheimer's disease. *Cortex, 44*(2), 185–195.

Wyszynski, A. A., Bruno, B., Ying, P., Chuang, L., Friedlander, M., & Rubenstein, B. (2005). The HIV-infected patient. In A. A. Wyszynski & B. Wyszynski (Eds.), *Manual of psychiatric care for the medically ill* (pp. 171–200). Washington, DC: American Psychiatric Publishing.

CHAPTER 6

Concerns of Special Populations

6.1 ADOLESCENTS

1. Description of the community
   a. Adolescence is a gradual and variable process from onset of puberty until maturity.
   b. For clinical purposes, adolescence extends from ages 12 to 21 years.
   c. Legally, adolescents are minors (under the age of majority) until age 18 in 47 states and age 19 in Alabama, Nebraska, and Wyoming.
   d. A *mature minor,* covered by mature minor doctrine, can understand the benefits and risks of treatment and is able to give informed consent.
   e. An *emancipated minor* is married, serving in the armed forces, or living apart from parents and managing own financial affairs.
   f. A *medically emancipated* minor is, in addition to the previous, above a specified age, a minor parent or runaway, deemed able to provide informed consent and to seek care for a condition that, if left untreated, could jeopardize the health of self or others (e.g., consent for pregnancy-related care, including contraceptive care; diagnosis and treatment of sexually transmitted diseases [STDs], including HIV; treatment for substance abuse).
   g. Demographics
   i) According to the Centers for Disease Control and Prevention (CDC), half of all new HIV infections in 2005 occurred in people between the ages of 13 and 25, reflecting an increase in transmission due to high-risk behaviors (CDC, 2005).
   ii) Geographic variation includes higher rates in urban areas, especially the Northeast and South.
   iii) African American and Hispanic adolescents have been disproportionately affected by HIV infection. Between the ages of 13 and 19, African Americans and Hispanics accounted for 66% and 21%, respectively, of the reported AIDS cases in 2003 (CDC, 2005).
2. Common health issues
   a. Adolescence is a time of growth and experimentation, a stage of striving for independence/autonomy, and a time of feeling curious and invulnerable. All of these factors may lead to sexual and drug-related risk behaviors that increase exposure to HIV (Neinstein, Gordon, Katzman, Rosen, & Woods, 2008). Social skills and negotiating skills are still evolving.

b. Adolescents generally are concrete thinkers, especially those under age 18; therefore, they are unlikely to think of the long-term consequences of their actions. Teens process information differently from adults or children.

c. Denial is a strong defense mechanism, and peer groups are major directives of behavior.

3. HIV/AIDS in the adolescent community

   a. Transmission, risk behaviors, and prevention issues

     i)   Most adolescents are unaware of their HIV status and may unknowingly transmit the virus.

     ii)   Primary identifiable mode of HIV transmission among adolescents is sexual activity, mainly heterosexual in females and homosexual in males. Most adolescents do not personalize risk or threat of HIV infection.

     iii) According to the *2007 Youth Risk Behavior Survey,* sexual intercourse was reported in almost half of all high school students, but only 63% reported condom use during their last encounter. Additionally, almost half of the students surveyed had used alcohol in the last 30 days and 38% had used marijuana (CDC, 2008).

     iv)   In a study of African American and Latina adolescent females with older male partners (3 years older or more), both gender and age power imbalance were found to increase young women's HIV risk (UCSF Center for AIDS Prevention Studies and AIDS Research Institute, 1999).

     v)   Twenty-three percent of sexually active high school students nationwide had drunk alcohol or used drugs before their last sexual intercourse (CDC, 2008).

     vi)   Adolescents at highest risk are those out of their homes (e.g., teens in foster care, or incarcerated, runaways, transient/homeless youth), school dropouts, young adolescent women, men having sex with men and those exploring same-sex relationships, sexually abused adolescents, teens in a high-prevalence community, and HIV-affected teens or those orphaned by the death of HIV-infected parent.

     vii) The risk of HIV transmission increases considerably in the presence of an STI (National Institute of Allergy and Infectious Diseases, 2006).

     viii) In early puberty, physiologic immaturity of the female cervical transformation zone increases vulnerability. A study by the Pediatric AIDS Clinical Trials Group, protocol 219C, found that 47.5% of the study population of girls aged 13 and older had abnormal cervical cytology, including atypical cells of undetermined significance, low-grade squamous intraepithelial lesions (SIL), and high-grade SIL (Brogly et al., 2007).

     ix)   Barriers to prevention programs include the following:

       (1) Parents, community organizations, and school systems often refuse to support HIV/AIDS educational offerings due to their denial, homophobia, and inadequate training.

       (2) A lack of social marketing exists; most teens report not knowing how or where to get tested.

       (3) Many adolescents at highest risk are the most difficult to reach; 10–15% of youth have dropped out of school (U.S. Department of Health and Human Services, Health Resources and Services Administration, HIV/AIDS Bureau, 2001a).

       (4) Many adolescents know about transmission, but fewer know to prevent infection or lack the skills to practice safer behaviors.

       (5) Half of teens believe parental permission is needed to get tested, which is often not true. Confidentiality is essential to ensure use of testing and treatment facilities by adolescents. Adolescents have the same right to confidentiality as adults have.

b. Access to care, treatment, and research

  i) Barriers include the following:

     (1) HIV care often is provided to adolescents by people with no training in adolescent health; few providers are trained to serve the specific sexual needs of minority youth.

     (2) The largest gap in health services is the treatment of adolescents with mental health or alcohol and substance-abuse problems.

     (3) Health care is not a top priority for most adolescents; many deny any health threat.

     (4) One in three youths, 18–24 years old, has no public or private health insurance.

     (5) There is a lack of youth-centered services that are accessible, convenient, and confidential.

     (6) There is a lack of a unified support community.

     (7) Adherence barriers related to developmental stage or specific psychosocial issues include chaotic lives, competing interests, fear of disclosure to family or friends, lack of support, conflict between dependency on adults and need to challenge authority for independence, acceptance of treatment when feeling well, and understanding of complex regimens (U.S. Department of Health and Human Services, Health Resources and Services Administration, HIV/AIDS Bureau, 1999).

     (8) Clinical research is impacted by small numbers of HIV-infected adolescents in care.

     (9) Institutional review boards that examine research proposals to ensure participant safety, confidentiality, and informed consent must weigh potential value of information about youth versus the vulnerability of youth.

    (10) Healthcare providers of HIV-infected youth are often not knowledgeable about opportunities for participation in research.

4. Specific care approaches

a. Individual

  i) Build and maintain a trusting relationship based on confidentiality. Assess family disclosure and dysfunction, social relationships, sexual orientation, mental health, parenting/pregnancy, job, school, and shelter.

  ii) Assess risk of STDs, alcohol and drug use, and incidents of abuse or violence. Use peer health educators/counselors; teens are more receptive to input from respected peers than from authoritarian adults.

  iii) Provide information to correct misconceptions (e.g., HIV is transmitted only if sick).

  iv) Promote routine, voluntary, and confidential HIV counseling and testing.

    v)   Build communication and negotiation skills.

    vi)   Provide risk reduction with condom demonstration and application practice.

 b. Community

    i)   HIV-prevention programs are most successful when appropriate adolescents (e.g., appropriate age range and sexual orientation, culturally competent) are involved in the planning and implementation.

    ii)   Prevention programs need to be implemented, sustained, and reinforced before practice of risky behavior (before early teen years).

    iii) Include information on sexual practices; most sexual intercourse is spontaneous rather than planned.

    iv) Provide easy access to condoms.

    v)   Provide easy access to information on drug use: Alcohol and recreational drugs impair judgment and promote high-risk behaviors.

    vi)   Prevention programs should involve various groups, such as media, schools, parents, and community organizations.

    vii) Outreach for those not in home or school include venues such as mobile vans, residential childcare facilities, shopping malls, recreation centers, youth shelters, and detention centers; ORASURE, HIV antibody test by oral swab, or OraQUICK Rapid HIV Antibody Test by finger stick should be available at these venues.

    viii) Each visit for health care should include STD and pregnancy prevention counseling (CDC, 2000).

    ix)   Prevention programs must be linked to HIV counseling and testing, comprehensive health care with support and legal services, and access to research on a continuum.

    x)   Use recognized adolescent models as guides for developing teen programs (e.g., U.S. Department of Health and Human Services, Health Resources and Services Administration, HIV/AIDS Bureau, 2001b).

REFERENCES

Brogly, S. B., Watts, D. H., Ylitalo, N., Franco, E. L., Seage, G. R., Oleske, J., et al. (2007). Reproductive health of adolescent girls perinatally infected with HIV. *American Journal of Public Health, 97*(6), 1047–1052.

Centers for Disease Control and Prevention (CDC). (2000). *Most teens not provided STD or pregnancy prevention counseling during check-ups.* Retrieved November 21, 2008, from www.thebody.com/cdc/std/teen_checkup.html

Centers for Disease Control and Prevention (CDC). (2005). *HIV/AIDS surveillance report: HIV infection and AIDS in the United States and dependent areas, 2005.* Retrieved November 21, 2008, from http://www.cdc.gov/hiv/topics/surveillance/basic.htm#hivaidsage

Centers for Disease Control and Prevention (CDC). (2008). *Youth risk behavior surveillance—United States, 2007.* Retrieved November 21, 2008, from http://www.cdc.gov/mmwr/preview/mmwrhtml/ss5704a1.htm

National Institute of Allergy and Infectious Diseases. (2006). *HIV infection in adolescents and young adults: NIAID fact sheet, May 2004.* Retrieved November 21, 2008, from http://www.niaid.nih.gov/factsheets/hivadolescent.htm

Neinstein, L. S., Gordon, C. M., Katzman, D. K., Rosen, D. S., & Woods, E. R. (2008). *Adolescent health care: A practical guide* (5th ed.). Philadelphia: Lippincott Williams & Wilkins.

USCF Center for AIDS Prevention Studies and AIDS Research Institute. (1999). *What are adolescents' HIV prevention needs?* San Francisco: Author.

U.S. Department of Health and Human Services, Health Resources and Services Administration, HIV/AIDS Bureau. (1999). *Helping adolescents with HIV adhere to HAART, 1999.* Washington, DC: Author.

U.S. Department of Health and Human Services, Health Resources and Services Administration, HIV/AIDS Bureau. (2001a). *Youth and HIV/AIDS.* Washington, DC: Author.

U.S. Department of Health and Human Services, Health Resources and Services Administration, HIV/AIDS Bureau. (2001b). *Lessons learned.* Washington, DC: Author.

White House Office of National AIDS Policy. (2000). *Youth and HIV/AIDS 2000: A new American agenda.* Washington, DC: Author.

6.2 THE BLIND AND VISUALLY IMPAIRED COMMUNITY

1. Description of the community
   a. Visual impairment occurs when vision is not fully corrected by ordinary prescription lenses, medical treatment, or surgery; it includes conditions ranging from the presence of good usable vision, to low vision, to the complete absence of sight.
   b. Blindness is lack of usable sight.
   c. Legal blindness defines visual conditions that, when present, connote eligibility for government or other benefits and services. An individual who is legally blind has a visual acuity of 20/200 or less in the better eye with the best correction, or a visual field of no more than 20 degrees and cannot read the big *E* on the Snellen eye chart.
   d. Low vision: Vision is not corrected to normal vision with standard eyeglasses or contact lenses, medications, or surgery, although some good usable vision remains. People with low vision can learn to make the best use of the vision available to them.
   e. Although estimates vary, there are approximately 20 million people with significant visual loss in the United States (American Foundation for the Blind, 2008).
   f. Approximately 1.3 million Americans are legally blind (American Foundation for the Blind, 2008).
   g. Approximately 109,000 people with visual impairments in the United States use long canes for mobility. Slightly more than 7,000 Americans use guide dogs (American Foundation for the Blind, 2008).
   h. Of all Americans who are blind or visually impaired, approximately 80% are White, 18% are Black, 8% are Hispanic, and 2% are other races (American Foundation for the Blind, 2008).
   i. Currently 42% of Americans with visual disabilities are married, 33% are widowed, 13% are separated or divorced, and 13% have never been married (American Foundation for the Blind, 2008).
   j. Approximately 46% of adult Americans with visual impairments are employed, whereas 32% of working-age Americans with blindness are employed. People with visual disabilities do not have the same range of opportunities available to them as sighted people (American Foundation for the Blind, 2008).
   k. Barriers to employment include poverty; discrimination; lack of education, resources, and necessary technology; and employer's lack of awareness.
   l. Forty-five percent of individuals with severe visual impairment or blindness have a high school diploma, compared with 80% of fully sighted individuals. Among high school

graduates, those with severe visual impairment or blindness are about as likely to have taken some college courses as those who are sighted, but they are less likely to have graduated (American Foundation for the Blind, 2008).

m. Of people with visual impairments, approximately 62% of Whites complete high school or higher education, compared with 41% of Blacks and 44% of Hispanics (American Foundation for the Blind, 2008).

2. Common health problems
   a. People with visual impairment suffer from a lack of understanding and research about visual impairment and the idea by sighted people that people with blindness are also deaf and mute.
   b. Adults over 55 years of age have more psychological and physical problems, such as depression, because of loss, isolation, and inability to maintain quality of life and activities of daily living.
   c. Due to lack of funding, only 1% of the elderly with visual impairment who need assistance and education are able to get help.
   d. Access to health care is an issue.
      i) Access to health care is difficult to assess. Most studies focus on either children (those younger than 21 years of age) or adults over 55 years when discussing psychosocial effects of blindness.
      ii) Lack of employment leads to lack of private insurance coverage.
      iii) Lack of own transportation leads to reliance on public transportation, family, or friends, which leads to a lack of independence.
      iv) Children have less mobility difficulties and adapt more quickly to their surroundings. More are being mainstreamed in public schools to prevent social isolation.

3. HIV/AIDS and visual impairment
   a. It is estimated that 50% to 75% of all HIV/AIDS clients will be affected at some point with ocular complications (Kestelyn & Cunningham, 2001).
   b. Causes of ocular complications include the following:
      i) Cytomegalovirus (CMV) retinitis (leading cause) tends to occur in advanced HIV infection, usually once the CD4+ T-cell count has fallen below 50 cells/mm^3. The combination of highly active antiretroviral therapy (HAART) and effective anti-CMV drugs, such as ganciclovir, foscarnet, and cidofovir, has vastly improved the visual prognosis for patients with CMV retinitis and has dramatically reduced the risk of developing bilateral blinding disease in the industrialized world (Kestelyn & Cunningham, 2001).
      ii) Progressive outer retinal necrosis and acute retinal necrosis: Non-CMV retinitis is a much rarer cause of retinal infection in HIV/AIDS patients. Progressive outer retinal necrosis, a disease caused mainly by varicella zoster virus, is characterized by fulminant, progressive retinal necrosis with relatively little vitreous inflammation. Herpes simplex virus may produce an identical clinical picture, often following or in association with viral encephalitis (Kestelyn, 2000).
      iii) HIV-related ischemic microvasculopathy and cotton-wool spots, the hallmark of HIV retinopathy, are probably the most common ocular manifestation of HIV infection occurring in about 50% of patients with HIV/AIDS. Like CMV retinitis, HIV

retinopathy tends to occur in advanced HIV disease, usually once the CD4+ T-cell count has fallen below 50 cells/mm^3. The etiology of HIV retinopathy is obscure, but it rarely develops after HAART (Cunningham & Margolis, 1998).

iv) Ocular syphilis is the most common bacterial intraocular infection in HIV-infected patients. Vision loss in patients with syphilis occurs most frequently as a result of either uveitis or optic nerve disease (Cunningham & Margolis, 1998).

v) Tuberculosis is the single most important HIV-related opportunistic infection in developing countries. Given the huge number of patients with both HIV/AIDS and active TB in developing countries, it is probable that ocular complications of TB occur more frequently than has been recognized (Havlir & Barnes, 1999).

vi) Cryptococcal meningitis is the most common life-threatening fungal pathogen that affects patients with AIDS. If left untreated, cryptococcal meningitis is always fatal (Kestelyn & Cunningham, 2001).

vii) Allergic drug reactions, sometimes known as Stevens-Johnson syndrome, are part of a spectrum of skin and mucous membrane diseases caused by a hypersensitivity reaction to various drugs or toxins, of which sulfa drugs are the most common (Coster, 1997).

c. It is difficult to assess the contribution of HIV/AIDS to blindness. Most studies have been carried out in industrialized countries, although more than 90% of all HIV sufferers live in developing countries. The CDC does not consider blindness to be a reportable demographic.

d. At present most patients with HIV/AIDS in developing countries who lose their vision have a very limited life expectancy. As antiretroviral therapy makes its way to these countries, life expectancy related to HIV/AIDS can be expected to increase.

4. Common problems
  a. Specific issues
    i) Transmission, risk behavior, and prevention
      (1) Gaps in sexual education, including HIV/AIDS and STDs
      (2) Lack of educational material for visually impaired
  b. Specific approaches
    i) Individual
      (1) Points of etiquette when interacting with a person who is blind or visually impaired include the following:
        (a) Introduce yourself using your name and position, especially if you are wearing a name badge containing this information.
        (b) Speak directly to the person who is blind or visually impaired, not through a companion, guide, or other individual.
        (c) Speak using a natural conversational tone and speed. Do not speak loudly or slowly, unless the person also has a hearing impairment.
        (d) Address the person by his/her name when possible. This is especially important in crowded areas.
        (e) Immediately greet the person when he or she enters a room or a service area. This allows you to let the person know you are present and ready to assist, and it eliminates uncomfortable silences.

(f) Indicate the end of a conversation to avoid the embarrassment of leaving a person speaking when no one is actually there (especially for those who are totally blind).

(g) Feel free to use words that refer to vision, such as *look, see,* and *watch;* they are part of everyday verbal communication. The words *blind* and *visually impaired* are also acceptable in conversation.

(h) Be precise and thorough when you describe people, places, or things to people who are totally blind. Don't leave things out or change a description because you think it is unimportant or unpleasant.

(i) Feel free to use visually descriptive language. Making reference to colors, patterns, designs, and shapes is perfectly acceptable.

(j) Offer to guide people who are blind or visually impaired by asking if they would like assistance. Offer them your arm. It is not always necessary to provide guided assistance; in some instances it can be disorienting and disruptive. Respect the desires of the person.

(k) Guide people who request assistance by allowing them to take your arm just above the elbow when your arm is bent. Walk ahead of the person you are guiding. Never grab a person who is blind or visually impaired by the arm and push him or her forward.

(l) Do not leave a person who is blind or visually impaired standing in free space when you serve as a guide. Always be sure that the person has a firm grasp on your arm or is leaning against a chair or a wall if you have to be separated momentarily.

(m) Guide dogs are working mobility tools. Do not pet them, feed them, or distract them while they are working.

(n) Be calm and clear about what to do if you see a person who is blind or visually impaired about to encounter a dangerous situation. For example, if a person is about to bump into a stanchion in a hotel lobby, calmly and firmly call out, "Wait there for a moment; there is a pole in front of you."

ii) Community

(1) Sexual education is generally acquired from conferences.

(2) Programs should assist individuals with visual impairments to be able to access conferences and conference material.

(3) Outreach efforts need to include people with visual impairments and other disabled groups.

REFERENCES

American Foundation for the Blind. (2008). *Statistical snapshots.* Retrieved January 29, 2008, from http://www.afb.org/Section.asp?SectionID=15

Coster, D. J. (1997). Stevens-Johnson syndrome. *Developments in Ophthalmology, 28,* 24–31.

Cunningham, E. T., Jr., & Margolis, T. P. (1998). Ocular manifestations of HIV infection. *New England Journal of Medicine, 339*(4), 236–244.

Havlir, D. V., & Barnes, P. F. (1999). Tuberculosis in patients with human immunodeficiency virus infection. *New England Journal of Medicine, 340*(5), 367–373.

Kestelyn, P. G. (2000). AIDS and the eye in developing countries. In S. Lightman (Ed.), *HIV and the eye* (pp. 237–263). London: Imperial College Press.

Kestelyn, P., & Cunningham, E. (2001). HIV/AIDS and blindness. *Bulletin of the World Health Organization, 79*(3), 208–213.

6.3 COMMERCIAL SEX WORKERS

1. Description of the community
   a. Sex industry workers are men, women, or transgendered individuals who exchange sexual services for money, gifts, drugs, a place to sleep, or other needs. General work locations include the street, massage parlors, escort services, and brothels.
   b. Economic need is the driving force behind entry into the industry. Individuals remain in this job until their economic situation changes, substance abuse issues are resolved, or individuals are able to leave coercive relationships or domination by other persons (e.g., pimp, madam). As in other professions, the more autonomy the worker has, the less vulnerable he or she is to stressors. For example, a number of peer organizations have been formed around the world that function to keep sex workers informed about health and other issues.
2. Common health issues
   a. Sex industry workers are often from oppressed groups (e.g., youth; women; ethnic or racial minorities; gay, lesbian, bisexual, transgendered people; homeless people with mental illness; or people living with addiction).
   b. Psychosocial issues include low educational or vocational skills, poor social support or connectedness with caring adults, complex social entanglements, and likelihood of criminalized lifestyle.
   c. Psychological issues including low self-esteem, low self-efficacy, decreased assertiveness, depression, posttraumatic stress, hopelessness, and multiple losses of support can affect persons with HIV and will often place individuals at risk for increased risk-taking behaviors. In addition, different patterns of stigma also can have an impact on behavior (Ross, Timpson, Williams, Amos, & Bowen, 2007).
   d. There is often a history of living with violence and sexual and physical abuse during childhood. Sex industry workers continue to be victims of violent crimes by patrons, employers, partners, police, and vigilantes.
3. HIV/AIDS in the sex industry worker community
   a. Transmission, risk behaviors, and prevention issues
      i) Sex workers who use IV drugs or crack cocaine are at very high risk for infection, transmission, and risk-taking behavior.
      ii) Risk for workers is often higher than it is for patrons because workers have multiple contacts and are more likely to perform higher risk receptive acts (e.g., patrons will often pay 2 to 3 times normal rates for unprotected sex).
      iii) There is an increased risk of partner being an IV drug user.
      iv) Sex industry workers are at increased risk for acquiring and transmitting multidrug resistant viral species.

     v) Sex industry workers are at increased risk of transmitting HIV infection, if not on anti-retrovirals, due to high HIV viral loads.

    vi) There is an increased risk of contracting and transmitting multiple HIV subtypes, opportunistic infections (OIs), and sexually transmitted diseases (STDs).

  b. Access to care, treatment, and research

     i) Barriers to care include financial issues, such as lack of health insurance, and a knowledge deficit concerning how to access the healthcare system. When the worker does not work, there is no income to pay for care.

    ii) Addiction and mental illness may be barriers to healthcare access.

   iii) Self-care efficacy may be decreased.

   iv) Fear and avoidance by healthcare workers and health systems related to stigma of sex work.

    v) Society and healthcare providers may be indifferent to women, substance users, and marginalized groups.

   vi) There may be limited access to experimental and complementary therapies that may improve quality of life.

  vii) Poor treatment outcomes are affected by numerous factors, including barriers to health care, late diagnosis and treatment of HIV disease and OIs, and chaotic interaction with healthcare system (e.g., lack of consistent care, incomplete treatment regimens, poor baseline health/nutritional status).

4. Specific care approaches

  a. Individual

     i) Establish trust through open, nonjudgmental exploration of lifestyle, issues related to substance use, and health history. Obtain an in-depth sexual history, which many sex industry workers do not want to disclose to healthcare providers.

    ii) Allow time for relationship to develop, be patient, and ask direct questions.

   iii) Foster hope and independence while recognizing functional and social limitations.

   iv) Assess legal history and current legal problems, and be aware of current laws related to sex work and HIV. Provide referrals when necessary.

    v) Assess knowledge of and provide education about healthy lifestyles, safer sex practices, and harm-reduction modalities (if pertinent). Provide written educational resources at fifth-grade reading level.

   vi) Assess connection to financial support systems, such as Social Security.

  vii) Social assistance and other forms of financial assistance may allow sex workers to stop working. HIV diagnosis can increase eligibility for financial assistance.

  viii) Refer for educational and career counseling when appropriate.

   ix) Discuss available support services with the client to reduce isolation and hopelessness and to begin the healing process.

    x) Refer to a peer group for support if one is available or if the patient has access to the Internet.

   xi) Refer to family, psychiatric, or addiction services and drug treatment if appropriate, preferably with a primary care provider who is able to provide sensitive, consistent care. Knowledge of working hours and substance abuse habits can assist in making appointments that can be kept.

b. Community
   i)   Use outreach teams to provide education about safer sex and safer substance use, and provide a connection to health care, legal services, and drug treatment.
   ii)   Use outreach workers recruited from the community of former sex industry workers because they are familiar with the community and culture.
   iii)   Organize a multidisciplinary team of healthcare providers educated about the needs of this population and implement consciousness raising regarding possible bias.
   iv)   Services and supplies (e.g., female and male condoms) should be accessible, affordable, accompanied with negotiation skills, and modeled by peers (Witte, Takeshi, El-Bassel, Gilbert, & Wallace, 2000).
   v)   The goal is to reduce risky behavior through the provision of needed healthcare services that include, but are not limited to, counseling to reduce drug abuse and sexual and physical abuse, and to support those seeking alternative employment opportunities.
   vi)   Work with law enforcement to provide useful interventions when sex workers are incarcerated.
   vii)   Direct education and outreach to sex industry consumers about risks related to HIV infection and transmission.
   viii) Focus on using a holistic approach to care by providing integrated programs that include substance abuse treatment (e.g., needle exchanges, drug treatment, methadone maintenance programs), abuse counseling, and the provision of basic primary care from a single care facility.
   ix)   Expand use of community-based clinics, mobile units, and home care nursing to provide services in the areas where sex workers live and work.

REFERENCES

Ross, M. W., Timpson, S. C., Williams, M. L., Amos, C., & Bowen, A. (2007). Stigma consciousness concerns related to drug use and sexuality in a sample of street-based male sex workers. *International Journal of Sexual Health, 19*(2), 57–67.

Witte, S. S., Wada, T., El-Bassel, N., Gilbert, L., & Wallace, J. (2000). Predictors of female condom use among women exchanging street sex in New York City. *Sexually Transmitted Diseases, 27*(2), 93–100.

6.4 THE GAY AND BISEXUAL MALE COMMUNITY

1. Description of the community
   a. Risk categorization
      i)   Although the label *men who have sex with men (MSM)* continues to be used as a risk category in statistical reporting of HIV/AIDS, many gay and bisexual men consider it offensive and reductionistic, connoting mere physicality during sexual encounters between men. One's sexual identity development and sexual behaviors are more complex, necessitating a holistic appreciation of same-sex intimacy, emotional attachment, and bonding.

ii) The gay and bisexual male community may include males who (a) identify as gay (i.e., engage or affiliate with the gay community as an element of their identity), (b) are bisexual (i.e., have erotic responses to both men and women, and may or may not identify with the gay community), and (c) have sex with men (MSM) but do not self-identify as gay or bisexual (whether or not they have sex with women). Additional terms such as *queer*, *questioning*, or *curious* may be used to denote varying degrees of how individuals align sexual behaviors with self-identification.

b. Sexual identity

i) A man's sexual identity is influenced by physical, emotional, and spiritual relationships with his partners; varying levels of affiliation with the gay culture and community may impact individual identity and behaviors through stereotypes, social expectations and opportunities, and/or peer pressure; and a man's personal comfort with his sexual identity is also impacted by familial, social, and political pressures that may be negative (e.g., stigma, legal discrimination) or positive (e.g., partner welcomed into family, same-sex unions legally recognized).

c. Diversity in the community

i) Gay and bisexual men are not a homogenous or monolithic group. They are diverse in age, race, ethnicity, socioeconomics, political affiliations, and religious beliefs; they may be impoverished, homeless, or orphaned. Gay and bisexual men may use injection drugs, have hemophilia, or live a life of celibacy. They may be single, partnered, married, or divorced and may have children. Hence, the interventions developed for HIV prevention, treatment, and care must be specifically targeted to meet the needs of a diverse group of men.

2. Common health issues

a. Stereotypes

i) Nurses, physicians, and other healthcare providers may embrace erroneous stereotypes, unfair biases, and a moral disdain of gay and bisexual men (Lobaugh, Clements, Averill, & Olguin, 2006; Northen, 2008).

ii) Programs need to educate providers and readjust attitudes if the providers are to be comfortable discussing sexuality and effective in meeting health needs (Harding, 2007).

iii) Providers need to be familiar with the complex emotional, interpersonal, and sociopolitical influences on personal sexual behaviors and the impact of healthcare worker prejudices.

b. Mental health

i) Mental health care professionals are often uneducated and insensitive to the internal struggles common to the coming-out process.

ii) Men who keep their sexual orientation secret may be distressed by compartmentalizing their personal life from their workplace persona or keeping details of their love life from their family members.

iii) Gay and bisexual men frequently do not inform their providers of their sexual orientation for fear of moral judgment and/or loss of confidentiality. Mental health providers may be ill equipped to counsel men who have experienced multiple losses of partners, friends, and acquaintances to AIDS.

c. Sexually transmitted infections

i)   The presence of a sexually transmitted infection (STI) facilitates the transmission of HIV to uninfected partners.

ii) Gay and bisexual men have disproportionately high rates of STIs (Stolte, de Wit, Kolader, Fennema, Coutinho, & Dukers, 2006). The incidence of syphilis among MSM remains high in the United States and is significantly associated with HIV coinfection (Taylor, Aynalem, Smith, Bemis, Kenney, & Kerndt, 2004).

iii) The emergence of multidrug-resistant, community-acquired methicillin-resistant *Staphylococcus aureus* (MRSA) infections among MSM across the United States may be sexually transmitted between same-sex partners (Diep et al., 2008).

d. Stigma

i)   Perceived stigma may be a barrier to the prevention and treatment of sexually transmitted diseases and HIV testing. Stigma interferes with HIV-positive men accessing resources and services for self-care management of their disease (Chenard, 2007).

e. Comorbid addictions

i)   Rates of alcoholism and tobacco use are high among gay men; the use of illicit and recreational drugs by young MSM increases HIV-related sexual risk behaviors.

ii) The recreational use of (crystal) methamphetamine among gay and bisexual men has reached epidemic proportions; "meth" is highly addictive and significantly associated with sexual disinhibition and multiple sexual partnering, which increases risks for acquiring HIV infection (Halkitis & Jerome, 2007).

3. Transmission, risk behaviors, and prevention

a. Disproportionately infected and affected

i)   The combined reported risk categories of MSM and MSM who use injection drugs accounted for 47% of the adolescent/adult AIDS cases reported in the United States in 2005, more than 70% of the cumulative number of adolescent/adult AIDS cases reported in the United States since the beginning of the epidemic, and approximately 68% of all AIDS-related deaths in the country (CDC, 2007).

b. Seroprevalence rates

i)   Population-based estimates of HIV seroprevalence among MSM have ranged from 11–17.7% in New York City (Manning et al., 2007) to 26.8% in San Francisco (Osmond, Pollack, Paul, & Catania, 2007).

c. Differential risk perception

i)   Gay men use condoms more often with partners with whom they have an intimate relationship than with males with whom they engage in casual sexual encounters (Sanchez et al., 2006).

ii) Nearly a third of HIV-positive men who knew their serostatus had unprotected anal intercourse (UAI) with a steady male partner; UAI was associated with positive men who identified as heterosexual, use crack cocaine, have lower education, and have a partner of "unknown" HIV status (Denning & Campsmith, 2005). MSM who are traveling on vacation have significantly more UAI than when not on vacation (Benotsch et al., 2006).

d. Men of color

i)   Men of color—particularly Black (not Hispanic/Latino men)—are disproportionately represented in new HIV infections, new cases of AIDS, and among deaths due to no treatment. Men of color may be less likely to self-identify as gay, bisexual, or even as an MSM in response to peer pressure, social stigmas, and/or cultural mores; hence, prevention, care, and treatment information may not be perceived as relating to them. Men of color may not perceive sufficient support from the "gay community" to initiate and maintain safer sexual behaviors.

e. Alcohol, tobacco, and other drugs (ATODs)

   i)   The associations between the use of ATODs illustrate the risks of mood-altering substances that lower sexual inhibitions and increase risk of unsafe sexual behaviors. The "recreational" use of drugs to enhance and extend erections (i.e., prescribed for men with erectile dysfunction conditions) is widespread and associated with engaging in unprotected anal intercourse (Benotsch et al., 2006).

f. Social barriers

   i)   Gay and bisexual men confront stigma, ridicule, discrimination, and interpersonal violence as a result of predominant social and religious prejudices. In addition, the illegality of male–male sexual behaviors in many states, the lack of relationship recognition (i.e., marriage or partner rights), and an apathy among law enforcement and judicial systems to protect the rights of gay and bisexual men contributes to an environment in which sexuality is often hidden and encounters may be clandestine.

g. Entrée into community

   i)   Each individual MSM has a unique "entrée" into the community; there are no official orientation programs or social rituals (e.g., dating expectations, prom night traditions) to guide men. Hence, initial (or ongoing) sexual encounters may be clandestine and clouded by shame. Men who seek anonymous sexual partners to maintain confidentiality may sacrifice the ability to explore intimacy and relationship building. Same-sex coupling either assumes a heterosexual framework or proceeds by trial and error; this may add to the stress associated with "coming out."

h. Bisexual men

   i)   There is scant literature differentiating the healthcare or HIV prevention needs of bisexual men from gay and other MSM. Men who have sex with men and women (MSMW) confront challenges in disclosure and misunderstanding of their sexual orientation. Bisexual behavior is highly contextual, varies by culture, and intersects with concepts of masculinity, homophobia, and socioeconomic factors (Stokes, Miller, & Mundhenk, 1998).

   ii)   Injection drug using men who have sex with men and women (IDU-MSMW) reported similar rates of insertive unprotected anal intercourse (UAI) with women as MSM (exclusively), but were only half as likely to report receptive UAI with male sexual partners (Knight et al., 2007).

   iii)   Models used to understand bisexual White men may not be appropriate for men of color; HIV prevention interventions need to be tailored to the needs of specific groups (Stokes, Miller, & Mundhenk, 1998).

4. Access to Care, Treatment, and Research

  a. Disparities in health

     i)   Subgroups are often marginalized through subtle or overt means. Collect data from expert informants to reassess practical barriers to accessing care and treatment (e.g., lack of translators) as well as perceived barriers (e.g., staff insensitivity with transgendered clients).

ii) Sensitive outreach and engagement may encourage marginalized subgroups to engage in research activities. Provide opportunities for HIV-negative gay and bisexual men to engage in intervention research (as controls or participants).

b. Health literacy skills

i) Educational and support materials directed toward the gay and bisexual male community often wrongly assume that they have a fundamental understanding of health promotion, self-care behaviors, and the ability to navigate the healthcare system. Developing multimedia materials (e.g., print, digital, online, DVDs) for a wide-ranging audience may be more effective in recruiting clients into care and treatment.

5. Specific care approaches

a. Individual

i) Information

(1) In addition to printed brochures, advertisements, and posters, HIV prevention approaches may include one-on-one counseling, personal skill-building activities, and group discussions. Pilot test materials with gay and bisexual men to avoid unanticipated stereotypes or offensive terminology. Reevaluate educational approaches and materials for their applicability to the target audience (e.g., younger vs. older).

ii) Psychosocial

(1) Provide education, networking, counseling, and support for gay men "coming out of the closet" to reduce internalized homophobia, increase self-esteem, and build skills in negotiating safer sex.

(2) The unique issues for HIV-negative gay men (e.g., survivor guilt, social isolation, anxieties about becoming infected) have been diminished and undervalued; prevention programs must address these issues openly and assist uninfected gay men to manage the complexities of their emotional and sexual lives.

iii) Targeting prevention interventions

(1) Targeted, and culturally appropriate, prevention services for men in minority populations and other marginalized subpopulations of the gay community (e.g., gay men with visual or hearing impairments, teens, bisexual men) need to be developed.

(2) Gay men who seek casual sexual partners via Internet sites are more likely to engage in unprotected anal intercourse; effective prevention messages could be designed for online dissemination (Taylor et al., 2004).

(3) Men who believe it is "inevitable" that they will acquire HIV need intensive, innovative, and sensitive HIV prevention programs.

iv) Outreach to young MSM

(1) Developing targeted prevention services for young men who have sex with men must integrate substance use as a facilitator of UAI (Celentano et al., 2006) and consider the issues of homelessness and sex-for-money among youth.

(2) Internet chat rooms may provide young men of color with opportunities to find sexual partners; they may also provide innovative approaches to prevention messages (Fields et al., 2006).

v) Addressing personal stressors

(1) Disclosing one's HIV status is an ongoing stressor for both HIV-positive and HIV-negative men; interventions that assist men in using disclosure as another

prevention tool must target men by their method of finding sexual partners (Riet-meijer, Lloyd, & McLean, 2007). HIV-positive gay men were more likely to be diagnosed with rectal gonorrhea (RG) than HIV-negative gay men (or men who did know their serostatus); rates of RG were higher for men reporting "safer sex fatigue" (Stolte et al., 2006).

   vi) Peer educators and support networks

      (1) Gay men have experienced unprecedented levels of AIDS-related death, grief, and bereavement. The traumatic effects of the epidemic losses may affect prevention behaviors and erode the individual's resolve to remain uninfected; HIV prevention programs can facilitate grief, acknowledge the traumas, and explore the effects on the health and well-being of HIV-negative gay men.

  b. Community

    i) Engage the community

      (1) Employ gay and bisexual men as outreach workers, clinicians, and counselors. Recognize social relationships by collaborating with community leaders and utilizing the community media.

    ii) Gay community versus HIV community

      (1) After decades of high HIV seroprevalence in the gay and bisexual community, it may be difficult to distinguish between supports for MSM and supports for (specifically) HIV-positive MSM. For young gay and bisexual men, it is important to promote a same-sex identity without becoming HIV infected. Continue to develop programs that neither ostracize nor demonize HIV-positive persons; inclusive and supportive approaches will support all members.

REFERENCES

Benotsch, E. G., Seeley, S., Mikytuck, J. J., Pinkerton, S. D., Nettles, C. D., & Ragsdale, K. (2006). Substance use, medications for sexual facilitation, and sexual risk behavior among traveling men who have sex with men. *Sexually Transmitted Diseases, 33*(12), 706–711.

Celentano, D. D., Valleroy, L. A., Sifakis, F., MacKellar, D. A., Hylton, J., Thiede, H., et al. (2006). Associations between substance use and sexual risk among very young men who have sex with men. *Sexually Transmitted Diseases, 33*(4), 265–271.

Centers for Disease Control and Prevention (CDC). (2007). *HIV/AIDS surveillance report, 2005* (Vol. 17). Atlanta, GA: U.S. Department of Health and Human Services, Centers for Disease Control and Prevention.

Chenard, C. (2007). The impact of stigma on the self-care behaviors of HIV-positive gay men striving for normalcy. *Journal of the Association of Nurses in AIDS Care, 18*(3), 23–32.

Denning, P. H., & Campsmith, M. L. (2005). Unprotected anal intercourse among HIV-positive men who have a steady male sex partner with negative or unknown HIV serostatus. *American Journal of Public Health, 95*(11), 152–158.

Diep, B. A., Chambers, H. F., Graber, C. J., Szumowski, J. D., Miller, L. G., Han, L. L., et al. (2008). Emergence of multidrug-resistant, community-associated, methicillin-resistant *Staphylococcus aureus* clone USA300 in men who have sex with men. *Annals of Internal Medicine, 148*(4), 249–257.

Fields, S. D., Wharton, M. J., Marrero, A. I., Little, A., Pannell, K., & Morgan, J. H. (2006). Internet chat rooms: Connecting with a new generation of young men of color at risk for HIV infection who have sex with other men. *Journal of the Association of Nurses in AIDS Care, 17*(6), 53–60.

Halkitis, P. N., & Jerome, R. C. (2007). A comparative analysis of methamphetamine use: Black gay and bisexual men in relation to men of other races. *Addictive Behaviors, 33*(1), 83–93.

Harding, T. (2007). The construction of men who are nurses as gay. *Journal of Advanced Nursing, 60*(6), 636–644.

Knight, K. R., Shade, S. B., Purcell, D. W., Rose, C. D., Metsch, L. R., Latka, M. H., et al. (2007). Sexual transmission risk behavior reported among behaviorally bisexual HIV-positive injection drug-using men. *Journal of the Acquired Immune Deficiency Syndrome, 46*(Suppl. 2), S80–S87.

Lobaugh, E. R., Clements, P. T., Averill, J. B., & Olguin, D. L. (2006). Gay-male couples who adopt: Challenging historical and contemporary social trends toward becoming a family. *Perspectives in Psychiatric Care, 42*(3), 184–195.

Manning, S. E., Thorpe, L. E., Ramaswamy, C., Jajat, A., Marx, M. A., Karpati, A. M., et al. (2007). Estimation of HIV prevalence, risk factors, and testing frequency among sexually active men who have sex with men, aged 18–64 years—New York City, 2002. *Journal of Urban Health, 84*(2), 212–225.

Northen, S. (2008). Pride and prejudice. *Nursing Standard, 22*(22), 18–20.

Osmond, D. H., Pollack, L. M., Paul, J. P., & Catania, J. A. (2007). Changes in prevalence of HIV infection and sexual risk behavior in men who have sex with men in San Francisco: 1997–2002. *American Journal of Public Health, 97*(9), 1677–1683.

Rietmeijer, C. A., Lloyd, L. V., & McLean, C. (2007). Discussing HIV serostatus with prospective sex partners: A potential HIV prevention strategy among high-risk men who have sex with men. *Sexually Transmitted Diseases, 34*(4), 215–219.

Sanchez, T., Finlayson, T., Drake, A., Behel, S., Cribbon, M., DiNenno, E., et al. (2006). Human immunodeficiency virus (HIV) risk, prevention, and testing behaviors—United States, National HIV Behavioral Surveillance System: Men who have sex with men, November 2003–April 2005. *Morbidity and Mortality Weekly Report, 55*(SS-6), 1–16.

Stokes, J. P., Miller, R. L., & Mundhenk, R. (1998). Toward an understanding of behaviorally bisexual men: The influence of context and culture. *The Canadian Journal of Human Sexuality, 7*(2), 101–113.

Stolte, I. G., de Wit, J. B. F., Kolader, M., Fennema, H., Coutinho, R. A., & Dukers, N. H. T. M. (2006). Association between "safer sex fatigue" and rectal gonorrhea is mediated by unsafe sex with casual partners among HIV-positive homosexual men. *Sexually Transmitted Diseases, 33*(4), 201–208.

Taylor, M., Aynalem, G., Smith, L., Bemis, C., Kenney, K., & Kerndt, P. (2004). Correlates of Internet use to meet sex partners among men who have sex with men diagnosed with early syphilis in Los Angeles County. *Sexually Transmitted Diseases, 31*(9), 552–556.

6.5 HIV-INFECTED HEALTHCARE WORKERS

1. Description of the community (CDC, 2003)
   a. Through December 2002, 486,826 AIDS cases in the United States were reported for whom occupational information is available. Of these cases, 24,844 (5.1%) were employed in health care, and 5,378 were nurses.
   b. Most of these healthcare workers were infected from nonoccupational exposure to HIV. There have been 57 occupationally acquired HIV infections among healthcare workers (26 have developed AIDS); 24 of these cases involved nurses, 16 involved laboratory workers, 6 involved in physicians, 2 involved surgical technicians, 1 involved a dialysis technician, 1 involved a respiratory therapist, 1 involved a health aide, 1 involved an embalmer/morgue technician, and 2 involved housekeepers/maintenance workers. Since December 2001, no new documented cases of occupationally acquired HIV/AIDS cases have been reported.
2. Common health issues
   a. Physical concerns
      i) Dealing with HIV-related fatigue while at work (evaluate sleep patterns, anemia, medications, and inadequate nutrition; Association of Nurses in AIDS Care, 2001)
      ii) Pushing too hard to prove one is healthy and can perform job responsibilities
      iii) Limiting exposure to opportunistic infections in the workplace (see "Work issues" section, p. 238)

   iv)   Remembering to take care of self (e.g., getting an annual flu vaccine, eating a bal-
         anced diet, exercising, getting plenty of sleep; ANAC, 2001)
 b. Psychosocial concerns
   i)   Avoiding overidentification with own HIV patients' physical and psychosocial issues
   ii)   Needing to be attentive to issues of grief overload, including loss of roles and
         changes in body image
   iii) Balancing the amount of HIV/AIDS work and volunteering
   iv)   Allowing self to be the patient, not the nurse, with healthcare providers involved in
         own care
   v)   Adjusting to having friends and colleagues who are now one's caregivers
   vi)   Allowing self to be a receiver rather than solely a giver of care
   vii) Working with own state nurses' association and ANAC chapter
   viii) Learning to know when, how, and what to ask for regarding own needs
 c. Financial/legal concerns
   i)   Deciding when to go on disability (earlier vs. later in course of illness); changing
         from full- to part-time employment, which may affect insurance eligibility or cost of
         premiums for health, life, and disability insurance
   ii)   Resolving confidentiality issues if employed at the same place where one receives
         health care
   iii) Handling insurance issues
         (1) Preexisting condition clauses on new policies
         (2) How to pay premiums when no longer working
   iv)   Determining the requirements to report HIV status to regulatory/licensing authorities
         (1) Become familiar with laws.
         (2) Bring a support person to any formal meetings regarding reporting HIV status or
             proposed restrictions on practice.
 d. Work issues
   i)   Deciding whom to tell (e.g., supervisor/manager, employee health department,
         coworkers, infection control practitioner)
         (1) It may be helpful to practice first, talking it through with someone outside of
             place of employment.
         (2) Pros of telling include scheduling flexibility and avoidance of exposure to oppor-
             tunistic and other infections.
         (3) Evaluate whom one can trust with this sensitive information.
   ii)   Working to develop practice guidelines to protect nurses from infections in patients
         and vice versa; using Centers for Disease Control and Prevention (CDC) and Occu-
         pational Safety and Health Administration (OSHA) guidelines such as *Universal
         (Blood and Body Fluid) Precautions* and *Isolation Techniques for Use in Hospitals*
   iii) Dealing with coworker issues: potential nonacceptance of HIV status, helplessness,
         not knowing how to help, and overprotectiveness
   iv)   Becoming familiar with the Americans with Disabilities Act (ADA) and employer
         compliance (WHO, 1999)

     v)   Determining continued ability to work (e.g., fatigue, mental slowing)

3. HIV in the infected healthcare worker community

   a. Transmission, risk behaviors, and prevention issues

     i)   Healthcare personnel living with HIV infection have a right to continue working as healthcare providers and to be assured of confidentiality about their HIV status in all cases. Healthcare workers with HIV infection should not be required to disclose their HIV status to their patients (ANAC, 1999).

     ii)   The Centers for Disease Control and Prevention did not document a single case of HIV transmission from 63 HIV-infected healthcare workers to any of their more than 22,000 patients (Gostin, 2000).

     iii) Based on the lack of any confirmed cases, the risk of transmission of HIV from provider to patient is judged to be so small that practice restrictions do not appear warranted.

     iv) All healthcare workers should be informed about mechanisms of transmission and preventative strategies for blood-borne pathogens, and these should be universally applied.

   b. Access to care, treatment, and research (WHO, 1999)

     i)   Seek care where confidentiality can be maintained.

     ii)   Maintain medical appointments.

     iii) Seek counseling when necessary to maintain health and well-being.

4. Specific care approaches

   a. Individual

     i)   Nurses caring for or working with an HIV-positive colleague

        (1) Be aware of your own feelings of discomfort.

           (a) If you feel any awkwardness, and it seems appropriate to talk about this, acknowledge this with your colleagues.

           (b) Failure to recognize your own feelings may lead to isolation of or withdrawal from your colleagues.

           (c) Sometimes saying, "I don't know what to say or do; how can I help?" may be very supportive or helpful.

        (2) Respect the right of your colleague not to talk about her or his health status or not to want support; your colleague needs to be the one to decide when and from whom to get support.

        (3) If your colleague is also your patient, be particularly cautious about protecting confidentiality (e.g., access to medical records, disclosure of medical information, informal conversations in the elevators or other public areas).

        (4) Be supportive without being overprotective.

        (5) Make reasonable accommodations when making work assignments.

     ii)   Nursing manager supervising an HIV-positive nurse

        (1) Be aware of the implications of the ADA and the need for reasonable accommodations.

        (2) Refer HIV-positive or other staff members to employee assistance if appropriate and available.

(3) Know that job expectations and performance need to be fair and equitable for all employees; difficulties may arise if other coworkers feel they are not treated in the same manner as their HIV-positive colleague.

b. Community

   i) Encourage involvement with HIV-positive healthcare workers for support and information.

   ii) Refer to resources, if appropriate, such as *HIV+ Nurse,* the newsletter of the HIV+ Nurses Committee of the Association of Nurses in AIDS Care, retrievable at http://www.nursesinaidscare.org/i4a/pages/index.cfm?pageid=3334.

REFERENCES

Association of Nurses in AIDS Care (ANAC). (1999). *Position paper: Discrimination protections for people with HIV infection: Reviewed and revised by the ANAC board August 14, 1999.* Retrieved March 24, 2009, from http://www.nursesinaidscare.org/files/public/PS_Discrimination_Protections_Rev_08_08.pdf

Association of Nurses in AIDS Care (ANAC). (2001). Work issues for the HIV+ nurse. *HIV+ Nurse, 2*(3), 1–4.

Centers for Disease Control and Prevention (CDC). (2003). *Surveillance of healthcare personnel with HIV/AIDS, as of December 2002.* Retrieved June 6, 2008, from http://www.cdc.gov/ncidod/dhp/bp_hiv_hp_with.html

Gostin, L. (2000). National policy on HIV-infected healthcare workers questioned. *Journal of the American Medical Association, 284,* 1965–1970.

World Health Organization (WHO). (1999). Managing work and HIV. *HIVFrontline, 38,* 1–8.

6.6 THE DEAF COMMUNITY

1. Definition of the community

a. Approximately 28 million persons in the United States have a significant hearing loss in one or both ears. Approximately 2 million Americans identify American Sign Language (ASL) as their primary language. The Deaf community is characterized by a unique culture with common language, beliefs, customs, and social norms. The use of ASL bonds the community.

b. The Deaf culture is often misunderstood by outsiders who fail to appreciate the unique personal, interpersonal, and social aspects of this subpopulation and the richness of American Sign Language (ASL).

c. Deaf persons often reject the label of *disabled* (deficit model), preferring to have pride in the richness and diversity of the Deaf culture.

   i) Degrees of hearing loss vary from minor to profound. If the hearing impairment is congenital—or its onset predates the learning of language—the individual may have considerable difficulty building vocabulary, mastering an oral language, or interacting with peers, family, and others until an effective communication method is established. Deafness usually assumes little or no ability to utilize auditory input for activities of daily living. Being hard of hearing (HOH) suggests less severe hearing loss and permits the learning of language with the use of hearing aids or related technological devices.

ii) Social affiliation often correlates with self-identification. Persons with significant hearing loss who don't self-identify or socialize with the Deaf community are often referred to as *deaf;* persons who mainly communicate in sign language and identify as culturally Deaf are called *Deaf* (capital *D*). Both deaf and Deaf (usually termed *d/Deaf*) persons have a high risk for acquiring HIV infection.

2. Common health issues
   a. Deaf children may be at higher risk for victimization by pedophiles and less able to effectively communicate their victimization to adults.
   b. Substance abuse is higher (1 in 7) among d/Deaf persons than among hearing (1 in 10), and d/Deaf persons have limited access to support groups or drug programs.
   c. Many d/Deaf persons have experienced discrimination, marginalization, and/or abuse in the healthcare setting that has resulted in a distrust of healthcare providers.
   d. Healthcare providers rarely use sign language interpreters with d/Deaf clients; many of the health-related educational materials are written at a level above the average fifth-grade reading level of d/Deaf adults; many d/Deaf persons are unfamiliar with basic facts about sexually transmitted diseases, safer sex strategies, or medication adherence principles.
   e. Many d/Deaf persons have only minimal anatomy and physiology knowledge necessary to comprehend the complexities of HIV/AIDS.

3. Social issues and problems
   a. Stigma, discrimination, and denial within the Deaf community are barriers.
      i) They often comprise small, tightly knit communities in which confidentiality is often lost, leading to denial and secrecy.
      ii) Homophobia contributes to LGBTQ individuals being ostracized and stigmatized.
      iii) Deaf people may be unempowered, have poor self-esteem, lack adequate skills in written and spoken English, and lack negotiation skills; behaviors common in Deaf culture are often misinterpreted by non-deaf persons (e.g., direct communications that are misunderstood as aggressive or rude).
   b. Marginalization and isolation of d/Deaf persons occur due to real and perceived barriers in healthcare communications.
   c. Deaf persons have limited or nonexistent access to HIV prevention, family planning, mental health, STD, and substance abuse resources; one study revealed that 94% of AIDS service organizations surveyed provided no services for deaf persons.
   d. Published research on the d/Deaf experience in health care is virtually nonexistent.
   e. Erroneous beliefs about the deaf/hearing impaired are a barrier to effective care. Healthcare workers may believe the following:
      i) Hearing impairment equals intellectual impairment.
      ii) The deaf cannot learn like hearing people.
      iii) Writing back and forth is effective communication and fosters comprehension.
      iv) Anyone who knows even a little sign language can act as an interpreter.
   f. Ninety percent (90%) of d/Deaf persons were born to hearing parents; parents may not accept their child's deafness, respect the Deaf culture, or learn their child's sign language and are likely to hide or deny the child's deafness by forbidding the use of sign language.
      i) Deaf persons often develop a "family of choice" with other Deaf persons; conflicts with family of origin may surface in the healthcare setting.

4. HIV/AIDS issues
    a. Impact of HIV/AIDS
        i)   Precise numbers of deaf persons with HIV/AIDS are unknown; CDC does not collect data on numbers of deaf persons with AIDS, and a sampling frame is unavailable.
        ii)   Only the state of Maryland compiles basic data to estimate the HIV seroprevalence rates of d/Deaf persons through its counseling and testing sites. HIV seroprevalence is higher among persons with hearing loss than the general population; infection rates for deaf gay men are as high as—or higher than—hearing (non-deaf) gay men.
    b. Transmission/risk behaviors/prevention
        i)   Transmission modes are similar to hearing (non-deaf) persons.
        ii)   d/Deaf gay men are isolated from Deaf community and marginalized from gay community, resulting in few skills to negotiate safer sex and manage risk behaviors.
        iii) d/Deaf access to counseling and treatment for substance use problems/addiction services is severely limited.
    c. Access to care/treatment or research protocols
        i)   d/Deaf persons with HIV infection are a minority within a minority community and lack necessary support structures to successfully manage their treatment.
        ii)   The complexities of contemporary healthcare systems require a minimal level of health literacy; d/Deaf persons may be left confused and frustrated when attempting to access services.
        iii) Acute care hospitalizations can be frightening and unpredictable if interpreters are not available; d/Deaf persons experience difficulty describing their symptoms effectively, and providers have equal difficulty providing equitable information about care options and legal/ethical aspects of health care for respectful, autonomous patient decision making. Further, d/Deaf partners and families may not receive appropriate education and support for maintaining the patient's health upon discharge.
        iv)   Communication barriers limit access to care/treatment or research protocols.
        v)   Low employment rates for the d/Deaf persons translate to less private insurance coverage and fewer options for personal transportation to attend appointments.
    d. Treatment outcomes
        i)   d/Deaf persons may be diagnosed with HIV late in disease (when symptomatic) and die sooner than hearing counterparts due to a decreased comprehension of HIV disease, limited assistance with medication adherence, and inadequate social support systems.
        ii)   d/Deaf persons may not understand the concept of taking medicines before getting sick (prophylaxis), the specificity of medications (e.g., mistakenly assuming all antibiotics can be used interchangeably), or the importance of adherence to HAART regimens.
5. Specific approaches
    a. Individual-level interventions
        i)   Assure professional interpreting services; interpreters vary according to linguistic abilities of the deaf person (i.e., minimal language skills, American Sign Language).
        ii)   Research telephone relay systems; these can provide d/Deaf clients with access to providers via the telephone.

    iii)   Identify potential deaf counselors/peer educators whenever possible and provide train-the-trainer skills building and ongoing support mechanisms.

    iv)   Use visual aids for comprehension, and encourage peer discussion for skills building.

    v)   Encourage emotional expression and facilitate grieving.

    vi)   Offer guidance/support in navigating the healthcare system.

    vii)   Empower individuals to take responsibility for actions and understand consequences of personal decision making.

    viii)   Role-play negotiating safer sex.

    ix)   Don't assume understanding of crucial vocabulary; explain all terminology and validate by encouraging d/Deaf person to explain concepts back to counselor.

b. Community-level interventions

    i)   Provide interpreting services at community forums and prevention/care sites.

    ii)   Involve d/Deaf persons at high risk in all levels of planning for HIV/AIDS prevention, treatment, and care services; involve d/Deaf persons in development and implementation of pertinent research projects that support the community.

    iii)   Maximize advances in online technologies and video and digital imaging to enhance communications in local settings and across distances.

    iv)   Support the development of policies to protect d/Deaf children from sexual abuse.

    v)   Develop an appreciation for the richness of Deaf culture, and identify beliefs, values, and needs; develop a culturally appropriate approach to providing HIV prevention and clinical care services.

    vi)   Recruit, educate, and hire deaf peer counselors to provide services, perform outreach activities, and build capacity through train-the-trainer models.

    vii)   Develop targeted services for specific subgroups in the population (e.g., deaf gay men, deaf women, deaf IDUs, deaf African Americans).

READER RESOURCES

AIDS Education/Services for the Deaf (AESD)
  A project of the Greater Los Angeles Council on Deafness (GLAD)
  2222 Laverna Avenue
  Los Angeles, CA 90041
  TTY/voice: (213) 550-4250
  Fax: (213) 550-4255
CDC National AIDS Hotline TTY Service
  TTY: (800) AIDS-TTY (same as 1-800-243-7889)
HIV InSite UCSF Center on Deafness
  3333 California Street, #10
  San Francisco, CA 94118
  http://hivinsite.ucsf.edu/InSite?page=li-06-17
  (415) 476-4980
"HIV/AIDS in the Deaf and Hard of Hearing" (April 2001, HRSA Care ACTION)
  Health Resources and Services Administration, HIV/AIDS Bureau
  http://hab.hrsa.gov
  (301) 443-6652

Housing Works!
  57 Willoughby Street, 2nd Floor
  Brooklyn, NY 11201
  http://www.housingworks.org
  (347) 473-7400
Laurent Clerc National Deaf Education Center
  Gallaudet University
  800 Florida Avenue, NE
  Washington, DC 20002
  http://clerccenter.gallaudet.edu/
Perlman, T., & Leon, S. C. (2006). Preventing AIDS in Chicagoland: The design and efficacy for culturally sensitive HIV/AIDS prevention education materials for deaf communities. *Deaf Worlds, 22*(1). Available at http://www.forestbooks.com/pages/deafwld.htm
Schmaling, C., & Monaghan, L. (Eds.). (2006). HIV/AIDS and deaf communities (DWHIV). *Deaf Worlds, 22*(1). Available at http://www.forestbooks.com/pages/Categories/Books/0946252610.html
What Are Deaf Persons' HIV Prevention Needs? (Fact sheet from the Center for AIDS Prevention Studies at the University of CA, San Francisco). Available at http://www.caps.ucsf.edu/pubs/FS/deaf.php

---

REFERENCES

Bisol, C. A, Sperb, T. M., & Moreno-Black, G. (2008). Focus groups with deaf and hearing youths in Brazil: Improving a questionnaire on sexual behavior and HIV/AIDS. *Qualitative Health Research, 18*(4), 565–578.
Job, J. (2004). Factors involved in the ineffective dissemination of sexuality information to individuals who are deaf or hard of hearing. *American Annals of the Deaf, 149*(3), 264–273.
Jones, E. G., Mallinson, R. K., Phillips, L., & Kang, Y. (2006). Challenges in language, culture, and modality: Translating English measures into American Sign Language. *Nursing Research, 55*(2), 75–81.
Mallinson, R. K. (2004). Perceptions of HIV/AIDS by deaf gay men. *Journal of the Association of Nurses in AIDS Care, 15*(4), 27–36.

6.7 PEOPLE WITH HEMOPHILIA

1. Description of the community
   a. Hemophilia is a sex-linked genetic disorder characterized by an absence or deficiency of a plasma-clotting protein; because of inheritance patterns, most people with hemophilia are male. Additionally, there are numerous other inherited bleeding disorders, such as von Willebrand disease, which are generally less severe in nature.
   b. Types of hemophilia
      i) Hemophilia A (classic hemophilia) is caused by deficiency of clotting protein factor VIII; it is 4 times more prevalent than hemophilia B.
      ii) Hemophilia B (Christmas disease) is caused by a deficiency of clotting protein factor IX.
   c. Hemophilia A and B are characterized by the severity of the clotting disorder (normal factor level is approximately 100%).
      i) Severe hemophilia: < 1% baseline clotting factor level
      ii) Moderate hemophilia: 1% to 5% baseline clotting factor level
      iii) Mild hemophilia: 6% to 50% baseline clotting factor level

d. U.S. incidence: 1 in 7,500 live male births; there are approximately 20,000 people with hemophilia in the United States (National Hemophilia Foundation, 2002a).

e. Many people with hemophilia have been instructed in self-infusion with factor concentrates to immediately treat bleeding episodes. Thus, they are very knowledgeable about recognition of bleeding episodes and infusion techniques.

f. Between 1978 and 1985, people with hemophilia were exposed to HIV through infusions of plasma-derived factor concentrates used to treat hemorrhages. It is estimated that approximately 8,000 people with hemophilia or other bleeding disorders became HIV-infected through plasma factor products (National Hemophilia Foundation, 2002b).

g. In 1982, the Centers for Disease Control and Prevention (CDC) reported the first case of AIDS in a person with hemophilia (CDC, 1982).

h. As of June 2007, 5,712 people with inherited bleeding disorders have been diagnosed with AIDS in the United States (CDC, 2007). Of these, 230 were < 13 years old when diagnosed. An additional 652 individuals are HIV-infected, but do not carry an AIDS diagnosis.

i. It is estimated that 50% of those infused with clotting factors between 1978 and 1985, and that 70–80% of those with severe hemophilia (baseline factor level < 1%) acquired HIV infection (Augustyniak et al., 1990; National Hemophilia Foundation, 2008) because of the amount of infected infusion products used. Many of those affected have subsequently died; it is estimated that currently 10–15% of persons with hemophilia are living with HIV infection or AIDS.

j. Some HIV-infected people with hemophilia subsequently transmitted the virus to their sexual partners.
   i) Between 15% and 30% of the sexual partners of people with hemophilia acquired HIV infection. As of June 2007, 611 sexual partners of persons with hemophilia have been diagnosed with AIDS (CDC, 2007).
   ii) Vertical transmission has also occurred.

k. The CDC reported two cases of HIV transmission occurring from one HIV-infected person with hemophilia to another person residing in the same household. One case occurred through IV or percutaneous exposure from home infusion (CDC, 1992). In the second case, the mechanism of exposure was from an unrecognized or unreported incident of blood contact (CDC, 1993).

l. Viral inactivation of all factor concentrates began in 1984; since 1987, through surveillance methods, no new infections have been identified from factor infusions that have been virally inactivated and donor screened (Frick et al., 1992).

m. As with other people who have a chronic illness, people with hemophilia do not want to be identified by a disease (i.e., "hemophiliacs") but rather as people with a disease.

2. Common health issues
   a. Hemarthrosis, a complication of hemophilia, may affect treatment for HIV (e.g., painful arthropathy is commonly treated with ibuprofen; however, the combination of antiretrovirals and ibuprofen may cause bleeding; Ragni et al., 1988).
   b. HIV therapies that are known to cause thrombocytopenia may be contraindicated or need to be monitored more cautiously.

    c. It is extremely important to consider the underlying bleeding disorder if procedures are planned that may induce bleeding, such as biopsies, arterial punctures, and bronchoscopy. Hemophilia treatment center staff should be consulted prior to any planned procedures.

    d. People with hemophilia are more likely to experience significant bleeding if they develop immune thrombocytopenia purpura (ITP) because of their underlying bleeding disorder.

    e. Septic arthritis may develop in joints previously damaged by hemarthrosis and in joints with arthroplasties.

    f. Lymphomas may present as pseudohematomas.

3. HIV/AIDS in the hemophilia community

    a. Transmission, risk behaviors, and prevention issues

       i) Sexual partners of HIV-seropositive people with hemophilia are at risk for HIV infection and need to cope with changing their sexual practices to incorporate safer sex practices.

    b. Access to care, treatment, and research

       i) During the early 1980s, people with hemophilia lived in constant fear of their HIV infection becoming known and of being associated with a high-risk group; stigma presented a significant barrier to care.

       ii) In the 1980s, people with hemophilia frequently lacked access to clinical trials because of the geographic location of research sites or exclusion from particular trials because of elevated liver function tests associated with complications of hemophilia, particularly hepatitis C.

       iii) Historically, the National Hemophilia Foundation coordinated the AIDS Clinical Trials Unit (ACTU) Without Walls to coordinate and monitor NIAID research protocols at hemophilia treatment centers nationwide (Kramer & Brownstein, 1990). Today, HIV-infected people with hemophilia are referred to local resources for research opportunities.

       iv) The National Hemophilia Foundation continues to advocate for research protocol inclusion criteria considerations so as not to exclude people with hemophilia.

       v) Most people with hemophilia are already connected to a hemophilia treatment center for coordination of their bleeding disorder; thus, many also have access to HIV care coordination through their established nurse coordinator.

4. Specific care approaches

    a. Individual

       i) Counsel about standard precautions to prevent viral transmission, including the handling and disposal of infusion products and equipment.

       ii) Refer patient to local hemophilia support groups and services.

       iii) Teach and reinforce safer sex practices.

    b. Community

       i) Promote hemophilia support services and programs, including peer programs.

       ii) Participate in public policy discussions about access to hemophilia and HIV care, treatment, and advocacy in schools and other public institutions or in community-based organizations that provide services to people with HIV infection.

REFERENCES

Augustyniak, L., Kramer, A. S., Frick, W., Brownstein, A. P., & Evatt, B. (1990, June). *Regional seropositivity rates for HIV infection in patients with hemophilia.* Paper presented at the Sixth International Conference on AIDS, San Francisco.

Centers for Disease Control and Prevention (CDC). (1982). Update on acquired immunodeficiency syndrome (AIDS) among patients with hemophilia. *Morbidity and Mortality Weekly Report, 31*(48), 644–646.

Centers for Disease Control and Prevention (CDC). (1992). HIV infection in two brothers receiving intravenous therapy for hemophilia. *Morbidity and Mortality Weekly Report, 41*(14), 228–231.

Centers for Disease Control and Prevention (CDC). (1993). HIV transmission between two adolescent brothers with hemophilia. *Morbidity and Mortality Weekly Report, 42*(49), 948–951.

Centers for Disease Control and Prevention (CDC). (2007). *HIV/AIDS surveillance report.* Atlanta, GA: U.S. Department of Health and Human Services, Public Health Service.

Frick, W., Augustyniak, L., Laurence, D., Brownstein, A., Kramer, A., & Evatt, B. L. (1992). Human immunodeficiency virus infection due to clotting factor concentrates: Results of the Seroconversion Surveillance Project. *Transfusion, 32*(8), 707–709.

Kramer, A., & Brownstein, A. P. (June, 1990). *ACTU without walls.* Paper presented at the Sixth International Conference on AIDS, San Francisco.

National Hemophilia Foundation. (2002a). *Hemophilia A: What is it?* Retrieved January 29, 2008, from http://www.hemophilia.org.bdi/bdi_types1.htm

National Hemophilia Foundation. (2002b). *Nurses' guide to bleeding disorders.* New York: Author.

National Hemophilia Foundation. (2008). *HIV/AIDS.* Retrieved January 29, 2008, from http://www.hemophilia.org/NHFWeb/MainPgs/MainNHF.aspx?menuid=43&contentid=39&rptname=bloodsafety?

Ragni, M. V., Tama, G., Lewis, J. H., & Ho, M. (1988). Increased frequency of haemarthroses in haemophiliac patient treated with zidovudine. *Lancet, 1*(8600), 1454–1455.

6.8 HOMELESS PERSONS

1. Description of the community
   a. The Stewart B. McKinney Homeless Assistance Act (1988) defines the homeless as an individual or family who meet the following criteria:
      i) Lack(s) a fixed, regular, and adequate nighttime residence, which includes such situations as living temporarily with friends or relatives
      ii) Has/have a primary nighttime residence that is supervised, such as a publicly or privately operated shelter
      iii) Use(s) a public or private place not designed for or ordinarily used as a regular sleeping accommodation for human beings
      iv) Use(s) a place for shelter that is designed to provide temporary living, such as welfare hotels, congregate shelters, or transitional housing for the mentally ill
   b. HIV/AIDS is 3 times higher in homeless compared with nonhomeless populations, and HIV/AIDS is even higher among the mentally ill. One-third to one-half of AIDS cases are among the homeless or those at risk of being homeless (Song & HRSA, 2000).
   c. Diverse factors that contribute to homelessness include the following:
      i) Unemployment/underemployment, lack of affordable housing, failure of the social safety net, and poverty

     ii)   Indigence following overwhelming medical cost for care of physical disabilities or chronic illness

     iii)   Abusive/neglectful home environments that force women, children, and adolescents onto the streets without shelter or social support

     iv)   Problems related to drug and alcohol use

     v)   Problems related to mental illness (an estimated 30% to 49% of homeless people suffer some degree of mental illness; they are easily victimized and unlikely to receive appropriate treatment; Song & HRSA, 2000)

     vi)   Dual or multiple diagnoses of addiction, mental illness, HIV, tuberculosis, and hepatitis C

     vii) Stigmatization related to any of the previous conditions

     viii) Discriminatory treatment by healthcare and service providers

     ix)   Illegal immigrant status

2. Common health issues

  a. Common comorbidities (e.g., respiratory, foot, skin, parasitic intestinal infections, dental and periodontal disease, infestations, tuberculosis, hepatitis C)

  b. No or limited access to hygiene facilities (toilets, bathrooms, shower, laundry); inadequate clothing in inclement weather

  c. Poor diet (inadequate caloric and nutrient intake reduces resistance to illness and ability to regain health)

  d. Few opportunities for purposeful activity, leading to boredom, low self-esteem, and an exacerbation of existing mental problems

  e. Special concerns of homeless families include the following:

     i)   Number of teen pregnancies higher in the homeless adolescent population

     ii)   Homeless people lack support structures for child rearing.

     iii)   Homeless people are more likely to drop out of school or miss school due to a chaotic lifestyle.

     iv)   Homeless people engage in minimal health maintenance (e.g., immunizations, especially for hepatitis; early detection of HIV; recognition of early developmental problems).

     v)   Homeless people, both adults and children, receive little or no teaching concerning safer sexual practices and problems arising from drug use.

  f. Social issues of homeless individuals include, but are not limited to, the following:

     i)   There is a high incidence of trauma-related injuries.

     ii)   Medications are often stolen or lost.

     iii)   There is a high incidence of physical and sexual abuse.

     iv)   Client-centered services are frequently unavailable.

     v)   Low-cost housing is unavailable in areas adjacent to available services.

     vi)   Programs that deal with addiction (e.g., needle exchange, methadone, detoxification) are inadequate.

     vii) Few service resources are available to assist with child rearing and education.

     viii) Fewer shelters are available in rural areas.

3. HIV/AIDS in the homeless community

  a. Transmission, risk behaviors, and prevention issues

i) The longer a person is homeless, the greater the likelihood he or she will fall into one or more high-risk behaviors, such as sharing needles and engaging in unsafe sexual practices (e.g., sex with multiple partners, exchanging sex for money).

ii) Homeless teens' intention to use condoms is based on present needs, social connectedness, self-efficacy, and lack of resources for condoms (Rew, Fouladi, & Yockey, 2002). Homeless teens do not receive social support of caring adults to guide decision making. They often use sex to acquire the bare necessities (e.g., food, shelter, drugs, companionship). They have decreased self-care because of despair, hopelessness, and untreated mental illness, and they lack social and assertive skills that might help reduce their risk for HIV.

iii) Sexual and physical abuse rates are disproportionately high, contributing to poor self-care.

iv) All activities of daily living, including consensual and nonconsensual sex, take place in unsafe and unclean conditions.

v) Lack of housing leads to affronts to the immune system due to extremes in temperatures.

vi) Food and shelter become first priority, leaving few economic resources for condoms.

vii) Infrequent access to health care may delay diagnosis of multiple health problems, including HIV, tuberculosis, hepatitis C, and sexually transmitted diseases, which in turn may increase rates of transmission, including vertical transmission.

b. Access to care, treatment, and research

i) Barriers include lack of health insurance and inability to pay for care, primarily due to having no fixed address and inability to receive social and medical entitlements.

ii) Fifty-six percent of homeless people have no regular source of health care, which contributes to poor continuity (Song & HRSA, 2000).

iii) Homeless people are not able to navigate the difficult and confusing healthcare system without assistance.

iv) Homeless people are not able to tolerate long waits for care due to substance use, mental illness, and risk of losing belongings or place in food or shelter lines.

v) Homeless people lack knowledge of where to go for care and lack transportation (or the means to pay for it).

vi) Homeless people do not trust the healthcare system because of previous negative experiences of discriminatory treatment by care providers.

vii) Homeless people have a limited ability to adhere to research protocols because of a chaotic lifestyle.

viii) Treatment outcomes are affected by lack of continuity of care because homeless people may use the emergency room instead of a doctor's office when seeking care. The lack of continuity of care may also be the reason that researchers have found that the costs of admissions for acute care are higher for homeless people (Nosyk, Li, & Anis, 2007).

ix) Homeless people may have poor adherence to medication schedules due to a chaotic lifestyle (e.g., cannot pay, unable to wait to have prescriptions filled, might have prescriptions stolen), mental illness, substance abuse and treatment failure due to developing resistance to medications, interactions with street drugs, or failure to take medications consistently. Homeless people's lack of refrigeration restricts choices of antiretroviral medications that require special diets or cooling.

4. Specific care approaches
   a. Individual
      i)   Establish trust through open, direct, nonjudgmental exploration of individual's beliefs, risk factors, and perceived needs and barriers to care.
      ii) Use client-centered approach to care and treatment.
      iii) Relationship may take time to develop; complete history may not emerge for weeks or months due to mistrust; be patient.
      iv) Listen carefully to what clients are trying to say; ask direct questions to clarify.
      v)   Assess cultural, legal, social service, and daily living needs; be aware that shelter, food, money, and drug and alcohol needs often take priority over health care; be prepared to assist with meeting basic needs first.
      vi) Assess financial support and eligibility for financial benefits: general assistance, Social Security income, AIDS Drug Assistance Program, and AFDC can help get homeless people off the street, but there may be little left over for food or other essentials. Stable housing improves appointment keeping.
      vii) Base interventions on realistic picture of individual's lifestyle, daily needs, and functional capabilities. Homeless people often do not keep calendars or wear watches; drop-in hours are more appropriate than strictly scheduled appointments.
      viii) Use multidisciplinary team approach to ensure all needs are being addressed.
           (1) HIV education
           (2) Immunizations to protect from hepatitis and other infections
           (3) Dental care
           (4) Nutrition: food pantries, emergency meal, or voucher programs
           (5) Harm reduction
           (6) Confidentiality
           (7) Consistency of services through nursing case management
           (8) Plan of care development
           (9) Referrals for education, skills building, and so on as individual is ready
   b. Community
      i)   Explore the perceptions and reported needs of homeless people in the community (individuals and families) to identify geographic location, social and community support, and available resources.
      ii) Use culturally representative outreach workers to gain entrance and trust in the community and to provide consistent presence, care, and messages within the community.
      iii) Expand use of community-based clinics, mobile units, and home care or public health nursing to increase accessibility to health care.
      iv) Incorporate services that meet the housing, legal, financial, and healthcare (including mental health) needs into existing community clinic structures to provide one-stop health care or housing facilities.
      v)   Provide appropriate, comprehensive mental health services and treatment centers to expand care options.

vi) In areas where a need for services for the homeless is not being met, consider the possibility of providing mobile services to meet the need (i.e., take the service to the client).

vii) Use models that have worked to develop new programs (U.S. Department of Health and Human Services, Health Resources and Services Administration, HIV/AIDS Bureau, 2001).

  (1) Interdisciplinary teams composed of a registered nurse, an addiction counselor, and a peer leader

  (2) Health advocate to liaison within clinic with healthcare provider and client

  (3) Flexibility to modify organizational structure and goals when needed

  (4) Engaged and challenged client, using stages of change (transtheoretical model)

  (5) Links with community agencies and learning to coexist with different services

  (6) Collaboration with public individuals who are homeless

  (7) Support for continued needle-exchange and free or affordable methadone maintenance programs

  (8) Support for day programs to provide stimulus to relieve boredom and build skills around activities of daily living

  (9) Support for programs to help integrate persons who have been homeless back into the workforce

---

REFERENCES

Nosyk, B., Li, X., & Anis, A. H. (2007). Psychological and socio-medial aspects of AIDS/HIV. *AIDS Care, 19*(4), 546–553.

Rew, L., Fouladi, R. T., & Yockey, R. D. (2002). Sexual health practices of homeless youth. *Journal of Nursing Scholarship, 34*(2), 139–145.

Song, J., & Health Resources and Services Administration (HRSA). (2000). *HIV/AIDS and homelessness: Recommendations for clinical practice and public policy.* Washington, DC: Bureau of Primary Health Care and HIV/AIDS Bureau, Health Resources and Services Administration.

The Stewart B. McKinney Homeless Assistance Act. (1988). *General definition of homeless individual.* U.S. Code: Title 42, Chapter 119, Subchapter 1, 11302—General Provisions. Retreived January 15, 2008, from http://www4.law. cornell.edu/uscode/html/uscode42/usc_sec_42_00011302——000-.html

U.S. Department of Health and Human Services, Health Resources and Services Administration, HIV/AIDS Bureau. (2001). *Lessons learned.* Washington, DC: Author.

6.9 INCARCERATED PERSONS

1. Background
   a. The term *incarcerated* refers to inmates in federal prisons, state prisons, and county or city jail systems; prisoners within jail systems are either being detained prior to trial or serving sentences.
   b. At the end of 2007, over 7 million (1 in 32 Americans) adults were incarcerated or on parole, giving the United States the highest incarceration rate worldwide.
   c. In 2006, 1.6% of male and 2.4% female inmates were known to be HIV positive or have confirmed AIDS (Maruschak, 2006).

    d. For many inmates, their first opportunity for access to health care is through the prison health service (Coffey, 2007).

    e. Risky behaviors such as unsafe substance use by sharing syringes or other injection equipment, and high-risk sexual practices may lead to incarceration and put inmates at risk for HIV and HCV infection. Chronic hepatitis B infection and tuberculosis are more common in the incarcerated population than the general population (Coffey, 2007).

    f. HIV disproportionately affects minority populations, and minorities are overrepresented in jails and prisons; in 2005, 60% of state and federal inmates were African American or Hispanic (AIDSAction, 2007).

    g. Incarcerated women

        i) Incarcerated women are more likely to be living with HIV than incarcerated men. In 2005, 2.3% of state and federal female inmates were HIV positive compared to 1.8% of men (AIDSAction, 2007).

        ii) HIV-infected female inmates have more HIV risk factors than men, some of which may have contributed to their incarceration. The risk factors include the following:

            (1) History of childhood sexual abuse and neglect

            (2) History of sex work with increased frequency for forced, unprotected sex

            (3) High rates of STDs

            (4) High rates of mental illness

            (5) History of IVDU and/or sex partners with IVDU history

            (6) Poverty

        iii) Many incarcerated women receive their first gynecologic care while in prison, and 10% entering facilities are pregnant (Coffey, 2007).

2. Prevention and testing

    a. Transmission

        i) Sexual activity among male inmates in not uncommon, but the frequency of homosexual rape is difficult to estimate.

        ii) Other modes of transmission among inmates include the following:

            (1) Violence, such as fights involving lacerations, bites, or bleeding

            (2) IVDU sharing injection equipment that may be made from resources available to them

            (3) Sharing of toothbrushes or shaving equipment

            (4) Tattooing and body piercing performed using nonsterile instruments (Kantor, 2006).

    b. Prevention

        i) Programs for primary prevention of HIV and other infectious diseases should encompass education, peer-based approaches, and access to means of prevention and harm reduction measures (Hammett, 2006).

            (1) Education programs must provide accurate and adequate information for the staff and inmates. They should include information on transmission, prevention, treatment and management (Kantor, 2006; Coffey, 2007).

            (2) Peer-led programs are effective in the prison system, as inmates can receive information from respected members of their community (AIDSAction, 2007).

        ii) Condoms

      (1) Availability of condoms is a major issue in the prison system. Condoms are available in most European prisons. In the United States, some state prisons offer them, and studies have found few incidents of improper use and safer sex by self-report (Kantor, 2006).

      (2) Condom use in prisons also addresses transmission from inmates to their sexual partners in the general population. Many inmates self-identify as heterosexual despite high prevalence of same-sex contact while incarcerated. These inmates often return to heterosexual relations when released (Hammett, 2006).

   iii) Harm reduction

      (1) Needle exchange programs have been discussed as a means to prevent HIV transmission, but have not been implemented in any U.S. prison. Some European prisons have set up needle exchange programs with positive outcomes and decreased transmission of HIV and hepatitis B and C. In addition, prison needle exchange programs have been associated with stability of drug use and decline in sharing of injection equipment without reports of security problems (Kantor, 2006; Hammett, 2006).

      (2) Information regarding safer injecting practices should include the provision of bleach for cleaning syringes. Some prison systems in the United States do provide bleach, but it is not systematic (Kantor, 2006).

      (3) Addiction and mental health treatment for inmates can decrease post-release criminal activity, drug use relapse, and recidivism (amfAR, 2008).

   iv) Post-exposure prophylaxis for HIV has shown promise in correctional facilities and should be considered as part of a comprehensive prevention program (Hammett, 2006).

  c. Testing

   i) HIV testing policies vary among local, state, and federal facilities. Some facilities require testing on admission, release, or both. Others perform testing based on clinical indication or risk exposure, while others implement random, voluntary, or mandatory testing (Coffey, 2007; Maruschak, 2006).

   ii) Because corrections facilities are the first interaction with health care for many high-risk individuals, they play an important role in HIV testing and identifying those already infected (Coffey, 2007).

   iii) It is important that inmates receive their HIV test results in a timely manner, whether they are positive or negative (amfAR, 2008).

   iv) Prisoners often require more information and education then the general population to make informed decisions about testing. Because inmates often bargain for privileges, it is important for them to understand the institutional consequences of a positive test result (Kantor, 2006).

3. Treatment

  a. Between 2001 and 2005, AIDS-related deaths declined from 10.3% to 5.3% of all prison deaths (Maruschak, 2006).

  b. HIV healthcare services are expensive, encompassing the costs of medications, lab tests, and staff. This expense creates an enormous fiscal burden for prisons and jails. Many prisons contract with facilities that can provide HIV treatment from specialists.

   c. The standard of care for HIV treatment in the prison system consists of antiretroviral ther-apy; however, there is no current requirement to adhere to established guidelines or stan-dards. Unfortunately, prisons and jails frequently fail to provide health services at the necessary level for patients with HIV.

   d. Prison conditions often undermine the consistent antiretroviral dosing schedules required for long-term effectiveness. Interruptions in treatment occur due to transfers within or among facilities, court appearances, punitive detention, and/or release (Kantor, 2006).

   e. Two medical policies for medication dispensing exist in the prison system.

      i) Directly Observed Therapy (DOT)

         (1) Advantages

            (a) More frequent interactions with the prison health team, so side effects and other issues can be recognized earlier

            (b) Better adherence

         (2) Disadvantages

            (a) Requires frequent visits to the medical unit, which may be a distance from the inmate's unit

            (b) Potential loss of confidentiality due to the large number of pills and frequent visits to the medical unit

            (c) Does not foster self-sufficiency in adhering to medications

      ii) Keep on Person (KOP)

         (1) Allows inmates to obtain a monthly supply of medications and keep them in their cell to take independently

         (2) Increases privacy and confidentiality about HIV status

         (3) Allows self-sufficiency regarding adherence to medications

         (4) Decreases contact with medical staff that may delay interventions for side effects or other issues (Coffey, 2007)

4. Confidentiality/disclosure

   a. Confidentiality of HIV status is difficult to maintain in the prison system due to the large number of people who handle the information.

   b. Once information is released, it travels rapidly throughout the system.

   c. Infected inmates whose serostatus is known to others are often subjected to discrimination pertaining to housing, segregation, work assignments, and visiting privileges.

   d. Some states require disclosure of inmates' HIV serostatus to correctional administrators (Kantor, 2006).

   e. Measures are needed to reduce stigma and discrimination. Implementation and enforce-ment of procedures by prison staff to ensure confidentiality of inmates' medical informa-tion is essential (amfAR, 2008).

5. Specific care approaches

   a. Individual

      i) Counsel inmates individually about ways to reduce the risk of HIV transmission, and allow time for questions.

      ii) Encourage participation in peer education classes.

      iii) Educate inmates about preventive health behaviors, disease processes, medications, and adherence (Coffey, 2007).

iv) Discharge planning

    (1) Treatment failure as evidenced by increased viral load has been shown to occur after release from prison in inmates who were well-controlled while incarcerated. Therefore, discharge planning is critical to decrease recidivism and ensure continuity of HIV care, including adherence to antiretroviral therapy (Stephenson et al., 2005).

    (2) Offenders require referrals and linkages with medical and psychiatric services, and other social services to assure subsistence needs are met. Also, issuance of legal identification and assistance with Medicaid eligibility should be included in the discharge planning (amfAR, 2008; Stephenson et al., 2005).

    (3) Whenever possible, copies of medical records and an adequate supply of medications should be provided.

    (4) Transitional services are also beneficial for many inmates who are released and return to the community (Hammett, 2006).

    (5) Unfortunately, unplanned releases from court appearances jeopardize the best plans.

b. Correctional facilities

    i) Implement policies that enforce the incarcerated inmate's constitutional right to health care for HIV, as well as for all medical and psychological illnesses (amfAR, 2008).

    ii) Consult with HIV specialists to assure the patient is receiving proper care. This is especially important because HIV care is complicated and many prison medical providers lack experience in treating HIV-infected persons (Coffey, 2007).

    iii) Work with community and public health authorities to assure that all inmates, not only those with HIV, receive appropriate and consistent care while incarcerated and after release (amfAR, 2008).

    iv) Provide HIV education at all levels of staff and inmates regarding HIV prevention, transmission, treatment, stigma, and discrimination.

    v) Develop policies that reduce barriers to medication administration to ensure the highest quality of care. This includes policies regarding DOT and KOP, HIV clinical trials, food restrictions, and activities that interfere with administering medications (Babudieri, Aceti, D'Offizi, Carbonara, & Starnini, 2000).

    vi) Apply public health practices to reduce transmission of HIV, tuberculosis, and STDs, including harm reduction (Gaiter, Jurgen, Mayer, & Hollibaugh, 2000).

REFERENCES

AIDSAction. (2007). *Policy brief: The criminal justice system and HIV/AIDS.* Retrieved August 8, 2008, from http://www.aidsaction.org/communications/publications/HIV%20Incarceration.pdf

Babudieri, S., Aceti, A., D'Offizi, G. P., Carbonara, S., & Starnini, G. (2000). Directly observed therapy to treat HIV infection in prisoners. *Journal of the American Medical Association, 284*(2), 179–180.

Coffey, S. (Ed.). (2007). Section 9: Correctional settings. *Clinical manual for management of the HIV-infected adult, 2006 edition.* AIDS Education and Training Centers. Retrieved August 8, 2008, from http://aidsetc.org/aidsetc?page= cm-801_corrections

The Foundation for AIDS Research (amfAR). (2008). *Issue brief: Summary of recommendations: HIV in correctional settings: Implications for prevention and treatment policy.* Retrieved August 7, 2008, from http://www.amfar.org/uploadedFiles/In_the_Community/Publications/HIV%20In%20Correctional%20Settings.pdf

Gaiter, J., Jurgen, R., Mayer, K., & Hollibaugh, A. (2000). Harm reduction inside and out: Controlling HIV in and out of correctional facilities. *AIDS Reader, 10*(1)*,* 45–52.

Hammett, T. M. (2006). HIV/AIDS and other infectious diseases among correctional inmates: Transmission, burden, and an appropriate response. *American Journal of Public Health, 96*(6), 974–978.

Kantor, E. (2006). HIV transmission and prevention in prisons. *HIV InSite Knowledge Base* [online textbook]. Retrieved August 11, 2008, from http://hivinsite.ucsf.edu/InSite?page=kb-07-04-13

Maruschak, L. M. (2006). *HIV in prisons, 2006.* Retrieved August 8, 2008, from http://www.ojp.usdoj.gov/bjs/pub/html/hivp/2006/hivp06.htm

Stephenson, B. L., Wohl, D. A., Golin, C. E., Tien, H., Stewart, P., & Kaplan, A. H. (2005). Effect of release from prison and re-incarceration on the viral loads of HIV-infected individuals. *Public Health Reports, 120*(1), 84–88.

6.10 LESBIANS AND BISEXUAL WOMEN

1. Description of the community
   a. Lesbian: female who is primarily attracted emotionally and physically to other females
   b. Bisexual woman: woman who identifies self as emotionally and physically attracted to males and females
      i)   Women who have sex with women (WSW) may self-identify as heterosexual or may not identify at all as lesbian for various reasons related to culture, ethnicity, occupation, or peer support.
      ii) Women, especially women of color or of non-White cultural backgrounds, may not identify themselves for fear of rejection by their family and cultural supports.
2. Common health issues
   a. Sexual orientation identity does not predict sexual behaviors.
   b. WSW are visible to society as women with the same gender biases, and women who fear social retaliation may not identify themselves as lesbian.
   c. Access to health care and quality of care is a major concern of WSW.
      i)   Many use complementary healthcare providers to seek care that is more holistic and less discriminatory.
      ii) Healthcare practices emerge from heterosexual assumptions with perspectives that neglect to address lesbian concerns, which establish alienating practices.
      iii) Providers should use unbiased language and questions.
      iv) Lack of sexual history that includes sexual orientation fails to assess risk behaviors (e.g., toys, sexual play during menses, other specific sexual risks).
   d. A social history is important in making appropriate recommendations about preventive health screenings, preventive behaviors, and treatment options. Social history should include the following:
      i)   Substance use and abuse history
      ii) Physical or emotional abuse
      iii) Social systems and employment
      iv) A complete history that assesses behavior placing women at risk for HIV transmission
   e. Clinicians should take a careful sexual history.

i) It is important to include history of sexual activity with men because past and current sexual partners may not be limited to women. Of WSW, 53% to 99% report having had sex with men, and 20% to 30% continue to have sex with men as well as women (Marrazzo, Koutsky, & Handsfield, 2001). Unprotected sexual activity with men increases the likelihood of risk for past acquisition of chronic viral STD, such as HIV, HSV, and HPV.

ii) Sexual history should also include the following:

(1) Use of words about sexual behaviors that are understandable to the client

(2) Prior sex with gay, bisexual, or IV drug using men and women

(3) Number of lifetime male sex partners

(4) Exchange of sex for drugs or money

(5) Age at first vaginal or anal intercourse

(6) Unprotected anal intercourse

(7) Use of condoms

(8) How sex toys are cleaned and whether they are shared

(a) Whether there is sex during menses

(b) Whether there are other sex behaviors placing women at risk for HIV transmission

3. HIV/AIDS in the lesbian and bisexual community of women

a. Transmission, risk behaviors, and prevention issues

i) Through December 2004, 7,381 of the 246,461 women reported with AIDS are reported to have had sex with women; however, most had other risk factors.

ii) Of the 7,381 women, 534 reported having had sex only with women, and 91% of them had another risk factor, mainly IV drug use (CDC, 2006).

iii) Information regarding WSW is missing in more than 60% of the 246,461 reports, which is possibly due to lack of solicitation of information by the provider or lack of self-disclosure by the woman (CDC, 2006).

iv) Female-to-female transmission is uncommon; however, the possibility exists, though other behaviors can mask it. Further research is needed in this area, and a high priority for follow-up is given to reports of transmission of HIV to women who report their risk of transmission as WSW (CDC, 2006).

v) Transmission of STDs, such as herpes simplex virus, *Trichomonas vaginalis, Gardnerella vaginalis,* and human papillomavirus, has been reported from woman to woman (Marrazzo, Coffey, & Bingham, 2005).

vi) Transmission of HIV in women whose only risk factor is sex with women is still possible despite the lack of confirmed cases (CDC, 2006). There is also a belief among lesbian women of "lesbian immunity" to HIV— that they are not at risk for contracting HIV (Fishman & Anderson, 2003).

vii) Researchers suggest transmission is biologically and reasonably possible; however, the following factors were noted to hinder transmission:

(1) Lack of traumatic sex (for many WSW)

(2) Lowered rate of sex in lesbian couples

(3) Lower risk in lesbian sexual practices

(4) Lower level of HIV in cervicovaginal secretions

(5) Efficacy of defensive biological mechanisms

(6) Higher attention to risk practices (Raiteri, Baussano, Giobbia, Fora, & Sinicco, 1998)

viii) Modes of HIV transmission among WSW include the following:

(1) IV drug use (most common mode of transmission)

(2) Donor insemination for pregnancy through fresh and frozen semen

(3) Sexual risk behaviors for WSW

(4) Unprotected oral, anal, or vaginal intercourse with an HIV-infected partner (male or female)

(5) Sharing toys and razors

(6) Sex during menses

(7) Brushing/flossing immediately before sex

(8) Any sadomasochistic sex behavior that causes breaks in the skin (Fishman & Anderson, 2003)

(a) WSW, like heterosexual women, engage in a wide variety of sexual behaviors and practices.

(b) Some factors can increase the chance of transmission. These factors include concurrent STDs, especially ulcerative conditions; sores on the lips and mouth; cuts on the hands; and transfer of fluid by hand, glove, toy, or insertion device.

(c) Sex toys or other insertion devices may play a role in transmission. These objects can cause trauma, which may become a portal of entry for HIV during activities; cause exchange of infected fluids if they are shared without disinfection; draw blood or cause abrasion if used in traumatic or sadomasochistic activities; and transfer virus through contact with urine, feces, or menstrual blood on partner's broken skin or mucous membranes.

ix) Spermicides added or found on condoms can kill HIV and STDs; however, they can increase inflammation, which can increase transmission.

x) Douches and enemas may irritate vaginal and rectal linings and cause microscopic tears or abrasions, which increase risk.

4. Specific care approaches

a. Individual

i) Use of universal precautions and latex barriers during traumatic or sadomasochistic activities.

ii) Avoid use of semen from HIV-infected men and avoid using fresh semen unless donor has been properly screened.

iii) Precautions should be used to avoid sexual transmission.

(1) Use protective barriers during cunnilingus or anilingus.

(2) Use dental dams.

(3) Condoms may be cut at the tip and the side to lie flat as a barrier.

(4) Plastic wrap, such as Glad Wrap or Saran Wrap, are unofficially advocated as body fluid barriers. Effectiveness of these methods has not been researched.

iv) Wear protective gloves (latex or polyurethane) on hands during mutual masturbation to avoid sharing of body fluids, especially during menstruation.

   v)   Use female condom with sex toys in the vagina or for anal sex. Do not use female condoms for cunnilingus because they do not cover the entire vaginal opening.

   vi)   Use precautions with toys and devices. Partners should have their own toy or device, and condoms should be applied on dildos or other toys at each use. Disinfect toys and devices using the following procedure:

     (1) Wash with soap and water, then rinse.

     (2) Boil the toy for 20 minutes (except for electric and battery-operated devices, such as vibrators).

     (3) Soak in isopropyl alcohol for 30 minutes and rinse with water.

     (4) Rinse three times with full-strength bleach, then rinse with water.

b. Community

   i)   Screening programs targeted toward women of all sexual orientations and socioeconomic levels for early identification and management of HIV disease

   ii) Assistance accessing health care

   iii) Increasing awareness among all nurses and healthcare providers regarding HIV risks among lesbian and bisexual women

   iv) Increasing awareness among lesbian and bisexual women regarding risk factors for HIV transmission

REFERENCES

Centers for Disease Control and Prevention (CDC). (2006, June). *CDC HIV/AIDS fact sheet: HIV/AIDS among women who have sex with women*. Retrieved March 26, 2009, from http://www.cdc.gov/hiv/topics/women/resources/factsheets/pdf/wsw.pdf

Fishman, S. J., & Anderson, E. H. (2003). Perception of HIV and safer sexual behaviors among lesbians. *Journal of the Association of Nurses in AIDS Care, 14*(6), 48–55.

Marrazzo, J., Coffey, P., & Bingham, A. (2005). Sexual practices, risk perception and knowledge of sexually transmitted disease risk among lesbian and bisexual women. *Perspectives on Sexual and Reproductive Health, 37*(1), 6–12.

Marrazzo, J. M., Koutsky, L. A., & Handsfield, H. H. (2001). Characteristics of female sexually transmitted disease clinic clients who report same-sex behavior. *International Journal of STD and AIDS, 12*(1), 41–46.

Raiteri, R., Baussano, I., Giobbia, M., Fora, R., & Sinicco, A. (1998). Lesbian sex and risk of HIV transmission. *AIDS, 12*(4), 450–451.

6.11 MIGRANT/SEASONAL FARM WORKERS AND DAY LABORERS

1. Description of the communities

   a. Migrant/seasonal farm workers (MSFW) are agricultural laborers who cultivate and harvest crops and migrate to other areas following the growing seasons.

   b. There are three major streams of MSFWs in the United States.

     i)   The East Coast stream, which runs from New England to the southern states, consists of native African Americans and Latinos.

     ii) The Central stream, running through the central states, is populated by Mexicans and Mexican Americans.

     iii) The West Coast stream, from Washington to California, is made up primarily of Mexicans.

    c. The largest number of MSFWs are employed in California, Texas, Florida, North Carolina, and Washington.

    d. Due to the transient nature of their livelihood, it is difficult to know the actual numbers of MSFWs. However, it has been estimated to be over 4 million.

    e. The majority of MSFWs are in their 20s and male. They live away from their families (i.e., partners/spouses and children) in rural camps near the farms that employ them.

    f. Day laborers are manual laborers who are hired for the day by local suburban contractors in the construction and lawn maintenance industries.

    g. They aggregate in parking lots or street corners, waiting to be "hired" and then transported to the job site in vans or trucks.

    h. The individuals are usually residents of neighboring communities, sometimes residing with family or living with other day laborers. Like the MSFWs, many are undocumented immigrants.

2. Common health issues

    a. Most live in poverty.

    b. Education and literacy may be limited in their native language.

    c. Stressors include the following:

        i) Substandard and/or overcrowded living conditions

        ii) Inadequate diet and difficulty adhering to dietary restrictions and medication regimens

        iii) Limited sanitation facilities at the job site

        iv) Isolation (due to immigration status and language barriers)

        v) Long working hours in sometimes extreme weather conditions

        vi) Often are cheated out of wages

    d. Cultural and language barriers to care are present.

    e. Other access to care barriers are lack of knowledge of healthcare facilities and inability to qualify or pay for services.

    f. Misconceptions about HIV/AIDS may delay testing.

3. HIV/AIDS in the MSFW/day laborer communities

    a. Transmission, risk behaviors, and prevention issues

        i) HIV/AIDS prevalence is estimated to be much higher than in the general population.

        ii) Unprotected sexual activity is the major mode of HIV transmission.

        iii) MSFWs and day laborers who are away from their regular partners may frequent sex workers.

        iv) Condom use is inconsistent at best, and some are unable to properly use them.

        v) Self-injection of antibiotics and vitamins is common and considered more potent than the oral route.

        vi) Injection needles/syringes are often unclean, reused, shared, and improperly disposed.

    b. Access to care, treatment, and research

        i) Due to their extended work hours, many are unable to access prevention education programs and some healthcare services.

        ii) Following the jobs makes continuity of care and adherence to complex treatment regimens extremely challenging.

iii) Community-based outreach programs can be effective means to reach this population (Hovey, Booker, & Seligman, 2007).

iv) There may be delays in accessing HIV counseling, testing, and care.

v) Complex regimens and diet restrictions will affect the ability to work and decrease earning potential.

4. Approaches to care

   a. Individual level

   i)   Care should be culturally sensitive and gender specific.

   ii) Incorporate current healing, self-care practices.

   iii) Client may need to learn new skills to earn money or may wish to return to place of origin.

   iv) If client remains able to work, treatment needs to be coordinated between healthcare sites or agencies.

   b. Community level

   i)   Programs should consider the level of acculturation of the individuals, any generational differences, and the mobility of the population.

   ii) Short and effective interventions are needed that include HIV testing and counseling (Hovey, Booker, & Seligman, 2007).

   iii) Farmworker Health Services, Inc., provides outreach and education to MSFWs by creating and maintaining linkages between the MSFWs and existing local healthcare providers, including lay health workers.

   iv) User-friendly and language-appropriate services, such as mobile units and extended hours, would increase accessibility to care.

REFERENCES

Hovey, J. D., Booker, V., & Seligman, J. D. (2007). Using theatrical presentations as a means of disseminating knowledge of HIV/AIDS risk factors to migrant farm workers: An evaluation of the effectiveness of the Infórmate program. *Journal of Immigrant Health, 9*(2), 147–156.

6.12 OLDER PERSONS

1. Description of the community

   a. For years, the Centers for Disease Control and Prevention (CDC) grouped all cases of middle-aged and older adults AIDS cases into one category of age 50 or older (Stark, 2007). In 2005, the number of new AIDS cases in persons aged 50 and older was 7,767 (CDC, 2008a), and 13% of all new HIV cases were in persons aged 50 to 64 years (CDC, 2008b). Sociodemographic characteristics of older persons living with HIV/AIDS reflect the population of their country of origin (Nokes et al., 2006).

2. Common health issues

   a. The incidence of chronic illnesses increases with aging. The interaction of chronic illnesses (such as diabetes and hypertension) with HIV results in complex health management plans. Antiretrovirals can further complicate treatment plans already consisting of numerous medications (Nokes & Emlet, 2006).

   b. With increased age, there is decreased organ functioning.

   c. Older injecting drug users often have acquired injection-related chronic illnesses, such as kidney problems, cardiac changes, and blood-borne infections, such as hepatitis and HIV. Older adults with or at risk for co-infection with HIV and HCV are at higher risk for insulin resistance (Howard et al., 2007).

   d. Antiretroviral-associated dyslipidemia and insulin resistance are particularly problematic in middle-aged and older persons already at increased risk for heart disease, stroke, and diabetes. African Americans are at even higher risk for these health problems.

   e. Early work indicated that mortality rates after an AIDS diagnosis were twice as high for persons ages 50 and older, compared with younger persons, but this may be due to complications from the multiple comorbidities.

3. HIV/AIDS in the middle-aged and older community

   a. Transmission, risk behaviors, prevention issues

     i) Prevention messages do not target this age group and their unique needs, sending the message that HIV is a problem that affects only younger people.

     ii) In the United States, the life expectancy for women exceeds that of men. Heterosexual women are at particular disadvantage if they desire sexual activity due to the lower number of potential male partners in their age cohort. Middle-aged and older women may have lost a steady partner to death or divorce and are reentering the dating scene with few skills in condom negotiation and facing fierce competition for an attractive, sexually competent male partner.

     iii) Older adults disclose their HIV status to fewer persons.

       (1) Heightened fear of stigmatization and rejection after disclosure and stigma was significantly higher in older African Americans as compared to Whites (Emlet, 2007).

       (2) There are fewer persons in the middle-aged and older person's social network, and older persons are more likely to live alone (Emlet, 2006).

     iv) Middle and older age is a period in which people have ideally acquired wisdom based on life experiences and education. There is an assumption that, unlike younger people, older people should know better and control their urges to prevent exposure to HIV.

     v) The two major risk behaviors for HIV infection are unprotected male–male sex and injection drug use, presenting unique challenges for middle-aged and older persons in the gay male and injection drug use communities. Cooperman, Arnsten, and Klein (2007) found that substantial numbers of older HIV-infected and at-risk men were putting themselves or others at risk for HIV infection by having unprotected sex or multiple partners, or participating in the exchange of sex for money or drugs.

     vi) Substance abuse presents several issues.

       (1) Substance abusers often have a history of incarceration that limits their employment opportunities, and they may have strained relationships with their non-drug-using social support network.

        (2) Persons with a family history of drug use are more likely to have a drug use is-sue; older adolescent and younger adult children may be repeating the patterns of their parents, which causes much pain, guilt, and regret.

   vii) Middle-aged and older men may experience erectile dysfunction, which makes con-dom application difficult because the penis may not sustain an erection. Medications to treat erectile dysfunction, such as sildenafil, have resolved the problem of condom application, but use of these drugs is associated with high-risk sexual practices (Cooperman et al., 2007).

  viii) Middle-aged and older women are experiencing the symptoms of menopause, which usually includes decreased vaginal secretions. The lack of lubrication may increase microabrasions that would increase the possibility of HIV infection during unpro-tected sex. Although there are a variety of strategies that women can use to increase vaginal lubrication, they are not tied to an HIV prevention message.

   ix) Healthcare providers may be reluctant to screen middle-aged and older adults for risky sexual and drug use behaviors because they fear offending the older person and may feel embarrassed to ask personal questions of clients who may remind them of their parents or grandparents. The CDC recommends voluntary HIV screening for all persons over age 13 but states, "because persons age 65 and older comprise less than 2% of new HIV infections, CDC recommends 64 as the cut-off age for screening in persons without risk factors for HIV" (CDC, 2008b). This paradoxical recommenda-tion seems to be an example of age discrimination and raises the question of whether the policy is based more on economics than seroprevalence. If the policy were actu-ally based on the number of possible cases, then it is not clear why CDC isn't recom-mending routine voluntary screening for persons starting at age 20: The number of new HIV cases in 2005 for persons aged 13 to 19 was only 533 compared to 801 for persons aged 65 and older (CDC, 2008a). Because the average life expectancy in the United States is 78 years, a newly infected 65-year-old could hope to live an addi-tional 13 years.

  b. Access to care, treatment, and research

    i) There are very few healthcare providers who have expertise both in HIV treatment and biological changes associated with aging. Using multiple providers results in fragmented health care. When middle-aged and older persons fail to disclose their HIV status to providers who are treating their aging problems, unexpected and possi-bly dangerous outcomes of treatment can result.

    ii) Medications are metabolized differently as people age, yet there are no guidelines for HIV medication protocols for middle-aged and older persons. HAART-induced im-mune reconstitution may be diminished in older patients (Andrade et al., 2007).

   iii) Studies to explore the interrelationship of menopause treatment and HIV disease in aging women have been small and uncontrolled.

4. Specific care approaches

  a. Individual

    i) Healthcare providers need to anticipate that these individuals may need more activity of daily living supports to maintain themselves at home. Functional impairments

related to activities, such as walking up steps and carrying groceries, occur more often in older persons. Also, because many older persons live alone, they might need
more frequent visits and intensive follow-up if they start to miss appointments.

   ii) Middle-aged and older adults reported that they want to be respected for their age
and sometimes find it difficult to be lectured by health and social service providers
who are their children's age. A fine balance needs to be achieved because the
younger provider has knowledge and skills needed by the older person, but these
contributions must be conveyed in a manner that promotes acceptance. As one ages
with HIV, the synergistic effects on chemosensory (olfactory and gustatory abilities)
declines may be profound and influence quality of life including mood, cognition,
and overall enjoyment (Vance & Burrage, 2006).

  b. Community

   i) Middle-aged and older adults with HIV/AIDS may play a pivotal role in an extended
family network. They may be the grandparent, parent, significant other, and friend
who comforts, cooks, and nurtures. Illness of this significant hub in the social network may destabilize the social equilibrium of the network.

   ii) The gay and lesbian communities have created social supports that provide vital services that cannot be accessed from the broader, heterosexual community because of
real or perceived stigma. These services are often provided free of charge, and the
more widespread use of the Internet has facilitated access to resources for gay and
lesbian persons who live in more remote areas. Telephone support groups have been
found helpful for older isolated and/or physically challenged persons living with
HIV/AIDS.

REFERENCES

Andrade, R., Lima, P., Filhho, R., Hygino, J., Milczanowski, S., Andrade, A., et al. (2007). Interleukin-10-secreting CD4
cells from aged patients with AIDS decrease in-vitro HIV replication and tumour necrosis factor alpha production.
AIDS, 21(13), 1763–1770.

Centers for Disease Control and Prevention (CDC). (2008a). *AIDS cases by age.* Retrieved February, 19, 2008, from
http://www.cdc.gov/hiv/topics/surveillance/basic.htm#aidsage

Centers for Disease Control and Prevention (CDC). (2008b). *Questions and answers for professional partners: Revised
recommendations for HIV testing of adults, adolescents and pregnant women in healthcare settings.* Retrieved March
26, 2009, from http://www.cdc.gov/hiv/topics/testing/resources/qa/qa_professional.htm

Cooperman, N., Arnsten, J., & Klein, R. (2007). Current sexual activity and risky sexual behavior in older men with or
at-risk for HIV infection. *AIDS Education and Prevention, 19*(4), 321–333.

Emlet, C. (2006). An examination of the social networks and social isolation in older and younger adults living with
HIV/AIDS. *Health & Social Work, 31*(4), 299–308.

Emlet, C. (2007). Experiences of stigma in older adults living with HIV/AIDS: A mixed-methods analysis. *AIDS Patient
Care and STDs, 21*(10), 740–752.

Howard, A., Lo, Y., Floris-Moore, M., Klein, R., Fleishcher, N., & Schoenbaum, E. (2007). Hepatitis C virus infection
is associated with insulin resistance among older adults with or at risk of HIV infection. *AIDS, 21*(5), 633–641.

Nokes, K., & Emlet, C. (2006). Health care strategies for older adults with HIV/AIDS. In P. M. Burbank (Ed.), *Vulnerable older adults: Health care needs and interventions* (pp. 235–250). New York: Springer.

Nokes, K., Rivero-Mendez, M., Valencia, C., Tsai, Y., Bunch, E., Coleman, C., et al. (2006). Socio-demographic and other
characteristics in persons 50 years and older with HIV/AIDS in five countries. *Global Ageing: Issues and Action, 4*(2),
5–13.

Stark, S. (2007). The aging face of HIV/AIDS. *American Nurse Today, 2*(6), 30–34.

Vance, D., & Burrage, J. (2006). Chemosensory declines in older adults with HIV: Identifying interventions. *Journal of Gerontological Nursing, 32*(7), 42–48.

6.13 RURAL COMMUNITIES

1. Description of the community
   a. Rural versus urban (U.S. Department of Agriculture, 2002)
      i)   Often referred to as a nonmetropolitan area
      ii) Rural residents represent 21% of the U.S. population
      iii) Rural areas have fewer than 2,500 residents.
      iv) Urbanized areas have over 50,000 residents.
   b. Characteristics of a rural community (Bushy, 2000; Leight, 2003; Ricketts, 1999)
      i)   The South has the largest proportion of rural residents, and the Northeast has the smallest.
      ii) People in rural communities often have better access to extended family than urban residents.
      iii) Rural residents value self-reliance and independence.
      iv) People in rural communities have strong, informal support resources (family members and friends).
      v)   Insiders are long-time residents, and outsiders are newcomers.
      vi) Rural communities are characterized by a lack of anonymity (lack of privacy).
      vii) The population is not homogeneous as there are large proportions of other special populations in some areas (e.g., Native Americans, Hispanics, seasonal migrant farm workers).
      viii) Employment rates in agriculture, forestry, and fishing are higher in rural than in urban areas and are declining. Most employment is in manufacturing and services.
2. Common health issues
   a. Residents are generally poorer, older, less insured, have higher rates of unemployment, and are less educated than residents in urban areas.
   b. Residents experience isolation due to geographical remoteness.
   c. There is often difficulty receiving health care due to lack of a nearby public transportation system.
   d. Rural residents often delay seeking health care until gravely ill.
   e. Rural residents are less likely to practice preventive behaviors (e.g., immunizations) than urban residents. They are also less likely to practice health promotion or to receive regular physical examinations.
   f. Fewer healthcare providers, especially specialists (including HIV specialists), practice in rural areas.
   g. Higher rates of chronic disease and infant mortality occur in rural than in urban areas.
3. HIV/AIDS in the rural community
   a. Transmission, risk behaviors, and prevention issues (National Rural Health Association, 2004)
      i)   New cases of HIV/AIDS in rural areas are increasing at a higher rate than in urban areas.

    ii)   The South is disproportionately affected, and comprises 68% of all rural AIDS cases.

    iii)   African Americans and Latinos are disproportionately affected by HIV in rural areas; African Americans represent 50% of all rural AIDS cases.

    iv)   Most rural cases are among men (75%), but rates among women are increasing. The incidence of HIV/AIDS is higher in rural women than urban women. Some states report a 170-fold increase in incidence over a 10-year period among rural African American women (Crosby, Yarber, Diclemente, Wingood, & Myerson, 2002).

    v)   Most rural women are infected through heterosexual contact.

    vi)   Men who have sex with men (MSM) represent the largest number of rural AIDS cases in males.

  b. Access to care, treatment, and research

    i)   There are a number of barriers to care in rural communities (Hall, Li, & McKenna, 2005):

       (1) Distance to care and lack of transportation

       (2) Gaps in the healthcare system. There is a limited healthcare infrastructure with fewer facilities and providers. Providers have less experience with HIV treatment protocols.

       (3) Individuals with HIV/AIDS likely to be under-/uninsured.

       (4) Individuals with HIV/AIDS fear their confidentiality will not be protected.

       (5) Limited HIV/AIDS related resources and services are available in rural communities, as well as integrated case management systems and professional networks to assist individuals and families.

       (6) Rural residents perceive themselves to be at low risk for HIV transmission. Rural women are more likely than their urban counterparts to accept partner statements regarding risk or testing.

    ii)   According to Bushy (2000), the following conditions contribute to the continued spread of HIV in rural communities:

       (1) Rural residents are less likely to seek testing, and healthcare providers are less likely to test for HIV.

       (2) Stigma prevents people from seeking care and increases social isolation.

       (3) HIV/AIDS education is not well received, particularly in the schools.

       (4) Two high-risk groups in rural areas who are difficult to monitor are migrant farm workers and newly released prisoners.

4. Specific care approaches

  a. Individual

    i)   Adopt culturally sensitive care because rural communities often contain people of different cultures.

    ii)   Acknowledge social isolation, and ensure that appropriate referrals are made for care, services, and resources.

    iii)   Increase frequency of contact through outreach from experts who use telephone callbacks and telephone education and support systems through the use of telehealth/telemedicine technology, if available, and visiting nurses.

  b. Community

    i)   Identify appropriate HIV educational Web sites that the community can use.

ii) Use HIV care delivery techniques that have been successful in rural areas (National Rural Health Association, n.d.). Federal resources such as the Ryan White Program and state funding are critical to support HIV care in rural areas.

    (1) Individuals willing to take the lead: A clinician is often willing to put in extra time, travel to special clinics, and serve as a resource to others. Information on leaders and resources is available from the NRHA (http://www. ruralhealthweb.org).

    (2) Integrate HIV care with general health care: HIV specialty care is a luxury for rural areas. Because of the myriad of other health problems and conditions experienced by individuals with HIV disease, it is advantageous for them to receive all of their care where general rural medical services are provided. HIV guidelines are available to assist in planning the care.

    (3) Consultations and co-management: HIV experts or clinics provide consultation to non-HIV practitioners. Phone consultations can be informal and done on an as-needed basis or as prescheduled conference calls. There is also a National Clinician's Consultation Center that can be contacted at 800-933-3413. There are a number of protocols on HIV care available from the National Quality Center and the Ryan White Program. HIV specialists can also do chart reviews to help clinics improve patient care.

    (4) Traveling clinics: Vans with a multidisciplinary staff are driven to areas to provide HIV care at certain sites at set times. Temporary clinics may provide care in various locations (a community center or a church). Also, an HIV specialist may provide care at general care clinics on certain days.

    (5) Centers for expertise: Clinics with HIV care expertise serve as consultative centers for others. They are often supported through Ryan White funding.

    (6) Providing services: Clinics in rural areas must provide on-site services or appropriate referrals to other agencies. Providing multiple services is often difficult or impractical, so partnerships and referral networks must be established.

    (7) Case-management: These services ensure that individuals' health and service needs are addressed and coordinated. Nurses and/or social workers serve as case managers.

    (8) Peer support: Peer counselors are used in many rural programs to provide extra advice and help to clients. Usually they are current patients who have received special training and are supervised in their various tasks. They are from the community and understand the client culture.

    (9) Schedule adjustment: Clinic schedules (days, times, etc.) at many clinics are adjusted to fit the needs of the patients.

iii) Education and prevention

    (1) AIDS service organizations (ASOs) provide valuable prevention and educational programs in rural areas.

    (2) Sensitivity to confidentiality, disclosure, and stigma are essential in successful education, prevention, and outreach programs.

    (3) Collaboration among ASOs, local health departments, health providers, and other service agencies are necessary to reach diverse, targeted groups (Zuniga, Buchanan, & Chakravorty, 2005).

(4) Community groups can be educated about the needs of local HIV/AIDS populations (e.g., the faith-based organizations).

(5) Local social gathering spots (e.g., elders, diners, grange, beauty shops, 4H,
church) can be identified and then targeted for prevention efforts.

REFERENCES

Bushy, A. (2000). HIV/AIDS: The silent enemy within rural communities. In A. Bushy (Ed.), *Orientation to nursing in the rural community* (pp. 141–154). Thousand Oaks, CA: Sage.

Crosby, R. A., Yarber, W. L., DiClemente, R. J., Wingood, G. M., & Meyerson, B. (2002). HIV-associated histories, perceptions and practices among low-income African-American women: Does rural residence matter? *American Journal of Public Health, 92*(4), 655–659.

Hall, H. I., Li, J., & McKenna, T. (2005). HIV in predominantly rural areas of the United States. *Journal of Rural Health, 21*(3), 245–253.

Leight, S. B. (2003). The application of a vulnerable populations conceptual model to rural health. *Public Health Nursing, 20*(6), 440–448.

National Rural Health Association. (n.d.). *Rural HIV/AIDS care.* Retrieved March 3, 2009, from http://www.ruralhealthweb.org/go/left/programs-and-events/programs-and-events-overview/rural-hiv/aids-resource-center/rural-hiv/aids-resource-center

National Rural Health Association. (2004). *HIV/AIDS in America: Disproportionate impact on minority and multicultural populations* (Issue Paper). Virginia: Author.

Ricketts, T. C. (Ed.). (1999). *Rural health in the United States.* New York: Oxford University Press.

U.S. Department of Agriculture. (2002). *Measuring rurality: What is rural?* Retrieved January 16, 2008, from http://www.ers.usda.gov/Briefing/Rurality/WhatisRural/

Zuniga, M. A., Buchanan, R. J., & Chakravorty, B. J. (2005). HIV education, prevention, and outreach programs in rural areas of the southeastern United States. *Journal of HIV/AIDS & Social Services, 4*(4), 29–45.

6.14 THE AFRICAN AMERICAN COMMUNITY

1. Description of the community
   a. The majority of African Americans are descendants of West Africans living in the western hemisphere. This definition includes African descendants in the West Indies, Canada, Cuba, Central and South America, and Mexico. The terms *African American* and *Black* are used interchangeably to include those individuals who self-identify as either. Generally speaking, for people of the older generation, the word *Black* is more widely acceptable, whereas the younger generation might prefer the term *African American.*
   b. According to Census 2000, 36.4 million people, or 12.9% of the total population, reported being Black or African American. About 60% live in 10 states that contain almost half of the total U.S. population (U.S. Census Bureau, 2001).
2. Common health issues
   a. Disparities in health and illness experienced by African Americans, compared with the U.S. population as a whole, are varied, and despite efforts to improve the health of African Americans disparities persist (National Center for Health Statistics, 2006).
      i) Heart disease is the leading cause of death for all racial and ethnic groups. African Americans are 30% more likely to die of heart disease than are Whites. This occurs

despite the fact that 9.6 percent of African Americans have heart disease versus 12.2 percent of Whites.

ii)   Diabetes is the fourth leading cause of death for this population. On average, African Americans are 1.8 times more likely to have diabetes as non-Hispanic Whites of similar age (National Institute of Diabetes and Digestive and Kidney Diseases, 2005).

iii)   African Americans have the highest mortality rate of any racial and ethnic group for all cancers combined and for most major cancers. Death rates for all major causes of death are higher for African Americans than for Whites, contributing to a lower life expectancy for both African American men and African American women.

iv)   African Americans are almost twice as likely to have a first-time stroke as Whites. They are almost one and a half times more likely to die from the condition.

v)   According to the 2001 Surgeon General's report (DHHS, 2001) on mental health, the prevalence of mental disorders is believed to be higher among African Americans than among Whites, and African Americans are more likely than Whites to use the emergency room for mental health problems.

3. HIV/AIDS in the African American community
    a. Transmission, risk behaviors, and prevention issues
        i)   The rate of AIDS diagnoses for Black adults and adolescents was 10 times the rate for Whites and nearly 3 times the rate for Hispanics. The rate of AIDS diagnoses for Black women was nearly 23 times the rate for White women. The rate of AIDS diagnoses for Black men was 8 times the rate for White men (CDC, 2005a).

        ii)   Each year, more than 50% of the new HIV infections occur in African Americans (CDC, 2005b).

        iii)   Of all ethnic populations, the African American community has the largest number of people living with AIDS.

        iv)   Black Americans express concern about HIV/AIDS, and are the only racial/ethnic group to name it as the number one health problem in the United States. However, half (49%) say the United States is "losing ground" on the domestic AIDS epidemic; half also say that HIV/AIDS is a more urgent problem in their community than it was a few years ago (Kaiser Family Foundation, 2006).

        v)   Subgroups in the African American community are overrepresented in the epidemic.
            (1)   African American women comprise 12% of the U.S. population, and in 2005 represented 66% of the reported AIDS cases in women.
            (2)   African American teens (13–19 years old) comprise 16% of the U.S. population and account for 69% of the reported AIDS cases in teenagers.
            (3)   African American infants comprise 65% of perinatal infections (CDC, HIV/AIDS Reporting System, unpublished data, December 2006).
            (4)   For African American men ages 25–44 years, HIV infection is the fourth leading cause of death and the third most common cause of death for African American women.

        vi)   Anemia is a frequent complication of HIV disease and is an independent predictive marker for disease progression and death in HIV-infected patients. Blacks are almost twice as likely as Whites to have non-drug-related anemia (Sullivan, Hanson, Chu,

Jones, & Ward, 1998). The factors associated with this finding have not been elucidated.

vii) The highest mortality from HIV-related illness occurs in African American men and women.

viii) The vast majority of African Americans are aware of the basics of HIV and how the virus is transmitted. There does continue to be some misconception about the transmission of HIV through casual contact, such as kissing and sharing a drink with an HIV-infected person (Kaiser Family Foundation, 2006).

ix) A national survey showed that the median age at first vaginal intercourse for African American men is lower than that of Whites (15 years vs. 17 years). In the same study, coital frequency did not differ significantly by race (Billy, Tanfer, Grady, & Klepinger, 1993).

x) Sexually transmitted diseases are reported more often in African Americans than in Whites and remain an important biological risk factor for the transmission of HIV.

xi) African Americans are much more likely to be tested late in the course of HIV disease (Wortley et al., 1995).

b. Access to care, treatment, and research

i) Being African American or of any race is not a risk factor for AIDS, but social determinants such as poverty, discrimination, social segregation, and lower quality of HIV care have contributed to the continued spread of the disease.

ii) Multiple barriers to care exist in the African American community:

(1) Studies have found that African Americans continue to be discriminated against in a variety of areas, ranging from face-to-face interactions, housing, employment, and health and social services (Klonoff & Landrine, 1999).

(2) African Americans are less likely than other groups to have health insurance and correspondingly are less likely to benefit from early intervention and preventive treatment.

(3) A national study found that inferior patterns of HIV care were seen for many of the measures studied in Blacks and Latinos compared with Whites and in the uninsured and Medicaid-insured compared with the privately insured. Even with multivariate adjustment, many differences remained statistically significant. Even by early 1998, fewer Blacks, women, and uninsured and Medicaid-insured persons had started taking antiretroviral medication (CDC, 2005a; Shapiro et al., 1999).

(4) African Americans are underrepresented in AIDS research. Researchers have difficulty recruiting African Americans into clinical trials.

(a) Many African Americans still believe that HIV is an artificially created virus designed by the federal government to exterminate the Black population. Interestingly, this belief was most associated with those of higher levels of education. Men rather than women are likely to hold this view (Bogart & Thorburn, 2005; Klonoff & Landrine, 1999).

(b) In one study of Blacks of unknown HIV status, more than half disagreed with the U.S. government's involvement in AIDS research as being beneficial to the African American community. Two-thirds of the respondents

(n = 301) had heard of the Tuskegee Study (in which Black men were knowingly not treated for syphiiis) and often cited this as the reason why Blacks do not participate in clinical trials. Of those, 50% reported that today's AIDS scientists are more honest and respectful of Blacks than their Tuskegee counterparts (Sengupta et al., 2000).

   iii)   Researchers have established that the stigma associated with AIDS is more negative among minorities than among Whites (Herek & Capitanio, 1993).

4. Specific care approaches
  a. Individual
     i)   Appreciate the role racism has played and continues to play in the lives of African American patients. Nurses of all ethnic origins must understand and accept their own values to effectively work with others from different cultures.
     ii)   Do a client cultural assessment that includes beliefs, values, biases, taboos, customs, traditions, language, and relationships with family and community.
     iii)   Recent evidence has demonstrated that about one-third of men with a sexually transmitted disease are never tested for HIV. The nurse must ensure that individuals at high risk for HIV are appropriately tested (Ciesielksi & Boghani, 2002).
     iv)   Studies demonstrate that culture-sensitive risk education and interventions are effective in promoting greater use of condoms and reducing risky behaviors (Jemmott, Jemmott, Fong, & McCaffree, 1999). Long-term studies are needed to see if the effects of the interventions are sustained.

  b. Community
     i)   Beliefs surrounding AIDS-conspiracy theories among Blacks must be acknowledged and addressed in culturally tailored AIDS prevention and education programs.
     ii)   The continued spread of HIV in the African American community is multifactorial. One social theory suggests that when residential, educational, and social segregation exists, African Americans are more likely to engage in sexual and drug-use behaviors that may lead to HIV transmission with other African Americans than with members of other racial groups (Smith et al., 2000).
     iii)   Systematic social support has been demonstrated to be influential in controlling the epidemic in certain groups (e.g., the gay community). Adequate and effective support mechanisms are essential if epidemic control is to occur in this and other communities (e.g., injection drug users).
     iv)   Throughout the 20th century, the Black church has promoted education, business, and political activism within the Black community. The church is an ideal setting in which to offer health promotion activities for African Americans (Markens, Fox, Taub, & Gilbert, 2002).

REFERENCES

Billy, J. O. G., Tanfer, K., Grady, W. R., & Klepinger, D. H. (1993). The sexual behavior of men in the United States. *Family Planning Perspective, 25*(2), 52–60.

Bogart, L. M., & Thorburn, S. (2005). Are HIV/AIDS conspiracy beliefs a barrier to HIV prevention among African Americans? *Journal of the Acquired Immune Deficiency Syndrome, 38*(2), 213–218.

Centers for Disease Control and Prevention (CDC). (2005a). Health disparities experience by black or African-Americans—United States. *Morbidity and Mortality Weekly Report, 54*(1), 1–3.

Centers for Disease Control and Prevention (CDC). (2005b). *HIV/AIDS Surveillance Report, 2005*. Retrieved September 29, 2007, from http://www.cdc.gov/hiv/topics/surveillance/resources/reports/2005report/pdf/2005SurveillanceReport.pdf

Ciesielski, C., & Boghani, S. (2002, March). *HIV infection among men with infectious syphilis in Chicago 1998–2000*. Paper presented at the Ninth Annual Retrovirus Conference, Seattle, WA.

Herek, G. M., & Capitanio, J. P. (1993). Public reactions to AIDS in the United States: A second decade of stigma. *American Journal of Public Health, 83*(4), 574–577.

Jemmott, J. B., Jemmott, L. S., Fong, G. T., & McCaffree, K. (1999). Reducing HIV risk-associated sexual behavior among African American adolescents: Testing the generality of intervention effects. *American Journal of Community Psychology, 27*(2), 161–187.

Kaiser Family Foundation. (2006, May). *2006 Kaiser Family Foundation Survey of Americans on HIV/AIDS*. Retrieved September 29, 2007, from http://www.kff.org/kaiserpolls/pomr050806pkg.cfm

Klonoff, E., & Landrine, H. (1999). Do blacks believe that HIV/AIDS is a government conspiracy against them? *Preventive Medicine, 28*(5), 451–457.

Markens, S., Fox, S. A., Taub, B., & Gilbert, M. L. (2002). Role of Black churches in health promotion programs: Lessons from the Los Angeles Mammography Promotion in Churches Program. *American Journal of Public Health, 92*(5), 805–810.

National Center for Health Statistics (2006). *Health, United States, 2006 with chartbook on trends in the health of Americans*. Retrieved September, 29, 2007, from http://www.cdc.gov/nchs/data/hus/hus06.pdf

National Institute of Diabetes and Digestive and Kidney Diseases. (2005). *National diabetes statistics, November 2005*. Retrieved September 29, 2007, from http://diabetes.niddk.nih.gov/dm/pubs/statistics

Sengupta, S., Strauss, R. P., DeVellis, R., Quinn, S. C., DeVellis, B., & Ware, W. B. (2000). Factors affecting African-American participation in AIDS research. *Journal of Acquired Immune Deficiency Syndromes & Human Retrovirology, 24*(3), 275–284.

Shapiro, M. F., Morton, S. C., McCaffrey, D. F., Senterfitt, J. W., Fleishman, J. A., Perlman, J. F., et al. (1999). Variations in the care of HIV-infected adults in the United States: Results from the HIV Cost and Services Utilization Study. *Journal of the American Medical Association, 281*(24), 2305–2315.

Smith, D. K., Gwinn, M., Selik, R. M., Miller, K. S., Dean-Gaitor, H., Ma'at, P. I., et al. (2000). HIV/AIDS among African Americans: Progress or progression? *AIDS, 14*(9), 1237–1248.

Sullivan, P. S., Hanson, D. L., Chu, S. Y., Jones, J. L., & Ward, J. W. (1998). Epidemiology of anemia in human immunodeficiency virus (HIV)-infected persons: Results from the multistate adult and adolescent spectrum of HIV disease surveillance project. *Blood, 91*(1), 301–308.

U.S. Census Bureau. (2001). *Profiles of general demographic characteristics: 2000 census of population and housing, United States, 2000*. Retrieved September, 29, 2007, from http://www.census.gov/prod/cen2000/dp1/2khus.pdf

U.S. Department of Health and Human Services (DHHS). (2001). *Mental health: Culture, race, and ethnicity supplement*. Rockville, MD: Author.

Wortley, P. M., Chu, S. Y., Diaz, T., Ward, J. W., Doyle, B., Davidson, A. J., et al. (1995). HIV testing patterns: Where, why, and when were persons with AIDS tested for HIV? *AIDS, 9*(5), 487–492.

6.15 PREGNANT WOMEN

1. Description
   a. With the advances in HIV care and treatment, many HIV+ women are living longer, healthier lives. As they think about the future, some of these women are deciding to have the babies they have always wanted.
   b. Approximately 80% of women infected with HIV are of childbearing age (Anderson, 2005).

c. Almost one-third of HIV-infected men and women receiving medical care in the United States desire children in the future (Chen et al., 2001).

d. Approximately 20% of serodiscordant couples would practice unsafe sex in order to conceive (Klein et al., 2003).

e. Vertical or perinatal transmission refers to pregnant women with HIV transferring HIV to their unborn children.

    i)   Vertical transmission rates are 15–25% in industrialized countries, such as the United States and Western Europe.

    ii)   In developing countries, vertical transmission rates are 25–45%.

    iii)   Perinatal HIV transmission is the most common route of HIV infection in children and is now the source of almost all AIDS cases in children in the United States (CDC, 2007).

f. HIV can be transmitted antepartally, intrapartally (during delivery), and postpartally through breastfeeding; the majority of all infections are thought to occur late in pregnancy (20–33%) or during delivery (45–80%), with breastfeeding adding an additional 15–35% globally (Newell, 1998; Rouzioux et al., 1995; Dabis & Ekpini, 2002).

2. Common heath issues

a. Reproductive decisions of HIV-infected women are similar to uninfected women.

b. Pregnancies are often unplanned in both HIV-infected and uninfected women. In 2001, approximately one-half of pregnancies in the United States were unintended (Finer & Henshaw, 2006). In the Women's Interagency Health Study (WIHS), 3.5% of HIV-infected women versus 9% of uninfected women had unplanned pregnancies (Wilson et al., 1999).

c. Women are often economically dependent on men and unable to leave abusive relationships. Children often represent bonding in intimate or coercive relationships between a man and woman. Abuse increases during pregnancy, especially in women in relationships with a history of domestic violence. It is important to assess the client's safety and ability to access care, which is often decreased in this population.

3. HIV/AIDS in pregnant women

a. Transmission, risk behaviors, and prevention issues

    i)   For serodiscordant couples (one HIV-seronegative and one HIV-seropositive partner), conception counseling is often omitted by healthcare professionals for fear of medical legal repercussions should the HIV-uninfected partner seroconvert.

    ii)   Failure to discuss risks associated with unsafe sex or to provide guidance as to how to reduce or minimize HIV transmission risks actually places discordant couples at an increased risk for unsafe behavior. HIV transmission risks should be discussed often with both individuals present, and the discussion needs to be documented. It is important to know your institution's policy on this topic before providing counseling.

    iii)   Explore options such as adoption, in vitro fertilization (IVF), intracytoplasmic sperm injection (ICSI), or intrauterine insemination. These methods have low to no HIV transmission reported. Economics and insurance will dictate most options.

    iv)   If the woman is HIV infected, reduce the partner's risk of contracting HIV by considering intrauterine insemination or self-insemination. Self-insemination methods include fertility timing and turkey basting (Macaulay et al., 1995; Pinn, 2008). Turkey basting is an unconventional method in which unsafe sex is recommended during ovulation and is an affordable option for many. It is essential that the HIV viral load is undetectable. It is believed that reducing unsafe sexual practices from 30 days/month to 1–2 days/month reduces overall risks significantly. Maintaining menstrual calendars for at least 3 months with basal body temperatures can assist in identifying ovulation and should be kept prior to attempting conception. Safer sex must be encouraged during this time and at nonfertile times.

v)   If the man is HIV infected, consider sperm donation. Recent studies with sperm washing or the previously mentioned alternatives have been encouraging (Ball, 2000; Bujan et al., 2007; Gilling-Smith, 2000).

vi)   Preconception counseling for men should include education regarding the impact of antiretroviral therapy (ART) on HIV concentration in semen. HIV levels in semen are twice as high as levels in plasma. Most men believe that an undetectable HIV plasma level indicates that HIV is undetectable in the semen, and as a result may abandon safer sex practices (Kalichman et al., 2002). After 6 months of ART therapy 15–34% of men had detectable HIV in the semen. After 18 months of ART, most men have undetectable semen HIV; however, one study found several men to still have detectable HIV after 2 years of ART treatment (Leruez-Ville, 2001; Zhang et al., 1998).

vii)   Infertility issues related to HIV can complicate a woman's desire for pregnancy.
  (1)   If not on antiretroviral therapy, HIV increases spontaneous abortions, stillborns, and preterm delivery (Olaitan et al., 1996; Shapiro et al., 2000; Anderson, 2005).
  (2)   There is an increased incidence and severity of pelvic inflammatory disease with HIV (6.7–22%), which causes blocked fallopian tubes.
  (3)   Substance use (marijuana, cocaine, heroine, methadone, alcohol, and central nervous system agents, such as barbiturates and PCP) can disrupt the hypothalamic-pituitary-ovarian (HPO) axis, altering fertility at various levels (Goeders, 1997). Chemical toxins, such as those found in plastics manufacturing, farming, and lead smelters, can also alter the HPO, altering fertility (Silbergeld & Flaws, 1999).
  (4)   HIV-infected partners may have decreased sperm count or impaired sperm motility, especially if CD4 cell count is less than 200 (Muller, Coombs, & Krieger, 1998; Umapathy, Simbini, Chipata, & Mbizvo, 2001).

viii)   Some states (e.g., New York and Connecticut) have mandatory prenatal testing for all women.
  (1)   CDC guidelines recommend universal counseling and voluntary HIV testing for all pregnant women. The "One Test, Two Lives" campaign from the CDC focuses on ensuring that all women are tested for HIV early in their pregnancy (CDC 2007; Branson et al., 2006). HIV screening should be included in the routine panel of prenatal screening tests for all pregnant women.
  (2)   HIV screening is recommended after the patient is notified that testing will be performed unless the patient declines (opt-out screening).
  (3)   Separate written consent for HIV testing should not be required; general consent for medical care should be considered sufficient to encompass consent for HIV testing.

      (4)   Repeat screening in the third trimester is recommended in certain jurisdictions with elevated rates of HIV infection among pregnant women.

      (5)   Many women learn their seropositivity during pregnancy.

b. Access to care, treatment, and research

  i)   Early prenatal care has significantly reduced morbidity and mortality associated with pregnancy. Early detection of maternal HIV infection, along with intervention and prenatal care, can significantly reduce vertical transmission.

  ii) Prenatal care includes the following:

      (1)   Assess knowledge about perinatal transmission, partner's HIV status, and patient's HIV status. Is partner notification necessary? (Refer to state laws regarding this issue.) Pregnancy does not lower CD4 cell counts (vanBenthem, Vernazza, Coutinho, & Prins, 2002).

      (2)   Stabilize all chronic illnesses, including HIV and anemia, to maximize maternal and fetal outcomes. This includes assessing HIV disease, CD4 cell counts, and viral load. Screen and treat sexually transmitted diseases and obtain a Pap smear.

      (3)   Screen for mental illness (including substance abuse), which presents challenging problems in that many psychiatric medications are contraindicated during pregnancy, which can then compromise adherence to ART and prenatal appointments.

      (4)   Immunize for hepatitis, influenza, tetanus and diptheria, and pneumonia as appropriate prior to conception.

      (5)   Screen for rubella titers, blood type, and hemoglobin levels.

      (6)   Place patient on folate 0.4 mg PO prior to conception and 0.4 mg to 0.8 mg daily during pregnancy. Higher doses may be necessary if woman is taking trimethoprim-sulfmethoxazole (AETC, 2007).

      (7)   Initiate and manage ART, which does not differ between HIV-pregnant and HIV-nonpregnant women, with the exception of contraindicated medications. Women who have not initiated ART and do not have an impending need to begin therapy may wish to delay therapy until the second trimester, when organogenesis is complete.

      (8)   Assess readiness for ART or evaluate current ART regimen, modifying ART as necessary (Anderson, 2001).

      (9)   Emphasize the importance of adherence to the ART regimen to reduce risk of transmission to the infant.

     (10) Recommend antiretroviral therapy or antiretroviral prophylaxis for prevention of perinatal HIV transmission during the antepartum period to all pregnant, HIV-infected women regardless of plasma HIV RNA copy number or CD4 cell count (PHSTF, 2008).

     (11) Suggest beginning of ART by second trimester. Although monotherapy is not recommended, adding zidovudine (ZDV) to current three-drug combination antiretroviral regimens is the current recommendation unless there is severe toxicity or documented resistance. If antenatal ZDV use is not possible, at least one agent with known transplacental passage should be part of the antiretroviral regimen (PHSTF, 2008).

        (12) Report all pregnancies and suspected adverse ART events to the Antiretroviral Pregnancy Registry (phone: 800–258–4263; address: 1410 Commonwealth Drive, Wilmington, NC 28403).

        (13) Note ARTs that are contraindicated during pregnancy: efavirenz (Sustiva), hydroxyurea.

        (14) Use the following medications with caution and careful monitoring: indinavir (Crixivan), d4T (Zerit), ddi (Videx).

  c. Factors contributing to perinatal (vertical) transmission

    i) Maternal risk factors with strong evidence-based support include individuals with advanced HIV disease as evidenced by decreased CD4 cell count or CD4-CD8 ratio, or HIV viral load greater than 1,000 copies/mL. Individuals not on ART are at highest risk for transmitting HIV to their unborn child.

    ii) Maternal risk factors with limited evidence include individuals with vitamin A deficiency, sexually transmitted diseases, active genital herpes simplex virus lesion if in labor, anemia, genetic factors, illicit drug use, smoking, and seroconversion.

    iii) Obstetrical risk factors for transmitting HIV to the unborn child include prolonged rupture of membranes ($>$ 4 hrs), with a 2% increased risk for each hour until delivery (Read et al., 2000), vaginal delivery, and lack of ART during labor and delivery. Additionally, chorioamnionitis, invasive fetal procedures, and episiotomies may also contribute to increased rates of HIV transmission.

    iv) Characteristics of those who were least likely to complete zidovudine therapy included older maternal age, CD4 counts greater than 500, preterm birth, smoking or alcohol use, and cocaine or heroin use during pregnancy, especially at birth (Orloff et al., 2001).

4. Specific care approaches

  a. Individual

    i) Hold frank discussions about the pros and cons of pregnancy, being HIV infected and pregnant, risk of HIV transmission to the unborn child, and to discordant partners. All discussions should be documented.

    ii) Provide basic education about fertility and ovulation, including how to time conception.

    iii) Keep menstrual calendar for 3–6 months.

    iv) Discuss guardianship issues and support of partner, family, and friends.

    v) Discuss safer sex and contraception postpartum.

    vi) Educate regarding stages of pregnancy, intrapartum and postpartum.

    vii) Assess obstetrical history, outcomes, and any children born HIV-seropositive. Are children living with patient or have they been lost to protective services or adoption?

    viii) Assess need for parenting classes.

    ix) Assess nutritional intake, economic ability to buy food, histories of eating disorders, obesity or underweight issues, and housing (ability to prepare food and bottles and to bathe an infant).

    x) Assess stability of housing and whether or not housing is needed.

    xi) Provide social work and nutrition referrals.

    xii) Provide mental health and substance abuse referrals as needed with appropriate harm reduction when needed.

xiii) Assess smoking history and encourage cessation program prior to conception.

xiv) Refer to primary care provider for routine HIV care and to obstetrics/gynecology for Pap smear, sexually transmitted disease screening, and prenatal care. If patient has cervical dysplasia, refer for colposcopy and biopsy prior to pregnancy because biopsies cannot be done during pregnancy.

xv) Assess partner's HIV status and involvement in the pregnancy or desire for pregnancy, including discussions about discordant couples and disclosure issues.

xvi) Counsel regarding cesarean section at delivery with all women. Current studies have shown no difference in perinatal transmission rates between women on ART who had vaginal (5.5%) versus cesarean section (4.5%) deliveries (Patel et al., 2002). There is no evidence of cesarean section benefit if the women is in labor or has ruptured membranes. Cesarean section is only beneficial if viral load is $\geq$ 1,000 copies/ml near term, even if on ART, or with women who are not on ART (Watts, 2002). The risk of morbidity is increased with cesarean versus vaginal deliveries, especially with low CD4 cell counts.

b. Community

i) Continue to educate healthcare providers and policymakers about the importance of voluntary HIV testing for pregnant women.

ii) Encourage and support outreach to all women in a variety of community places for the purposes of early HIV identification and HIV education.

iii) Educate community-based organizations and peer advocates about the importance of early prenatal care to reduce vertical transmission.

iv) Educate healthcare providers and related ancillary professionals regarding management of HIV in pregnancy.

REFERENCES

AIDS Education & Training Centers (AETC). (2007). *Care of HIV-infected pregnant women.* Retrieved March 26, 2009, from http://www.aidsetc.org/aidsetc?page=cm-306_pg_tx

Anderson, J. R. (Ed.). (2001). *A guide to the clinical care of women with HIV.* Rockville, MD: U.S. Department of Health and Human Services, Health Resources and Services Administration.

Anderson, J. R. (2005). *A guide to the clinical care of women with HIV/AIDS, 2005 edition.* Rockville, MD: U.S. Department of Health and Human Services, Health Resources and Services Administration, HIV/AIDS Bureau.

Ball, S. C. (2000). Addressing the issue of childbearing in heterosexual couples discordant for HIV. *AIDS Reader, 10*(3), 144–145.

Branson, B. M., Handsfield, H. H., Lampe, M. A., Janssen, R. S., Taylor, A. W., Lyss, S. B., et al. (2006, September 22). Revised recommendations for HIV testing of adults, adolescents, and pregnant women in health-care settings. *Morbidity and Mortality Weekly Report, 55*(RR14), 1–17.

Bujan, L., Hollander, L., Coudert, M., Gilling-Smith, C.,Vucetich, A., Guibert, J., et al. (2007, September). Safety and efficacy of sperm washing in HIV-1-serodiscordant couples where the male is infected: Results from the European CREAThE network. *AIDS, 21*(14), 1909–1914.

Centers for Disease Control and Prevention (CDC). (2007). *HIV/AIDS surveillance report, 2005* (Vol. 17, Rev. ed., pp. 1–54). Atlanta, GA: U.S. Department of Health and Human Services, CDC.

Chen, J. L., Philips, K. A., Kanouse, D. E., Collins, R. L., & Miu, A. (2001). Fertility desires and intentions of HIV-positive men and women. *Family Planning Perspectives, 33*(4), 144–152, 165.

Dabis, F., & Ekpini, E. R. (2002). HIV-1/AIDS and maternal and child health in Africa. *Lancet, 359*(9323), 2097–2104.

Finer, L. B., & Henshaw, S. K. (2006). Disparities in rates of unintended pregnancy in the United States. *Perspectives on Sexual and Reproductive Health, 348*(2), 90–96.

Gilling-Smith, C. (2000). Assisted reproduction in HIV-discordant couples. *AIDS Reader, 10*(10), 581–587.

Goeders, N. E. (1997). Stress, the hypothalamic-pituitary-adrenal axis, and vulnerability to drug use. *NIDA Research Monograph, 169,* 83–104.

Kalichman, S. C., Rompa, D., Cage, M., Austin, J., Luke, W., Barnett, T., et al. (2002). Sexual transmission risk perceptions and behavioural correlates of HIV concentrations in semen. *AIDS Care, 14*(3), 343–349.

Klein, J., Pena, J. E., Thornton, M. H., & Sauer, M. V. (2003). Understanding the motivations, concerns, and desires of human immunodeficiency virus 1-serodiscordant couples wishing to have children through assisted reproduction. *Obstetrics and Gynecology, 101*(5 pt. 1), 987–994.

Leruez-Ville, M., Dulioust, E., Costabliola, D., Salmon, D., Tachet, A., Finkielsztein, L., et al. (2001). Decrease in HIV-1 seminal shedding in men receiving highly active antiretroviral therapy: An 18 month longitudinal study (ANRS EP012). *AIDS, 16*(3), 486–488.

Macaulay, L., Kitzinger, J., Green, G., & Wight, D. (1995). Unconventional conceptions and HIV. *AIDS Care, 7*(3), 261–276.

Muller, C. H., Coombs, R. W., & Krieger, J. N. (1998). Effects of clinical stage and immunological status on semen analysis results in human immunodeficiency virus type 1-seropositive men. *Andrologia, 30*(Suppl. 1), 15–22.

Newell, M. L. (1998). Mechanisms and timing of mother-to-child transmission of HIV-1. *AIDS, 12*(8), 831–837.

Olaitan, A., Reid, W., Mocroft, A., McCarthy, K., Madge, S., & Johnson, M. (1996). Infertility among human immunodeficiency virus-positive women: Incidence and treatment. *Journal European Society of Human Reproduction and Embryology, 11*(12), 2793–2796.

Orloff, S. L., Bulterys, M., Vink, P., Nesheim, S., Abrams, E. J., Schoenbaum, E., et al. (2001). Maternal characteristics associated with antenatal, intrapartum, and neonatal zidovudine use in four cities, 1994–1998. *Journal of Acquired Immune Deficiency Syndromes, 28*(1), 65–72.

Patel, J., Melville, S., Heath, C., Sukalac, K., Dominguez, M. G., Fowler, I., et al. (2002, February). *Role of combination antiretroviral therapy and mode delivery in perinatal HIV transmission (PHT): Pediatric Spectrum of Disease Project (PSD) United States, 1995–2000.* Paper presented at the Ninth Conference on Retroviruses and Opportunistic Infections, Seattle, WA.

Pinn, V. W. (2008, January). *HIV/AIDS in girls and women* (Podcast 8: Pinn Point on women's health). Office of Research on Women's Health (ORWH). Available at http://videocast.nih.gov/rss/orwh.asp

Public Health Service Task Force (PHSTF), U.S. Department of Health and Human Services (DHHS) Panel on Treatment of HIV-Infected Pregnant Women and Prevention of Perinatal Transmission. (2008, July 8). *U.S. Public Health Service Task Force recommendations for use of antiretroviral drugs in pregnant HIV-infected women for maternal health and interventions to reduce perinatal HIV transmission in the United States.* Retrieved March 30, 2009, at http://aidsinfo.nih.gov/contentfiles/PerinatalGL.pdf

Read, J. S., Tuomala, R., Kpamegan, E., Zorrilla, C., Landesman, S., Brown, G., et al. (2001). Mode of delivery and postpartum morbidity among HIV-infected women: The Women and Infants Transmission Study. *Journal of Acquired Immune Deficiency Syndromes, 26*(3), 236–245.

Rouzioux, C., Costalgliola, D., Burgand, M., Blanche, S., Mayaux, M. J., Griscelli, C., et al. (1995). Estimated timing of mother-to-child human immunodeficiency virus type 1 (HIV-1) transmission by use of a Markov model. The HIV Infection in Newborns French Collaborative Study Group. *American Journal of Epidemiology, 142*(12), 1330–1337.

Shapiro, D., Tuomala, R., Samelson, R., Burchett, S., Ciupack, G., McNamara, J., et al. (2000, January). *Antepartum antiretroviral therapy and pregnancy outcome in 462 HIV-infected women in 1998–1999 (PACTG 367).* Paper presented at the Seventh Conference on Retroviruses and Opportunistic Infections, San Francisco. Retrieved March 30, 2009, from http://www.retroconference.org/2000/Abstracts/664.htm

Silbergeld, E. K., & Flaws, J. A. (1999). Chemicals and menopause: Effects on age at menopause and on health status in the postmenopausal period. *Journal of Women's Health, 8*(2), 227–234.

Umapathy, E., Simbini, T., Chipata, T., & Mbizvo, M. (2001). Sperm characteristics and accessory sex gland functions in HIV-infected men. *Archives of Andrology, 46*(2), 153–158.

U.S. Department of Health and Human Services (DHHS), Panel on Antiretroviral Guidelines for Adults and Adolescents. (2008, January 29). *Guidelines for the use of antiretroviral agents in HIV-1-infected adults and adolescents* (pp. 1–128). Bethesda, MD: Author.

vanBenthem, B. H. B., Vernazza, P., Coutinho, R. A., & Prins, M. (2002). The impact of pregnancy and menopause on CD4 lymphocyte counts in HIV-infected women. *AIDS, 16*(6), 919–924.

Watts, G. H. (2002). Management of human immunodeficiency virus infection in pregnancy. *New England Journal of Medicine, 346*(24), 1879–1891.

Wilson, T. E., Massad, L. S., Riester, K. A., Barkan, S., Richardson, J., Young, M., et al. (1999). Sexual, contraceptive, and drug use behaviors of women with HIV and those at high risk for infection: Results from the Women's Interagency HIV Study. *AIDS, 13*(5), 591–598.

World Health Organization (WHO). (2004). *HIV transmission through breastfeeding: A review of available evidence.* Geneva, Switzerland: Author.

Zhang, H., Dornadula, G., Beumont, M., Livornese, L. Jr., Van Uitert, B., Henning, K., et al. (1998). Human immunodeficiency virus type 1 in the semen of men receiving highly active antiretroviral therapy. *New England Journal of Medicine, 339*(25), 1803–1809.

6.16 RECENT IMMIGRANTS

1. Definition of the community
    a. An immigrant is a person who is foreign born, and who is not a citizen of the country in which he/she is currently residing. This person may have entered the country with or without official documentation from either the country of origin or the country of residence.
    b. In 2003, 33.5 million foreign-born residents were in the United States. They comprised 11.7% of the total population (Levsen, 2004).
    c. Percentage of documented immigrants in the United States (Levson, 2004)
        i)   Latin American (includes Central American, Caribbean, and South American): 53.3%
        ii)   Asian (includes Chinese [Cantonese, Mandarin, and Fukinese], Vietnamese, Korean, Cambodian, Filipino, Thai, Japanese, and Laotian): 25%
        iii) European: 13.7%
    d. In 2006, over 1,200,000 deportable aliens (undocumented immigrants or those whose visas have expired) were located in the United States (Chertoff, 2007).
        i)   The visa quotas imposed by the United States and/or countries of origin and the long waits for official documents lead some individuals to find other ways to enter the country.
        ii)   Because Canada and Mexico share U.S. borders, both countries serve as conduits for undocumented immigrants entering the United States, some of whom are from countries that don't border the United States. Examples include El Salvador, Guatemala, Haiti, the Philippines, the Dominican Republic, and China.
        iii) Persons seeking to enter the United States without documents take extreme measures. They endure great physical hardships, such as stowing away on ships, trucks, trains, and planes, without food or water and in extreme temperatures (e.g., refrigerated holds). Some die before they reach the United States.
        iv)   They may also pay/promise exorbitant fees to brokers in exchange for shepherding them into the country. Some are enslaved or indentured upon entry into the United States and are forced to hand over their earnings, become sex workers in brothels, or work as servants. Immigrants and their families may be threatened with bodily harm and/or death.
    e. More than 24.6% of immigrants live below the poverty line (Levsen, 2004).

2. Common health issues
   a. Immigrants face many cultural, economic, and political barriers to healthcare access in the United States.
      i)   Up to 52% of immigrants lack health insurance (The Kaiser Family Foundation, 2007).
      ii)   Many immigrants hold jobs that do not offer health insurance. Low incomes make it difficult to purchase health insurance.
      iii) Many immigrants are unfamiliar with the healthcare system of this country.
      iv)   Some immigrants may be unsure of Western healthcare practices, preferring instead to seek care from traditional healers. Unscrupulous people, posing as traditional healers, may take advantage of them.
      v)   Both documented and undocumented immigrants fear being reported to the Department of Homeland Security.
   b. Immigration and the law
      i)   The Immigration and Nationality Act (INA) of 1952 bars admission to the United States by individuals infected with dangerous contagious diseases. In 1987, HIV infection was added to that list.
      ii)   Various attempts have been made to remove all sexually transmitted diseases from the list of communicable diseases in the INA, but to no avail. Beginning in 1990, permissions were granted for entry into the United States by HIV-infected individuals on a case-by-case basis for conference and sporting events (such as United Nations assemblies, the 2002 Salt Lake City Olympics).
      iii) Currently there is a proposal to streamline the process by which travel visas are granted and to permit entry into the United States by HIV-infected individuals for business or pleasure for up to 30 days (Chertoff, 2007).
      iv)   The INS does allow HIV-infected immigrants to apply for individual asylum status based on past or possible persecution upon return to the country of origin. However, inadequate medical care and social ostracism related to HIV infection are not deemed to be persecution (Chertoff, 2007).
      v)   An HIV-infected immigrant already living in the United States cannot be deported if he/she maintains legal status.
      vi)   All immigrants applying for legal permanent status must be tested for HIV infection. HIV counseling is often unavailable. The immigrant may be denied residency status if found to be HIV positive. However, a waiver may be granted if the immigrant has close family ties in the United States or has applied for asylum.
      vii) Medical facilities have no legal right or obligation to report undocumented immigrants to the DHS.
3. HIV/AIDS in the immigrant community
   a. Transmission, risk behaviors, and prevention issues
      i)   Transmission modes vary among immigrant populations, dependent upon risk factors. They are the same as for the United States (unprotected sexual contact, and use of infected injection equipment). However, there is an increased risk of transmission from contaminated blood products and perinatal transmission.
      ii)   Unique risk factors include the following:

(1) Condom use may be limited due to cultural norms and multiple sexual partners (of either sex).

(2) Injection equipment may be shared for medications and vitamins taken in the homes. Injected medications are believed to be more potent than oral forms.

(3) Prophylaxis for perinatal transmission is not commonly used because of the costs involved.

(4) Breastfeeding is more commonly practiced in other countries for both cultural and sanitary reasons.

(5) Blood products may not be screened for HIV and other blood-borne pathogens. Monetary compensation for blood donation is still practiced.

b. Access to care, treatment, and research

i) Immigrants may arrive in poor health (sometimes due to the dangerous nature of their journey to the United States) and seek medical care only when seriously ill.

ii) Immigrants may have infectious diseases that are endemic to their countries of origin, such as tuberculosis, hepatitis, and parasitic diseases.

iii) Some immigrants may mistakenly believe that HIV is a gay, White male disease of U.S. citizens and do not see themselves at risk.

iv) Because in their cultures of origin HIV is associated with unaccepted behaviors (homosexuality and drug use), HIV-infected individuals will not disclose their status to others and they will isolate themselves in shame.

v) For research and statistical purposes, some immigrants are ethnically and racially misclassified as "other" because of misunderstanding of the criteria.

4. Specific approaches

a. Individual

i) Awareness of cultural characteristics and health beliefs is important in developing an individualized plan of care.

ii) Clinic office hours should be accessible to clients who work long hours.

iii) Assistance with access to social and legal services should be provided as necessary for the uninsured or undocumented.

b. Community

i) Efforts should be made to create linkages with social service and legal agencies that specialize in the particular needs of undocumented immigrants.

ii) Prevention efforts should include materials that are culturally appropriate and utilize peers for outreach.

REFERENCES

Chertoff, M. (2007, November). *Issuance of a visa and authorization for temporary admission into the United States for certain nonimmigrant aliens infected with HIV* (72 FR 62593; FR 59-07). Washington, DC: U.S. Department of Homeland Security. Retrieved March 27, 2009, from http://www.dhs.gov/xlibrary/assets/hiv_waiver_finalrule.pdf

The Kaiser Family Foundation. (2007, October). *The Kaiser Commission on Medicaid and the uninsured: Health insurance coverage in America, 2006 data update.* Retrieved February 4, 2008, from http://www.kff.org/uninsured/upload/7651.pdf

Levsen, L. J. (2004). *The foreign born population in the United States: 2003 current population reports* (P20-551). Washington, DC: U.S. Census Bureau.

U.S. Department of Homeland Security. (2007, October). *2006 Yearbook of Immigration Statistics.* Washington, DC: Author.

6.17 SUBSTANCE USERS

1. Description of the community
   a. People who use legal or illegal substances with the intent to alter consciousness; *addiction, substance abuse,* and *substance misuse* are terms generally applied when use becomes harmful or uncontrolled.
   b. Compared to non-substance users, substance users have less access to ambulatory medical care for their HIV infection, less access to highly active antiretroviral therapy (HAART) and worse adherence to HAART. HIV-infected substance users have poorer health outcomes than other HIV risk groups (Cunningham, Sohler, Berg, Shapiro, & Heller, 2006).
   c. Substance use exists on a continuum from minimal to maximal impact and within a social context that is value laden and tends to marginalize and criminalize users.
   d. Types of substance users and their relation to HIV disease
      i) Injecting drug users (IDUs)
          (1) IDUs currently make up more than 26% of total AIDS cases and 21.9% of HIV cases; many pediatric HIV cases are related to mothers who are IDUs (Lieb et al., 2006).
          (2) High rates of substance abuse, mental illness, marginal employment, and inadequate housing may make it particularly difficult for HIV-positive IDUs to access and utilize health care (Purcell et al., 2004).
          (3) Previous use also has implications for care (e.g., possibilities for relapse, pain control, stress management).
          (4) Heroin, amphetamines, and cocaine are the most commonly injected drugs. Each substance has specific psychological, social, and physical effects on the user and requires providers to tailor patient care plans specific to the patient's drug use.
          (5) HIV-positive IDUs often live in socially and economically disadvantaged communities characterized by health and psychosocial problems (Mizuno et al., 2006).
      ii) Non-IDUs
          (1) Crack cocaine is highly addictive and is associated with many infections. Smoking increases the risk of pulmonary conditions, such as asthma and many different pneumonias (e.g., aspergillus pneumonia, asthma).
          (2) Volatile nitrites have been reported to ease the pain of receptive anal intercourse through relaxation of the sphincter muscles (Romanelli, Smith, Thorton, & Pomeroy, 2004). Lastly, drugs such as ketamine and gamma hydroxyl butyrate (GHB) could also have effects of decreasing physically painful experiences (Drumright, Patterson, & Strathdee, 2006).

(3) Given the chronic relapsing nature of drug use and addiction, it is important for clinicians to help prevent initial drug use and identify early relapse by thorough explanation and communication about drug use behavior (Sohler, Wong, Cunningham, Cabral, Drainoni, & Cunningham, 2007).

(4) Use of non-injectable drugs has been increasingly recognized as a risk factor in the transmission of HIV due to its potential indirect effects on HIV transmission. Substance use is moderately correlated with risky sex for men (Klinkenberg & Sacks, 2004).

2. Common health issues

a. There is a high prevalence of substance abuse and psychiatric disorders among HIV-infected individuals. Importantly, drug and alcohol use disorders are frequently comorbid with depression, anxiety, and severe mental illness (Chander, Himelhoch, & Moore, 2006).

b. Race, ethnicity, gender, sexual preference, and socioeconomic status affect drug use, health, and access to health care.

c. Criminalization of lifestyle leads to marginalization and a distrust of authority and institutions; access to housing, food, and health care is often compromised by restrictions on serving active users. The Americans with Disabilities Act prohibits withholding of health services to people who are addicts.

d. Adverse health effects of substance use

   i) Infections (e.g., abscesses; sepsis; endocarditis; central nervous system [CNS], hepatic, and renal infections) related to unclean injection equipment, unsafe techniques, and impurities in substances injected

   ii) Organic syndromes related to direct effect of substances/impurities on tissues; affects skin, muscular, CNS, hepatic, renal, and vascular systems

   iii) Causation or exacerbation of depression, psychosis, suicidal tendencies, isolation from social support systems, stigmatization, and poor self-esteem

   iv) Self-medication with illicit substances to manage pain or mental illness often masks underlying problems and precludes their diagnosis.

   v) Associated risks of substance abuse include malnutrition, homelessness, and poor coping mechanisms. These added risks increase the challenges healthcare providers face in delivering care to these clients. In addition, because HIV-positive substance-abusing patients traditionally use the emergency department as their usual source of care, the emergency departments may be an appropriate setting to coordinate services for these vulnerable patients (Masson, Sorensen, Phibbs, & Okin, 2004).

   vi) Poor health related to lifestyle and substance abuse adds to the challenges in providing care. Adherence issues become a problem when the treatment plan is believed to be incompatible with street and prescribed drugs. Nonadherence leads to poor response to therapy, as well as viral drug resistance and cross-resistance, making current treatment ineffective and future treatment potentially unsuccessful (Haug, Sorensen, Lollo, Gruber, Delucchi, & Hall, 2005).

   vii) Substance use places individuals at increased risk for HIV and other infectious diseases, such as tuberculosis, sexually transmitted diseases (STDs), and hepatitis.

viii)   Substance use, particularly rational or moderate, may provide positive coping strategies for some and improve quality of life; some substance use (e.g., marijuana, opiates) may provide symptom relief as well as have positive effects on mental status or sense of well-being.

3. HIV/AIDS in the substance abuse community
   a. Transmission, risk behaviors, and prevention issues
       i)   Substance use may increase a person's risk of contracting HIV and transmitting it to others.
       ii)   The risk increases because the person engages in risk behaviors (e.g., trading sex, money, and drugs, having multiple partners, having unprotected sex, and not being treated for sexually transmitted diseases) while high or in exchange for substances (Mark et al., 2006).
       iii) Drug cravings may lead to risky practices, such as unsafe sexual practices, unsafe injection practices, and interpersonal violence.
   b. Access to care, treatment, and research
       i)   Structural barriers such as insurance, finances, and knowledge deficit may create a confusing healthcare system.
       ii)   Substance users are often labeled as immoral, noncompliant, manipulative, and drug seeking. This puts an undue burden on the client to access appropriate care.
       iii) Users are often disorganized due to lifestyle and altered mental status; appointments, records, and medication refills may be lost, not kept, or stolen.
       iv)   Conflicts over pain medication often undermine relationships with provider. Pain management is often undertreated.
       v)   Restrictions, rules, and requirements for persons to be clean and sober deter users from accessing care while using substances.
       vi)   Users of illicit substances may fear arrest and thus may have distrust of authority including medical institutions.
       vii) Providers often refuse to treat active users who are mentally ill.
       viii) Active users are usually denied access to clinical trials for experimental treatments.
       ix)   Addiction (craving) must be addressed by user before other needs, especially those involving stress (stress triggers craving), are met. According to researchers, buprenorphine is safer than methadone, because it is a partial opioid agonist and has a lower potential to induce respiratory depression (Luty, O'Gara, & Sessay, 2005).
       x)   Barriers to care often prevent diagnosis of HIV disease and related problems until it is too late for treatment.
       xi)   Interactions between street drugs and prescribed medications are poorly understood. However, some amounts of alcohol in nelfinavir may be a contraindication for recovering addicts and alcoholics. Efavirenz does give the sensation of being high for some individuals and is often abused by active addicts.
           (1) Efavirenz and nevirapine have been found to induce the metabolism of methadone and may precipitate opioid withdrawal in individuals chronically maintained on methadone (Basu, Chwastiak, & Bruce, 2005; Bruce et al., 2006).

(2) Methadone increases area under the curve (AUC) for delavirdine and fluconazole; decreases AUC of abacavir, amprenavir, efavirenz, lopinavir, nelfinavir, ritonavir, phenytoin, rifabutin, and rifampin; has no effect on didanosine (ddI), stavudine (d4t), and zidovudine (AZT).

4. Specific care approaches
   a. Individual
      i) Provider needs to have working knowledge of substance-use culture; ask questions if you do not know.
      ii) Establish trust through open, nonjudgmental exploration of substance use.
      iii) Users will often cover or minimize use until trust is established; allow time for relationship to develop (can be months to years).
      iv) User may not perceive substance use as primary problem; assess immediate needs and offer assistance.
      v) Understand the user's relationship with substances, and work to provide safer alternative.
         (1) Harm reduction is a model that attempts to reduce or eliminate risk of HIV infection/transmission by changing high-risk sex and substance-use behaviors (e.g., teaching safe injection use/techniques, initiating needle/syringe exchange programs; Patten, Vollman, & Thurston, 2000). The most commonly described programs that use a harm reduction approach include pretreatment counseling and drop-in counseling. Outreach and education, case management, residential programs, and acupuncture detoxification are other services provided in a harm reduction model (Tobias, Wood, & Drainoni, 2006).
         (2) Abstinence is one option in a multifaceted approach.
         (3) Peer programs such as Alcoholics Anonymous (AA) and Narcotics Anonymous (NA) are free and have high success rates.
      vi) Provide information on demand drug treatment programs that are accessible, flexible, and noncoercive.
      vii) Acknowledge difficulty accessing health care; express willingness to work to overcome barriers.
      viii) Discuss benefits of substance use for person as well as costs; substance use is often related to primary coping mechanisms; do not attempt to remove this coping mechanism without providing a substitute.
      ix) Comprehensive substance use history may take time to complete; be patient.
      x) Substance users are capable of making decisions concerning treatment and quality-of-life issues; respect their ability to do so.
      xi) Construct interventions with substance users' culture in mind: Be aware that users often do not keep appointments (drop-in schedules and rescheduling several times may be necessary), and do not schedule appointments that coincide with peak use times (beginning and midmonth when person gets paid) because appointments will usually not be kept.
      xii) Offer drug treatment/detoxification regularly after trust is established; avoid making recovery a requirement for continued care.

xiii) Manipulation and scamming are survival tools for many users; expect and acknowledge this. Do not take it personally if you are scammed. Respect, trust, and negotiation are the best tools to minimize manipulation.

xiv) Assess support networks and family relationships; remember that dysfunctional relationships are sometimes better than none.

xv) Interventions in the acute setting
    (1) Assess substance use and most recent use.
    (2) Anticipate and treat withdrawal symptoms; know that opiate and alcohol withdrawal are better understood and treated than amphetamine and cocaine withdrawal.
    (3) Users expect to be judged and treated punitively; anticipate this, and reassure them that this will not happen.
    (4) Stress, fear, and poor coping mechanisms without drugs potentiate cravings.
    (5) Despite best attempts, users may leave against medical advice (AMA); begin discharge planning early. Provide medications and referrals if possible.
    (6) Attempt referral to home care agencies to complete IV therapy and provide follow-up.
    (7) Primary care/community-based agency referrals are important to break the cycle of using the ER and hospital as the only source of health care.

xvi) Clear, reasonable, firm limits help patient understand expectations.

xvii) Patient advocacy remains central to the nurse's role in caring for the substance user with HIV disease.

xviii) A team approach with excellent communication reduces impact of attempts to split and manipulate.

xix) Assess and treat pain adequately (often the precipitating factor in users leaving AMA).

b. Community
  i) Expanded services for substance users
    (1) Day treatments in which the client can still work in the evening or return to home provide advantages to the drug user.
    (2) Outreach clinics and services in areas populated by users are more easily accessed.
    (3) Drug treatment centers need childcare services for single parents.
    (4) Develop alternatives to prison for nonviolent drug-related offenses, especially for women and individuals from lower socioeconomic levels (Freudenberg, Wilets, Greene, & Richie, 1998).
    (5) Needle exchange programs (NEPs) are designed to stem the spread of HIV and other blood-borne pathogens among IDUs by providing sterile needles in exchange for contaminated ones (Huo, Bailey, Hershow, & Ouellette, 2005).
    (6) Expand access to drug treatment and detox. Methadone HIV treatment services have been successfully integrated into some methadone maintenance treatment programs. These treatment programs, despite their considerable success in treating opiate dependence, have been tightly regulated in the United States, so that as few as 15% of opiate-dependent people can access these services at present (Basu, Smith-Rohrberg, Bruce, & Altice, 2006).

(7) Develop housing options for active users. Active users are often restricted from subsidized AIDS housing.

(8) Expand use of community-based clinics, walk-in clinics, mobile vans, and public health and home care nursing to provide as much health care as possible in the neighborhoods where users live. Integrating trauma and substance abuse services may lead to improvement in intermediate outcomes, such as reducing drug use and increased relationship power (Amaro et al., 2007).

(9) Expand harm reduction services to meet people where they are; for example, IDUs often require wound care services, so nurses could provide harm reduction at the same time.

ii) Design outreach and case management programs targeting substance users in a multidisciplinary approach to connect them with housing, food, health care, and financial support.

iii) Rework the traditional model of hospice and palliative care to accommodate the needs of substance users with HIV disease; this would include adequate pain control.

iv) Expand research into treatment of withdrawal and detoxification from cocaine and amphetamines.

v) Educate professionals and patients about available resources such as the following:

(1) Alcoholics Anonymous: http://www.alcoholics-anonymous.org

(2) Al-Anon/Alateen: http://www.al-anon.alateen.org

(3) Harm Reduction Coalition: http://www.harmreduction.org. East Coast Office, 22 West 27th Street, 5th floor, New York, NY 10001; phone: 212-213-6376; fax: 212-213-6528; email: hrc@harmreduction.org.

(4) Harm Reduction Training Institute: New York Office, 22 West 27th Street, 5th Floor, New York, NY 10001; phone: 212-683-2334; fax: 212-213-6582; email: hrti@harmreduction.org. West Coast Office, 1440 Broadway, Suite 510, Oakland, CA 94612; phone: 510-444-6969; fax: 510-444-6977; email: hrcwest@harmreduction.org.

(5) Narcotics Anonymous: http://www.na.org

(6) National Institute on Drug Abuse: http://www.nida.nih.gov

(7) SAMHSA's National Clearinghouse for Alcohol and Drug Information (NCADI): http://ncadi.samhsa.gov

(8) Web of Addictions: http://www.well.com/user/woa

(9) World Health Organization: http://www.who.int.en

REFERENCES

Amaro, H., Larson, M., Zhang, A., Acevedo, A., Dai, J., & Matsumoto, A. (2007). Effects of trauma intervention on HIV sexual risk behaviors among women with co-occurring disorders in substance abuse treatment. *Journal of Community Psychology, 35*(7), 895–908.

Basu, S., Chwastiak, L., & Bruce, R. (2005). Clinical management of depression and anxiety in HIV-infected adults. *AIDS, 19*(18), 2057–2067.

Basu, S., Smith-Rohrberg, D., Bruce, R., & Altice, F. (2006). Models for integrating buprenophrine therapy into the primary HIV care setting. *Clinical Infectious Diseases, 42*(5), 716–721.

Bruce, R., Altice, F., Gourevitch, M., & Friedland, G. (2006). Pharmacokinetic drug interactions between opioid agonist therapy and antiretroviral medications: Implications and management for clinical practice. *Journal of Acquired Immune Deficiency, 41*(5), 563–572.

Chander, G., Himelhoch, S., & Moore, R. (2006). Substance abuse and psychiatric disorders in HIV-positive patients. *Drugs, 66*(6), 769–789.

Cunningham, C., Sohler, N., Berg, K., Shapiro, S., & Heller, D. (2006). Type of substance use and access to HIV-related health care. *AIDS Patient Care, 20*(6), 399–407.

Drumright, L., Patterson, T., & Strathdee, S. (2006). Club drugs as causal risk factors for HIV acquisition among men who have sex with men: A review. *Substance Use and Misuse, 41*(10–12), 1551–1601.

Freudenberg, N., Wilets, I., Greene, M. B., & Richie, B. E. (1998). Linking women in jail to community services: Factors associated with rearrest and retention of drug-using women following release from jail. *Journal of American Women's Association, 53*(2), 89–93.

Haug, N., Sorensen, J., Lollo, N., Gruber, V., Delucchi, K., & Hall, S. (2005). Gender differences among HIV-positive methadone maintenance patients enrolled in a medication adherence trial. *AIDS Care, 17*(8), 1022–1029.

Huo, D., Bailey, S., Hershow, R., & Ouellette, L. (2005). Drug use and HIV risk practices secondary and primary needle exchange users. *AIDS Education and Prevention, 17*(2), 170–184.

Klinkenberg, W., & Sacks, S. (2004). Mental disorders and drug abuse in persons living with HIV/AIDS. *AIDS Care, 16*(Suppl. 1), S22–S42.

Lieb, S., Rosenberg, R., Arons, P., Mallow, R., Liberti, T., Maddox, L., et al., (2006). Age shift in patterns of injection drug use among the HIV/AIDS population in Miami-Dade County, Florida. *Substance Use and Misuse, 41*(10–12), 1623–1635.

Mark, H., Nanda, J., Davis-Vogel, A., Navaline, H., Scotti, R., Wickrema, R., et al. (2006). Profiles of self-reported HIV risk behaviors among injection drug users in methadone maintenance treatment, detoxification, and needle exchange programs. *Public Health Nursing, 23*(1), 11–19.

Masson, C., Sorensen, J., Phibbs, C., & Okin, R. (2004). Predictors of medical service utilization among individuals with co-occurring HIV infection and substance abuse disorders. *AIDS Care, 16*(6), 744–755.

Mizuno, Y., Wilkinson, J., Santibanez, S., Rose, C., Knowlton, A., Handley, K., et al. (2006). Correlates of health care utilization among HIV-seropositive injection drug users. *AIDS Care, 18*(5), 417–425.

Patten, S., Vollman, A., & Thurston, W. (2000). The utility of the Transtheoretical Model of behavior change for HIV risk reduction in injection drug users. *Journal of the Association of Nurses in AIDS Care, 11*(1), 57–66.

Purcell, D., Metsch, L., Latka, M., Santibanez, S., Gomez, C., Eldred, L., et al. (2004). Interventions for seropositive injectors—research and evaluation: An integrated behavioral intervention with HIV-positive drug users to address medical care, adherence, and risk reduction. *Journal of Acquired Immune Deficiency Syndrome, 37*(Suppl. 2), S110–S118.

Romanelli, F., Smith, K., Thornton, A., & Pomeroy, C. (2004). Poppers: Epidemiology and clinical management of inhaled nitrite abuse. *Pharmacotherapy, 24*(1), 69–78.

Sohler, N., Wong, M., Cunningham, W., Cabral, H., Drainoni, M., & Cunningham, C. (2007). Type and pattern of illicit drug use and access to health care services for HIV-infected people. *AIDS Patient Care and STDs, 21*(Suppl. 1), S68–S76.

Tobias, C., Wood, S., & Drainoni, M. (2006). Ryan White Title I survey: Services for HIV-positive substance users. *AIDS Patient Care and STDs, 20*(1), 58–67.

6.18   TRANSGENDER/TRANSSEXUAL PERSONS

1. Description of the community
   a. Transgender is an umbrella term that includes intersex, transsexual, transvestite, transgender, and other nontraditional presentations.
   b. Persons of transgender experience reflect society at large. The members of this community are not a homogenous group; they come from all possible backgrounds.

   c. Many people of trans experience also belong to other disenfranchised groups (e.g., unemployed, sex workers, homeless, racial/ethnic minorities), which creates additional hurdles to optimizing care.

   d. Lexicon for transgender community is diverse and growing; *trans* is considered the most inclusive term.

      i) It is not necessary to have genital surgery to define oneself as trans, and many such people have no intention to have the surgery.

      ii) Conversely, many people who have had sexual reassignment surgery (SRS) obtain all legal documentation in the new gender and no longer consider themselves trans.

   e. The trans community has been affected disproportionately from the beginning of the HIV epidemic in the United States.

   f. Statistical reporting of HIV transmission risk has not included trans identity as a category; supposition is that most data are subsumed into men who have sex with men (MSM) data (Millet et al., 2007).

   g. Two broad categorizations exist within trans community.

      i) Female-to-male (FTM; transmen): born phenotypically female, seeking masculine identity/presentation.

      ii) Male-to-female (MTF; transwomen): born phenotypically male, seeking feminine identity/presentation. This group has a higher rate of HIV prevalence (Kenagy, 2002).

2. Common health issues

   a. Social stigma is associated with trans identities.

   b. Public disdain, verbal harassment, even physical violence may be directed at the trans community/individuals (i.e., transphobia; Freedberg, 2006).

   c. There is a scarcity of employers willing to support persons during time of transition or when not deemed "fully passing" by employer.

   d. Some people need to hide gender identity to preserve employment, family, social relationships, and religious affiliations.

   e. There may be a lack of acceptance by other marginalized communities (i.e., lesbian and gay populations).

   f. Entrance and orientation to trans culture is often clandestine, guilt laden, and occasionally dangerous.

   g. Lack of access to culturally competent medical and social service providers

   h. Minimal access can lead to purchase of illicit hormones, which can lead to needle-sharing, metabolic/mood disorders, and other avoidable side effects of hormone therapy (see below).

   i. If there is insurance coverage, it is most likely under birth gender, so most of the indicated prescriptions are not covered, leading to out-of-pocket expenses.

   j. For under- or unemployed persons, commercial sex work is often used to pay for medications and procedures.

   k. Desire to pass in society can lead to seeking unsupervised surgical procedures (i.e., facial sculpting), which are often performed in foreign countries to reduce the cost.

   l. Rate of alcoholism, illegal drug use, and sex work is understood to be disproportionately high in trans community (Edwards et al., 2007).

3. HIV/AIDS in the trans community
   a. Transmission, risk behaviors, and prevention issues.
      i)   There have been almost no behavior-change "risk reduction" programs specifically targeting the trans communities, MTF or FTM (Nemoto et al., 2004).
      ii)   Healthcare professionals remain uncomfortable with trans sexuality and are largely unaware of the complex sexual, emotional, and personal issues affecting prevention.
      iii) Effective prevention efforts must account for myriad gender presentations and sexual practices, and this complicates the dissemination of the message.
      iv)   Mandatory name reporting for HIV testing (in most states) is incongruent with need to hide gender from society.
      v)   It is difficult to target prevention messages for trans people if they are not self-identified, or, if self-identified, they may be isolated from the larger community.
   b. Access to care, treatment and research
      i)   Historically, the medical professions have not respected the trans experience, leading to distrust and avoidance.
      ii)   Reliable and evidence-based information about trans care is difficult to locate.
      iii) Healthcare workers maintain social stereotypes and prejudices of trans experience; programs to educate and adjust attitudes are limited.
      iv)   Mental healthcare professionals are often uneducated and insensitive to trans issues and the psychological/sociological needs.
            (1) Training is required to distinguish trans experience from incidental findings (e.g., depression, personality disorders).
            (2) Few mental health providers are trained/equipped to counsel around routine concerns (e.g., clearance letters for SRS).
      v)   Pursuit of hormones (over HIV care) is major entry point into medical care for transgender persons (Melendez et al., 2006).
      vi)   There are no known treatment or research protocols regarding the HIV-positive trans community.
      vii) Public assistance to the uninsured is most often awarded only under legal name and gender; this may no longer reflect the person's reality and prevent/limit the person from accessing benefits.
4. Specific care approaches
   a. Individual
      i)   Cross-gender hormone therapy (CGHT)
            (1) Several established organizations have issued guidelines related to CGHT (CLCHC, 2002; TWHC, 2006; WPATH, 2001).
            (2) Both feminizing and masculinizing hormone treatments impact on interpretation of standard lab data (e.g., hemoglobin, hematocrit, lipid profile).
            (3) Estrogen therapy will lower hemoglobin/hematocrit to normal female range. If lab report is labeled *male*, it may be flagged as abnormal and lead to an unnecessary workup for anemia.
            (4) Conversely, testosterone therapy will increase these same levels and possibly lead to unnecessary workup for polycythemia.

(5) Persons with hepatitis-related liver disease (the aforementioned needle-sharing has led to a high rate of hepatitis C infection in the trans community) may need adjusted hormone doses or use of delivery systems that bypass the liver (e.g., transdermal).

(6) Consistently elevated estrogen levels do not supersede genetics to cause greater breast growth, and can even lead to endogenous testosterone production.

ii) HIV-positive people of trans experience may not initially reveal trans identity to healthcare providers, appearing in clothing, hairstyle, and so forth of the legal gender until trust is established.

(1) Physical exam/nursing assessment

(a) Intake: Validate client's experience with gender as personally and socially important.

(i) Ask and then offer to use client's preferred name and gender expression to the fullest extent allowed by charting and medical-legal restrictions.

(ii) Reassure the client of your intention to be sensitive, despite your own lack of training or experience with people of trans experience.

(iii) Full exam may need to be done in trust-building stages over several visits, especially the genital exam.

(b) Monitoring

(i) Help client interpret lab reports in appropriate normal ranges for gender.

(ii) Patient education related to possible outcomes of surgeries and importance of post-op self-care is of high priority.

(iii) Assess need for referrals, especially for mental health, substance abuse, and needle exchange, in an ongoing manner (Boggs, 2007).

(2) Minimal data related to effects of antiretroviral medications on hormones, and vice versa, are available.

(a) It is known that most protease inhibitors decrease the biotransformation of estrogens, whereas NNRTIs can increase it (Jaworsky et al., 2007).

(b) To date no dose adjustments of HAART medications or hormone therapies have been recommended.

iii) Cosmetic surgeries (e.g., breast enlargement or removal, body sculpting) may be pursued separate from SRS, and they are often performed by surgeons/practitioners not in communication with the client's primary health center/provider.

(1) There are many, often overlapping, reasons:

(a) Stigma

(b) Cost of procedures in the United States

(c) Refusal of U.S. surgeons to perform procedures difficult to reverse

(d) Reluctance of client to disclose HIV status

(2) Healing may be compromised by a low CD4 count/high viral load (especially if unknown to surgeon), or by recuperation in a country with decreased access to standard hygiene measures.

iv) Provide education, networking, counseling and support for transmen and -women to reduce internalized transphobia and increase self-efficacy.

    v)   Identify trans-friendly healthcare providers to create a referral network.

    vi)   Offer to monitor/prescribe CGHT for client, especially as part of harm reduction measures.

    vii) Provide additional counseling and education about long-term effects of CGHT (Leon, 2002).

        (1) Infertility: This applies especially, but not only, after SRS.

        (2) There may be a lack of erection function (may be partially reversible with PDE-5 inhibitors, if desired by client).

        (3) Educate MTF clients that estrogen therapy may increase risk of DVT and PE, especially if also a smoker.

        (4) Help set realistic expectations about limits of CGHT to affect desired body changes (e.g., body hair, voice, fat redistribution).

    viii) Revisit topic of relevant safer sex practices as level of trust, needs, and client's body changes.

    ix)   Offer legal counseling/referrals as needed.

b. Community approaches

    i)   Transphobia must be identified, exposed, and publicly denounced; provide education and training for clinicians and staff.

    ii)   Reevaluate safer sex messages for culturally appropriate language and absence of moral judgments.

    iii) Prevention messages must acknowledge people of trans experience, not only as individuals but also as social beings with complex family, group, and community roles and relationships.

    iv) Explore medical–legal issues related to feminization/virilization within practice setting.

    v)   Employ people of trans experience, especially as outreach workers.

    vi)   Use existing trans media (e.g., Web sites, periodicals) regularly to educate and reach the community to build trust and familiarity.

    vii) Develop outreach projects to access the trans population, such as mobile van.

    viii) Work with trans-identified community-based organizations, if available.

REFERENCES

Boggs, W. (2007). HIV incidence among needle-exchange users explained by risk profiles. *Reuters Health Information.* Retrieved March 30, 2009, from http://www.modernhealthinc.com/cd_3884.aspx

Callen-Lorde Transgender Team (CLCHC). (2002). *Protocols for the provision of hormone therapy.* Michael Callen-Audre Lorde Community Health Center, New York.

Edwards, J., Fisher, D., & Reynolds, G. (2007). Male-to-female transgender and transsexual clients of HIV service programs in Los Angeles County, California. *American Journal of Public Health, 97*(6), 1030–1033.

Freedberg, P. (2006). Health care barriers and same-sex intimate partner violence: A review of the literature. *Journal of Forensic Nursing, 2*(1), 15–24, 41.

Jaworsky, D., Antoniou, T., & Loutfy, M. (2007). Considerations regarding antiretroviral therapy in HIV-positive women. *Future HIV Therapy, 1*(2), 203–213.

Kenagy, G. P. (2002). HIV among transgender people. *AIDS Care, 14*(1), 127–134.

Leon, W. (2002). *HIV and transgender persons.* Lecture presented at Hunter School of Nursing, New York.

Melendez, R., Exner, T., Ehrhadt, A., Reimen, R., Rotheram-Borus, M., Lightfoot, M., et al. (2006). Health and health care among male-to-female transgender persons who are HIV-positive. *American Journal of Public Health, 96*(6), 1034–1037.

Millet, G., Flores, S., Peterson, J., & Bakeman, R. (2007). Explaining disparities in HIV infection among black and White men who have sex with men: A meta-analysis of HIV risk behaviors. *AIDS, 21*(15), 2083–2091.

Nemoto, T., Operario, D., Keatly, J., Han, L., & Soma, T. (2004). HIV risk behaviors among male-to-female transgender persons of color in San Francisco. *American Journal of Public Health, 94*(7), 1193–1199.

Tom Waddell Transgender Team (TWHC). (2006). *Protocols for hormonal reassignment of gender.* Tom Waddell Health Center, San Francisco.

The World Professional Association for Transgender Health, Inc. (WPATH), formerly Harry Benjamin International Gender Dysphoria Association (HBIGDA). (2001). *Standards of care for gender identity disorders, sixth version.* Retrieved February 4, 2008, from http://wpath.org/Documents2/socv6.pdf

6.19 WOMEN

1. Description of the community
   a. The percentage of female AIDS cases has risen from 7% in 1985 to 27% in 2006 (CDC 2008a).
   b. As of 2004, AIDS was the fifth leading cause of death among all U.S. women aged 35 to 44 years (decreasing from the third leading cause of death, reflecting the HAART era) and the leading cause of death for Black women (including African American women) aged 25–34 years. The only diseases causing more deaths among women were cancer and heart disease (CDC, 1999, 2000, 2008a).
   c. Annual cases of new HIV infections among women have declined from approximately 12,000 in 2001 to 9,700 in 2005 (CDC, 2008a). However, between 1999 and 2003, the annual number of estimated AIDS cases increased 15% among women but only 1% among men (NWHRC, 2006).
   d. In 1993, the Centers for Disease Control and Prevention (CDC) expanded its AIDS surveillance case definition for adolescents and adults. The expanded definition included invasive cervical carcinoma, thus increasing sensitivity in identifying HIV disease manifestations in women.
   e. Poor women of color disproportionately account for 79% of AIDS cases, and Hispanic women account for 21% (AIDSAction, 2002). In 2006, the HIV diagnosis rate for Black females (56.2 per 100,000) was more than 19 times the rate for White females (2.9 per 100,000). The rate for Hispanic women was 15.1, more than 5 times that for White females (CDC, 2008a).
   f. There is significant geographic variability in the prevalence of AIDS in women. Most of the women with CDC-defined AIDS live in large cities on the U.S. coasts, principally in the Northeast. The number of women with AIDS in rural areas and smaller communities continues to grow, particularly in the Southeast.
2. Common health issues
   a. Most opportunistic infections (OIs) are seen equally in men and women, with the exception of Kaposi's sarcoma, which occurs in only 2% of women.
   b. There is a greater incidence of *Candida* esophagitis among women.
   c. Vaginal candidiasis is more persistent than in uninfected women, especially as the CD4 cell counts drop.

d. Cervical dysplasia is the most prominent and problematic OI.

e. Sexually transmitted diseases (STDs) and pelvic inflammatory disease (PID) are more severe and difficult to treat than in uninfected women.

f. Women not on antiretroviral therapy (ART) were twice more likely than women on ART to have anemia (Levine et al., 2001). Although anemia is a common condition for HIV-infected women, it often goes unrecognized and untreated. If left untreated, anemia is strongly associated with HIV disease progression and an increased risk of death (Margolese, 2004).

g. Impact of HIV on hormonal levels (Cu-Uvin et al., 2000; Greenblatt, Ameli, Grant, Bacchetti, & Taylor, 2000)

   i)   Normal levels of progesterone and estradiol

   ii) Luteinizing hormone (LH) may increase CD4 cells.

   iii) Follicle-stimulating hormone (FSH) may decrease CD4 cells while increasing CD8 cells.

   iv) Interactions within the hypothalamic-pituitary-ovarian axis (HPO) can be altered or suppressed by OIs, HIV medications, and opiates (prescription and illicit drugs), including methadone. In HIV-infected women, there is a three-fold increased risk for amenorrhea, especially with lower CD4 counts, serum albumin less than 3, or current use of amphetamine or heroine (Levine et al., 2001). Lower CD4 counts appear to contribute to anovulation in 48% of HIV-infected women (Clark et al., 2001).

   v)   Generally, intermenstrual bleeding occurs more commonly in AIDS than in HIV disease, although when hepatitis C and cervical dysplasia are concomitant, it can occur in both stages (Cohen et al., 1996; Ellerbrock et al., 1996; Levine et al., 2001, NIAID, 2006).

   vi) Infected women on average enter menopause at age 47, whereas the average age of onset for uninfected women is 51 (Clark et al., 2001). Hot flashes occurred twice as frequently in women with CD4 counts greater than 500 (54%) as in women with CD4 counts less than 200 (Clark et al., 2000).

3. HIV/AIDS and women

   a. Transmission, risk behaviors, and prevention issues

      i)   The incidence of woman-to-woman transmission of HIV is low (less than 0.04% contact from oral–vaginal, oral–anal, and digital penetration); larger studies of lesbians with HIV have found that other risk factors (e.g., injecting drug use, sex with men, transfusions) could not be ruled out as the mode of disease acquisition (Anderson, 2001; CDC, 2006).

      ii) By 1995, heterosexual transmission surpassed injecting drug use (IDU) transmission as the leading mode of HIV acquisition in women diagnosed with AIDS in the United States and is now the predominant mode of transmission worldwide. Women who have IDU partners are at increased risk for HIV transmission.

      iii) Power imbalances (economic, gender, cultural) make it difficult for women to negotiate safe sexual relationships (CDC, 2008b; Gollub, 1999; UNAIDS, 2006; Wyatt et al., 2002).

      iv) Drug dependence may increase women's exposure to unsafe situations (e.g., needle use, sex, multiple partners, exchanging sex for money) and decrease the ability to negotiate safe ones.

v) Domestic violence rates among HIV-infected women are approximately 67%, and women are less likely than men to disclose HIV status in these relationships (Browne, Miller, & Maguin, 1999; Cohen et al., 2000; El-Bassel, Witte, Wada, Gilbert, & Wallace, 2001; Zierler et al., 2000).

vi) Heterosexual women (who may believe that monogamy means they are not at risk) may have partners with past or current hidden risks. There is a lack of a sense of vulnerability or risk for HIV, particularly for women unaware of their partner's current or past risk behaviors (Espinoza et al., 2007). Women who are reentering the sexual arena after a long hiatus may lack knowledge about the risks of acquiring HIV (Rich, 2001).

vii) Acquiring and transmitting HIV is enhanced by the following circumstances:

(1) Both circulating and prescription hormones contribute to HIV transmission. Progesterone is present in hormonal contraceptives and megestrol acetate (Megace, Crowley-Nowick, Douglas, & Moscicki, 2002; Sager et al., 2002). HIV-1 RNA shedding is lowest just prior to the LH surge, and a rapid increase occurs from the LH surge to menses (Hawes, Critchlow, Redman, Sow, & Kiviat, 2002).

(2) Transmission risk increased during menses, postpartum, and post-abortion, and following cervical biopsies.

(3) Douching disturbs the vaginal ecosystem, making transmission of HIV and other sexually transmitted infections easier.

(4) Non-oxynol 9 (N-9) use tends to create vaginal abrasions and facilitates HIV transmission (DeZoysa, 2000).

(5) Presence of STDs facilitates HIV transmission four-fold.

viii) No single prevention strategy will work with this heterogeneous group because different subgroups require discrete prevention efforts; women are at risk through IDU or sexual contact. Age, gender, and cultural considerations must be applied.

b. Access to care, treatment, and research

i) Access to treatments may be impaired by socioeconomic/lifestyle barriers, lack of transportation or child care, employment that grants no sick leave or healthcare benefits, or active drug use. Disorganized lifestyles may reduce drug users' ability to follow through with care needs; health care may be a low priority.

ii) Women with stigmatized lifestyles or who are illegal immigrants may shy away from contact with mainstream providers or may not fully disclose relevant information.

iii) Some women are dependent on unsupportive or abusive partners.

iv) Psychosocial/cultural barriers may impair access. Women may have a tendency to take care of themselves last: Caregiving responsibilities as a mother or primary care provider for other HIV-infected family members may consume all available time and energy. As many as 35% of HIV-infected women report another family member (sibling, husband, child) as also being HIV-infected (Fiore et al., 2001). Women may not understand the language or medical vocabulary of educators and providers. Health-care environments may not be sensitive to women, and some primary care provider(s) are untrained in HIV/AIDS and related issues.

v) Women are underrepresented in experimental HIV/AIDS protocols. They may be barred from participation in protocols by virtue of gender, presence of a uterus, or lack of surgical sterilization.

(1) Female AIDS Clinical Trials Group (ACTG) participants between 1987 and 1990 represented 6.7% of all participants. Nearly half were White, with different socioeconomic and demographic profiles from most HIV-infected women. Only 22.6% had a history of IDU (Levine, 1999).

(2) Women comprise approximately 17% of clinical trial participants, and the small numbers may jeopardize identifying specific gender differences in ART.

4. Specific care approaches
   a. Individual
      i) Response to ARV
         (1) ART has extended survival time—twice as long in men as in women—and may reflect initiating therapy later in their disease and poorer access to care.
         (2) Protease inhibitors can impact the menstrual cycle (Barlett & Gallant, 2001): Viracept (nelfinavir) and Norvir (ritonavir) may cause menorrhagia (i.e., prolonged and heavy menses). About 23% of women taking Crixivan (indinavir) or Invirase (saquinavir) report menstrual changes.
         (3) ART can impact hormonal contraceptives. Other contraceptive methods or medication adjustments may be necessary (Barlett & Gallant, 2001).
         (4) The following reduce the area under the curve (AUC) for estrogen: Viracept (nelfinavir, by 47%, and progesterone, 18%); Norvir (ritonavir; by 40%); Viramune (nevirapine; by 20%); Kaletra (LPV/RTV; by 42%). The following increase estrogen AUC: Crixivan (indinavir; by 24%, and progesterone, 26%) and Sustiva (efavirenz; by 37%).
         (5) Proportionately, fewer women than men receive ARV. This was reflected in 1997, when there was a 3% increase in deaths among women while other categories declined (CDC, 1999).
         (6) Gender differences in ARV metabolism may explain increased side effects, increased risk of lactic acidosis and hyperglycemia, and higher plasma concentrations of delavirdine and ritonavir as compared to men (Currier, Yetzer, Potthoff, Glassman, & Heath-Chiozzi, 1997; Currier et al., 2000; Hader, Smith, Moore, & Holmberg, 2001; Project Inform, 2001).
         (7) Fat maldistribution occurring in women both on and off ARV generally results in increased breast size and abdominal girth compared to men.
      ii) Survival rates of women with HIV
         (1) Early studies found shorter survival rates in women than in men, with HIV diagnosis at decreased CD4 counts, socioeconomic status, lack of access to treatment, and later initiation of ART being major contributors (Hader et al., 2001).
         (2) CD4 counts are generally higher in healthy women than they are in men. CD4 counts often drop faster in women but then level off similar to men; however, women tend to be diagnosed with AIDS with higher CD4 counts than men, and have higher CD4 counts at death (Anastos et al., 1999; Junghans, Ledergerber, Chan, Weber, & Egger, 1999). Higher CD4 counts may be more predictive of survival in women than low HIV RNA (viral load). Women generally have lower HIV RNA than do men, with similar CD4 counts, especially in early infection (Anastos et al., 2000; Farzadegan et al., 1998; Rompalo et al., 1999). Hormonal

variance may be a contributing factor. No changes in prophylaxis or initiation of ART are indicated at this time because the findings of studies are mixed.

   iii) Don't assume heterosexuality; ask directly about relationships and sex with both men and women to develop an appropriate plan of care (Morrow & Allsworth, 2000).

   iv) Facilitate empowerment of women to assist them in making healthy and safe choices. Assist in developing positive life skills that can alter negative appraisal related to HIV illness (Bova, 2001). This includes education about sexuality, anatomy, and physiology, as well as STDs and HIV disease. Reframing negative appraisals of illness, which are often linked to cultural health beliefs, can assist in managing symptoms and adjusting to chronic illness (Bova, 2001). Provide assistance to heal from interpersonal violence to increase self-care practices (Leenerts, 1999).

   v) The client's relationship with her provider is the most significant factor in predicting adherence to medical regimes, including ART (Carr, 2001; Roberts, 2002).

   vi) Discuss long-term planning for minor children.

b. Community

   i) Coordinate clinical care and services when possible to facilitate one-stop shopping for HIV care, gynecologic services, and HIV care for children. Arrange clinic times to allow for visits by women with school-age children. Make provisions for child care in clinic.

   ii) Have other resources that women use frequently (e.g., drug treatment, colposcopy, support groups, family planning, case management, legal services) available for immediate referral.

   iii) Discuss clinical drug trials with all women and need for contraception if of reproductive age.

   iv) Educate healthcare providers regarding the special needs of women with HIV, including research.

REFERENCES

AIDSAction. (2002). *Communities of color and HIV/AIDS.* Retrieved January 11, 2002, from www.aidsaction.org

Anastos, K., Gange, S. J., Lau, B., Weiser, B., Detels, R., Giorgi, J. V., et al. (2000). Association of race and gender with HIV-1 RNA. *Journal of Acquired Immune Deficiency Syndrome, 24*(3), 218–226.

Anastos, K., Kalish, L. A., Hessol, N., Weiser, B., Melnick, S., Burns, D., et al. (1999). The relative value of CD4 cell count and qualitative HIV-1 RNA in predicting survival in HIV-1-infected women: Results of the women's interagency HIV study. *AIDS, 13*(13), 1717–1726.

Anderson, J. R. (Ed.). (2001). *A guide to the clinical care of women with HIV.* Rockville, MD: U.S. Department of Health and Human Services, Health Resources and Services Administration.

Barlett, J. G., & Gallant, J. E. (2001). *2001–2002 medical management of HIV infection.* Baltimore: Johns Hopkins University Press.

Bova, C. (2001). Adjustment to chronic illness among HIV-infected women. *Journal of Nursing Scholarship, 33*(3), 217–223.

Browne, A., Miller, B., & Maguin, E. (1999). Prevalence and severity of lifetime physical and sexual victimization among incarcerated women. *International Journal of Law and Psychiatry, 22*(3–4), 301–322.

Carr, G. S. (2001). Negotiating trust: A grounded theory study of interpersonal relationships between persons living with HIV/AIDS and their primary health care providers. *Journal of the Association of Nurses in AIDS Care, 12*(2), 35–43.

Centers for Disease Control and Prevention (CDC). (1999). *HIV/AIDS surveillance report* (Vol. 11). Atlanta, GA: U.S. Department of Health and Human Services, Public Health Service.

Centers for Disease Control and Prevention (CDC). (2000). *HIV/AIDS surveillance report.* Atlanta, GA: U.S. Department of Health and Human Services, Public Health Service.

Centers for Disease Control and Prevention (CDC). (2006, June). *HIV/AIDS among women who have sex with women.* CDC HIV/AIDS Facts Sheet. Retrieved March 30, 2009, from http://www.cdc.gov/hiv/topics/women/resources/factsheets/pdf/wsw.pdf

Centers for Disease Control and Prevention (CDC). (2008a, May). *Estimated number and proportion of AIDS cases among female adults and adolescents 1985–2006—United States and dependent areas.* Retrieved March 30, 2009, from http://www.cdc.gov/hiv/topics/surveillance/resources/slides/women/slides/Women.pdf

Centers for Disease Control and Prevention (CDC). (2008b, August). *HIV and AIDS in the United States: A picture of today's epidemic.* Retrieved March 30, 2009, from http://www.cdc.gov/hiv/topics/surveillance/united_states.htm

Clark, R. A., Cohn, S. E., Jarek, C., Craven, K. S., Lyons, C., Jacobson, M., et al. (2000). Perimenopausal symptomatology among HIV-infected women at least 40 years of age. *Journal of Acquired Immune Deficiency Syndrome, 23*(1), 99–100.

Clark, R. A., Mulligan, K., Stamenovic, E., Chang, B., Watts, J. A., Squires, K., et al. (2001). Frequency of anovulation and early menopause among women enrolled in selected adult AIDS clinical trials group studies. *Journal of Infectious Diseases, 184*(10), 1325–1327.

Cohen, M., Deamant, C., Barkan, S., Richardson, M., Young, M., Holman, S., et al. (2000). Domestic violence and childhood sexual abuse in HIV-infected women and women at risk for HIV. *American Journal of Public Health, 90*(4), 560–565.

Cohen, M. H., Greenblatt, R., Minkoff, H., Barkan, S. E., Burns, D., Denenberg, R., et al. (1996, July). *Menstrual abnormalities in women with HIV infection.* Paper presented at the Eleventh International Conference on AIDS, Vancouver, British Columbia.

Crowley-Nowick, P., Douglas, D., & Moscicki, A. B. (2002, July). *Hormonal contraceptive use and IL-12 concentration in cervical secretions are associated risks for high grade squamous intra-epithelial lesion.* Paper presented at the Fourteenth International AIDS Conference, Barcelona, Spain.

Currier, J. S., Spino, C., Grimes, J., Wofsky, C. B., Katzenstein, D., Hughes, M., et al. (2000). Differences between women and men in adverse events and CD4+ responses to nucleoside analogue therapy for HIV infection. *Journal of Acquired Immune Deficiency Syndromes, 24*(4), 316–324.

Currier, J. S., Yetzer, E., Potthoff, A., Glassman, H., & Heath-Chiozzi, M. (1997, May). *Gender differences in adverse events on ritonavir: An analysis from the Abbott 247 study.* Paper presented at the First National Conference on Women and HIV, Pasadena, CA.

Cu-Uvin, S., Wright, D. J., Anderson, D., Kovacs, A., Watts, D., Cohn, J., et al. (2000). Hormonal levels among HIV-1 seropositive women compared with high-risk HIV-seronegative women during the menstrual cycle. *Journal of Women's Health and Gender Based Medicine, 9*(8), 857–863.

DeZoysa, I. (2000, July). *Non-oxynol 9 (M-9) significantly increases heterosexual transmission to women.* Paper presented at the Thirteenth International AIDS Conference, Durban, South Africa.

El-Bassel, N., Witte, S. S., Wada, T., Gilbert, L., & Wallace, J. (2001). Correlates of partner violence among female street-based sex workers: Substance abuse, history of child abuse, and HIV risks. *AIDS Patient Care and STDs, 15*(1), 41–51.

Ellerbrock, T. V., Wright, T. C., Bush, T. J., Dole, P., Brudney, K., & Chiasson, M. A. (1996). Characteristics of menstruation in women infected with human immunodeficiency virus. *Obstetrics and Gynecology, 87*(8), 1030–1034.

Espinoza, L., Hall, H. I., Hardnett, F., Selik, R. M., Ling, Q., & Lee, L. M. (2007). Characteristics of persons with heterosexually acquired HIV infection, United States 1999–2004. *American Journal of Public Health, 97*(1), 144–149.

Farzadegan, H., Hoover, D. R., Astemborski, J., Lyles, C. M., Margolick, J. B., Markham, R. B., et al. (1998). Sex differences in HIV-1 viral load and progression to AIDS. *Lancet, 352*(9139), 1510–1514.

Fiore, T., Flanigan, T., Hogan, J., Cram, R., Schuman, P., Schoenbaum, E., et al. (2001). HIV infection in families of HIV-positive and at-risk HIV-negative women. *AIDS Care, 13*(2), 209–214.

Gollub, E. B. (1999). Human rights is a U.S. problem, too: The case of women and HIV. *American Journal of Public Health, 89*(10), 1476–1485.

Greenblatt, R, M., Ameli, N., Grant, R. M., Bacchetti, P., & Taylor, R. N. (2000). Impact of the ovulatory cycle on virologic and immunologic markers in HIV-infected women. *The Journal of Infectious Diseases, 181*(1), 82–90.

Hader, S. L., Smith, D. K., Moore, J. S., & Holmberg, S. D. (2001). HIV infection in women in the United States: Status at the millennium. *Journal of the American Medical Association, 285*(9), 1186–1192.

Hawes, S., Critchlow, C. W., Redman, M., Sow, P., & Kiviat, N. (2002, February). *A longitudinal study of the detection of human immunodeficiency virus (HIV) type-1 and type-2 RNA in vaginal secretions among Senegalese women.* Paper presented at the Ninth Conference on Retroviruses and Opportunistic Infections. Seattle, WA.

Junghans, C., Ledergerber, B., Chan, P., Weber, R., & Egger, M. (1999). Sex differences in HIV-1 viral load and progression to AIDS. *Lancet, 353*(9152), 590–591.

Leenerts, M. H. (1999). The disconnected self: Consequences of abuse in a cohort of low-income white women living with HIV/AIDS. *Health Care for Women International, 20*(4), 381–400.

Levine, A. (1999). HIV disease in women. *HIV Clinical Management, 9,* 8–11.

Levine, A. M., Berhane, K., Masri-Lavine, L., Sanchez, M., Young, M., Augenbraun, M., et al. (2001). Prevalence and correlates of anemia in a large cohort of HIV-infected women: Women's interagency HIV study. *Journal of Acquired Immune Deficiency Syndromes, 26*(1), 28–35.

Margolese, S. (2004). *Women and anemia.* Retrieved August 16, 2008, from http://www.thewellproject.org

Morrow, K. M., & Allsworth, J. E. (2000). Sexual risk in lesbians and bisexual women. *Journal of the Gay and Lesbian Medical Association, 4*(4), 159–165.

National Institute of Allergy and Infectious Diseases (NIAID). (2006, May). *HIV infection in women.* Retrieved March 30, 2009, from http://www3.niaid.nih.gov/topics/HIVAIDS/Understanding/Population+Specific+Information/womenHiv.htm

The National Women's Health Resource Center (NWHRC). (2006). *Health topic: HIV/AIDS.* Retrieved March 30, 2009, from http://www.healthywomen.org/healthtopics/hivaids

Project Inform. (2001, March). Women & pharmacology. *PI Perspective.* Retrieved March 30, 2009, from http://www.projectinform.org/info/pip/32/09.shtml

Rich, E. R. (2001). Negotiation of HIV preventive behaviors in divorced and separated women reentering the sexual arena. *Journal of the Association of Nurses in AIDS Care, 12*(4), 25–35.

Roberts, K. J. (2002). Physician-patient relationships, patient satisfaction, and antiretroviral medication adherence among HIV-infected adults attending a public health clinic. *AIDS Patient Care and STDs, 16*(1), 43–50.

Rompalo, A. M., Astemborski, J., Schoenbaum, E., Schuman, P., Carpenter, C., Holmberg, S. D., et al. (1999). Comparison of clinical manifestations of HIV infection among women by risk group, CD4+ cell count, and HIV-1 plasma viral load. *Journal of Acquired Immune Deficiency Syndrome and Human Retrovirology, 20*(5), 448–454.

Sager, R., Lavreys, L., Baeten, J., Richardson, B., Mandaliya, K., Kreiss, J., et al. (2002, February). *Correlates of viral diversity in primary HIV-1 infection in women.* Paper presented at the Ninth Conference on Retroviruses and Opportunistic Infections, Seattle, WA.

UNAIDS, The Global Coalition on Women and AIDS. (2006). *Increase women's control over HIV prevention: Fight AIDS, 4.* Retrieved August 16, 2008, from http://data.unaids.org/pub/BriefingNote/2006/20060530_FS_Women%27s%20HIV%20Prevention%20Control_en.pdf

Wyatt, G. E., Myers, H. F., Williams, J. K., Kitchen, C. R., Loeb, T., Carmona, J. V., et al. (2002). Does a history of trauma contribute to HIV risk for women of color? Implications for prevention and policy. *American Journal of Public Health, 92*(4), 660–665.

Zierler, S., Cunningham, W. E., Andersen, R., Shapiro, M. F., Nakazono, T., Morton, S., et al. (2000). Violence victimization after HIV infection in U.S. sample of adult patients in primary care. *American Journal of Public Health, 90*(2), 208–215.

6.20 INDIVIDUALS WITH INTELLECTUAL AND DEVELOPMENTAL DISABILITIES (I/DD)

1. Description of community
   a. Intellectual and developmental disability (I/DD) is a current term for what is also called mental retardation, a term no longer accepted internationally (Prabhala, 2007).

b. I/DD is defined as significant limitations in both intellectual functioning (generally an IQ below 70) and in adaptive behavior as expressed in conceptual, social, and practical adaptive skills. The disability originates before the age of 18.

c. The *DSM–IV–TR* classifies four different degrees of I/DD: mild, moderate, severe, and profound. Mild I/DD generally involves an IQ of 55–70, and moderate I/DD involves an IQ 35–54 (APA, 2000).

d. Approximately 7.6 per 1,000 individuals age 6–64 in the United States have I/DD (CDC, 1996). Mild I/DD is about 3 times as common as other levels of I/DD (CDC, 2004).

e. I/DD is caused by conditions that impair brain development before or during birth or during childhood.

f. Major causes are Down syndrome, fetal alcohol syndrome, and Fragile X syndrome. Only in about 25% of cases are the causes known. Among the many other causes are maternal infections, childhood infections and accidents, lead poisoning, exposure to toxins, and other genetic syndromes such as Williams syndrome, Prader-Willi syndrome, and Rett syndrome (Rauch, 2005).

2. HIV infection can cause I/DD

a. HIV-induced encephalopathy can cause I/DD and is the direct effect of the virus on the brain or neuromuscular system; it is not the result of an opportunistic infection (Gonzalez-Scarano & Martin-Garcia, 2005).

b. HIV encephalopathy involves various cytokines, chemokines, and neurotransmitters that promote ongoing inflammation, excitation, and overstimulation; this subsequently leads to neuronal injury and death secondary to apoptosis, astrocytosis, and dendritic and synaptic damage.

c. HIV encephalopathy among perinatally infected children in the United States was initially defined by a classic triad of findings that included the following:

  i) Developmental delay

  ii) Secondary or acquired microcephaly

  iii) Pyramidal tract neuromotor deficits

d. The most severe HIV encephalopathy cases are highly correlated with young children who developed rapidly progressive disease together with profound immunosuppression and *Pneumocystis jiroveci* pneumonitis (Mitchell, 2006).

3. Common health issues

a. Seizure disorders

b. Mental health and behavioral disorders

c. Sensory impairments

d. Health problems often associated with specific syndromes

  i) With Down syndrome, individuals have increased risk of hypothyroidism, heart problems, atlantoaxil subluxation, early-onset Alzheimer's disease, and leukemia.

  ii) With Williams syndrome there is increased risk for heart and blood vessel problems, hypercalcemia, kidney problems, and dental problems.

  iii) With Prader-Willi, individuals have increased risk of obsessions with food, morbid obesity, diabetes, and heart disease.

4. HIV/AIDS in individuals with I/DD

    a. Demographics of HIV-infected I/DD individuals is severely limited.

       i) One New York City study of HIV-infected adults with I/DD found the following correlations:

- More likely to be female
- More likely to be African American
- More likely to have acquired infection via injection drug use

       ii) Approximately 1.4% ($N = 119$) of adult HIV-infected Medicaid recipients in New Jersey were reported to have I/DD (Walkup, Sambamoorthi, & Crystal, 1999).

    b. Transmission, risk behaviors, and prevention issues include the following:

       i) Limited knowledge, misinformation, lack of basic social skills, poor judgment, and low self-esteem are common and increase vulnerability to HIV infection (Birch & Marti, 1995).

       ii) May lack control and choice in sexual relations including what to do, when, and with whom (McCarthy, 1999)

       iii) May have poor understanding of consent and the difference between consenting and nonconsenting partners (McCarthy, 1999)

       iv) High risk of sexual abuse (McCarthy & Thompson, 1997), which may be related to culture of obedience, different caretakers, need for personal care, lack of sexual knowledge, and lack of knowledge of normal social and sexual limits (Aylott, 1999)

    c. Barriers to prevention programs

       i) Hesitance on part of caregivers to address sexuality of this population

       ii) May have had limited or no sexual education

       iii) Limited cognitive abilities

5. Access to care, treatment, and research

    a. Providers often feel uncomfortable or unsure how to provide care to this population. Few professional healthcare programs provide specific experience.

    b. Individuals with I/DD often have advanced disease (with any condition) before it is diagnosed.

    c. Individuals with I/DD are often specifically excluded from research.

6. Specific care approaches

    a. Communication: Know the best way to communicate with the client. If the client is nonverbal, ask the caregiver/escort the best way to communicate.

    b. Talk to the client and caregiver (if available). Even if the client is nonverbal, make sure to address the client.

    c. Keep language simple.

7. Special considerations

    a. Guardianship: Individuals with I/DD often have legal guardians. However, do not assume that someone accompanying the person to a health visit is the guardian and can give consent.

    b. Participation in care: Research shows that most individuals with mild I/DD and approximately half with moderate I/DD could participate in choices for elective health treatment (Cea & Fisher, 2003). Even if the client has a guardian, encourage participation in care to the extent possible.

    c. End-of-life care: Individuals with mild or moderate I/DD are able to participate in choices related to end-of-life care (Tuffrey-Wijne, Bernal, Butler, Hollins, & Curfs, 2007).

d. Caregivers: may be elderly, may be a parent, sibling, other relative, or may be staff at a residential agency.

e. Living situation: May live with family or in residential agencies. In 2005, over 400,000 lived in residential placement, a 30% increase over the previous decade (Lakin, Prouty, & Coucouvanis, 2006).

   i) If living with family, caregivers may be elderly parent(s).

   ii) If living with a residential agency, high staff turnover is a chronic problem.

f. Insurance: If insured, are likely to have Medicaid and Medicare.

g. Medications: May need assistance with complicated medication regimes.

   i) Family caregivers may be elderly.

   ii) If in residential care, medications are supervised. Depending on the setting, medication supervision may be provided by unlicensed staff.

h. Disease transmission: Depending on cognitive level, personal hygiene issues, and tendencies to behaviors such as self-injurious behaviors and biting, there may be legitimate concerns about risk of transmission to others.

i. Incarceration: A small percentage of individuals with I/DD are incarcerated; individuals with I/DD may make up a disproportionate percentage of the prison population (Human Rights Watch, 2001).

REFERENCES

American Psychiatric Association (APA). (2000). *Diagnostic and statistical manual of mental disorders* (4th ed., text rev.). Washington, DC: Author.

Aylott, J. (1999). Preventing rape and sexual assault of people with learning disabilities. *British Journal of Nursing, 8*(13), 871–876.

Birch, D. A., & Marti, R. (1995). *HIV/AIDS education for students with special needs: A guide for teachers.* Reston, VA: Association for the Advancement of Health Education.

Cea, C. D., & Fisher, C. B. (2003). Health care decision-making by adults with mental retardation. *Mental Retardation, 41*(2), 78–87.

Centers for Disease Control and Prevention (CDC). (1996). State-specific rates of mental retardation—United States, 1993. *Morbidity and Mortality Weekly Report, 45*(3), 61–65. Retrieved March 30, 2009, from http://www.cdc.gov/mmwr/preview/mmwrhtml/00040023.htm

Centers for Disease Control and Prevention (CDC). (2004). *Intellectual disability/Mental retardation.* Retrieved March 30, 2009, from http://www.cdc.gov/ncbddd/dd/ddmr.htm

Gonzalez-Scarano, F., & Martin-Garcia, J. (2005). The neuropathogenesis of AIDS. *Nature Reviews, Immunology, 5*(1), 69–81.

Human Rights Watch. (2001). Beyond reason: The death penalty and offenders with mental retardation. *Human Rights Watch Reports, 13*(1). Retrieved March 30, 2009, from http://www.hrw.org/reports/2001/ustat/index.htm#TopOfPage

Lakin, K. C., Prouty, R., & Coucouvanis, K. (2006). Changing patterns in size of residential settings for persons with intellectual and developmental disability, 1977–2005. *Mental Retardation, 44*(4), 306–309.

McCarthy, M. (1999). *Sexuality and women with learning disabilities.* London: Jessica Kingsley.

McCarthy, M., & Thompson, D. (1997). A prevalence study of sexual abuse of adults with intellectual disabilities referred for sex education. *Journal of Applied Research in Intellectual Disabilities, 10*(2), 105–124.

Mitchell, C. D. (2006). HIV-1 encephalopathy among perinatally infected children: Neuropathogenesis and response to highly active retroviral therapy. *Mental Retardation and Developmental Disabilities Research Reviews, 12*(3), 216–222.

Prabhala, A. (2007). Mental retardation is no more—new name is intellectual and developmental disabilities. Retrieved March 30, 2009, from http://www.sath.org/index.php?id=10130&sec=741

Rauch, D. (2005). Mental retardation. *Medline Plus.* Retrieved March 30, 2009, from http://www.nlm.nih.gov/medlineplus/ency/article/001523.htm

Tuffrey-Wijne, I., Bernal, J., Butler, G., Hollins, S., & Curfs, L. (2007). Research methodology: Using nominal group technique to investigate the views of people with intellectual disabilities on end-of-life care provision. *Journal of Advanced Nursing, 58*(1), 80–89.

Walkup, J., Sambamoorthi, U., & Crystal, S. (1999). Characteristics of persons with mental retardation and HIV/AIDS infection in a statewide Medicaid population. *American Journal on Mental Retardation, 104*(4), 356–363.

6.21 LATINOS

1. Definition of community
   a. *Latino(a)* is a term used to describe an individual who is of Latin American or Spanish-speaking origin, regardless of race, who resides in the United States. This term is often used interchangeably with *Hispanic*, a demographic term coined by the U.S. government in the 1970s.
   b. In 2006, it was estimated that Latinos comprise 14.8% of the U.S. population (U.S. Census Bureau, 2007). Not included in this estimate are the undocumented immigrants, the vast majority of whom are Latino.
   c. Latinos have been a significant part of what is now the United States since the settling of the western hemisphere by the Europeans. Major portions of the some of the most populous states (California, Texas, and Florida) were originally settled by the Spanish and were a part of New Spain.
      i) Latinos are ethnically, culturally, and racially mixed. The dominant language comes from Spain, but many indigenous languages are still spoken. The Latin American countries have been host to the Europeans, Africans, Middle Easterners, and Asians as well as the indigenous peoples (Aztecs, Incans, Mayans, and Taínos).
   d. Latinos have varying levels of acculturation. Some with Spanish surnames have descended from people who have lived in the United States for generations. Some Latinos do not speak Spanish as their first language or even at all. Some are recent immigrants struggling with their children's moving away from their culture. Some frequently travel between their countries of origin and their homes in the United States (Elder et al., 2005).
   e. For those Latinos who exclusively speak Spanish, their job opportunities are often limited to positions in the service sector that may not offer benefits, such as health or disability insurance, or withhold taxes, which could affect eligibility for federal benefits (Medicare).
   f. Some Latinos are migrant/seasonal farmworkers and day laborers. If their families still reside in the country of origin, the workers often send significant portions of their salaries to them (Hovey et al., 2007).
   g. Most Latinos practice religions based in Christianity (Roman Catholicism, Protestantism, and Santeria, a fusion of the Yoruba and Catholic religions). Latinos also practice indigenous religions, Judaism, Eastern religions, and so forth.
   h. Two cultural concepts observed by some Latinos are *marianisma* and *machismo* (Moreno, 2007).
      i) Marianisma emphasizes the respect that women in the family are due as the physical representative of the Virgin Mary. Mothers, wives, sisters, daughters, nieces, and granddaughters are treated respectfully.

     ii) Machismo emphasizes the responsibility of the male figure to provide for his family and the respect due to him. Fathers, husbands, brothers, sons, nephews, and grandsons are deferred to in all things regarding the family.

     iii) The dichotomy of these concepts impacts the lives of Latinos because women in the family are expected to be virginal and maternal and a woman outside of the family is to fulfill sexual desires. The activities of men outside of the home are expected to be tolerated. Being the dominant figure in the home, the man is permitted to emphasize his masculinity by having extramarital affairs and even becoming physically violent with those who challenge him (Moreno, 2007).

     iv) Homosexuality is not accepted in the dichotomy of marianisma and machismo, because it goes against the accepted gender roles. Gays, lesbians, bisexuals, and transgenders raised with these cultural concepts are forced to hide their true selves or leave their families.

     v) Within machismo, a man is permitted to have insertive anal sex and still preserve his masculinity; receptive anal sex is not compatible with the macho identity. *Maricón* is a derogatory term used to describe the person who engages in receptive anal sex.

     vi) Latinos have issues with envy (*envidia*), and shame (*vergüenza*), and consequently there may be problems with connecting with others outside of and within the accepted social circles (Bathum & Baumann, 2007).

2. Common health issues

  a. Latinos are at greater risk for some health conditions, such as diabetes. Also to be considered is the racial makeup of the individual, which would also indicate certain health risks (e.g., black Latinos may have sickle cell anemia or carry the sickle cell trait).

  b. Latinos in the United States have dietary concerns related to the availability of traditional foods. Latinos in their countries of origin have a more diverse and balanced diet than Latinos in the United States.

  c. Some Latinos work in extreme conditions (long hours, outdoors in inclement weather, etc.)

  d. Degree of acculturation has been noted to have an impact on the health of Latinos. As they become more acculturated, they adopt more of the health habits of the United States. They are more likely to consume a high-fat, high-calorie, high-carbohydrate diet. They are more likely to engage in behaviors that increase their risk of HIV infection. Latinas are more likely to develop depression (Elder et al., 2005; Loue et al., 2004).

  e. Language, culture, health insurance (none or limited), and health literacy issues can impact Latinos' access to care.

  f. To manage their health issues, Latinos may prefer to consult *curanderos* (traditional healers) for herbal remedies or *santeros* (spiritualists) for spiritual advice. The concepts of balance, hot and cold foods, and the power of the intentions of others heavily influence Latino health beliefs (Spector, 2004).

3. HIV/AIDS risk

  a. In 2005 the number of new AIDS cases in the Latino community was 7,676, whereas the cumulative number of AIDS cases was 155,179 (CDC, 2007). The incidence of AIDS among Latinos was 18.0 per 100,000 people, which is 3 times the rate for Whites (CDC, 2007; Espinoza et al., 2007). The number of Latinos living with AIDS was 78,064. This represents 18.9% of the total AIDS cases (421,873; CDC, 2007), even though in 2006 Latinos accounted for only 14.8% of the total U.S. population (U.S. Census Bureau, 2007).

   b. The main risk factors for HIV transmission for Latinos are unprotected sexual intercourse (both MSM and heterosexual) and sharing injecting equipment (illegal drugs, vitamins, and medications). Different nationalities have varying distributions of risk (Espinoza et al., 2007).

   c. Frequent travel by some Latinos to and from their countries of origin have created "air bridges" for the virus.

4. Specific approaches to care

   a. Individual

      i)   The provider should perform a cultural assessment to ascertain the acculturation level and health beliefs of the individual (Elder et al., 2005; Loue et al., 2004).

      ii) The provider should sensitively ascertain the HIV risk behavior(s) of the client and provide information regarding risk reduction.

      iii) Care should be provided in a nonjudgmental and confidential manner to respect concerns of *envidia* and *vergüenza*.

      iv) The provider should incorporate the client's traditional healing practices into the plan of care (Spector, 2004).

      v)   The provider should be aware of the immigration and insurance status of the client.

   b. Community

      i)   Programs should be culturally sensitive, taking into account that there are issues with racism and classism within the Latino community (Bathum & Baumann, 2007).

      ii) The various dialects in Spanish and the health literacy of the target group should be considered during the planning process.

      iii) The use of peer educators can help to deliver subtle contextual messages.

      iv) Planners should be aware of the fear of deportation among members of the target group.

REFERENCES

Bathum, M. E., & Baumann, L. C. (2007). A sense of community among immigrant Latinas. *Family and Community Health, 30*(3), 167–177.

Centers for Disease Control and Prevention (CDC). (2007). *HIV/AIDS surveillance report: HIV infection and AIDS in the U.S. and dependent areas: 2005.* Washington, DC: Author. Retrieved February 5, 2008, from http://www.cdc.gov/hiv/topics/surveillance/basic.htm#aidsrace

Elder, J. P., Broyles, S. L., Brennan, J. J., Zúñiga de Nuncio, M. L., & Nader, P. R. (2005). Acculturation, parent-child acculturation differential, and chronic disease risk factors in a Mexican-American population. *Journal of Immigrant Health, 7*(1), 1–9.

Espinoza, L., Dominguez, K. L., Remaguera, R. A., Hu, X., Valleroy, L. A., & Hall, H. L. (2007, October 12). HIV/AIDS among Hispanics—United States, 2001–2005. *Morbidity and Mortality Weekly Report, 56*(40), 1052–1057.

Hovey, J. D., Booker, V., & Seligman, J. D. (2007). Using theatrical presentations as a means of disseminating knowledge of HIV/AIDS risk factors to migrant farm workers: An evaluation of the effectiveness of the Infórmate program. *Journal of Immigrant Health, 9*(2), 147–156.

Loue, S., Cooper, M., Traore, F., & Fielder, J. (2004). Locus of control and HIV risk among a sample of Mexican and Puerto Rican women. *Journal of Immigrant Health, 6*(4), 155–165.

Moreno, C. (2007). The relationship between culture, gender, structural factors, abuse, trauma and HIV/AIDS for Latinas. *Qualitative Health Research, 17*(3), 340–352.

Spector, R. E. (2004). Health and illness in the Hispanic population. In *Cultural diversity in health and illness* (pp. 253–272). Upper Saddle River, NJ: Prentice Hall.

U.S. Census Bureau. (2007). *2006 American community survey.* Washington, DC: Author. Retrieved March 30, 2009, from http://www.factfinder.census.gov

CHAPTER 7

Clinical Management of the HIV-Infected Infant and Child

7.1 PERINATAL TRANSMISSION OF HIV INFECTION

1. Prevention of perinatal transmission
   a. Treatment with antiretroviral (ARV) medications during pregnancy, labor, and delivery, and treatment of the newborn, reduces the risk of mother-to-child, or perinatal transmission, of HIV from 25% to as low as 2% (PHSTF, 2008).
   b. Results of PACTG 076, a study of 477 pregnant women randomly assigned to receive a placebo or zidovudine (ZDV) during pregnancy and intravenously (IV) during labor and delivery (the newborns received treatment for 6 weeks), showed that treatment reduced transmission from 22.6% to 7.6% (Connor et al., 1994).
   c. In resource-poor countries, shorter course regimens with ZDV and other ARVs have been shown to reduce perinatal transmission significantly. A study in Thailand found that a short course of ZDV—oral ZDV given to a pregnant woman from 36 weeks' gestation and during labor in a non-breastfeeding population—reduced transmission from 50% to 9.4% (Shaffer et al., 1999). The PETRA study in four African breastfeeding countries found that oral ZDV/3TC given pre-, intra-, and postpartally, or intra- and postpartally only, significantly reduced perinatal transmission (Petra Study Team, 2002). The HIVNet 012 study, also in a breastfeeding population, found that a single dose of nevirapine to the mother at the onset of labor and to the newborn in the first 72 hours of life could reduce transmission to 12% compared with 21% for a short course ZDV regimen (Guay et al., 1999). The simplicity and low cost of the HIVNet 012 regimen makes it particularly applicable to low resource settings. However, NVP-resistance mutations have been detected in both mothers and infants for 1 year and longer after the single dose, which may reduce the efficacy of this regimen for subsequent pregnancies (Flys et al., 2005). A retrospective study in New York State found that intrapartal-only or postpartal-only ZDV treatment significantly reduced the risk of transmission. Transmission rates were 10% with only intrapartum ZDV and 9.8% if only the newborn was treated for 6 weeks, compared with a 26.6% transmission rate if no treatment was initiated (Wade et al., 1998).
   d. The U.S. Public Health Service Perinatal HIV Guidelines Working Group routinely updates guidelines for maternal health and for reducing perinatal transmission. Current guidelines are available at http://www.hivatis.org.
2. Breastfeeding

    a. Breastfeeding increases the risk of HIV transmission to newborns by 12% to 16% (Fowler, Simonds, & Roongpisuthipong, 2000; Mbori-Ngacha et al., 2001).

    b. Studies suggest that most transmission occurs in first few weeks and months of life (Miotti et al., 1999; Nduati et al., 2000).

    c. Mechanism of transmission is thought to be frequent and prolonged exposure of the infant's oral and gastrointestinal (GI) tract to breastmilk that is infected with HIV.

    d. Women with HIV infection in the United States and other countries where safe substitute feeding is available are urged not to breastfeed.

    e. Breastfeeding is the norm among many cultural groups in the United States, particularly among recent immigrants from developing countries. Decisions not to breastfeed may raise issues regarding confidentiality of a mother's HIV diagnosis and require sensitivity and supportive interventions (National Pediatric and Family HIV Resource Center, 2002).

3. Diagnosis and evaluation of the HIV-exposed infant

    a. All infants born to mothers with HIV infection will have transplacentally acquired HIV antibody (Nielsen & Bryson, 2000; Working Group on Antiretroviral Therapy and Medical Management of HIV-Infected Children, 2001).

    b. Maternally acquired antibody can be present for up to 18 months of age (Working Group on Antiretroviral Therapy and Medical Management of HIV-Infected Children, 2001).

    c. Diagnosis of HIV in infants should be made using virologic assays that identify the presence of the HIV antigen (Nielsen & Bryson, 2000).

    d. HIV polymerase chain reaction (PCR) has a sensitivity of 90% at 3 months and nearly 100% at 6 months of age (Nielsen & Bryson, 2000).

        i) Presumptive diagnosis of HIV infection can be made on one positive HIV PCR and definitive diagnosis with a confirmatory test on a different blood sample (Working Group on Antiretroviral Therapy and Management of Children with HIV Infection, 1998).

        ii) HIV can be reasonably excluded with two negative HIV PCR results on different samples if both are obtained after 1 month of age and the second is after 4 months of age; some clinicians also use a confirmatory negative ELISA at > 18 months of age (Working Group on Antiretroviral Therapy and Management of Children with HIV Infection, 1998).

    e. Children > 18 months of age can be diagnosed with a positive HIV ELISA and confirmatory Western blot (Working Group on Antiretroviral Therapy and Management of Children with HIV Infection, 1998).

    f. AIDS can be diagnosed based on clinical symptoms in conjunction with laboratory evidence of dysfunction of humoral and cellular immunity using the 1994 Centers for Disease Control and Prevention (CDC) Pediatric HIV Classification System (CDC, 1994).

REFERENCES

Centers for Disease Control and Prevention (CDC). (1994). Revised classification system for human immunodeficiency virus infection in children less than 13 years of age. *Morbidity and Mortality Weekly Review, 43*(RR-12), 1–10.

Connor, E., Sperling, R., Gelber, R., Kiselev, P., Scott, G., O'Sullivan, M., et al. (1994). Reduction of maternal-infant transmission of human immunodeficiency virus type 1 with zidovudine treatment. *New England Journal of Medicine, 331*(18), 1173–1180.

Flys, T., Nissley, D. V., Claasen, C. W., Jones, D., Shi, C., Guay, L. A., et al. (2005). Sensitive drug-resistance assays reveal long-term persistence of HIV-1 variants with the K103N nevirapine (NVP) resistance mutation in some women and infants after the administration of single-dose NVP: HIVNET 012. *Journal of Infectious Diseases, 192*(1), 24–29.

Fowler, M. G., Simonds, R. J., & Roongpisuthipong, A. (2000). Update on perinatal HIV transmission. *Pediatric Clinics of North America, 47*(1), 21–38.

Guay, L. A., Musoka, P., Fleming, T., Bagenda, D., Allen, M., Nakabiito, C., et al. (1999). Intrapartum and neonatal single-dose nevirapine compared with zidovudine for prevention of mother-to-child transmission of HIV-1 in Kampala, Uganda: HIVNET 012 randomized trial. *Lancet, 354*(9181), 795–802.

Mbiori-Ngacha, D., Nduti, R., John, G., Reilly, M., Richardson, B., Mwatha, A., et al. (2001). Morbidity and mortality in breastfed and formula-fed infants of HIV-1-infected women: A randomized clinical trial. *Journal of the American Medical Association, 286*(19), 2413–2420.

Miotti, P. G., Taha, T. E., Kumwenda, N. I., Broadhead, R., Mtimavalye, L., Van der Hoeven, L., et al. (1999). HIV transmission through breastfeeding: A study in Malawi. *Journal of the American Medical Association, 282*(8), 744–749.

National Pediatric and Family HIV Resource Center. (2002). *HIV and pregnancy: Managing mother and baby—A curriculum for providers.* Newark, NJ: The National Pediatric & Family HIV Resource Center.

Nduati, R. W., John, G. L., Mbori-Ngacha, D., Richardson, B., Overbaugh J., Mwatha, A., et al. (2000.) Effect of breastfeeding and formula feeding on transmission of HIV-1: A randomized clinical trial of breast feeding and formula feeding. *Journal of the American Medical Association, 283*(9), 1167–1174.

Nielsen, K., & Bryson, Y. J. (2000). Diagnosis of HIV infection in children. *Pediatric Clinics of North America, 47*(1), 39–63.

Petra Study Team. (2002). Efficacy of three short-course regimens of zidovudine and lamivudine in preventing early and late transmission of HIV-1 from mother to child in Tanzania, South Africa, and Uganda (Petra study): A randomised, double-blind, placebo-controlled trial. *Lancet, 359*(9313), 1178–1186.

Shaffer, N., Chuachoowong, R., Mock, P. A., Bhadrakom, C., Siriwasin, W., Young, N., et al. (1999). Short-course zidovudine for perinatal HIV-1 transmission in Bangkok, Thailand: A randomized controlled trial. *Lancet, 353*(9155), 773–780.

U.S. Public Health Service Task Force (PHSTF). (2008). *Recommendations for use of antiretroviral drugs in pregnant HIV-1 infected women for maternal health and interventions to reduce perinatal HIV-1 transmission in the United States.* Retrieved March 30, 2009, from http://www.aidsinfo.nih.gov/ContentFiles/PerinatalGL.pdf

Wade, N. A., Birkhead, G. S., Warren, B. L., Charbonneau T. T., French, P. T., Wang, L., et al. (1998). Abbreviated regimens of zidovudine prophylaxis and perinatal transmission of the human immunodeficiency virus. *New England Journal of Medicine, 339*(20), 1409–1414.

Working Group on Antiretroviral Therapy and Medical Management of HIV-Infected Children. (2001). *Guidelines for the use of antiretroviral agents in pediatric HIV infection.* Retrieved February 22, 2009, from http://www.aidsinfo.nih.gov/ContentFiles/pediatricGuidelines.pdf

7.2 CLINICAL MANIFESTATIONS AND MANAGEMENT OF THE HIV-INFECTED INFANT AND CHILD

1. Initial visit: The initial visit provides an opportunity to obtain a comprehensive history and physical examination. The quantity and quality of the historical information obtained may be dependent on the age of the child, as well as the relationship of the child to the guardian.
   a. Health history
      i)   Birth history: includes the maternal history, including the mother's antiretroviral history, CD4 count and viral load at the time of delivery, and any significant maternal illnesses that occurred during the pregnancy or any preexisting chronic conditions.

Intrauterine drug exposure to other prescription and nonprescription medications, as well as alcohol, tobacco, and illicit drugs, should also be included. If available, the infant's gestational age at birth; birth parameters, such as weight, length, and head circumference; and the route of delivery should be documented. Results of any neonatal screenings are also useful historical information.

ii)   Medical history: Because of their potential to result in ongoing health concerns for the child, all illnesses, including respiratory, infectious, metabolic, neurologic, renal, and cardiac problems, should be included in the medical history. For chronic illnesses, the dates of onset should be recorded, and for episodic illnesses onset and resolution dates are useful if available. Additionally, dates and reasons for hospitalizations are also significant components of the health history. Document CDC classification and route of transmission (e.g., perinatal, sexual abuse, etc.).

iii) Surgical history: All surgical procedures, whether extensive or minor, and their outcomes should be recorded during the initial health history and intake.

iv)   Medication history: A detailed medication history, including the initiation and discontinuation of all medications, is essential. Chronic and episodic medications, including those used for infections, HIV prophylaxis, nutritional supplementation, or chronic conditions such as asthma or dermatitis, along with medication allergies, are included in a thorough pediatric medication history.

v)   Childhood illnesses and immunizations: During the initial history, it is essential to obtain accurate information on diseases of childhood, such as varicella, including dates of illness and a description of the disease course. The most up-to-date record of immunizations should also be obtained to determine if a catch-up immunization schedule is needed.

vi)   Family history: If possible, a detailed family medical history should be obtained to determine the child's risk of certain inherited physical and mental conditions. HIV status of parents and siblings should be determined. Testing options should be provided if they are at risk and have not been tested.

vii) Psychosocial history: Any history of substance abuse and housing or financial issues should be elicited. A clear determination of the family constellation, members of the household, and key involved members of the extended family or community must also be identified. Any history of school or behavior problems should be identified. In addition, involvement in social service or foster home placement should be noted.

viii) Nutrition history: Serial measurements of weight and height should be documented to assess growth. Additionally, a detailed diet history and food preferences, as well as food allergy information, may inform future dietary and adherence-related interventions.

b. Review of systems
i)   General review: A thorough review of systems should be completed at each visit with a notation of the onset and course of the problem so far. Particular attention should be paid to new problems, problems associated with fever, and those that have not responded as expected to prescribed therapies. Growth parameters should be reviewed regularly. Pay special attention to abnormal growth curves for height and weight.

ii) Skin: Make note of all dermatological complaints, including rashes, skin discoloration, ulceration, itching, or bruising.

iii) Head: Problems of the scalp, including areas of hair loss, scaling, flaking, oozing, and any swellings should be noted.

iv) Eyes: Any history of visual disturbances, eye pain, discharge, floaters, or trauma should be noted.

v) Ears: Hearing disturbances, including diminished hearing or tinnitus, as well as ear pain or discharge, should be noted.

vi) Nose and sinuses: Information about the quantity and quality of any nasal discharge, as well as sinus pain or tenderness, assists in the diagnosis of infectious upper airway processes and should be noted in the review of systems.

vii) Mouth and throat: A history significant for oral problems, such as bleeding, pain, ulceration, lesions, discharge, drooling, difficult or painful swallowing, and problems with dentition and decreased oral intake seemingly related to any of these factors, may indicate serious HIV-related disease processes in infants and children.

viii) Respiratory: Characteristics and duration of respiratory symptoms, including wheezing, cough, sputum production, shortness of breath, chest pain, and exposure to others with similar symptoms, are frequently reported among infants and children with HIV infection and may be representative of common childhood illnesses or more serious underlying HIV-related illnesses.

ix) Cardiovascular: A history of pallor, cyanosis, shortness of breath, murmur, edema, or irregular heartbeat, if identified, should be documented and in some cases followed with a detailed cardiology workup.

x) Gastrointestinal: Of note in the section of the review of systems is any report of abdominal pain, bloating, or cramping. Nausea, vomiting, diarrhea, and the history that preceded the onset of the symptoms should also be noted. Frequency of symptoms, exacerbating and mitigating factors, as well as quality and quantity of stool, should also be noted. Exposure to family members or other children with similar complaints is also of significance.

xi) Genitourinary: Notable symptoms and complaints often consistent with genitourinary infection or renal problems include any history of urgency, frequency, pain on urination, lower back pain, or strong-smelling or discolored urine, including urine containing blood.

xii) Gynecologic: When age appropriate, menstrual history and onset and norms (duration, pain, clotting) should be ascertained. Pregnancy history, including live births, miscarriages, and abortions, may also be pertinent for adolescent females. Any history of vaginal discharge, pain, or lesions should also be documented.

xiii) Musculoskeletal: Muscle aches, pains and cramps, joint pain, stiffness, swellings, history of trauma, and any events and activities that precede or exacerbate symptoms should be noted.

xiv) Neurologic: Neurological changes, including alterations in level of consciousness, failure to obtain or loss of developmental milestones, or change in general neurologic function, are often hallmark signs of HIV disease progression or an infectious process. Onset and specific symptoms identified in the review of systems (e.g., ataxia, memory loss, seizure) assists with further diagnostic workup of these complaints.

   xv) Nutrition assessment: Any history of significant nutritional deficiencies, eating disorders, lead toxicity, other dietary problems, including problems with food intake, and a dietary recall are contained in this component of the review.

   xvi) Psychiatric and emotional: Significant problems uncovered in this portion of the review of systems may include symptoms of depression, acting-out behavior at home or at school, interpersonal relationships with family members and peers, school performance, and knowledge of HIV diagnosis.

c. Physical examination: In general, unless there is an extremely specific reason for the healthcare visit, infants and children with HIV infection should have a complete physical examination at each healthcare encounter. This approach assists with the monitoring of ongoing problems and allows for the early diagnosis of new health issues as they emerge.

   i) General: Growth parameters and vital signs are essential components of every examination because they are often the first indicator of significant underlying HIV and non-HIV-related problems.

   ii) Growth and development: An initial screening of growth and development is indicated for every infant and child entering HIV services. This assessment may be performed by a developmental specialist or by providers trained in the administration of tests, such as the Denver Developmental Screening Test, to establish a developmental baseline against which future assessments can be compared.

   iii) Neurological examination: Because HIV is a disease that can especially affect the neurological functioning of infants and children, a comprehensive neurological exam is warranted at the initial visit. Particular attention should be paid to cranial nerve, reflex, and developmental status to determine the extent of any current neurological problems and to provide comparison for future assessments.

   iv) Mouth and throat examination: Oral problems and oral health can have a significant impact on the growth and well-being of infants and children with HIV infection. Notable findings include lesions such as aphthous ulcers and oral thrush, dental caries, and herpetic lesions.

   v) Cardiovascular evaluation: HIV-related cardiomyopathy may present in infants and children with HIV infection; therefore, findings including cardiac murmurs and abnormalities of heart rate, rhythm, or blood pressure warrant further evaluation by a trained cardiology practitioner.

   vi) Respiratory examination: Viral and bacterial pneumonias, as well as asthma, bronchiectasis, and lymphoid interstitial pneumonitis (LIP), can be causes of diminished respiratory function in infants and children with HIV. Findings of cough, wheezing, shortness of breath, poor aeration, and crackles may be indicative of HIV-related diseases. LIP involves the diffuse lymphoid infiltration of the lung parenchyma. Inflammatory cells are recruited into the pulmonary interstitium, alveolar wall, and perialveolar tissues, producing an alveolitis. Symptoms may be absent or mild. Severe symptoms include dyspnea, fatigue, tachypnea, cough, wheezing, cyanosis, and clubbing of the digits.

vii) Abdominal examination: HIV-infected infants and children should be assessed for abdominal pain, masses, and organomegaly. These symptoms may represent advancing HIV-related illnesses.

viii) Musculoskeletal examination: Muscle tone and bulk, as well as range of motion and tenderness or swelling of joints, should be evaluated at each visit. Lipodystrophy can be the result of HIV infection and/or antiretroviral therapy. Common indicators are facial and extremity fat wasting or fat accumulation in the abdomen, breasts, or dorsum of the neck (buffalo hump).

ix) Skin examination: Infants and children with HIV infection are prone to various types of dermatological problems, including tinea, herpes zoster, eczema, staphylococcal skin infections, rashes resulting from adverse drug reactions, molluscom, papillomas, and various viral exanthems.

d. Laboratory and diagnostic evaluation: The initial visit provides the opportunity to obtain a comprehensive baseline laboratory profile, as well as determine immunologic and virologic status and history of exposure to infectious agents.

i) Immunologic profile: CD4+ T-lymphocyte counts and percentages should be obtained at baseline and compared with age-specific norms to assess the child's degree of immunocompromise and risk for opportunistic infection. Baseline measurements also allow for assessment of the effectiveness of therapeutic regimen changes.

ii) HIV RNA PCR (viral load): Obtained at baseline for comparison with subsequent values to determine the need for and the effectiveness of therapeutic antiretroviral regimens. A viral load that is not undetectable may indicate development of viral resistance and/or lack of medication adherence.

iii) Complete blood count (CBC) with differential and platelets: The CBC with differential and platelets is performed at the initial visit to screen for anemia, neutropenia, thrombocytopenia, and other hematologic abnormalities that may be HIV or treatment related.

iv) Comprehensive chemistry panel: Blood chemistries are useful in identifying pancreatic, liver, renal, cardiac, and electrolyte abnormalities in infants and children with HIV infection.

v) Urinalysis (UA): A screening UA is recommended at baseline to identify asymptomatic infection and other abnormalities, such as proteinuria or glucosuria, which may be indicative of other HIV- and non-HIV-related disease processes. Subsequently, annual UAs are recommended (Laufer & Scott, 2000). Certain antiretroviral medications may necessitate more frequent screening.

vi) Tuberculin skin test (TST): TST is recommended for children at or before age 9–12 months and yearly thereafter. Due to increased risk of the development of active tuberculosis (TB) in TB- and HIV-coinfected persons, this is an essential baseline screening test that should be repeated annually or more often if a question of exposure arises.

vii) Toxoplasmosis: Perinatally HIV-exposed infants born to women seropositive for toxoplasmosis should be evaluated for congenital toxoplasmosis. Some experts suggest baseline toxoplasmosis antibody titers for all HIV-infected children greater than 18 months of age. However, in the United States, routine screening for young children is not recommended because of low prevalence. On the other hand, HIV-infected adolescents and adults are at higher risk for acquiring toxoplasmosis disease than infants or children and should undergo serologic testing. Annual testing should be considered in persons with severe immune compromise (Subauste, 2006; USPHS/ISDA, 2002).

Persons who lack IgG antibody to toxoplasmosis should receive preventive counseling regarding high-risk behavior (e.g., washing hands well after changing litter box or having contact with soil, making sure all meat is well cooked and fruits and vegetables are washed well before ingestion).

viii) Cytomegalovirus (CMV): Perinatally HIV-exposed infants who are also exposed to CMV should be evaluated for congenital CMV. Some experts suggest baseline CMV antibody titers for all HIV-infected children older than 18 months of age. Baseline CMV titers should be obtained for all HIV-infected persons older than 18 months of age. Annual testing should be considered in those with severe immune compromise.

ix) Varicella serologic tests: Varicella titers are useful in establishing a child's potential immunity to this common childhood illness. Because varicella can have especially severe sequelae in HIV-infected children, knowledge of immune status is essential in identifying children most at risk for varicella disease. Commercial serologic tests may not be sufficiently sensitive to demonstrate a vaccine-induced antibody (i.e., it may not pick up an antibody that is actually present).

x) Syphilis screening–rapid plasma reagin (RPR) test: This test is recommended at baseline for sexually active individuals. Consideration should be given to testing infants with unknown maternal syphilis status. Sexually abused children should also be screened.

xi) Baseline lipid panel: The high incidence of elevated LDL cholesterol and triglycerides in children on certain types of antiretroviral therapy warrants a baseline assessment. Infants and children at risk should have a lipid panel repeated every 6 months or as needed.

xii) Hepatitis profile (A, B, C): Determination of a child's hepatitis exposure status, infection status, and immunity are a component of the initial diagnostic evaluation and staging of HIV infection.

(1) Hepatitis A testing should be performed for high-risk individuals upon diagnosis of HIV infection. If no history of hepatitis A is determined, the child should be vaccinated.

(2) Hepatitis B surface antigen testing should be evaluated for new patients who may have no immunity to hepatitis B and are at high risk for infection. Hepatitis B antibody status should be verified after immunization.

(3) Hepatitis C antibody testing should be performed annually for high-risk individuals (e.g., IV drug use or sexual activity).

2. Immunizations: Children who are HIV-infected should follow the immunization schedules recommended by the CDC, which can be found at http://aidsinfo.nih.gov/contentfiles/ Pediatric_OI.pdf. The following immunization considerations apply to HIV-infected children.

a. Inactivated polio vaccine (IPV) is recommended for routine childhood polio vaccination in the United States (CDC, 2008). Live attenuated viruses, such as oral polio, should not be given to persons with HIV infection or their household contacts. Although oral poliovirus vaccine (OPV) has been given to these patients without adverse effects, the live polioviruses in OPV can be excreted and transmitted to immunosuppressed contacts, creating an increased risk for paralytic poliomyelitis caused by vaccine virus infection (this is no longer a consideration in areas such as the United States in which only IPV is used).

b. Measles/mumps/rubella immunization should be given in HIV-infected children in CDC immunologic classification categories 1 and 2 and should be given as soon after the first birthday as possible. Children in CDC classification 3 should not receive this vaccine until their immune system has been restored. Cases of immunization-related disease have been reported in the severely immunocompromised patient.

c. Influenza vaccine is recommended annually for all HIV-infected children starting at age 6 months. Household contacts should be vaccinated as well.

d. Pneumococcal vaccination is recommended for all children. Children with HIV infection are at risk for invasive pneumococcal infection.

i) Heptavalent pneumococcal conjugate vaccine (PCV) is recommended for all children who are HIV-infected. If the child is older than 12 months at the first dose, refer to the CDC Catch Up Immunization Schedule. All newly diagnosed children older than age 5 should receive one dose of PCV.

ii) In addition, children 2 years and older should receive the 23 valent pneumococcal polysaccharide vaccine (PPV). A booster shot should be administered 3–5 years later. PCV should be administered 4–6 weeks prior to PPV, if possible.

e. Varicella vaccine: All HIV-infected children with CDC immunologic category 1 or 2 should be immunized according to the CDC immunization schedule. Children in CDC classification 3 should not receive this vaccine until their immune system has been restored. Cases of immunization-related disease have been reported in the severely immunocompromised patient. Children who have documented history of varicella or who are antibody positive are not required to be vaccinated.

f. Rotavirus: There are no safety or efficacy data for administration to HIV-infected infants. Use of the vaccine in this population raises potential risks and benefits. One significant risk to HIV-infected infants is rotavirus gastroenteritis, which may be prolonged and/or fatal. Many infants who are HIV-exposed will not have completed testing to rule out HIV infection before 12 weeks of age. The series should not be started after 12 weeks of age. When considering administration of rotavirus to an HIV-exposed infant, one must consider the potential for secondary exposure through feces to a family member with an impaired immune system. Most experts agree that vaccination of the infant outweighs the risk to family members. Good hand washing with diaper changes for a week after the first vaccine administration is recommended (American Academy of Pediatrics, 2006).

g. Meningococcal conjugate vaccine (MCV4): Children with HIV infection are at higher risk for invasive meningococcal disease. This vaccine should be administered to all HIV-infected children ages 2 and older (CDC, 2007).

3. Prophylaxis for opportunistic infections

a. Prophylaxis against *Pneumocystis jirovecii* pneumonia (PJP) is critical for HIV-exposed infants.

  i) PJP remains a common AIDS-defining illness in children (CDC, 2008).

  ii) All HIV-exposed infants should receive PJP prophylaxis starting at age 6 weeks and continue until HIV infection has been reasonably excluded (usually HIV DNA PCR done at 3–6 months; NIH, 2007).

  iii) Most infants present with PJP at 4–6 months of age. Risk for PJP in the 1st year of life for a perinatally infected infant not receiving prophylaxis is estimated at 12% (Abrams, 2000).

  iv) All HIV-infected infants from age 4 weeks to 12 months should receive PJP prophylaxis regardless of CD4 count. Prophylaxis should be continued past 12 months for severe immune compromise.

  v) Prophylaxis can be stopped after 8 weeks of age if virologic test is negative (CDC, 2008).

  vi) PJP prophylaxis for children older than age 1 year is based on adjusted CD4 count (USPHS/IDSA, 2002).
    (1) Ages 1–5 years: CD4 count < 500 uL or CD4 percentage < 15%
    (2) Age 6–12 years: CD4 count < 200 uL or CD4 percentage < 15%

  vii) All HIV-infected children treated for PJP should receive lifelong prophylaxis (USPHS/IDSA, 2002). No studies regarding discontinuation of secondary prophylaxis in children have been conducted. However, most experts agree that discontinuing secondary prophylaxis is safe after initiation of HAART and subsequent reconstitution of the immune system. PJP prophylaxis recommendations and regimens for infants and children can be found at http://aidsinfo.nih.gov/contentfiles/Pediatric_OI.pdf.

  viii) Trimethoprim sulfa/sulfamethoxazole (TMP/SMX) is the most common agent used for prophylaxis of PJP. Intolerance, allergic reactions, or adverse effects of TMP/SMX may necessitate the use of dapsone, atovaquone, or pentamidine for PJP prophylaxis.

b. Prophylaxis against *Mycobacterium avium* complex (MAC): HIV-infected children aged < 13 who have advanced immune suppression can experience disseminated MAC. Prophylactic treatment should be offered to persons with the following CD4 T-lymphocyte counts:

  i) Children < 12 months: < 750

  ii) Children ages 1–2 years: < 500

  iii) Children ages 2–6 years: < 75

  iv) Children ages ≥ 6 years: < 50

Azithromycin is the most common agent for prophylaxis of MAC. MAC prophylaxis recommendations can be found at http://aidsinfo.nih.gov/contentfiles/Pediatric_OI.pdf.

4. Counseling and educating the family and child

a. Every healthcare encounter represents an opportunity for ongoing disease counseling and education. The often overwhelming and complex nature of the information requires frequent assessment of the patient and family's understanding. The clinician may need to reinforce previously discussed information on an ongoing or episodic basis.

b. Comprehensive HIV education, including relaying information about modes of transmission, the effect of HIV on the immune system and other body systems, and issues of confidentiality and disclosure, is a process that continues over the course of the disease.

Information should be tailored to the readiness and developmental level of the learners as well as their emotional and psychosocial needs.

c. Families and children, as appropriate, should be educated regarding the guidelines for antiretroviral treatment in children with HIV infection as well as available clinical trial opportunities.

d. The frequency and complexity of HIV care visits often result in difficulty or reluctance on the part of families to continue seeing a primary care provider. The need for a primary care provider and discussions about how the primary care provider and the HIV specialist will collaborate are essential components of patient education. Families should be told which provider they should call for various types of problems that may arise.

e. The role of a balanced diet and adequate nutrient intake should be reiterated with patients and families at each visit.

5. First and subsequent healthcare follow-up visits: Follow-up visits are necessary for assessment of physical and laboratory evidence of disease progression. The main goals include assessing the infant, child, and family for new or potential issues related to HIV infection, its symptoms or treatment, and new or ongoing educational needs.

a. Review of previous visit and available diagnostic results: The follow-up visit affords an opportunity to revisit issues raised at the previous encounter and to reinforce issues or information of importance, such as prophylactic and nutritional needs, care of the child with HIV infection, immunization recommendations, and so on.

b. Review of systems: A comprehensive review of systems is an essential component of every visit. Particular attention should be paid to systems in which previous or ongoing problems have been reported.

c. Physical examination: A comprehensive physical examination is essential to identify emerging health issues and provide reassurance to patients and families.

d. Nutrition assessment: Dietary habits, height, weight, and growth percentiles are evaluated at each visit to allow for early identification of potential nutritional or growth problems.

e. Laboratory and diagnostic evaluation: Subsequent to the initial HIV healthcare visit, laboratory and diagnostic testing may be driven by accepted monitoring guidelines, symptomatology, history of exposure to certain infectious processes, or for the purposes of monitoring for toxicities of antiretroviral medications and prophylactic regimens.

f. Immunologic profiles: CD4 cell counts and percentages are routinely monitored every 3–4 months or more frequently if significant changes in values are noted or if there is a change in antiretroviral therapy (Working Group on Antiretroviral Therapy and Medical Management of HIV-Infected Children, 2008).

g. HIV RNA PCR (viral load): Viral load monitoring is routinely performed every 3–4 months. More frequent testing is indicated when initiating therapy to assess response to treatment, when viral load values are noted to be increasing, or if adherence problems are suspected (Working Group on Antiretroviral Therapy and Medical Management of HIV-Infected Children, 2008).

h. CBC with differential and platelets is performed every 3–4 months or more often as indicated for persons on HAART, as some medications affect the bone marrow. Testing every 6 months is acceptable for those off therapy. HIV may have adverse effects on the bone marrow. Routine screening may identify serious HIV sequelae.

    i. Comprehensive chemistry panel should be performed every 3–4 months or more often as indicated for persons on HAART, to identify medication toxicities. Testing every 6 months is acceptable for those off therapy. HIV infection may have adverse effects on the liver and kidneys. Routine screening may identify sequelae of HIV infection.

    j. Other diagnostics may be performed as indicated based on the need for follow-up of prior visit findings or for newly identified problems.

6. Interventions

    a. Follow-up of initiation of antiretroviral therapy: If antiretroviral therapy has been initiated, assessment of adherence, administration issues, and dosing are key components of each follow-up visit.

    b. Nutrition intervention: Nutrition education, recommendation of dietary changes or nutritional supplementation, and follow-up may be necessary components of each subsequent visit depending on the growth parameters and nutritional well-being of the infant or child.

    c. Counseling and education: Each healthcare visit should be seen as an opportunity to enhance the patient or family's knowledge of HIV infection, the patient's disease status, HIV treatment, and issues related to living with HIV infection.

REFERENCES

Abrams, E. (2000). Opportunistic infections and other clinical manifestations of HIV disease in children. *Pediatric Clinics of North America, 47*(1), 79–108.

American Academy of Pediatrics Committee on Infectious Diseases. (2007). Prevention of rotavirus disease: Guidelines for use of rotavirus vaccine. *Pediatrics, 119*(1), 171–182.

Centers for Disease Control and Prevention (CDC). (2007, December 7). Recommendation from the Advisory Committee on Immunization Practices (ACIP) for use of quadrivalent meningococcal conjugate vaccine (MCV4) in children aged 2–10 years at increased risk for invasive meningococcal disease. *Morbidity and Mortality Weekly Report, 56*(48), 1265–1266.

Centers for Disease Control and Prevention (CDC). (2008). *Guidelines for prevention and treatment of opportunistic infections among HIV-exposed and HIV-infected children.* Available at http://aidsinfo.nih.gov/contentfiles/Pediatric_OI.pdf

Laufer, M., & Scott, G. (2000). Medical management of HIV disease in children. *Pediatric Clinics of North America, 47*(1), 127–154.

National Institutes of Health (NIH). (2007, November 2). *Recommendations for use of antiretroviral drugs in pregnant HIV-1-infected women for maternal health and interventions to reduce perinatal HIV-1 transmission in the United States.* Retrieved February 22, 2009, from http://www.aids-ed.org/aidsetc?page=etres-display&resource=etres-105

Subauste, C. S. (2006). Toxoplasmosis. *HIV Insite Knowledge Base* [online textbook]. Available at http://hivinsite.ucsf.edu/InSite?page=kb-00&doc=kb-05-04-03

U.S. Public Health Service and the Infectious Diseases Society of America (USPHS/ISDA). (2002, June 14). *Guidelines preventing opportunistic infections among HIV-infected persons—2002.* Retrieved February 22, 2009, from http://www.cdc.gov/mmwr/preview/mmwrhtml/rr5108a1.htm

Working Group on Antiretroviral Therapy and Medical Management of HIV-Infected Children. (2008, July 29). *Guidelines for the use of antiretroviral agents in pediatric HIV infection* (pp. 1–140). Available at http://www.aidsinfo.gov/ContentFiles/PediatricGuidelines.pdf

7.3 MANAGING ANTIRETROVIRAL THERAPY IN HIV-INFECTED INFANTS AND CHILDREN

1. Antiretroviral (ARV) therapy

    a. Not all ARVs approved for adults are available to children.

i) Not all ARVs have FDA approval because of lack of clinical trial data for children. However, some ARVs that are not FDA approved for use in pediatrics are often used to treat pediatric HIV infection if other FDA-approved medications are not an option.

ii) Some ARVs pose a particular risk of adverse effects in children.

iii) Other ARVs are not available in a formulation appropriate for young children (e.g., liquid or tablet that can be crushed).

iv) Table 7.3a presents antiretroviral medications that are approved for children and infants as of July 2008.

Table 7.3a Antiretroviral Drugs in Children

Nucleoside Reverse Transcriptase Inhibitor (NRTI)

Drug	Pediatric Labeling	Liquid Formulation	Neonate/ Infant Dose
Zidovudine (ZDV)	Yes	Yes	Yes
Didanosine (ddI)	Yes	Yes	Yes
Stavudine (d4T)	Yes	Yes	Yes
Lamivudine (3TC)	Yes	Yes	Yes
Abacavir (ABC)	Yes	Yes	age > 3 months, yes
Tenofovir (TDF)	In trial	No	No

Nonnucleoside Reverse Transcriptase Inhibitor (NNRTI)

Drug	Pediatric Labeling	Liquid Formulation	Neonate/ Infant Dose
Nevirapine (NVP)	Yes	Yes	Yes
Efavirenz (EFV)	Yes	No	No
Etravirine (ETR)	No	No	No

Protease Inhibitor (PI)

Drug	Pediatric Labeling	Liquid Formulation	Neonate/ Infant Dose
Saquinavir (SQV)	In trial with another PI	No	No
Ritonavir (RTV)	Yes	Yes	age > 1 month, yes
Indinavir (IDV)	No	No	No
Nelfinavir (NFV)	Yes*	Yes	In trial
Fosamprenavir (f-APV)	age > 2 years, yes	Yes	No
Lopinavir/Ritonavir (LPV/RTV)	Yes	Yes	In trial
Atazanavir (ATV)	age ≥ 6 years and wt ≥ 15 kg, yes	Powder in trial	No
Tipranavir (TPV)	In trial	No	No
Darunavir (DRV)	No	No	No

continues

Table 7.3a Antiretroviral Drugs in Children (continued)

Entry and Fusion Inhibitors			
Drug	Pediatric Labeling	Liquid Formulation	Neonate/ Infant Dose
Maraviroc (MVC)	age ≥ 16 years, yes	No	No
Enfuvirtide (T-20)	age ≥ 6 years, yes	No	No

Integrase Inhibitor			
Drug	Pediatric Labeling	Liquid Formulation	Neonate/ Infant Dose
Raltegravir (RAL)	age ≥ 16 years, yes	No	No

*Although used in younger children, not labeled for children younger than 2 years.
Source: Working Group on Antiretroviral Therapy and Medical Management of HIV-Infected Children, 2008.

2. Prescribing guidelines
  a. Principles of general infectious disease treatment should be applied to pediatric HIV disease.
    i)   Early diagnosis and treatment optimize outcome.
    ii)   Changes in the quantity of the infectious agent measures the effectiveness of antimicrobial therapy.
    iii) The goal of therapy is to suppress the infectious agent or achieve a sustained decrease in replication.
    iv)   Combination antimicrobial therapy should be used because single-drug therapy leads to drug resistance.
    v)   Combination antimicrobial therapy should use drugs with different sites or mechanisms of action and nonoverlapping toxicities.
    vi)   If suppression of the infectious agent is not possible, therapy should be changed if the patient shows clinical or laboratory progression.
    vii) For potentially fatal infections, aggressive treatment and greater tolerance for adverse side effects are acceptable risks.
    viii) The goal of ARV therapy is to reduce viral load to undetectable levels with therapeutic regimens that support adherence to medications.
    ix)   Parents and children must be active participants in the decision making (Working Group on Antiretroviral Therapy and Medical Management of HIV-Infected Children, 2008).
  b. Goals of therapy
    i)   Reduce HIV-related morbidity and mortality.
    ii)   Restore and preserve immune function.
    iii) Maximally and durably suppress viral replication.

     iv)   Minimize drug-related toxicity.

     v)   Maintain normal physical growth and neurocognitive development.

     vi)   Improve quality of life.

c. Risks and benefits of therapy

     i)   Lack of adherence and subtherapeutic levels of ARV may drive the development of resistance.

     ii)   Children who receive combination therapy have decreased mortality (Gortmaker et al., 2001).

     iii)   Children who are treated before they reach Category C have slower disease progression (European Collaborative Study, 2001).

     iv)   Early aggressive treatment allows for preservation of immune function and minimizes the risk of ARV resistance (Palumbo, 2000).

     v)   Failure of a drug regimen may limit the ARV options available for treatment because of cross-resistance within classes of drugs.

     vi)   The risk of drug toxicity and side effects from ARVs pose potential risks for some patients.

d. Readiness to start treatment

     i)   A careful assessment of family readiness to start treatment in an infant or child with HIV infection is essential.

     ii)   A range of considerations from palatability to scheduling to family understanding of illness must be weighed before treatment is begun.

     iii)   The clinician and the family must work together as a team to ensure that the regimen chosen is appropriate for the child and the family.

3. Initiating therapy in infants and children: A working group of clinicians, researchers, and family representatives developed guidelines for antiretroviral management of children with HIV infection (Working Group on Antiretroviral Therapy and Management of Children with HIV Infection, 2008). Those guidelines, which include recommendations for initiating ARV and initial therapy regimens, are updated regularly and are available online at the HIV/AIDS Treatment Information Service Web site (http://www.aidsinfo.nih.gov/contentfiles/ pediatricGuidelines.pdf).

4. Changing antiretroviral therapy

a. Failure of ARV therapy may be based on the following:

     i)   Clinical, immunologic, or virologic parameters

     ii)   Toxicology or intolerance of the current therapy

     iii)   New data demonstrating that another regimen is superior to the current regimen

b. Clinical failure is demonstrated by evidence of one of the following:

     i)   Progressive neurodevelopmental deterioration

     ii)   Growth failure despite adequate nutritional support and with no other explanation

     iii)   Disease progression as evidenced by symptoms or conditions that are diagnostic for a more advanced clinical category

c. Immunologic failure is present when the following occur:

     i)   Laboratory findings lead to a change in immune classification.

     ii)   CD4 percentage in a child with severe immune suppression fails to increase by ≥ 5 percentage points above baseline.

    iii)   CD4 cell counts in severely immunosuppressed children ≥ 5 years fail to improve by ≥ 50 cells/mm³ above baseline within 1 year of starting treatment.

    iv)   For children with CD4 cell percentage of < 15%, the percentage shows a persistent decline of 5 points or more (e.g., 14% to 9%).

    v)   The child has evidence of a rapid and extensive decrease in absolute CD4 cell count.

  d. Virologic failure is suspected when the following occur:

    i)   Less than a minimally acceptable HIV RNA response after 8 to 12 weeks

      (1) Defined as < 10-fold (1.0 log) decrease from baseline when treated with HAART (triple ARV regimen)

    ii)   Lack of suppression of HIV RNA levels to undetectable by 6 months

      (1) Such suppression is not always achievable in children if they have complicated resistance patterns.

      (2) Baseline HIV RNA level and the level achieved should be taken into account when considering regimen change.

    iii)   Repeated detection of HIV RNA in children who initially had undetectable levels in response to ARV

      (1) Consider more frequent evaluation of HIV RNA.

      (2) Assess adherence and renew efforts at family education.

    iv)   Persistent rise in HIV RNA levels in a child who has had a significant and sustained decrease

5. Considerations when changing therapy due to toxicity/intolerance

  a. Choose drugs with a different toxicity profile.

  b. Change the offending drug or, in certain circumstances, reduce the dose within the therapeutic range.

6. Other considerations in changing therapy

  a. Assess adherence as a potential cause of failure. Often pediatric patients hide medications from their guardians. Assess whether the guardian watches child swallow medications.

  b. If the patient is adherent, change the regimen to include drugs with the least likelihood of resistance and therefore maximal activity. In general, it is recommended to change at least two drugs in a failing regimen.

  c. Review all other medications for possible drug interactions with the new regimen.

  d. When changing therapy because of disease progression, consider quality-of-life issues.

7. The use of ARV drug resistance testing in children

  a. HIV-resistance assays may prove useful in guiding initial therapy and in changing failing regimens.

  b. Resistance testing should be performed prior to starting therapy in antiretroviral-naïve children.

  c. Resistance testing should be performed prior to changing therapy for treatment failure.

  d. To be accurate, resistance testing should be done while the child is on ARV therapy.

  e. Resistance testing is recommended when the patient has a viral load > 1,000 copies/mL and the patient reports adherence to the regimen.

  f. The presence of viral resistance to a particular drug suggests that the drug is unlikely to suppress viral replication, but absence of resistance to a drug does not ensure efficacy.

  g. Consult with a pediatric HIV specialist for resistance assay interpretation.

8. Special considerations in pediatric antiretroviral therapy
   a. Pharmacokinetic issues
      i) Age-related differences between children and adults in body composition, renal excretion, and liver metabolism affect drug processing.
      ii) Potential for differences in drug distribution, metabolism, and clearance.
      iii) Age-related differences may affect drug dosing and toxicities.
   b. Diagnostic issues
      i) Early diagnosis of perinatally infected infants allows early initiation of ARV therapy and may lead to greater immune preservation.
   c. Natural history differences
      i) CD4 T-cell counts in healthy infants are much higher than in adults and slowly decline to adult levels by age 6 years.
      ii) CD4 percentage may be a better marker for HIV disease progression in infants and young children.
      iii) Age-adjusted CD4 counts should be used for ARV decisions.
   d. Adherence issues
      i) Pediatric patients often do not like taking medications daily or twice daily.
      ii) Encourage guardians to observe the child taking the medications so that adherence is verified.
      iii) Assess adherence at routine medical appointments.

REFERENCES

European Collaborative Study. (2001). Fluctuation in symptoms for human immunodeficiency virus-infected children: The first 10 years of life. *Pediatrics, 108*(1), 116–122.

Gortmaker, S. L., Hugh, M., Cervia, J., Brady, M., Johnson, J. M., Seage, G., et al. (2001). Effect of combination therapy including protease inhibitors on mortality among children and adolescents infected with HIV-1. *New England Journal of Medicine, 345*(21), 1522–1528.

Palumbo, P. (2000). Antiretroviral therapy of HIV infection in children. *Pediatric Clinics of North America, 47*(1), 155–169.

Working Group on Antiretroviral Therapy and Medical Management of HIV-Infected Children. (2008, July 29). *Guidelines for the use of antiretroviral agents in pediatric HIV infection*, pp. 1–140. Available at http://aidsinfo.nih.gov/ContentFiles/PediatricGuidelines.pdf

7.4 ADHERENCE TO MEDICAL REGIMENS FOR CHILDREN AND FAMILIES

1. Unique pediatric/family adherence issues
   a. Not all medications are available in palatable liquid formulations.
   b. Children may refuse strong and/or unusual tastes and/or smells.
   c. Children may have difficulty ingesting large volumes of liquid medications.
   d. Children may have difficulty swallowing secondary to large sizes of some tablets/capsules.
   e. Infants and young children eat more frequently, making it difficult to coordinate medications with or without food.

    f. Children are dependent on caregivers for their medications.

    g. Secrecy may limit when, where, and who gives the child medications.

2. Psychological issues of adherence

    a. HIV infection in children is a family and often multigenerational disease.

       i) A perinatally-infected child and mother may both be on antiretroviral therapy.

       ii) A parent may lack parenting skills to administer medications.

       iii) A parent may be too ill to manage a complex medication regimen.

       iv) Children and adolescents with HIV are often cared for by elderly grandparents struggling with their own chronic illnesses.

       v) After witnessing their own child die, grandparent guardians may associate antiretrovirals with dying.

       vi) Poverty, substance use, denial, secrecy, depression, and mental illness may contribute to an unstable or chaotic home environment, which makes adherence difficult (Gross et al., 1999).

       vii) Parent may be dealing with own feelings of guilt, making it more difficult to reinforce adherence.

       viii) Parent/guardian may lack social support system to help cope with issues related to medication administration.

3. Developmental issues

    a. Giving long-term medications to children can be stressful and difficult; child may refuse or vomit medications.

    b. Children who are given premature responsibility for taking antiretrovirals exhibit more nonadherence (Mellins et al., 2004).

    c. Adolescents face specific developmental issues.

       i) They want to feel independent; not taking medication can be seen as a way to be in control (Childs & Cincotta, 2006).

       ii) They may have difficulty understanding rationale for medication regimen when asymptomatic.

       iii) They may not be knowledgeable enough about medications, regimen, and adherence and their impact on resistance (Mellins et al., 2004).

4. Adolescent social issues related to adherence

    a. Adolescents may have unstructured, chaotic lifestyles, which may include homelessness, lack of access to proper nutrition and refrigeration, and lack of family social support (Martinez et al., 2000).

5. Readiness prior to initiating antiretroviral therapy

    a. Prior to initiating therapy, assess readiness to maintain long-term adherence.

    b. Assess the needs of the child and/or family (i.e., nursing, social, behavioral; Working Group on Antiretroviral Therapy and Medical Management of HIV-Infected Children, 2008).

    c. Educate the family about HIV, the purpose of antiretroviral therapy, and the importance of adherence.

6. Beginning antiretroviral therapy

    a. Educate the family about the possible side effects, such as nausea, vomiting, or diarrhea. Caregivers may stop treatment when faced with unexpected side effects. Educate them about how to help manage these side effects, what to call about, and who, where, and when to call. Educate about the self-limiting nature of most side effects. The more knowledgeable the caregiver, the better the adherence (Martin et al., 2007).

b. Stress the need to administer the medication to younger children, and directly observe older children and adolescents taking their antiretrovirals to optimize adherence (Martin et al., 2007). Need to stress the responsibility rests with the adult, particularly in an undisclosed child who has no means to understand the gravity of the situation.

c. Teach pill swallowing. Children as young as 4 years of age can learn.

d. Develop as simple a schedule as possible; the easier the regimen, the higher the degree of adherence (Dolin, Masur, & Saag, 2008).

e. Offer to set up home delivery or mail delivery of medications.

f. Educate about the need for monitoring the efficacy of the antiretroviral regimen by attending routine clinic visits.

g. Employ anticipatory problem solving (e.g., what to do if the child vomits the medication or has diarrhea, if a dose is 3 hours late, if a trip away from home or weekends change routine).

h. In instances of poor literacy, color-code bottles and syringes to match a written schedule. If possible, start the first dose under supervision.

i. Be accessible and follow up with a phone call, a home visit, or both in the first few days (Reddington et al., 2000). Many problems with medication adherence occur in the first few days of the regimen.

j. Educate the guardian to be cognizant of when the medication supply is running low. Call the pharmacy a few days prior to running out of medication to avoid lapses in administration.

k. Prepare the family for common developmental and behavioral issues that are likely to arise. Medication administration should be consistent. Developing a ritual for medication administration may help to improve adherence. In instances in which children are given responsibilities that may exceed their capabilities, provide supports such as a home nurse or school nurse for directly observed therapy, or engage another family member to supervise the child taking the medications. For very difficult situations, a gastrostomy tube may be an option (Shingadia et al., 2000). Consult a behavioral psychologist for behavioral problems.

7. Assessing family adherence

a. Assessment of adherence should be part of every clinic and home visit. The goals should be to identify problems, provide support, and help solve the family problem so they can become self-sufficient. Give permission for honesty.

  i) Do not assume a family understands their child's medication or regimen. Ask for name, dose, time, and reason for each medication. There is a positive correlation between caregiver regimen knowledge and adherence (Martin et al., 2007).

  ii) Display posters of medications, and use these in assessment.

  iii) Try to interview the child and the guardian separately regarding medication administration. Some question/interviewing techniques that may be helpful include the following:

    (1) How many pills did you take this morning? Last night?

        (2) Share an instance in which you may have had trouble adhering to a medication regimen yourself.

        (3) What are the reasons you typically forget to take a dose? Can offer suggestions:

            (a) Woke up late

            (b) Rushing to get out to school

            (c) Out with friends

            (d) Fell asleep

            (e) At different location for the weekend

            (f) Don't like the taste

            (g) I don't feel well after taking it.

            (h) I just don't want to take it.

    iv) Home visits, if planned around medication time, are a useful tool for assessing family adherence. Families are more relaxed in their own environment and are able to discuss problems and identify possible solutions.

    v) Review medications brought to appointments. Have the caregiver draw up liquid medications when there is possible confusion about the dose.

    vi) Methods to assess adherence include self-report, direct observation, refills, pill counts, bottle checks, electronic pill bottle caps, diaries, and calendars. Each method has limitations when used alone.

    vii) Review virologic and immunologic response to antiretroviral therapy. Rising viral load with a concurrent drop in CD4 count may be a good indication of poor adherence; however, other factors may contribute to treatment failure, such as poor or altered absorption, resistance, concomitant viral or bacterial infections, the strain of the virus, or compromised immune function.

8. Strategies to support adherence

    a. Education is key to optimal adherence. There is a strong association between caregiver regimen knowledge and adherence (Martin et al., 2007).

    b. Take into account the medication administrator's perceived potential barriers (pill burden, dosing frequency, noxious taste, etc.) when devising the "ideal" HAART regimen (Stone et al., 2004).

    c. Build a trusting relationship, and be available and accessible to families (Working Group, 2008).

    d. Make a medication sheet that lists the medication, the dose, and the time to administer.

    e. For liquid formulations, mark syringes with the correct dose. If there is a question about a caregiver's ability to measure liquid medications, have the pharmacy unit dose the medication.

    f. Suggest using pill boxes to avoid forgetting if a dose was taken or not.

    g. Use home visits and agencies, such as visiting nurses, to support adherence (Williams et al., 2006).

    h. Commend positive immunologic and virologic responses. Positive reinforcement can be a strong motivator.

    i. Call a few days after initiating or changing a regimen to determine if there are any barriers. Give reassurance about the transient nature of most side effects if they seem to be a deterrent.

j. When appropriate, suggest joining an adolescent support group. Hearing another adolescent's strategy may help develop one's own strategy.

k. Support disclosure to age/developmentally appropriate children and to select family and friends.

   i) Secrecy makes adherence difficult; medications cannot be stored openly or taken in front of others. Disclosure to a family member or friend may provide backup for giving medications to a child and support adherence (Byrne et al., 2002).

   ii) Disclosing to uncooperative children who cannot understand why they have to take medications may help adherence.

   iii) If morning dosing is an issue, consider disclosing to the school nurse, who can administer the morning dose.

REFERENCES

Byrne, M., Honig, J., Jurgau, A., Heffernan, S., & Donahue, M. (2002). Achieving adherence with antiretroviral medications for pediatric HIV disease. *The AIDS Reader, 12*(4), 151–154, 161–164.

Childs, C., & Cincotta, N. (2006). Pediatric HIV adherence: An ever-evolving challenge. *Social Work in Health Care, 42*(3/4), 189–208.

Dolin, R., Masur, H., & Saag, M. (2008). *AIDS therapy* (3rd ed.). Philadelphia: Churchill Livingstone.

Gross, E., Burr, C., Lewis, S., Storm, D., & Boland, M. (1999). Medication adherence in pediatric HIV: A provider survey of difficulties and strategies (abstract). *Proceedings of the Association of Nurses in AIDS Care Conference,* 196.

Martin, S., Elliot-DeSorbo, D. K., Wolters, P. L., Toledo-Tamula, M. A., Roby, G., Zeichner, S., et al. (2007). Patient, caregiver and regimen characteristics associated with adherence to highly active antiretroviral therapy among HIV-infected children and adolescents. *Pediatric Infectious Disease Journal, 26*(1), 61–67.

Martinez, J., Bell, D., Camacho, R., Henry-Reid, L. M., Bell, M., Watson, C., et al. (2000). Adherence to antiretroviral drug regimens in HIV-infected adolescent patients engaged in care in a comprehensive adolescent and young adult clinic. *Journal of the American Medical Association, 92*(2), 55–61.

Mellins, C., Brackis-Cott, E., Dolezal, C., & Abrams, E. (2004). The role of psychosocial and family factors in adherence to antiretroviral treatment in human immunodeficiency virus-infected children. *Pediatric Infectious Disease Journal, 23*(11), 1035–1041.

Reddington, C., Cohen, J., Baldillo, A., Toye, M., Smith, D., Kneut, C., et al. (2000). Adherence to medication regimens among children with human immunodeficiency virus infection. *Pediatric Infectious Disease Journal, 19*(12), 1148–1153.

Shingadia, D., Viani, R., Yogev, R., Binns, H., Danker, W., Spector, S. A., et al. (2000). Gastrostomy tube insertion for improvement of adherence to highly active antiretroviral therapy in pediatric patients with human immunodeficiency virus. *Pediatrics, 105*(6), 80–84.

Stone, V. E., Jordan, J., Tolson, J., Miller, R., & Pilon, T. (2004). Perspectives on adherence and simplicity for HIV-infected patients on antiretroviral therapy: Self-report of the relative importance of multiple attributes of highly active antiretroviral therapy (HAART) regimens in predicting adherence. *Journal of Acquired Immune Deficiency, 36*(3), 808–816.

Williams, A. B., Fennie, K., Bova, C. A., Burgess, J. D., Danvers, K. A., & Dieckhaus, K. (2006). Home visits to improve adherence to highly active antiretroviral therapy: A randomized controlled trial. *Journal of Acquired Immune Deficiency, 42*(3), 314–321.

Working Group on Antiretroviral Therapy and Medical Management of HIV-Infected Children. (2008). *Guidelines for the use of antiretroviral agents in pediatric HIV infection.* Retrieved March 30, 2009, from http://aidsinfo.nih.gov/contentfiles/PediatricGuidelines_PDA.pdf

CHAPTER 8

Symptomatic Conditions in Infants and Children with Advancing Disease

8.1 SYMPTOMATIC CONDITIONS IN INFANTS AND CHILDREN WITH ADVANCING DISEASE

Many of the symptomatic conditions that occur in adults can be manifested in HIV-infected infants and children. In this section, an overview of specific conditions will be presented. Reference will be made to the adult section where specific information is identical.

Symptomatic Conditions		
Anemia	Etiology/epidemiology	See adult section.
	Pathogenesis	See adult section.
	Clinical presentation	See adult section.
	Diagnosis	See adult section.
	Prevention/treatment	a. During the postneonatal period and in early infancy, children with anemia due to antiretroviral therapy (ART) seldom need cessation of treatment and often respond to erythropoietin if needed (Belperio & Rhew, 2004; Donato, 2005).
		b. Erythropoietin at a dose of 50–200 IU/kg/dose, 3 times/week is recommended. Regular transfusion may benefit if response to erythropoietin is unsatisfactory (DHHS, 2008).
	Nursing implications	a. Monitor lab work that is suggestive of anemia: complete blood count (CBC), red blood cell count (RBC), hemoglobin (Hbg), hematocrit (Hct), and reticulocyte count.
		b. Educate patients to recognize and report early signs of anemia, such as fatigue, shortness of breath, and amenorrhea.

c. Provide dietary counseling and nutritional support as needed. Iron is best absorbed from meat, fish, and poultry. Orange juice doubles the absorption of iron from an entire meal, whereas tea or milk reduces absorption to less than one half.

d. Patients receiving erythropoietin therapy should receive iron supplementation (DHHS, 2008).

Cardiomyopathy	Etiology/epidemiology	a. The cause of cardiomyopathy is not completely understood and may be related to primary HIV disease, infection, or antiretroviral (ARV) medications. b. Cardiac dysfunction rates in children with HIV infection have been reported to vary between 18% and 39% (Fisher et al., 2005) with a prevalence rate of more than 90% in pediatric patients (Dadlani & Lipshultz, 2006).
	Pathogenesis	a. The severity of cardiac disease in children with HIV infection may range from asymptomatic cardiac lesions to fatal disease with severity correlated to the degree of immune suppression (Laufer & Scott, 2000). Included are abnormalities in left ventricular performance, contractility, wall thickness, dilated cardiomyopathy, rhythm disturbances, myocarditis, and pericarditis (Dadlani & Lipshultz, 2006). b. With increased survival of HIV-infected patients, cardiovascular complications impact morbidity and mortality (Dadlani & Lipshultz, 2006).
	Clinical presentation	a. Most commonly, cardiomyopathy is associated with sinus tachycardia; however, other symptoms including dysrhythmias and blood pressure abnormalities may also be present. b. Problems seen in children with HIV infection include cardiomegaly, congestive heart failure, nonbacterial thrombotic endocarditis, cardiac tamponade, conductive disturbances, and sudden death.
	Diagnosis	a. Echocardiogram is the most commonly used diagnostic tool for detection of cardiac abnor-

		malities and should be routine for all HIV-infected children.
		b. Routine screening should include blood pressure, lipid panels, and blood markers of cardiomyopathy and myocardial injury.
	Prevention/treatment	a. Medications to improve cardiac output may be prescribed in collaboration with a cardiac specialist.
	Nursing implications	a. Patient and family education focuses on the possible cause of the abnormality and any limitations on activity that should be undertaken as well as monitoring needs, such as daily blood pressures or heart rate readings.
Dermatitis	Etiology/epidemiology	a. Dermatitis and other mucocutaneous manifestations are commonly seen in children with HIV infection.
		b. Frequency is related to the child's degree of immunosuppression.
	Pathogenesis	a. Most skin lesions in HIV-infected children are the result of secondary infections with viral, bacterial, or fungal organisms.
		b. Frequently seen noninfectious skin conditions include seborrheic dermatitis, atopic dermatitis, and eczema. These occur at similar rates to immune-competent patients.
	Clinical presentation	a. Infectious skin conditions often present as more severe forms than those seen in healthy children and may be more recalcitrant (Blauvelt, 2006).
		b. Some skin lesions may be signs of severe systemic infection or cancer (Blauvelt, 2006).
	Diagnosis	a. Diagnosis is commonly made by visual inspection of the area and characteristic primary and secondary skin changes.
	Prevention/treatment	Treatment is based on etiology.
	Nursing implications	Nursing care is based on etiology.
Diarrhea, recurrent or chronic	Etiology/epidemiology	a. Infection, noninfectious inflammatory processes, and anatomic abnormalities, as well as antiretroviral therapies, may cause diarrheal illness in HIV-infected children.

b. In children who are severely immunocompromised, causes may include AIDS-defining illnesses, such as *Cryptosporidium,* cytomegalovirus (CMV), and mycobacterium avium complex (MAC). Others causes include *Clostridium difficile, Giardia lamblia, Campylobacter, Salmonella*, and *Shigella* (Winter & Moye, 2006).

Pathogenesis

a. Diarrheal disease in children with HIV infection may be acute, recurrent, or persistent with persistent causes, such as infection with cryptosporidiosis, which may be more likely to cause severe dehydration and weight loss.

b. Diarrhea is a common clinical symptom resulting from immune system deterioration and viral load increase (Winter & Moye, 2006).

Clinical presentation

a. Abdominal pain, distention, frequent watery bowel movements, fever, dehydration, and weight loss may all be present in children with diarrhea.

Diagnosis

a. Diagnosis is made on the basis of symptoms.

b. More specific causes of diarrhea are diagnosed with stool collection for culture and sensitivity of suspect organisms.

c. Ongoing diarrheal illness not caused by medications and in the absence of identified enteric pathogenesis is presumed to be caused by direct HIV infection and replication in the intestinal tract.

Prevention/treatment

a. Prevention of diarrheal illness includes good nutritional practices, such as a healthy diet and appropriate food preparation techniques.

b. Immunocompromised patients should also be cautioned about the use of water supplies that may contain infectious organisms.

c. Treatment measures for diarrheal illness include treating any identifiable underlying infectious causes with appropriate courses of antibiotic therapy.

d. Treatment can also include bulk-forming diets, antiretroviral (ARV) medication changes or dose adjustments, and short-term use of antidiarrheal agents, such as loperamide.

	Nursing implications	a. Caretakers of children with HIV infection should be educated about diarrheal illness and when to report symptoms.
		b. Historical information, such as food intake and illnesses in other members of the household or among school and social contacts, should also be reported.
		c. Parents and children should be informed to anticipate some gastrointestinal symptoms with the initiation of or change in ARV medications.
		d. Antidiarrheal medication may be prescribed in advance when medication regimens are changed so that it can be taken as soon as symptoms begin.
Hepatitis	Etiology/epidemiology	a. For discussion of hepatitis A, B, and C, see Chapter 3.
		b. Successful vaccination of adults and children with HIV makes infection with hepatitis A and B rare.
		c. Hepatitis C is mainly acquired during childhood via true vertical transmission.
		d. The risk of acquiring hepatitis C is related to the presence and amount of RNA for hepatitis C virus (HCV) in mothers at the time of birth. The infection rate for the hepatitis C virus is higher in children from mothers who have tested positive for HIV.
		e. Vertical transmission of HCV is between 5% and 20% but varies according to the presence or absence of certain cofactors (particularly maternal coinfection with HIV) or medical conditions, or both (Abrams, Moon, Robinson, & Van Dyke, 2006).
		f. The average rate of HCV infection among infants born to women coinfected with HCV and HIV is 15% to 22%, higher than among infants born to women infected with HCV alone (Abrams et al., 2006)
	Pathogenesis	a. Data are limited on the natural history of HCV infection in children. For discussion on the natural history of hepatitis C, see Chapter 3.
	Clinical presentation	a. There is the absence or paucity of signs and symptoms of this disease in children.

Diagnosis	a. There are two types of tests used in HCV infection evaluation.
	  i) Tests measuring serum antibodies—an enzyme-linked immunoassay (EIA) and an immunoblot assay obtained through genetic recombination (RIBA)
	  ii) A test detecting the presence of HCV nucleic acid in plasma (PCR)
	b. For the child 18 months of age or younger, the presence of maternal anti-HCV IgG antibodies in the infant's serum necessitates the use of tests that detect plasma viral RNA with polymerase chain reaction (PCR) techniques. Due to a very low sensitivity in the newborn period, PCR should be performed after 4 to 6 weeks of age.
	c. In children 18 months of age or older, these tests are diagnostic for current or past infection with HCV, with a sensitivity of 97% and a specificity of 95%. HCV-RNA testing is necessary to confirm active infection.

Prevention/treatment	a. Testing for hepatitis C virus during pregnancy will also identify infants who require subsequent testing and follow-up. b. Antiviral drugs for chronic hepatitis C are not FDA approved for use in children under 18 years of age. Therefore, children should be referred to a pediatric hepatologist or similar specialist for management and for determination for eligibility in clinical trials. c. Children with HCV infection should be immunized for hepatitis A and B viruses. d. Adolescents should avoid unprotected sexual intercourse, body piercings, and intravenous drug use (Abrams et al., 2006).
Nursing implications	a. Standard precautions should be used on all patients. b. Patients with HCV should be screened for hepatitis A and B and immunized if indicated. c. Treatment with INF/ribaviran (if indicated) is associated with many adverse reactions (e.g., injection site reactions, anemia). Educate patients about adverse effects and monitor patient frequently.

		d. Provide patient and family teaching regarding prevention of disease and disease management (see Chapter 3).
Hepatomegaly	Etiology/epidemiology	a. A common finding in children with HIV infection and can be related to HIV replication, antiretroviral agents, and viral causes, such as the hepatotrophic virus
	Pathogenesis	a. Varies according to the etiology
	Clinical presentation	a. Hepatomegaly typically presents with other findings indicative of lymphoproliferation, such as lymphadenopathy. b. Palpation on physical examination may be the only finding in some children. c. In some children, abdominal distension and pain may be significant findings.
	Diagnosis	a. Initial laboratory testing to determine the cause of hepatomegaly includes liver function tests (LFTs), Epstein-Barr Virus (EBV) testing, and hepatitis panels. b. Follow-up includes serial LFT monitoring.
	Prevention/treatment	a. In general, no specific treatment is undertaken for otherwise asymptomatic hepatomegaly. b. Treatment may be specific to identified organism.
	Nursing implications	a. Nursing interventions primarily focus on patient and family education regarding the possible causes of hepatomegaly and the need for ongoing follow-up of laboratory studies, as well as drug toxicity monitoring.
Herpes simplex virus	Etiology/epidemiology	a. Transmission is primarily through infected oral secretions in HSV-1 and through infected genital secretions in HSV-2. b. Children living in lower socioeconomic conditions are at higher risk of contracting herpes simplex virus (HSV; Rutstein & Starr, 2006).
	Pathogenesis	a. After infection, the virus becomes latent and recurs in response to fever, menstruation, sun exposure, or trauma. b. Most commonly seen as herpes labialis, viremia and disseminated disease can develop in the severely immunosuppressed patient (Rutstein & Starr, 2006).

	Clinical presentation	a. Lesions erupt as painful vesicles evolving to crusted ulcerations. b. Patients experience fever, mucosal ulcerations, drooling, pain or burning at lesion site, and anorexia.
	Diagnosis	a. The diagnosis is often made on the basis of clinical presentation. b. The definite diagnostic test is viral isolation. Because HSV grows rapidly, it can be detected in tissue culture from 1 to 3 days (Rutstein & Starr, 2006).
	Prevention/treatment	a. Treatment: The drug of choice is acyclovir. Oral: maximum 80 mg/kg/day in 3–5 doses; IV: 250 mg/m2 q8h b. Secondary prophylaxis for HSV infection: oral, 80 mg/kg/day in 3–4 divided doses c. Topical (ointment): apply every 3 hours, 6 times/day
	Nursing implications	a. Local care of mucocutaneous lesion includes keeping lesions clean and dry by gently cleansing with mild soap and water. b. Teach child and parent that frequent hand washing will prevent the spread of infection to others. c. Pain can be severe, and analgesia should be administered as needed.
Leiomyosarcoma	Etiology/epidemiology	a. Leiomyosarcomas are included in Category B as a sign of a moderately symptomatic stage. b. They are described as high aggressive neoplasms arising from smooth muscle. c. The number of children with HIV infection who develop a malignancy is poorly defined. d. Although very rare, leiomyosarcomas are the second leading cancer of children with HIV infection (Pollock et al., 2003).
	Pathogenesis	a. There is an association with EBV in HIV disease.
	Clinical presentation	a. The clinical presentation varies according to the location of the tumor. Unusual localizations, such as spleen, pleural space, adrenal glands, and lungs, have been described, although they present most commonly in the gastrointestinal tract.

		b. May be characterized by fever, abdominal pain or obstruction, bloody diarrhea, and pulmonary infection unresponsive to antibiotics (Little, 2006).
	Diagnosis	a. The method of diagnosis varies according to the site of tumor.
	Prevention/treatment	a. Smooth muscle tumors are in general not very sensitive to chemotherapy or radiotherapy; local excision, if feasible, is the first line of therapy.
		b. The course of the disease is highly variable, with indolent tumors (more likely leiomyomas) that probably do not necessitate intervention in some children, and very aggressive, disseminated tumors in other children.
		c. Intensive and prolonged chemotherapy as used in noninfected patients is undefined (Little, 2006).
	Nursing implications	a. Provide education about the disease, specific therapies, and potential side effects and their management.
		b. Emphasize the importance of adequate rest and nutrition. In all diseased states, the body requires adequate rest and nutrition to heal.
		c. A diagnosis of cancer can be distressing to the family and child. Provide emotional support for the patient and the family and significant others. Assess the need for palliative care and hospice.
Lymphadenopathy	Etiology/epidemiology	a. High levels of viral replication in the lymphoid tissue associated with perinatally acquired HIV infection makes lymphadenopathy a common finding among children with HIV disease.
		b. Lymphadenopathy is typically a direct result of HIV replication but may also be caused by Epstein-Barr virus (EBV), cytomegalovirus (CMV), or mycobacterial infections, as well as malignancies.
	Pathogenesis	a. Varies according to the etiology
	Clinical presentation	a. There are a large number of diseases with which lymphadenopathy can be present; therefore, the detection of lymphadenopathy is common.

		b. Nodes less than 0.5 cm generally are not cause for concern.
		c. If nodes have grown rapidly and are suspiciously large (2–3 cm), mildly painful, or fixed, they should be investigated further. Bilateral findings count as one site.
	Diagnosis	a. Biopsy is the most definitive test to determine the etiology of enlarged lymph nodes.
	Prevention/treatment	a. Meticulous physical examination to detect abnormal lymph nodes is essential.
		b. Treatment varies according to the etiology of enlarged nodes.
	Nursing implications	a. See specific implications according to etiology of enlarged nodes.
Lymphoid interstitial pneumonia (LIP)	Etiology/epidemiology	a. LIP is considered an AIDS-defining condition, but because it is associated with a relatively benign course, favorable prognosis, and long-term survival, it has been placed in the B category of the Centers for Disease Control and Prevention's (CDC) classification system.
		b. LIP is more commonly seen in children with HIV infection than in adults and has been found in approximately 30%–40% of these children with pulmonary disease (Wood, 2006).
	Pathogenesis	a. LIP is a chronic lymphocytic infiltrative disease of the lung, and the cause is poorly understood.
		b. Non-infectious
	Clinical presentation	a. LIP is often seen in combination with other signs of lymphoproliferation, such as parotitis and hepatomegaly.
		b. It is characterized by its insidious onset, often with persistent cough, wheezing, and tachypnea that over time progresses to dyspnea and hypoxia with resultant finger clubbing.
		c. The clinical course is generally benign but can be highly variable (Wood, 2006).
	Diagnosis	a. Though the diagnosis is initially made clinically, serial chest X-rays or chest CT scan, or both, showing a reticulonodular pattern or interstitial infiltrates is used to confirm the diagnosis.

		b. Chest CT is used to confirm X-ray findings and monitor disease severity and extent. Biopsy is rarely used in diagnosis (Wood, 2006).
	Prevention/treatment	a. Prevention of LIP is dependent on controlling HIV replication through the use of HAART.
		b. Treatment of symptomatic LIP with hypoxia includes the use of prednisone at 2 mg/kg/day for 2–4 weeks on a tapering schedule, then continuing at 1 mg/kg/day until oxygen saturation improves. Complete weaning can be undertaken when a satisfactory response is observed. Repeated courses of steroids may be necessary.
		c. Bronchodilators, chest physical therapy, and, in some cases, diuretics may be useful.
	Nursing implications	a. Nursing interventions are supportive depending on the severity of the disease.
		b. Patient and family education as to the chronic and persistent nature of LIP and its associated symptoms is essential.
Nephropathy	Etiology/epidemiology	a. The incidence of glomerular disease in HIV-infected children is unknown (Tanawattanacharoen & Kopp, 2006), but virus-associated nephropathy (HIVAN) has become a common disease among those who are HIV infected (Herman & Klotman, 2003).
	Pathogenesis	a. The pathogenesis of HIV-associated nephropathy is a focal segmental glomerulosclerosis and is a result of viral replication within renal cells causing proliferation and apoptosis (Herman & Klotman, 2003).
		b. HIV nephropathy is typically associated with a higher degree of immune suppression and a higher mortality rate.
	Clinical presentation	a. May range from an asymptomatic proteinuria to symptomatic renal tubular acidosis, hematuria, and acute renal failure (Herman & Klotman, 2003).
	Diagnosis	a. In children, diagnosis is made by using the ratio of urine creatinine to protein. A creatinine–protein ratio of more than 0.2 is consistent with nephropathy.

	Prevention/treatment	a. Routine urinalysis
		b. Alkalinizing agents, such as sodium or potassium citrate, in addition to other mineral supplements, may be used to correct renal tubular acidosis.
		c. In severe cases, dialysis may be considered.
	Nursing implications	a. Dose adjustments on antiretroviral therapy (ART) and other drugs used to treat HIV associated diseases are often necessary.
		b. Nursing interventions focus on supportive care and education.
Neutropenia	Etiology/epidemiology	a. In some children, neutropenia represents manifestations of HIV disease and may improve with enhanced suppression of HIV with antiretroviral therapy (ART).
	Pathogenesis	a. Impaired myelopoieses due to HIV infection of accessory cells in the bone marrow
		b. Myelosuppression related to drugs, opportunistic infections, nutritional deficiencies, and malignancies
		c. Peripheral destruction of neutrophils due to hypersplenism and infection (Owen & Werner, 2006).
	Clinical presentation	a. Respiratory tract symptoms, such as cough and sputum production
		b. Urinary tract infection symptoms: frequency, urgency, burning
		c. Fever
		d. Adenopathy
		e. Organomegaly
	Diagnosis	a. Complete blood count (CBC) with differential reveals decreases in white blood cells (WBCs), including neutrophils, lymphocytes, and sometimes monocytes. Atypical lymphocytes may be seen.
	Prevention/treatment	a. If a child is clinically stable, but there is a significant and persistent absolute neutropenia, supportive treatment with granulocyte colony stimulating factor (G-CSF) or filgastrim should be initiated before modifying ART. The dosage for children is 5–10 mcg/kg/day (IV/SC): single daily dose for up to 14 days, then titrated to maintain ANC > 1000–2000/mm^3.

		b. If neutropenia does not improve within 1 week of initiating G-CSF, the dose can be increased.
		c. When no alternative etiology is identified and the response to G-CSF is not adequate, then interruption of ART should be considered but only for as brief a period of time as possible (American Academy of Pediatrics, 1998).
	Nursing implications	a. Few HIV-infected children suffer infectious complications of neutropenia. Severe and prolonged fever is suggestive of an infectious complication, thus teach the patient and family to report high and prolonged fevers immediately. When children are present in clinical settings, staff should use neutropenic precautions.
Otitis media, acute and recurrent	Etiology/epidemiology	a. This is a common finding in children with symptomatic HIV infection especially during first 2 years of life and recurs more often in this group (Wald & Dashefsky, 2006).
		b. Acute otitis media (AOM) is much more common in the pediatric HIV-infected patient when compared with noninfected patients.
	Pathogenesis	a. Frequency of infections may be related to immunological deficiencies or eustachian tube dysfunction resulting from lymphoproliferation.
		b. The pathogens encountered in recurrent otitis media do not differ from the general population. *Streptococcus pneumoniae, Haemophilus influenzae,* and *Moraxella catarrhalis* predominate.
	Clinical presentation	a. Fever and ear pain are the most common presenting symptoms.
		b. Examination of the ear demonstrates marked redness or distinct fullness or bulging of the tympanic membrane.
		c. Hearing loss may be present.
	Diagnosis	a. Made on the basis of history and physical examination, including assessment of tympanic mobility
		b. Selected use of tympanocentesis under following conditions: previous treatment failure; suppurative complications; suspicion of unusual pathogen; seriously ill patients with otitis

		media; and relief of severe pain (Wald & Dashefsky, 2006)
	Prevention/treatment	a. Treatment is dependent on suspected or cultured organism and may be highly individualized based on history.
		b. Chemoprophylaxis is recommended when there are three or more well-documented cases of AOM within 4 months or four cases within 12 months.
		c. Myringotomy and tube placement are recommended for patients when chemoprophylaxis does not reduce the incidence of disease or when there is significant hearing loss due to chronic middle ear effusion.
		d. Children younger than 2 years of age may be immunized with pneumococcal conjugate vaccine (PCV7; Wald & Dashefsky, 2006).
	Nursing implications	a. Families should be educated about the frequency of otitis media in children with HIV infection. Symptoms should be reported promptly, and adherence to antimicrobials is essential to minimize the chance of developing resistant organisms.
Parotitis	Etiology/epidemiology	a. Prevalence rate in controlled studies is 2–14% (Atkinson & O'Connell, 2006).
		b. Although it is the least-reported Category A event, parotitis can be difficult to treat and may be associated with life-threatening illnesses.
	Pathogenesis	a. Swelling of the parotid gland is generally a benign process associated with lymphoepithelial lesions, but it may also be the result of bacterial infections, malignant processes, or mumps.
		b. *Staphylococcus aureus* is the most common bacterial cause of acute suppurative parotitis and has been cultured in 50% to 90% of cases. Streptococcal species, including *Streptococcus pneumoniae* and *Streptococcus pyogenes* (beta-hemolytic streptococcus), as well as *Haemophilus influenzae,* have been recognized as common causes.
	Clinical presentation	a. Sudden onset of parotid pain and swelling.
		b. Symptoms may be exacerbated by meals.

	Diagnosis	a. Physical examination reveals induration, erythema, edema, and extreme tenderness over the cheek and angle of the mandible.
		b. With parotid swelling, the clinician should be suspicious for mumps, and HIV-infected children should be evaluated at appropriate ages (12 months, 4–6 years) for MMR (measles, mumps, rubella) immunization.
		c. Malignancy, especially lymphoma, should be considered in the differential diagnosis of rapid, progressive parotid swelling.
	Prevention/treatment	a. Antimicrobial therapy initially is directed toward the gram-positive and anaerobic organisms identified as common causes.
	Nursing implications	a. Attempts must be made to reverse salivary stasis and stimulate salivary flow by application of warm compresses, maximization of oral hygiene and mouth irrigations, and administration of sialogogues, such as lemon drops or orange juice.
		b. External or bimanual massage of the gland both intraorally and externally should be employed if the patient can tolerate these measures.
Sinusitis, recurrent	Etiology/epidemiology	a. Occurs more frequently in immunocompromised children as compared to their immunocompetent children, as high as 39% in one study (Wald & Dashefsky, 2006).
	Pathogenesis	a. Most infections caused by organisms commonly associated with sinusitis in immune competent hosts. Obstruction of sinus ostia caused by mucositis production.
	Clinical presentation	a. Nasal discharge lasting more than 2 weeks, persistent cough, which may be worse at night. Fever and facial pain may or may not be present.
	Diagnosis	a. Based on clinical history and examination.
		b. Radiographic studies may be useful in producing a definitive diagnosis.
		c. CT scans with contrast for persistent symptoms.

Prevention/treatment a. Antimicrobial therapy initially is directed toward the gram-positive and anaerobic organisms identified as common causes. The duration of antimicrobial therapy is individualized based on response to therapy and risk for complications (Wald & Dashefsky, 2006). For the use of chemoprophylaxis, see section on otitis media.

Nursing implications a. Families should be educated about the disease in children with HIV infection.

b. Symptoms not improved with treatment should be reported promptly to the healthcare provider.

c. Adherence to antimicrobials is essential to minimize the chance of developing resistant organisms.

REFERENCES

Abrams, E., Moon, R. Y., Robinson, L. G., & Van Dyke, R. B. (2006). Routine pediatric care. In S. L. Zeichner & J. S. Read (Eds.), *Handbook of pediatric HIV care* (2nd ed., pp. 134–176). London: Cambridge University Press.

American Academy of Pediatrics. (2008). Antiretroviral therapy and medical management of pediatric HIV infection. *Pediatrics, 102*(4), 1005–1065.

Atkinson, J. C., & O'Connell, A. (2006). Oral health and dental problems. In S. L. Zeichner & J. S. Read (Eds.), *Handbook of pediatric HIV care* (2nd ed., pp. 535–542). London: Cambridge University Press.

Belperio, P. S., & Rhew, D. C. (2004). Prevalence and outcomes of anemia in individuals with human immunodeficiency virus: A systematic review of the literature. *American Journal of Medicine, 116*(7), 27–43.

Blauvelt, A. (2006). Cutaneous diseases. In S. L. Zeichner & J. S. Read (Eds.), *Handbook of pediatric HIV care* (2nd ed., pp. 473–502). London: Cambridge University Press.

Dadlani, G. H., & Lipshultz, S. E. (2006). Cardiac problems. In S. L. Zeichner & J. S. Read (Eds.), *Handbook of pediatric HIV care* (2nd ed., pp. 554–566). London: Cambridge University Press.

Donato, H. (2005). Erythropoietin: An update on the therapeutic use in newborn infants and children. *Expert Opinion in Pharmacotherapy, 6*(5), 723–734.

Fisher, S. D., Easley, K. A., Orav, E. J., Colan, S. D., Kaplan, S., Starc, T. J., et al. (2005). Mild dilated cardiomyopathy and increased left ventricular mass predict mortality: The prospective P2C2 HIV Multicenter Study. *American Heart Journal, 150*(3), 439–447.

Herman, E. S., & Klotman, P. E. (2003). HIV-associated nephropathy: Epidemiology, pathogenesis, and treatment. *Seminars in Nephrology, 23*(2), 200–208.

Laufer, M., & Scott, G. B. (2000). Medical management of HIV disease in children. *Pediatric Clinics of North America, 47*(1), 127–153.

Little, R. F. (2006). Gastrointestinal disorders of HIV disease. In S. L. Zeichner & J. S. Read (Eds.), *Handbook of pediatric HIV care* (2nd ed., pp. 637–652). London: Cambridge University Press.

Owen, W. C., & Werner, E. J. (2006). Hematologic problems. In S. L. Zeichner & J. S. Read (Eds.), *Handbook of pediatric HIV care* (2nd ed., pp. 588–601). London: Cambridge University Press.

Pollock, B. H., Jensen, H. B., Leach, C. T., McClain, K. L., Hutchison, R. E., Garzarella, L., et al. (2003). Risk factors for pediatric human immunodeficiency virus-related malignancy. *JAMA, 289*(18), 2393–2399.

Rutstein, R. M., & Starr, S. E. (2006). Herpesvirus infections. In S. L. Zeichner & J. S. Read (Eds.), *Handbook of pediatric HIV care* (2nd ed., pp. 721–739). London: Cambridge University Press.

Tanawattanacharoen, S., & Kopp, J. B. (2006). Renal disease. In S. L. Zeichner & J. S. Read (Eds.), *Handbook of pediatric HIV care* (2nd ed., pp. 619–629). London: Cambridge University Press.

U.S. Department of Health and Human Services (DHHS). (2008). *Supplement II: Managing complications of HIV infection in HIV-infected children on antiretroviral therapy*. Washington, DC: Author.

Wald, E. R., & Dashefsky, B. (2006). Otitis media and sinusitis. In S. L. Zeichner & J. S. Read (Eds.), *Handbook of pediatric HIV care* (2nd ed., pp. 543–553). London: Cambridge University Press.

Winter, H. S., & Moye, J. (2006). Gastrointestinal disorders of HIV disease. In S. L. Zeichner & J. S. Read (Eds.), *Handbook of pediatric HIV care* (2nd ed., pp. 602–617). London: Cambridge University Press.

Wood, L. V. (2006). Pulmonary problems. In S. L. Zeichner & J. S. Read (Eds.), *Handbook of pediatric HIV care* (2nd ed., pp. 567–587). London: Cambridge University Press.

CHAPTER 9

Symptom Management of the HIV-Infected Infant and Child

9.1 PAIN

1. Etiology
   a. Advances in the treatment of HIV in children have resulted in a decrease in the incidence of opportunistic infections and other complications that cause pain. However, pain has been reported in children with HIV across the continuum of illness and should be assessed at every patient encounter (Hirschfeld et al., 1996; Lolekha et al., 2004; O'Hara & Czarniecki, 1997).
   b. Pain results in adverse physiologic effects that can result in increased morbidity and mortality (Gaughan et al., 2002).
   c. Reported adverse effects of pain include increased vital signs, release of adrenal stress hormones, decreased oxygen saturation, and decreased oxygen (Mitchell & Boss, 2002).
   d. Untreated pain in children with HIV can lead to decreased appetite, weight loss, refusal of medications, decreased activity level, and depression (Oleske & Czarniecki, 1999).
   e. Abdominal pain syndromes in the HIV-infected child
      i) Mycobacterium avium causes continuous periumbilical pain. As it advances, the pain can become severe. The proliferation of lymph tissue acts like a space-occupying lesion.
      ii) Cryptosporidiosis pain tends to be more intermittent and cramplike.
      iii) Acute pancreatitis, which can be related to the use of some antiretrovirals, has also been a source of abdominal pain.
   f. Oral, throat, and esophageal pain syndromes in children with HIV
      i) Candida, herpes, and cytomegalovirus (CMV) are agents responsible for causing thrush and esophagitis.
      ii) Dental caries, gingivitis, and aphthous ulcers are also sources of pain.
   g. Neurological sources of pain in children
      i) Cryptococcal meningitis causes headache.
      ii) HIV encephalopathy may cause hypertonicity and spasticity.
      iii) Postherpetic neuropathies may cause pain.
      iv) Peripheral neuropathy may be caused by some antiretroviral medications.
      v) Other sources of pain include musculoskeletal pain, chest pain, and total body pain.
   h. Treatment of HIV and procedures also are a source of pain.

      i) Diagnostic tests, such as venipuncture, lumbar puncture, skin testing, biopsies, and other invasive studies, are regular sources of pain for children with HIV.

      ii) Some antiretroviral medications have side effects that cause pain, particularly gastrointestinal discomfort and peripheral neuropathy.

  i. Pain in children with HIV is undertreated for various reasons.

      i) Clinicians caring for children with HIV are focused on controlling the virus, rather than alleviating symptoms.

      ii) HIV subspecialists lack education and training in pain management.

      iii) Pain is difficult to assess and treat in children with a complex disease such as HIV.

      iv) Pediatric clinicians often believe certain myths about pain in children that preclude their adequate management of it.

        (1) *Myth: Infants and young children do not experience pain as much as adults.* Multiple studies have demonstrated that infants and young children have the physiologic capacity to experience pain (Mitchell & Boss, 2002).

        (2) *Myth: All opioids are dangerous for infants and children.* Even premature infants can receive opioids safely as long as doses are titrated carefully and specific physiologic differences are taken into account.

        (3) *Myth: Opioids cause addiction.* It is estimated that the risk of addiction in children treated with long-term opioids is 1 in 30,000 (Connelly & Shanberg, 2006).

        (4) *Myth: Children make up pain reports to get attention.* Children's reports of pain have been found to be real.

        (5) *Myth: If a child can play or sleep, he or she has no pain.* Children use play as a distraction from pain and, when exhausted, even if in pain, can fall asleep.

2. Nursing assessment

  a. Subjective

      i) Ask the child and caregiver about pain at every encounter. Ask, "Have you had any pain since your last clinic (office, emergency room) visit?"

      ii) Always take the child's report of pain at face value.

      iii) Explain to the child and the caregiver the importance of reporting pain.

      iv) Teach the child how to use a pain assessment scale to indicate the severity of pain.

        (1) Useful scales for children include face scales, body charts to color, and, for older children, numerical scales (Hockenberry et al., 2003, pp. 1052–1053).

        (2) Consider family issues that might affect reports of child's pain (e.g., previous experience with pain in family, culture of family, experience with and fear of addiction).

  b. Objective

      i) Assess child for behavioral signs of pain, such as listlessness; crying; wincing; change in mood, sleep pattern, or activity level; and loss of concentration, playfulness, or interest in things usually enjoyed.

      ii) Consider a trial of pain medication when a child is unable to report pain but shows signs and symptoms of pain or had a problem that could be expected to cause pain.

3. Nursing diagnosis

  a. Pain

4. Goals
   a. Reduce incidence and severity of pain using pharmacologic and nonpharmacologic interventions.
   b. Achieve optimal level of patient comfort via the least invasive route.
5. Interventions and health teaching
   a. Nonpharmacological interventions
      i)   Nonpharmacological interventions should be used in conjunction with, not instead of, pharmacologic management.
      ii) These interventions can help children with episodic, chronic, and procedural pain.
      iii) Encourage parents to participate.
      iv) Take the time to teach the child and the caregiver about procedures and the intervention to be employed.
      v)   Assess the coping style of the child and family:
           (1) Attenders: those who must know everything that is happening to them. Help them to participate.
           (2) Distractors: those who do not want to know anything and prefer to look away. This is the group for whom nonpharmacologic/behavioral interventions work best.
      vi) Specific intervention types
           (1) Distraction: Blow bubbles, read pop-up books, look at "magic wands," sing, tell stories.
           (2) Guided imagery: Take a mental trip, use a "magic glove," use a mental TV pain knob to turn down pain.
           (3) Breathing and relaxation: Teach diaphragmatic breathing and muscle relaxation ("being like a rag doll").
           (4) Cutaneous stimulation: Use superficial heating and cooling, vibration, and massage (efficacy of these modalities has not been scientifically proven, but anecdotal evidence warrants their inclusion as possible options).
   b. Pharmacologic interventions
      i)   General principles
           (1) The backbone of good pain management is pharmacologic treatment (McCaffery & Pasero, 1999).
           (2) The choice of medication is dictated by the cause, type, and severity of pain, and previous use of pain medication.
           (3) The dose of medication is determined by the child's weight and severity of pain.
           (4) Predictable, recurrent, or chronic pain is best treated with around-the-clock dosing or continuous administration (preventive approach) as opposed to PRN, allowing a constant blood level to be maintained and thereby decreasing the total amount of medication needed to control pain (Schechter, Berde, & Yaster, 2002).
           (5) Injections should be avoided as a route of pain medication administration in children.
           (6) Opioids are safe for infants and young children (Connelly & Shanberg, 2006).
           (7) Monitor and treat side effects aggressively.
      ii) Pain medications: indications

(1) Mild pain: Use nonopioids, such as acetaminophen or ibuprofen. Some pain may need treatment with a nonanalgesic (e.g., antacid for stomach pain). If pain is not relieved or worsens, add an opioid.

(2) Moderate pain: Use a nonopioid and add another analgesic, such as codeine. If patient is unresponsive or pain worsens, change to a stronger opioid.

(3) Severe pain: Begin with a strong opioid, such as morphine.

(4) Procedural pain: Analgesia and anesthesia should be administered when doing any painful procedure. This minimizes trauma to the patient and prevents future procedure anxiety. The procedure can then be performed safely.

iii) Nonopioids

(1) Acetaminophen can achieve satisfactory pain relief in children (Korpela, Korvenoja, & Meretoja, 1999).

(2) There is a ceiling effect on the dose. Higher doses than recommended do not relieve more pain and can cause toxicity.

(3) When nonopioids no longer relieve pain, add opioids and keep the nonopioids. This can allow for a lower opioid dose because the pain is being targeted at both the peripheral and central levels. Examples of nonopioids include the following: ibuprofen, acetaminophen, naproxen, choline magnesium trisalicylate, aspirin, and ketorolac.

iv) Opioids

(1) Titrate dose to effect. Can increase by 25–50% to reach pain control. Maintaining a steady level is safer than bolus doses. There is no ceiling on how high opioid doses can go. The dose should be that which relieves pain with the least amount of undesirable side effects.

(2) Initiate pain control with a short-acting preparation to titrate dose. Once pain is stable, switch to a long-acting preparation.

(3) To switch opioids or routes, use the equianalgesic chart (McCaffery & Pasero, 1999, pp. 241–243).

(4) Prevent and treat side effects (nausea, vomiting, itching, constipation) aggressively.

(5) Addiction from use of opioids for pain is rare. Respiratory depression is a result of dosing errors and can be prevented with care and knowledge.

(6) Examples of opioids include the following: Morphine sulfate, codeine, hydrocodone, oxycodone, methadone, and fentanyl transdermal system.

v) Local analgesic: This can include eutectic mixture of local anesthetic (EMLA) or a mixed solution of tetracaine, adrenaline, and cocaine (TAC) for painful procedures, such as venipuncture and lumbar punctures.

vi) Adjuvants

(1) Adjuvants are medications that are indicated for non-pain conditions, but that have been found to relieve pain.

(2) Tricyclic antidepressants are effective for neuropathic pain. Use cautiously in children with cardiac problems.

(3) Anticonvulsants, such as gabapentin, pregabalin, topiramate, lamotrigine, and oxcarbazepine, are used for neuropathic pain.

(4) Clonidine can be used in the treatment of neuropathic pain and to potentiate the pain relief of opioids.

(5) Anxiolytics, such as benzodiazepines, relieve anxiety but do not relieve pain.

(6) Antihistamines can relieve vomiting and itching and potentiate the pain relief given by opioids. Laxatives can prevent and treat constipation. Patients started on opioids should be started on a bowel program.

  c. Alternative/complementary therapies

    i) Aromatherapy

    ii) Therapeutic touch/Reiki

    iii) Homeopathy

6. Evaluation

  a. Continually reassess the patient's pain to determine the efficacy of nursing and medical interventions.

  b. Adjust doses, routes, and schedules to achieve maximum pain relief.

REFERENCES

Connelly, M., & Shanberg, L. (2006). Opioid therapy for the treatment of refractory pain in children with juvenile rheumatoid arthritis. *Nature Clinical Practice Rheumatology, 2*(12), 636–637.

Gaughan, D. M., Hughes, M. D., Seage, G. R., III, Selwyn, P. A., Carey, V. J., Gortmaker, V. J., et al. (2002). The prevalence of pain in pediatric human immunodeficiency virus/acquired immunodeficiency syndrome as reported by participants in the Pediatric Late Outcomes Study (PACTG 219). *Pediatrics, 109*(6), 1144–1152.

Hirschfeld, S., Moss, H., Dragisic, K., Smith, W., & Pizzo, P. A. (1996). Pain in pediatric human immunodeficiency virus infection: Incidence and characteristics in a single-institution pilot study. *Pediatrics, 98*(3), 449–456.

Hockenberry, M., Wilson, D., Winkelstein, M., & Kline, N. (2003). *Wong's nursing care of infants and children.* Philadelphia: Mosby.

Korpela, R., Korvenoja, P., & Meretoja, O. (1999). Morphine-sparing effect of acetaminophen in pediatric day-case surgery. *Anesthesiology, 91*(2), 442–447.

Lolekha, R., Chanthavanich, P., Limkittikul, K., Luangxay, K., Chotpitayasunodh, T., & Newman, C. J. (2004). Pain: A common symptom in human immunodeficiency virus-infected Thai children. *Acta Paediatrica, 93*(7), 891–898.

McCaffery, M., & Pasero, C. (1999). *Pain clinical manual* (pp. 241–243). Philadelphia: Mosby.

Mitchell, A., & Boss, B. J. (2002). Adverse effects of pain on the nervous systems of newborns and young children: A review of the literature. *Journal of Neuroscience Nursing, 34*(5), 228–236.

O'Hara, M. J., & Czarniecki, L. (1997). Pain management in children with HIV/AIDS. *GMHC Treatment Issues, 11*(7–8), 38–40.

Oleske, J., & Czarniecki, L. (1999). Continuum of palliative care: Lessons from caring for children infected with HIV-1. *Lancet, 354*(9186), 1287–1291.

Schechter, N., Berde, C., & Yaster, M. (2002). *Pain in infants, children, and adolescents.* Philadelphia: Lippincott Williams & Wilkins.

9.2 ANOREXIA AND WEIGHT LOSS

1. Anorexia

  a. Definition: loss of appetite

    i) The first year of life is critical for adequate physical and psychological growth and development (Samour & King, 2005).

      ii)   Relative to body weight, the amount of nutrients needed is greater in infancy than at any other time (Dudek, 2006).

          (1) Protein, vitamins, and minerals are vital for normal growth and development.

          (2) Iron deficiency (anemia) is the most common nutritional deficiency in children; it is known to cause a delay in mental and physical development and can lower the body's resistance to infection (Samour & King, 2005).

      iii) Adolescence is a time of rapid growth, physically and psychologically, thus requiring additional nutrients, especially calories, protein, calcium, iron, and zinc (Dudek, 2006).

  b. Etiology

      i)   Side effects of medications

      ii)   Feeding aversions resulting from dislike of medication tastes

      iii) Oral candidiasis

      iv) Encephalopathy or discordant swallowing

      v)   Upper gastrointestinal disease or inflammation (Samour & King, 2005)

      vi)   Depression or psychological stress

      vii) Eating disorder

  c. Nursing assessment

      i)   Subjective: The parent or child reports loss of appetite, little interest in food, or the child not eating; the parent or child reports abdominal or oral pain or nausea on eating; familial attitude toward weight, thinness, and client's weight may be a factor.

      ii)   Objective: medication history, oral lesions, vomiting, diarrhea, flatus, gastrointestinal hypermotility, and change in affect/behavior. Nutritional assessment of adolescents should include eating patterns, use of vitamin/mineral supplements—type, amount, and frequency; use of alcohol, tobacco, and other drugs; use of fad diets, methods and patterns of dieting and age client began dieting, and any events associated with eating pattern; and the intensity and frequency of physical activity (Dudek, 2006).

  d. Nursing diagnosis: altered nutrition, less than body requirements

  e. Interventions and health teaching

      i)   Nonpharmacologic

          (1) A nutritional assessment should be done initially and at each visit.

          (2) If an eating disorder is suspected, appropriate referrals should be made to mental health professional for counseling and treatment.

          (3) Fresh air and activity may also increase or stimulate appetite.

          (4) Spicy, sweet, or highly flavored and favorite foods that are ethnically and age appropriate may stimulate the child's appetite.

          (5) All interventions must consider social and supportive concerns of eating with family and friends, and the child should be encouraged to participate in family and social meal activities.

      ii)   Pharmacologic

          (1) Evaluate all medications; treat oral/esophageal infections or lesions as per standard.

          (2) Appetite stimulants (e.g., megestrol acetate) have been used in treating appetite loss with consequent weight gain in children by increasing fat mass. Risk of ad-

renal suppression must be weighed against benefit of medication (Working Group on Antiretroviral Therapy and Medical Management of HIV-Infected Children, 2008).

   f. Evaluation (see following discussion on weight loss)

2. Weight loss
   a. Failure to gain weight is defined as wasting in children and meets the Centers for Disease Control and Prevention's definition of a Class C AIDS–defining condition when one of the following conditions is met:
- Downward crossing of 2 percentile lines on standard weight-for-age growth chart in children $>$ 1 year of age, or
- Persistent 10% loss of baseline body weight, or
- Weight $<$ 5% on growth chart on two consecutive measurements 30 days apart and associated with chronic diarrhea or persistent (30 days) documented fever (Working Group on Antiretroviral Therapy and Medical Management of HIV-Infected Children, 2008)

   b. Etiology
     i)   Anorexia
     ii) Opportunistic infections (e.g., oral/esophageal candidiasis, mycobacterium avium complex, cryptosporidium, *C. difficile; Salmonella, Shigella, Campylobacter,* and other enteric pathogens)
     iii) HIV encephalopathy or neurological complications leading to discordant suck and swallowing, inability to chew and swallow, and time demands for feeding
     iv) Pain associated with oral lesions, poor dental hygiene or significant dental caries, abdominal cramps, and constipation
     v) Fullness or discomfort related to organomegaly
     vi) Poor or inadequate food supply at home
     vii) Nausea and vomiting, particularly due to medication side effects
     viii) Fever (persistent, low grade)
     ix) Diarrhea (persisting $>$ 1 month with $\geq$ two loose stools daily)
     x) Poor absorption secondary to primary HIV infection in the gut
     xi) Endocrine abnormalities associated with HIV

   c. Nursing assessment
     i)   Subjective: The parent or child reports poor or prolonged feedings or that child has difficulty swallowing, has a poor appetite, or refuses food.
     ii) Objective
        (1) Accurate serial measurements of height and weight plotted on standard growth curves and assessment of growth in relation to height and age
        (2) Anthropometric data, body mass index (BMI), tricep skin-fold measurements (if available), and midarm circumference measurements
        (3) History of opportunistic infections, diarrhea, fever, food availability, and medications
        (4) Laboratory data, including chemistry panel, liver profile, Vitamin B_{12}, zinc, fasting glucose and lipids (especially critical in infants and children because weight loss is usually caused by decreased muscle mass rather than body fat; Pizzo & Wilfert, 1998)

       (5) Complete physical examination, including abdominal exam for masses or organomegaly, neurological exam, mental state, and oral and dental examinations

       (6) Esophagogastroduodenoscopy to rule out esophagitis, gastritis, or duodenitis (Pizzo & Wilfert, 1998)

  d. Nursing diagnosis: altered nutrition, less than body requirements

  e. Interventions and health teaching

    i) Nonpharmacologic

      (1) Refer patient to registered dietitian for full nutritional assessment and recommendations, including enteral or parenteral nutrition, or both.

      (2) Have the family complete a 2-day diet recall to assess caloric intake.

      (3) Evaluate to rule out opportunistic infections that may affect eating or swallowing or the gastrointestinal tract (e.g., esophageal candidiasis, cryptosporidium).

      (4) Evaluate to rule out malabsorption.

      (5) Provide nutritional support with high-calorie supplements if gut is functioning.

      (6) Decisions regarding interventions for weight gain and management should have clearly defined short- and long-term goals.

      (7) The family must be involved in the decisions because they will bear the burden and must be able to support such highly technical interventions.

    ii) Pharmacologic

      (1) Evaluate, diagnose, and treat opportunistic infections that interfere with oral intake or cause loss of food or fluids through diarrhea or malabsorption.

      (2) Consider use of nasogastric (NG) feedings prior to parenteral intervention.

        (a) NG feedings (bolus or continuous) can provide additional nutritional support or can be used as a main source of nutrition. For older and school-age children, this can be planned as a continuous feeding during sleep.

        (b) In cases of poor absorption, severe diarrhea, or malabsorption, total parenteral nutrition (TPN) should be considered for continued weight loss or during acute medical crises.

  f. Evaluation

    i) Perform nutritional assessment, measure weight, review diet and nutritional intake, interview the family and child regarding symptoms and food and eating behaviors, and observe the child eating.

    ii) Observe and interview the family and child to determine the extent and effectiveness of interventions.

REFERENCES

Dudek, S. G. (2006). *Nutrition essentials for nursing practice.* Philadelphia: Lippincott Williams & Wilkins.

Pizzo, P. A., & Wilfert, C. M. (1998). *Pediatric AIDS: The challenge of HIV infection in infants, children, and adolescents* (pp. 516–531). Baltimore: Williams & Wilkins.

Samour, P. Q., & King, K. (2005). *Handbook of pediatric nutrition* (3rd ed.). Sudbury, MA: Jones and Bartlett.

Working Group on Antiretroviral Therapy and Medical Management of HIV-Infected Children. (2008, July 29). *Guidelines for the use of antiretroviral agents in pediatric HIV infection,* pp. 1–134. Retrieved October 3, 2008, from http://aidsinfo.nih.gov/ContentFiles/PediatricGuidelines.pdf

9.3 COGNITIVE IMPAIRMENT AND DEVELOPMENTAL DELAY

1. Etiology
   a. Direct infection of the central nervous system (CNS)
      i) Cognitive, motor, language, and behavioral impairments in HIV-infected children are most often the result of direct infection of the CNS by the virus infecting macrophages and microglia, causing a release of toxic substances into the brain.
      ii) These processes are thought to result in damage to the white matter of the brain, de-myelination of nerve tracks, and alterations in the blood brain barrier, which cause cerebral atrophy; ventricular enlargements; calcifications in the basal ganglia, cerebellum, and subcortical frontal white matter; reduction in white matter; and a process of demyelination (Willen, 2006).
   b. Opportunistic infections, secondary to immunodeficiency: Although less common, neuro-logical deficits in children have been shown to be secondary effects of infections such as toxoplasmosis, herpes simplex, and cytomegalovirus (CMV; Mitchell, 2001).
   c. Neoplasms, strokes, metabolic abnormalities, and sensory impairments due to repeated infections (e.g., hearing loss; Armstrong, Seidel, & Swales, 1993)
   d. HIV progressive encephalopathy
      i) Associated with advanced disease; characterized by cognitive impairment, poor brain growth, abnormalities of motor function and tone, movement disorders, language impairment, and mood and behavioral problems (Burns, Hernandez-Reif, & Jessee, 2008)
      ii) Severe form: rapid deterioration and loss of previously acquired milestones; less severe form: developmental plateau or marked delays in acquiring milestones and progressive deterioration (Willen, 2006)
   e. Static encephalopathy: characterized by delayed brain development but without deterioration of previously acquired skills; more common than progressive encephalopathy. Cognitive abilities often range from low average to markedly impaired (Willen, 2006).
   f. Specific deficits: Many children will not exhibit global deficits or delays in their neurocognitive functioning; however, they can experience specific functional deficits in the areas of memory, processing speed, motor abilities, executive functioning (e.g., problem-solving ability, planning ability) visual-spatial and perceptual-organizational skills, language development, attention, and social-emotional regulation (Bisiacchi, Suppiej, & Laverda, 2000; Wachsler-Felder & Golden, 2002).
   g. Comorbid factors: Other risk factors often seen in HIV-infected children include prenatal drug exposure, poor or no prenatal care, birth complications or prematurity, poor nutrition, limited stimulation during critical periods of development, chronically or terminally ill parents, and maternal death (Armstrong et al., 1993).
2. Nursing assessment
   a. Subjective
      i) Parents report concerns about the child's rate of milestone achievement (e.g., delays in sitting up, crawling, walking, or talking for infants and toddlers); preschoolers not learning age-appropriate skills (e.g., ABCs; letter, number, or color recognition), lack of coordination, gait disturbance when walking, and poor communication skills (e.g., cannot communicate clearly, not using sentences to communicate).

  ii) Parents or school-age children, or both, report difficulty in school or difficulty paying attention in class.

b. Objective

  i) Many children will exhibit global deficits or delays in their developmental level or neurocognitive functioning. Others experience specific functional deficits in memory, processing speed, motor abilities, executive functioning, visual-spatial and perceptual-organizational skills, language development, attention, and social-emotional regulation.

  ii) Assess physical growth, serial head circumference in young children, viral load, and CD4 count, and screen hearing and vision.

  iii) For infants, toddlers, and preschoolers, assess acquisition of motor, language, cognitive, and social-emotional milestones through observation, Denver Developmental Screen, or parent interview. Observe child walking to assess for gait disturbance, toe walking, hyperreflexia and hypertonicity in lower extremities, spasticity, or clumsiness/poor coordination. Assess language development, including vocabulary, articulation, and clarity of speech. Evaluate current developmental status relative to previously achieved status, and assess for deterioration or loss of previously acquired milestones or slowed development of new skills.

  iv) For school-age children and adolescents, ask whether the child is having difficulty keeping up in school or completing class work and homework, failing any classes, or being held back a grade. Assess whether the child is having difficulty concentrating or focusing, sitting still, following directions, or staying on task. Ask the parent if any changes in child's processing speed, attention, memory, judgment, or problem-solving skills have been observed. Also assess for changes in motor functioning, including clumsiness, poor balance, or poor fine motor coordination.

3. Nursing diagnosis

  a. Alteration in growth and development and visual or auditory sensation or perception
  b. Impaired communication and physical mobility related to HIV infection or its complications

4. Goals

  a. Child has been appropriately evaluated by a clinical psychologist, speech pathologist, occupational and physical therapist (OT/PT), and other specialists as indicated to determine current level of developmental and neurocognitive functioning and to determine eligibility for intervention services.

  b. Child is receiving intervention services (e.g., educational intervention, speech therapy, OT/PT) as needed for developmental or neurocognitive delays.

  c. Child's pain has been evaluated and addressed with pain management strategies.

  d. Family has been educated about child's current level of functioning and appropriate expectations for child given any identified deficits.

  e. Child and family have been linked with mental health intervention to help them cope with the child's special needs, compromised physical or mental status, and psychosocial aspects of HIV disease.

  f. Child is receiving regular monitoring and evaluation to ensure that all developmental, behavioral, and emotional needs are being adequately addressed.

5. Interventions and health teaching
   a. Nonpharmacological
      i) Refer to clinical psychologist, speech pathologist, occupational and physical therapist, and other specialists as indicated to determine current level of developmental and neurocognitive functioning and to determine if intervention is needed.
      ii) For intervention services, infants through age 3, refer to early intervention program; for preschoolers, make referrals to special education preschool programs through their local school system; for school-age children and adolescents, refer children to the special education coordinator of their school to develop an individualized education plan (IEP) to address school interventions. Liaison with the school system and complete a 504 form if the child needs any nonacademic accommodations (e.g., rest periods/shortened day due to fatigue, classrooms close together to reduce walking, access to elevators, special transportation assistance).
   b. Pharmacological
      i) HAART to address declines in functioning
      ii) Pain medications as indicated
      iii) Psychostimulants to address attention problems
   c. Alternative/complementary therapies
      i) Behavioral strategies to address attention problems
      ii) After-school programs or supplemental tutoring to address delays
      iii) Educational computer programs or games, workbooks, flashcards, library programs
6. Evaluation
   a. Assess whether child is making gains developmentally or is improving in skills.
   b. Assess whether child is doing better in school with assistance or whether additional accommodations or interventions are needed.
   c. Assess whether child's attention and behavior are being managed or whether additional interventions are needed.
   d. Assess whether child's and family's emotional needs are being addressed or whether additional mental health intervention is indicated to help child cope with illness-related stressors and disabilities.
   e. Determine if additional advocacy is needed to assist family in obtaining services for child. If indicated, refer family to child advocacy program for assistance.

REFERENCES

Armstrong, F. D., Seidel, J. F., & Swales, T. P. (1993). Pediatric HIV infection: A neuropsychological and educational challenge. *Journal of Learning Disabilities, 26*(2), 92–103.

Bisiacchi, P. S., Suppiej, A., & Laverda, A. (2000). Neuropsychological evaluation of neurologically asymptomatic HIV-infected children. *Brain and Cognition, 43*(1–3), 49–52.

Burns, S., Hernandez-Reif, M., & Jessee, P. (2008). A review of pediatric HIV effects on neurocognitive development. *Issues in Comprehensive Pediatric Nursing, 31*(3), 107–121.

Mitchell, W. (2001). Neurological and developmental effects of HIV and AIDS in children and adolescents. *Mental Retardation and Developmental Disabilities Research Review, 7*(3), 211–216.

Wachsler-Felder, J. L., & Golden, C. J. (2002). Neuropsychological consequences of HIV in children: A review of the current literature. *Clinical Psychology Review, 22*(3), 441–462.

Willen, E. J. (2006). Neurocognitive outcomes in pediatric HIV. *Mental Retardation and Developmental Disabilities Research Reviews, 12*(3), 223–228.

9.4 FEVER

1. Etiology
   a. Fever is defined as an elevation in normal body temperature, which ranges from 97°F to 99°F orally (36°C to 37.2°C, 1° higher if the temperature is taken rectally).
   b. Equally important is recognizing that hypothermia (rectal temperature of less than 96.8°F or 36.0°C) in infancy can be associated with serious infectious diseases (Baraff et al., 1993).
   c. The evaluation of temperature in an HIV-infected child with an unexplained fever should be guided by the clinical presentation. Multiple infections may coexist concurrently in the HIV-infected child (Nicholas, 1991).
   d. Children with HIV infection are deficient in circulating antibodies. Even in children who are hypergammaglobulinemic, antibodies are not specific and do not function normally (Dorfman, Crain, & Bernstein, 1990).
   e. Some HIV-infected children have fever frequently (daily or several times per week) without any obvious underlying infection other than HIV (Nicholas, 1991).
   f. Fever heralds many HIV-related opportunistic infections (OIs), including infections of the respiratory and urinary tract and central nervous system, abscesses, gingivitis, gastroenteritis, drug reactions, and lymphoma, as well as noninfectious processes.
2. Nursing assessment
   a. Subjective
      i) Review of symptoms: vomiting, diarrhea, lethargy, rashes, cough, congestion, increased irritability, and temperature duration
      ii) Activity level: listlessness, increased sleep, lack of interest in play, and so on
      iii) Elimination patterns: diarrhea, vomiting, fewer wet diapers, and decreased urine output
      iv) Eating habits: decreased PO intake, not waking to eat
      v) Exposure history: infectious diseases, animals (cats, dogs, reptiles, farm animals, birds), molds, day care (large or small), well/city water at home, older/newer home; recent restaurant visits, exposure to anyone from a foreign country, incarceration, residence in a halfway house
      vi) Travel history: outside of the state (which states), outside of the country
      vii) Recent immunizations
      viii) Recent medications
   b. Objective
      i) Measure weight, height, temperature, pulse, respiration, and blood pressure (head circumference for children ≤ 12 months).
      ii) Assess general appearance.
      iii) Complete a physical examination.

     iv)   Take a complete blood cell count with differential.

     v)   Obtain a blood culture (if the child has a central venous catheter or port specimens, blood culture must be obtained from these sites as well).

     vi)   Other tests that should be considered include the following (Nicholas, 1991):

         (1)   Chest radiograph

         (2)   Pulse oximetry

         (3)   Urinalysis

         (4)   Urine culture (obtained by suprapubic aspiration or catheterization)

         (5)   Lumbar puncture

3. Nursing diagnosis: Include those for which the child/parent/guardian is at risk (Carpenito, 2002).

   a. Anxiety

   b. Risk for imbalanced body temperature

   c. Impaired comfort

   d. Risk for infection

4. Goals

   a. Stabilize patient clinically.

   b. Identify source of fever.

   c. Communicate test results and plan of care in a timely fashion to patient/parent/guardian.

5. Interventions and health teaching

   a. Nonpharmacological

     i)   The principal rationale for treating fever is relief of discomfort, and there is no general level of temperature that requires treatment (Whaley & Wong, 1999).

     ii)   Cooling procedures such as sponging or tepid baths have been shown to be ineffective in treating fever, either alone or in combination with antipyretics, and they inflict considerable discomfort on the child.

     iii) Repeat cultures to verify sterility and if fever persists or clinical deterioration occurs.

     iv)   Collect lab specimens and evaluate need for other diagnostic procedures.

     v)   Guidelines for parents of HIV-infected child with fever (Whaley & Wong, 1999): Call your primary care provider immediately in the following situations:

         (1)   Child is < 6 months of age.

         (2)   Fever is > 101°F for more than 24 hours.

         (3)   Child is crying inconsolably.

         (4)   Child is difficult to awaken.

         (5)   Child is confused or delirious.

         (6)   Child has had a seizure.

         (7)   Child has a stiff neck.

         (8)   Child has purple spots on the skin.

         (9)   Breathing is difficult and the child does not feel better after the nose is cleared.

        (10) Child is acting very sick.

   b. Pharmacological

     i)   Empirical treatments are best avoided but may be acceptable when both the clinical suspicion of infection is high and the risk from a delay in starting treatment is significant (Dorfman, Crain, & Berstein, 1990; Nicholas, 1991).

       ii)   Acetaminophen for discomfort

       iii)   Organism-specific antibiotics

   c. Alternative/complementary therapies

       i)   Reiki therapy: Universal life force energy is facilitated through the practitioner's hand and naturally goes to the places in the recipient's body in which it is needed. Universal life force energy is postulated to connect to the body's innate power of healing and to promote physical, mental, emotional, and spiritual self-healing (Nield-Anderson & Ameling, 2001).

       ii)   Touch therapy: This is used to promote relaxation, reduce pain, and accelerate the healing process (Wardell & Engebretson, 2001).

6. Evaluation

   a. Evaluate patient's response to the febrile symptoms and their treatment.

   b. Criteria for hospital admission (Nicholas, 1991)

       i)   Temperature $> 105°F$ ($40.5°C$)

       ii)   Marked leukocytosis (white blood cell count $> 25,000$ cells/mm^3)

       iii) Marked immature neutrophils

       iv)   The diagnostic procedures used to work up the patient depend on the presenting symptoms (Nicholas, 1991).

   c. Evaluation in the febrile HIV-positive child with focal findings

       i)   Meningeal signs: lumbar puncture

       ii)   Severe oral thrush: consider a barium esophagram

       iii) Respiratory distress: chest radiograph, pulse oximetry, or arterial blood gas; depending on the severity, consider gallium scan, bronchoalveolar lavage

       iv)   Diarrhea: stool smear for white blood cells, stool culture for bacteria, examination for ova and parasites

       v)   Dehydration: serum electrolytes

       vi)   Bone or joint pain: consider bone scan, radiographs, bone or joint aspirations

   d. Expand the diagnostic evaluation when a child's condition deteriorates or when the frequency or pattern of fever noticeably changes (Nicholas, 1991).

REFERENCES

Baraff, L., Bass, J., Fleisher, G., Klein, J., McCracken, G. H., Jr., Powell, K., et al. (1993). Practice guideline for the management of infants and children 0 to 36 months of age with fever without source. *Pediatrics, 92*(1), 1–12.

Carpenito, L. (2002). *Handbook of nursing diagnosis.* Philadelphia: Lippincott.

Dorfman, D., Crain, E., & Bernstein, L. (1990). Care of febrile children with HIV infection in the emergency department. *Pediatric Emergency Care, 6*(4), 305–310.

Nicholas, S. (1991). Guidelines for the care of children and adolescents with HIV infection. Management of the HIV-positive child with fever. *Journal of Pediatrics, 119*(1 Pt 2), S21–S24.

Nield-Anderson, L., & Ameling, A. (2001). Reiki: A complementary therapy for nursing practice. *Journal of Psychosocial Nursing, 39*(4), 42–49.

Wardell, D., & Engebretson, J. (2001). Biological correlates of Reiki touch healing. *Journal of Advanced Nursing, 33*(4), 439–445.

Whaley, L., & Wong, D. (1999). *Nursing care of infants and children.* St. Louis, MO: Mosby.

CHAPTER 10

Psychosocial Concerns of the HIV-Infected Infant and Child and Their Significant Others

10.1 DECISION MAKING AND FAMILY AUTONOMY

1. Decision-making styles vary among individuals, within and between groups (e.g., medical team vs. family), and may significantly impact the outcome of treatment. Therefore, be aware of decision-making styles and use them in assessing the effectiveness of a treatment plan.
2. Styles of decision making
   a. Autocratic or authoritarian (top-down) management: One individual makes all decisions without input from others.
      i) This style may fail to anticipate potential conflicts, impediments, or factors that can negatively impact treatment.
      ii) With one primary decision maker in a family, it is helpful to offer alternative viewpoints that may need to be considered. Suggest the inclusion of others who are perceived as helpful or supportive (a second in command).
   b. Inclusive management: An individual seeks input, assigns members to research issues prior to final decision making, attempts to identify problems, and suggests solutions before implementing a plan.
      i) Limited agreement (not necessarily consensus) is usually a goal.
      ii) There is potential for too much input, which can delay a needed decision. An identified primary person or consensus is needed.
   c. Passive management: An individual succumbs to outside influences (e.g., individuals, policies, money) without exploring resources or the impact those influences may have on treatment. This style can lead to feelings of ineffectiveness and may delay a decision until a crisis forces one.
3. Types of decisions common to HIV care
   a. Testing
      i) Often families learn that siblings need testing when one child in the family is diagnosed.
      ii) Decisions regarding testing include which tests to perform; communication decisions related to staff, family members, child welfare agencies, or all three; informed consent; and sharing of results and the meaning of those results.
      iii) Families need time to process how positive test results may impact their lives, and they need simple, clear, and practical written information about what to expect. The

prospect of caring for a potentially ill child can be overwhelming; some caregivers are reluctant to take on this role.

b. Treatment
   i)   Families with an HIV-infected child need to make decisions about available treatment options and whether those options are helpful given the health status of the child and the family supports.
   ii)   Single-parent households may need help identifying their support system or need assistance navigating institutional systems.
   iii) Factors that affect treatment decisions may include the caregivers' HIV status, their health beliefs, the support or resources available to them, and their sense of trust or mistrust of the clinician or team.
   iv)   Supports and resources can be family members, friends, hospital personnel, and clergy, who provide emotional, financial, physical, and concrete assistance when needed. The assistance may include attending clinic visits and providing or arranging transportation, food assistance, respite, or help with entitlement applications.

c. Antiretroviral therapy and other treatments
   i)   Families and clinicians struggle with when and if to start antiretroviral medications, particularly when the child is asymptomatic.
   ii)   Families may be reluctant to burden a child who appears healthy with daily medicines and possible side effects.
   iii) Respect family reluctance and acknowledge their confusion while educating them (in understandable terms) about disease progression and treatment options.
         (1) Explore beliefs about taking medication. Disagreements between clinician and family on starting treatment early may result in nonadherence and the development of viral resistance, which can compromise future treatment. Does the family have the resources (financial, emotional, etc.)? Is the household disorganized and chaotic, with little structure for getting routine tasks done? Do caregivers have a backup plan for giving medicine if they are unavailable? Would they be willing to involve a school nurse or extended family members?
         (2) Families must know when a medication is required (e.g., PCP prophylaxis) and the consequences of not adhering.

d. Quality of life issues
   i)   HAART has lessened the burden of HIV disease on children and caregivers. However, the dilemma for many families is whether the benefit of suppressing viral load outweighs the side effects, daily struggles with the child, and disruption of family life.

e. Enrollment in study protocols
   i)   The Tuskegee Syphilis Study has made African Americans and others wary of medical research and medical practitioners (Gamble, 1997).
   ii)   Families may be concerned that their children are being used as guinea pigs in studies. Open discussion of these concerns is critical for gaining the family's trust.
   iii) Families have the right to refuse to participate in studies and must be reassured that their refusal will not affect their child's care.

f. Complementary treatments

    i)   Many families use alternative or complementary medicines and therapies. This should be acknowledged early in the treatment relationship. Families should be encouraged to discuss what, if any, alternative treatments they use so that the effects of both treatments and possible interactions can be assessed.

  g. Disclosure

    i)   One of the most difficult decisions for parents/guardians is that of disclosure. The stigma of HIV/AIDS exists. Many parents fear that their child will be isolated, ostracized, made fun of, or discriminated against.

4. Family autonomy

  a. Families need independence from control of others (Barker, 1995).

  b. Most families have a sense of autonomy. However, when families receive care for chronic illness, it is quite easy for decision-making boundaries to be blurred. While recommendations regarding new treatments, medications, referrals to agencies, and interventions are perceived as helpful, each comes with loss of privacy and independence.

  c. Decision-making assistance

    i)   Boundaries

        (1) Many families rely on the advice of the clinician for medical decisions and social concerns.

           (a) It is not the provider's job to dictate treatment but to provide all available information in a way that is understandable, so the family can determine what is in their best interest.

           (b) Boundaries help define roles for both the family and the provider. For a family to maintain as much autonomy as possible, providers need to recognize boundaries. Providers who become too friendly in building rapport place undue burden on families. When a family feels that their provider is their friend, they may agree to things they would not normally agree to and may not be truthful to avoid disappointing the provider.

    ii)   Child welfare system issues

        (1) If and when it is necessary for a provider to inform the child protective agency of (suspected) physical, mental, or sexual abuse or neglect, the method of reporting can sustain or damage the rapport that has been established with the family. Families often feel angry and resentful about this interference in their life.

        (2) The family should be told that the referral was made out of concern for the child's well-being. Often when families see that providers are genuinely concerned about their child, an effective working relationship can be rebuilt. Document all attempts to educate families, make referrals, or provide assistance for needed services and the family's response. Document the physical and emotional state of the child at each visit as well as any missed appointments.

    iii) Obstacles to good decision making

        (1) Caregivers' mental state

           (a) Emotional and mental problems may block good parental decision making. Guardians suffering from depression or anxiety may have difficulty making decisions concerning their child. Recognize signs and symptoms of depression, anxiety, or other mental illness, and make referrals to the appropriate mental health professional.

    (2) Effective communication
      (a) Failure in communication usually involves a clinician who is too hurried or authoritarian or an explanation that is too long or technical.
      (b) Ask questions and get feedback from the patient and family to verify their understanding of what has been communicated.
      (c) Stress interferes with learning. Persons who have just been told that their child has a life-threatening illness will remember little else. Be prepared to repeat basic information and answer questions previously answered. Education of patients and family members is an ongoing process.
    (3) Substance abuse
      (a) Recognize signs and symptoms of drug or alcohol abuse, and address these with the child's guardian. If a child is solely in the care of a person demonstrating signs and symptoms of drug or alcohol abuse, it may be necessary to contact child protection services.
      (b) Document the behavior and what assistance was offered (e.g., referral to a rehabilitation center and any follow-up provided).
      (c) Decisions regarding the child's care should be discussed when the family member is not under the influence of any substances.
    (4) Need for support systems
      (a) Identify what supports the primary caregiver has. Invite the caregiver to bring other family members to the clinic to learn more about the disease and caring for the child.
  iv) Rapport building with families
    (1) Inquire about family/caregiver goals and expectations for their child's treatment.
    (2) Identify family/caregiver needs and assist them in getting them met. Listen and reflect on their thoughts and concerns. With each family, identify the best ways, and sometimes the best staff, to relay information.
    (3) Be patient; rapport building can take time. Families need to trust the clinician.
    (4) Respect and understand cultural differences and religious beliefs.
    (5) Be honest, genuine, and consistent. People need to know what to expect from their clinician and agency.
    (6) Work with the family in partnership.
  v) Empowerment of families
    (1) Empowerment is a gift for any person or family. HIV, like other chronic illnesses, leaves people feeling disempowered.
      (a) Help families recognize the opportunities to make decisions that can have a positive impact in their lives.
      (b) Help them realize that they do not need to have someone else do everything for them. Empowerment directs them to find resources for themselves and become responsible caregivers for themselves and their children.
      (c) Families who feel that they are legitimate partners in the decision-making process are more likely to work with the treatment team to develop creative solutions for solving problems. This includes the right to say something is not working.

vi) Case conference
    (1) The case conference is a very powerful tool in the decision-making process. It is used for anticipating difficulties, exploring options, and cooperatively implementing a treatment plan. Multidisciplinary discussions allow input and perspectives from each professional, providing exploration of various facets of a patient's life.

vii) Provision of resources
    (1) In urban areas or areas with a high HIV/AIDS incidence, numerous agencies provide support and assistance to families dealing with HIV.
    (2) In rural or low-incidence areas, HIV-specific resources may be organized on a regional basis. Examples of this assistance include federally funded HIV drug-assistance programs, housing for people with HIV/AIDS, and support groups for caregivers. A social worker should be knowledgeable about these resources.

REFERENCES

Barker, R. L. (1995). *The social work dictionary* (3rd ed.). Washington, DC: NASW Press.

Corlett, J., & Twycross, A. (2006). Negotiation of parental roles within family-centred care: A review of the research. *Journal of Clinical Nursing, 15*(10), 1308–1316.

Gamble, V. N. (1997). Under the shadow of Tuskegee: African Americans and health care. *American Journal of Public Health, 87*(11), 1773–1778.

Newton, M. S. (2000). Family-centered care: Current realities in parent participation. *Pediatric Nursing, 26*(2), 164–168.

Quill, T. E., & Brody, H. (1996). Physician recommendations and patient autonomy: Finding a balance between physician power and patient choice. *Annals of Internal Medicine, 125*(9), 763–769.

10.2 STRESS REDUCTION IN PEDIATRIC HIV

1. Psychological and emotional ramifications of chronic illness
   a. Typical response (APA, 1991)
      i) Cognitive: distressing dreams, poor attention span, and disorientation
      ii) Emotional: helplessness, frustration, feeling of abandonment, feeling of isolation, grief, irritability, numbness, and feelings of inadequacy
      iii) Interpersonal/social: child—lack of close peer group, loss of ability to participate in activities, ostracism by others, loss of family members or friends due to illness, activities focused only on illness; parent–child interactions—intrusive, overprotective, avoidant
      iv) Behavioral: withdrawn, excessive humor, and emotional outbursts
   b. Atypical response (APA, 1991)
      i) Mood disorders: depressed, elevated, expansive, or irritable mood, possibly caused by general medical condition
      ii) Anxiety disorders: symptoms of anxiety and fear avoidance
2. Stressors in children with HIV infection
   a. Chronic illness of a parent

   b. Increased instability of a child's world due to multiple losses, family disruption and separation, and changing roles of family members

   c. HIV effects on cognition and physical development

3. Stress response according to developmental stage

   a. Infant: increased crying, lethargy, elevated heart rate, tactile hypersensitivity, feeding issues, failure to thrive, emesis

   b. Toddler: temper tantrums, noncompliance, irritability, demanding behavior, attachment, separation issues, refusal to eat

   c. Preschool child: regression of toilet training; attachment issues; increased tantrums; reckless play; development of new fears or nightmares; misconceptions with treatments and care; stranger fear, especially with medical staff; language difficulty

   d. School-age child: noncompliance, disruption in school routine or formal learning, avoidance of school, need for information, misconceptions, regression of social behaviors, refusal of treatment, withdrawal

   e. Preteen child: separation from peer group, loss of independence, depression or withdrawal, coping with changes in physical appearance or abilities, risk-taking behavior, fear of peer rejection, aggressive behavior

   f. Teenager/adolescent: body image issues; withdrawal from peer group; loss of privacy; risk-taking behavior, such as substance abuse; psychosomatic complaints; sleep disturbances; increased dependence on parents

4. Strategies for helping families deal with the stress of having an HIV-positive child

   a. Assess support system during initial visit and at each consecutive visit.

   b. Tell the child about his/her disease.

     i) Infected child: Discussion needs to be developmentally appropriate. Be sensitive to parental guilt. Teach personal responsibility in relationship to containing blood, having safe sex, and informing potential sexual partners. Regarding disclosure, remember the importance of not telling everyone (Nehring, Lashley, & Malm, 2000). Help the child understand HIV and treatment effects.

     ii) Affected siblings: Discussion needs to be developmentally appropriate. Anticipate questions and help the family come up with creative solutions.

   c. Support family members in changing roles.

   d. Keep family intact as much as possible.

     i) Involve children in gradual transition to extended family situation.

     ii) Permanency planning is the process of anticipating the complexity of caregiver issues, including a discussion of who cares for the child if the caregiver is hospitalized or dies. If the parents are still alive, discuss guardianship issues prior to crisis situations (Ledlie, 2001).

   e. Review with parent/guardian developmentally appropriate behavior in relationship to their child (expected vs. unexpected).

   f. Discuss the importance of adherence to medication regimes, and acknowledge the complexity of treatment regimens.

   g. Acknowledge and discuss the complexities of raising an adolescent with HIV: relationship issues, dating, intimacy (e.g., help to develop scripts for future relationships), secrecy about their illness, realistic expectations for their future, asserting their need for independence with full knowledge of the consequences.

h. Acknowledge the impact of parental guilt.
   i) Administering a child's medication is a constant reminder of the child's illness.
   ii) Parents struggling to come to terms with their child's illness may forget to give the medication.
   iii) Failure to adhere to antiretrovirals may occur because of the complexity of the treatment regimens and because the child hates the way the medicine tastes (i.e., not wanting to fight with the child).
   iv) Parents may deny their own health needs, resulting in exhaustion, lack of nutrition, lack of adherence to their own antiretroviral regime, and hospitalization.
   v) The synergy of guilt and shame provides for more isolation than encountered with most other conditions.
   vi) Refer parents for counseling if the parents think it would be helpful to discuss their own personal guilt issues.
i. Recognize the complexities of disclosure.
   i) Discuss the difference between honesty and complete disclosure.
   ii) Support a family's choice to limit disclosure (Nehring, Lashley, & Malm, 2000).
   iii) Discuss the social stigma that is still attached to HIV/AIDS.
   iv) When a child discloses his or her HIV status, he or she may have to deal with the cruelty of classmates.
   v) Taking medications for HIV at school can be difficult for the child.
      (1) Taking medication singles the child out as different.
      (2) Lack of trained personnel to administer complex medication regimens might cause difficulties.
      (3) Children might have a difficult time dealing with what to say to classmates who inquire about medications.
j. Provide formal education for the HIV-infected child while being sensitive to his or her needs.
   i) Tailor education to the needs of the child (e.g., special education classes, tutoring, homebound teachers) for extended illnesses.
   ii) Understand that absences may occur due to illness, clinic visits, or hospitalization.
   iii) Encourage participation in team sports. The American Academy of Pediatrics (1999) recommends that children be allowed to participate in competitive sports to the extent that their health permits. Children with bleeding tendencies should be encouraged to choose sports other than high-contact sports, such as wrestling, boxing, and football (Dominguez, 2000).
k. Use complementary therapies, such as massage, creative visualization, Reiki, drumming, puppets, art therapy, and acupuncture (Nield-Anderson & Ameling, 2001; Wardell & Engebretson, 2001).

REFERENCES

American Academy of Pediatrics. (1999). Issues related to human immunodeficiency virus transmission in schools, child care, medical settings, the home, and community. *Pediatrics, 104*(2 Pt 1), 318–324.
American Psychiatric Association (APA). (1991). *Diagnostic and statistical manual of mental disorder* (4th ed.). Washington, DC: Author.

Dominguez, K. L. (2000). Management of HIV-infected children in the home and institutional settings. In M. Rogers (Ed.), *HIV/AIDS in infants, children, and adolescents: Pediatric clinics of North America* (Vol. 47). Philadelphia: W. B. Saunders.

Earls, F., Raviola, G., & Carlson, M. (2008). Promoting child and adolescent mental health in the context of the HIV/AIDS pandemic. *Journal of Child Psychology and Psychiatry, 49*(3), 295–312.

Hysing, M., Elgen, I., Gillberg, C., Lie, S. A., & Lundervold, A. J. (2007). Chronic physical illness and mental health in children: Results from a large scale population study. *Journal of Child Psychology and Psychiatry, 48*(8), 785–792.

Ledlie, S. (2001). The psychosocial issues of children with perinatally acquired HIV disease becoming adolescents: A growing challenge for providers. *AIDS Patient Care and STDs, 15*(5), 231–236.

Nehring, W., Lashley, F., & Malm, K. (2000). Disclosing the diagnosis of pediatric HIV infection: Mothers' views. *Journal of the Society of Pediatric Nurses, 5*(1), 5–14.

Nield-Anderson, L., & Ameling, A. (2001). Reiki: A complementary therapy for nursing practice. *Journal of Psychosocial Nursing, 39*(4), 42–49.

Wardell, D., & Engebretson, J. (2001). Biological correlates of Reiki touch healing. *Journal of Advanced Nursing, 33*(4), 439–445.

Wiener, L., Mellins, C. A., Marhefka, S., & Battles, H. B. (2007). Disclosure of an HIV diagnosis to children: History, current research, and future directions. *Journal of Developmental and Behavioral Pediatrics, 28*(2), 155–166.

10. 3 SOCIAL ISOLATION AND STIGMA

1. Social isolation refers to the lack of interaction with other people, usually outside of the immediate family. Social isolation, stigma, and disclosure issues are tightly entwined, for both families and children affected by HIV, as well as for adults. Factors promoting social isolation include the following:
   a. The illness, with its associated lack of energy and changes in appearance, which can interfere with social interactions
   b. The unpredictable course of the illness, with long absences or frequent interruptions in schooling and other activities outside the family
   c. Concerns about stigma and disclosure of HIV status, such as the following:
      i)   Fear of social rejection
      ii) Secrecy about HIV, making social interactions feel inauthentic, less satisfying
      iii) Preference for social isolation over having to be dishonest about HIV-status disclosure
2. Consequences of social isolation
   a. Loneliness
   b. Interference with developmental progress in socialization (at all ages), which is needed for development of intimate friendships and social skills
   c. Interference with development of a healthy self-concept and self-esteem
   d. Diminished resources for social support
   e. Isolation related to having HIV, which may be compounded by other problems that often affect families with HIV, including poverty, unstable living situations, multiple infected family members, multiple losses
3. Social isolation affects all members of the family, but with different emphases.
   a. For children with HIV, social isolation interferes with the following:
      i)   Development of social skills, including the ability to form intimate friendships and attachments
      ii) Formation of self-concept and self-esteem

       iii) Development of autonomy in relating to the outside world

   b. For adolescents, the lack of a peer group and close friendships can exacerbate feelings of not belonging. Concerns about being rejected may also be more intense for adolescents.

   c. For healthy siblings, the social isolation of the family as a whole can decrease their access to social interaction outside the family. Healthy children may also feel isolated within the family because of the amount of attention required by their ill sibling.

   d. For parents, the burden of care may absorb energy that would otherwise go toward generating social interactions. Concerns about protecting their children from stigma may dominate any considerations of social activities. Fear of infection may keep the family from engaging with others.

4. A stigma is a trait, attribute, or characteristic that society defines as highly undesirable (Goffman, 1963).

   a. Having such a trait makes a person vulnerable to stigmatization, which can cause the following:

       i) Changes in how the person is viewed by others (social identity)

       ii) Social rejection or decreased acceptance in social interactions

       iii) Limitation of opportunities (e.g., in housing, jobs, access to health care)

       iv) Feelings of shame and self-hatred if the person shares society's evaluation of what the trait means about its possessor

       v) Significant erosion of a person's quality of life

   b. The types of traits that can be stigmatizing include physical deformities, moral flaws (e.g., dishonesty or weak will), and tribal stigma, such as race, religion, or nationality. Stigma arising from having HIV can be influenced by all three of these categories.

   c. The intensity of the stigma produced by a trait is modulated by various factors (Jones et al., 1984), three of which are highly pertinent to HIV:

       i) How well the trait can be concealed from others

       ii) Who is responsible or who is to blame

       iii) The perceived danger of being around someone with the trait

   d. Stigmatization occurs when the undesirable meanings of the trait become attached to a person who possesses the trait. In addition to being stigmatized by others (enacted stigma), the person with HIV may stigmatize or denigrate himself or herself (felt stigma), resulting in feelings of self-blame or disempowerment.

   e. Interactions are often anxiety provoking for people with HIV because it is difficult to predict how others will respond once they know a person has HIV.

   f. Courtesy stigma, or associative stigma, occurs when the stigma applied to the person with the trait is also applied, though sometimes to a lesser extent, to those who are related to or associated with the person, even though they do not themselves possess the trait. Courtesy stigma related to HIV has been applied to family members, friends, healthcare providers, and volunteers and can affect the amount of social support available to these people as well.

5. Managing stigma generally means avoiding or minimizing enacted stigma.

   a. When HIV status is undisclosed, the person with HIV may "pass" (i.e., present oneself as not having HIV). This may involve disguising symptoms or hiding HIV medications, which can interfere with medication adherence. Passing can require considerable effort and energy (Ingram & Hutchinson, 1999). Many parents and families avoid disclosing that their child has HIV so that the child can pass and continue to be treated as a "normal" child.

b. If others know a person has HIV, the infected person may attempt to minimize enacted stigma by covering (i.e., making HIV-related symptoms or actions less noticeable or less obtrusive).

c. Avoiding social situations—limiting the circle of people that the person meets and interacts with—is another approach to managing stigma. The result is often social isolation and loneliness.

6. Prevalence of HIV-related stigma

   a. The prevalence and intensity of HIV-related stigma varies from country to country and, within a particular society, from group to group (Herek et al., 1998). Surveys in the United States and Europe of the general public (CDC, 2000) and nurses (Surlis & Hyde, 2001) continue to demonstrate stigmatizing attitudes toward people with HIV, although the proportion of people who stigmatize has decreased. Stigmatization of people with HIV is also widely reported in Africa and Asia.

   b. Rejection related to stigma is a pervasive theme in research on the psychosocial effects of HIV infection and includes subtle distancing as well as ostracism and discrimination.

   c. The proportion of people with HIV who experience stigma is not known. Many people with HIV are not stigmatized, but many others are, to devastating effect.

   d. The risk of experiencing HIV-related stigma can vary according to the following:
      i)   The imputed mode of transmission
      ii) Possession of other stigmatizing traits (e.g., homosexuality, injecting drug use)
      iii) Presence of visible physical changes that suggest HIV infection
      iv) The degree of anticipated physical contact
      v)   Individual characteristics of either party in the interaction (gender, cultural background, level of knowledge about HIV)
      vi) Geographical location (country, urban/suburban/rural location)

7. The experience of stigma for patients and families

   a. The degree to which having HIV can be concealed and the results of initial disclosures will influence the person's experience of stigma.

   b. For families affected by HIV, stigma is a group experience, which often includes social isolation.

   c. The potential for stigmatization may negatively affect many aspects of healthcare delivery, including confidentiality, willingness to be tested for HIV, and adherence to therapy.

8. Assessing the child and family for HIV-related stigma

   a. Individuals with HIV-related stigma may experience psychological sequelae, including depression, loneliness, anxiety, withdrawal, suicidal thoughts, and anger.

   b. HIV-related stigma for individuals and families can include the following:
      i)   Discrimination in job, housing, schools, health care, and insurance
      ii) Social isolation due to rejection, withdrawal, or both
      iii) Less-satisfying relationships due to lack of self-disclosure and increased social conflict
      iv) Loss of relationships that might have provided material support
      v)   Physical violence

    c. Nurses should ask directly about the following:
        i) Any changes in relationships or living situation since diagnosis
        ii) Problems at home, school, place of worship, or work
        iii) Unpleasant incidents, including physical or verbal assaults
        iv) Experiences or concerns about disclosing HIV status
9. Interventions for the child and family with HIV-related stigma include the following:
    a. Counseling
        i) Anticipatory counseling about issues of disclosure, possible discrimination and stigma, and social isolation should occur in conjunction with HIV testing and in treatment settings.
        ii) Tailor counseling individually.
    b. Recognition of the ongoing tension between wanting to disclose and fear of rejection and discrimination
    c. Discussion about ways to test the water with others (e.g., asking "How did you feel when you heard [name of someone famous] had HIV?")
    d. Exploration of previous experiences with stigma (related to sexual orientation or other traits); can strategies used previously be applied to managing HIV-related stigma?
    e. Education of patients, families, and partners about the following:
        i) Actual risk of transmission and safety of household members
        ii) The potential for HIV-related stigma
        iii) The importance of maintaining and developing new social contacts for all members of the family
    f. Referrals
        i) Ongoing counseling for the individual, the family, or both
        ii) Support groups, which may offer practical tips for managing or avoiding stigma in addition to chances for social interaction in a less-threatening situation

REFERENCES

Ahern, J., Stuber, J., & Galea, S. (2007). Stigma, discrimination, and the health of illicit drug users. *Drug and Alcohol Dependence, 88*(2–3), 188–196.

Bayer, R. (2008). Stigma and the ethics of public health: Not can we but should we. *Social Science & Medicine, 67*(3), 463–472.

Centers for Disease Control and Prevention (CDC). (2000). HIV-related knowledge and stigma—United States, 2000. *Morbidity and Mortality Weekly Report, 49*(47), 1062–1064.

Goffman, E. (1963). *Stigma: Notes on the management of spoiled identity.* New York: Simon & Schuster.

Herek, G. L., Mitnick, L., Burris, S., Chesney, M., Devine, P., Thompson Fullilove, M., et al. (1998). Workshop report: AIDS and stigma: A conceptual framework and research agenda. *AIDS and Public Policy Journal, 13*(1), 36–47.

Ingram, D., & Hutchinson, S. A. (1999). HIV-positive mothers and stigma. *Health Care for Women International, 20*(1), 93–103.

Jones, E. E., Farina, A., Hastorf, A. H., Markus, H., Miller, D. T., Scott, R. A., et al. (1984). *Social stigma: The psychology of marked relationships.* New York: W. H. Freeman.

Ostrom, R. A., Serovich, J. M., Lim, J. Y., & Mason, T. L. (2006). The role of stigma in reasons for HIV disclosure and non-disclosure to children. *AIDS Care, 18*(1), 60–65.

Stuber, J., Meyer, I., & Link, B. (2008). Stigma, prejudice, discrimination and health. *Social Science & Medicine, 67*(3), 351–357.

Surlis, S., & Hyde, A. (2001). HIV-positive patients' experiences of stigma during hospitalization. *Journal of the Association of Nurses in AIDS Care, 12*(6), 68–77.

Weiss, M., & Ramakrishna, J. (2006). Stigma interventions and research for international health. *Lancet, 367*(9509), 536–538.

10.4 SURROGATE CAREGIVERS

1. Why surrogates?
   a. Many children with HIV have been left without parents due to parental illness and death, incarceration, severe dysfunction related to drug abuse, or abandonment.
   b. Families of children perinatally infected with HIV by definition have mothers who have HIV infection, whereas the fathers may or may not be infected.
   c. A large percentage of HIV-involved families are headed by single parents (Burr & Lewis, 2000).
   d. Many abandoned infants in hospital nurseries and children in foster care have been exposed to HIV and require screening (Child Welfare League of America, 2002; HIV/AIDS Treatment Information Service, 2001).
      i) Child welfare concerns
         (1) Research has demonstrated that on measures of health and psychological and social well-being, children fare better in small, familylike groupings rather than in institutional care (Frank, Klass, Earls, & Eisenberg, 1996; Kaler & Freeman, 1994).
         (2) Child welfare reforms in the United States mandate that the states first attempt to reunite children with their biological families and, failing reunification within a specified time frame, attempt to locate extended family to care for the child (Adoption and Safe Families Act of 1997, P. L. 105-89). Although such efforts are made, children may be placed in foster care. Should these efforts fail (again, within a legally mandated time frame), the children must be legally cleared for adoption. Many states have adopted a dual track, in which simultaneous case plans are developed for reunification with immediate family and adoption. If reunification fails, adoption can be expedited.
2. Concept of family
   a. The nuclear family, consisting of a mother, a father, and their biological offspring, is only one of many possible examples of family.
   b. Other types of families include a child and his or her grandparents; a mother (or father), a stepfather (or stepmother), and several half-siblings; an aunt, uncle, and cousins; a single parent or two same-sex parents with older and/or younger siblings.
   c. Respecting and supporting the family that is caring for the patient is essential in developing a relationship of trust with a pediatric patient.
3. Who are the surrogate caregivers or guardians?
   a. Some surrogates may be family members (e.g., grandparents, aunts/uncles, older siblings, cousins).
   b. Minority families are more likely to provide surrogate care for their relatives' children rather than allowing the children to enter the child welfare system (Groce, 1995).

    c. Other surrogates may be foster or adoptive parents.

    d. The caregiver may be a friend of the family designated by the parent(s) but without any legal status in relation to the child. Every family has its unique history, style of coping, strengths, and weaknesses.

    e. Severely ill parents should be encouraged to create a legal document stating their wishes concerning custody and guardianship of their children after consultation with those named.

4. Extended family

    a. An extended family may consist of grandparents, aunts, uncles, older siblings, cousins, or more distant relatives and is the most common placement for children requiring surrogate caregivers.

    b. The extended family may voluntarily take children in or may be identified and approached by the local child welfare agency.

    c. The extended family may offer psychological and cultural benefits to the child but may present problems as well.

    d. Some families may have a cross-generational history of addictions, child neglect, or both. Extended family members may not be competent in caring for a chronically ill child.

    e. Members of the family know the biological parents and may know how HIV was contracted. They have formed opinions about the parents and have feeling and beliefs about this child and his or her parents that may impact on the child's care. They also have ideas about what it means to be sick, and these feelings need to be explored.

    f. Some families believe that it is important to keep the family together at all costs and may be financially overburdened, emotionally and mentally fatigued or bereft, or simply inundated with too many of their own family struggles.

    g. Many family members will not prevent children from having contact with the biological parents, even if the courts deny it.

    h. It is important to educate families about HIV and its treatment and transmission, so the child does not become isolated or ostracized out of fear of contamination. Having witnessed family members die of HIV, many families have strong beliefs about HIV treatment (e.g., some will refuse antiretroviral therapy) and may struggle to carry out the last wishes of a deceased parent.

    i. Some families see HIV as a conspiracy created in a lab to eliminate African Americans, and such beliefs may impair the provider–patient relationship. The provider must work hard to gain and maintain the family's trust and offer examples of successful treatment rather than confront this issue directly (Klonoff & Landrine, 1999).

5. Foster families

    a. Fostering is a legal relationship sanctioned by the child welfare agency.

    b. Foster parents may undergo specialized training to care for children with chronic medical conditions and HIV.

    c. Occasionally a family friend or other individual with some relationship to the child provides foster care (e.g., a teacher or nurse). Such individuals should be encouraged to formalize the relationship through legal guardianship or adoption when possible.

    d. Foster parents must be told the child's diagnosis prior to accepting the child for placement to ensure that appropriate medical care is provided. Clinicians who become aware that this information was omitted prior to placement should contact the child welfare agency immediately to facilitate appropriate disclosure.

6. Adoptive family
   a. Extended family members may choose to adopt the child they are caring for, but more often adoption involves a new, unrelated family for the child.
   b. Adoptive parents need to know the child has HIV infection or is HIV-exposed to determine whether they can provide for the child's needs and can cope with the uncertainties of having a child with a chronic and life-threatening illness.
   c. In unrelated adoptions, the prospective parents are most often White couples seeking a healthy, White infant. Therefore, children with HIV may be at the bottom of the list in terms of adoptability (Clark & Shute, 2001). When they do occur, such adoptions are often transracial. Gentle education about culture-specific needs (such as hair and skin care for African American children) and respect for the child's culture of origin is appropriate.

7. Fost-adopt
   a. Historically, foster parents were barred from adopting their charges and were even discouraged from forming strong attachments to the children. Increasingly, children are placed in foster families who may be willing to adopt them when and if they become legally cleared for adoption.
   b. This minimizes disruption in the child's relationships and provides the continuity now recognized as the foundation of healthy personality development.

8. Family constellation
   a. In any family situation there may be additional caregivers other than the legally designated ones who assist with daily care and medication administration.
   b. Good practice dictates determining who those other caregivers are and inviting them to attend clinic visits for education regarding the disease and its management.
   c. Although the child's specific medical needs must first be met, many families benefit from education concerning the notion that the child is not an AIDS patient but first a child, who happens to have HIV.
   d. Placing the disease in the proper perspective enables families to better attend to the business of being families, such as making sure children go to school, setting aside time for recreation, and providing appropriate guidance to all of the children in the household.

9. Understanding family history
   a. It is extremely useful for all clinicians to draw a genogram or family tree when encountering a new patient (Moore Hines & Boyd-Franklin, 1982).
   b. A genogram identifies family members and provides a snapshot of who is infected, which siblings may need to be screened, and which human resources are available for the family.
   c. Asking about medical history of extended family members, including alcoholism and drug dependence, will yield useful information.
   d. Ask about prior experiences in coping with stress and crises to gain a fuller picture of family functioning.

10. Contact with biological parents
   a. When biological parents are not the immediate caregivers, they may still have significant contacts with the child, and children may be aware of the health status of their parents.

b. Some extended families (and even some foster and adoptive families) are able to gracefully incorporate the biological parents into their lives.

c. Clinicians may be surprised to see a parent assumed absent at a clinic visit.

d. Pediatric patients routinely scrutinize clinicians' responses, and any display of disrespect toward the child's family will be noted and may jeopardize the clinician–patient relationship.

11. Supporting the child within the surrogate family

a. Educate the surrogate family concerning the disease and the management required for the individual patient.

b. Normalize the developmentally appropriate tasks and conflicts (e.g., some families may attribute any misbehavior to bad genes and may need to be educated about the power struggles inherent in the toddler and teen years).

c. Discuss any disagreements with caregivers' management of the child's illness outside of the hearing of the child, especially if under the age of 12.

d. Encourage teens to be part of the discussion because they will increasingly need to assume responsibility for their own care.

e. Assess the child's well-being within the surrogate family.

f. Recognize when the child's needs (medical, psychological, or other) are not being met within the surrogate family, and attempt to educate the surrogate family concerning the child's needs, referring the family to social services or the child protection authority, or both; documenting interactions is important in protecting and advocating for the child.

REFERENCES

Burr, C., & Lewis, S. (2000). *Making the invisible visible: Services for families living with HIV infection and their affected children.* Newark, NJ: National Pediatric & Family HIV Resource Center, University of Medicine and Dentistry.

Child Welfare League of America. (2002). *Factsheet: The health of children in out-of-home care.* Retrieved November 18, 2002, from http://www.cwla.org/programs/health/healthcarecwfact.htm

Clark, K., & Shute, N. (2001, March 12). The adoption maze. *U.S. News & World Report, 130*(10), 60–66, 69.

Frank, D. A., Klass, P. E., Earls, F., & Eisenberg, L. (1996) Infants and young children in orphanages: One view from pediatrics and child psychiatry. *Pediatrics, 47*(4), 569–578.

Groce, N. E. (1995). Children and AIDS in a multicultural perspective. In S. Geballe, J. Gruendel, & W. Andiman (Eds.), *Forgotten children of the AIDS epidemic* (pp. 95–106). New Haven, CT: Yale University Press.

HIV/AIDS Treatment Information Service. (2001). *Guidelines for the use of antiretroviral agents in pediatric HIV infection.* Retrieved April 1, 2009, from http://www.aidsinfo.nih.gov/contentfiles/PediatricGuidelines_PDA.pdf

Kaler, S. R., & Freeman, B. J. (1994). An analysis of environmental deprivation: Cognitive and social development in Romanian orphans. *Journal of Child Psychiatry and Psychology and Allied Disciplines, 35*(4), 769–781.

Klonoff, E. A., & Landrine, H. (1999). Do Blacks believe that HIV/AIDS is a government conspiracy against them? *Preventive Medicine, 28*(5), 451–457.

McKay, M., Block, M., Mellins, C., Traube, D. E., Brackis-Cott, E., Minott, D., et al. (2005). Adapting a family-based HIV prevention program for HIV-infected preadolescents and their families: Youth, families and health care providers coming together to address complex needs. *Social Work in Mental Health: The Journal of Behavioral and Psychiatric Social Work, 5*(93), 355–378.

Moore Hines, P., & Boyd-Franklin, N. (1982). Black families. In M. McGoldrick, J. K. Pearce, & J. Giordano (Eds.), *Ethnicity and family therapy* (pp. 8–107). New York: Guilford Press.

10.5 DISCLOSURE

1. Definition: Disclosure is the process of informing the child or youth of disease diagnosis, health changes, and opportunities that involve education, risks, benefits, adaptation, therapies, and responsibilities as they happen in the life continuum.
2. Issues surrounding chronic illness disclosure to children: HIV shares the threat of terminal illness with cancer, and the stigma of generational responsibility related to genetic disorders. Disclosure to the child should be done at a developmentally appropriate level chosen by family and health providers, with the family as active partners in the child's health decisions (American Academy of Pediatrics, 1999a).
3. Knowledge-based information needed in all chronic illnesses:
   a. Disease-specific education: individualized for child and family
   b. Associated challenges or problems: prospective identification to avoid crisis
   c. Community resources: assistance and support beyond healthcare needs
   d. Stressors: the impact they play in the lives of the child and family
4. Among children diagnosed with other illnesses, the literature suggests that failure to provide age-appropriate disclosure of diagnosis results in depression, poor self-esteem, acting out behaviors, and poor family social interactions (Gerson et al., 2001). Clinicians routinely encourage families to start the disclosure process early but families affected by HIV are often reluctant to disclose.
5. Families are reluctant to disclose the diagnosis for the following reasons (American Academy of Pediatrics, 1999b):
   a. Perception that the child is not ready to hear the diagnosis
   b. The burden of knowledge and loss of innocence
   c. Parent/caregiver not ready to reveal their own diagnosis
   d. Guilt and shame related to acquisition and transmission of the disease
   e. Fear of social rejection should the child tell others
   f. Social, financial, and housing discrimination
6. Factors that prompt families to disclose:
   a. Death of other family members
   b. School problems
   c. Medicine adherence problems
   d. Child's direct question
   e. Spiritual issues
   f. Healthcare team partnership with family
   g. Unexpected disclosure by family member, friend, or staff
7. Children's issues: Children's concepts of health and illness vary depending upon their development and chronological age.
8. The literature does not fully address the adaptation and functioning of the child after disclosure of the diagnosis of HIV, but qualitative research has identified the following factors (Gerson et al., 2001):
   a. Feelings of being different from peers
   b. Identification of trusted friends who will not tell
   c. Sadness related to taking medicines

  d. Need to ask questions of family members and healthcare providers for better understanding

  e. Identification of self with new label—HIV/sick

9. Specific approaches for disclosure in child's environment

  a. Family: Families may enlist the help of the healthcare team when sharing the diagnosis. Illness or death of a parent or grandparent caregiver may require disease disclosure to other family members.

  b. School: Disclosure of disease diagnosis is not necessary due to right of confidentiality. However, the child or teen may need special educational resources for academic achievement, and the disclosure of the diagnosis would facilitate the resources. Disclosure to school can be limited to principal, guidance counselor, and teacher with confidentiality maintained.

  c. Church: The child or family's decision to disclose to a pastor or church members is an individual one. More churches are offering health ministries and promoting understanding of HIV/AIDS.

  d. Community: HIV/AIDS awareness is growing in communities, but there is still discrimination, and families are often the best judge of the disease disclosure acceptance in their communities. More community agencies are addressing the needs of families affected by HIV. Multidisciplinary teams can provide the families with social agency referrals and local resources throughout the continuum of health care.

10. Interval interventions: Several developmentally appropriate interventions can be incorporated in the disclosure process. These interventions may be delivered by a multidisciplinary team that includes the healthcare provider/clinic staff, social worker, child life specialist, and psychologist.

  a. Play therapy techniques:

   i) Drawing virus (bad cells), T cells (good cells), and medicines (destroyers that are stronger than bad cells and helpers of the good cells)

   ii) Medical play for painful procedures

   iii) Support groups for families, children, and teens that provide safe environments for role playing

  b. Assess parental/caregiver knowledge base to build confidence.

  c. Assess familial cultural beliefs that may affect the child's understanding and acceptance.

11. Nursing implications:

  a. Assess parent/caregiver plans for disclosure.

  b. Discuss family's perceptions of risks and benefits of disclosure.

  c. Assess child's developmental level and understanding of health and illness. The two may be unrelated.

  d. Assess cultural beliefs and spirituality.

  e. Assess social support within the family and in the community.

  f. Facilitate forging a partnership between family members and multidisciplinary healthcare team to develop a disclosure plan that includes a disclosure event date.

  g. Monitor post-disclosure coping of child and family.

  h. Establish time intervals to assess the child's and family's understanding of disease diagnosis.

i. Update the child's or youth's understanding of disease diagnosis as the child develops and matures.

j. Document in progress notes the stages of diagnosis disclosure and diagnosis understanding of the child or youth at each visit.

REFERENCES

American Academy of Pediatrics. (1999a). Issues related to human immunodeficiency virus transmission in schools, child care, medical settings, the home and community. *Pediatrics, 104*(2), 318–324.

American Academy of Pediatrics. (1999b). Disclosure of illness status to children and adolescents with HIV infection. *Pediatrics, 103*(1), 164–166.

Gerson, A. C., Joyner, M., Fosarelli, P., Butz, A., Wissow, L., Lee, S., et al. (2001). Disclosure of HIV diagnosis to children: When, where, why, and how. *Journal of Pediatric Health Care, 15*(4), 161–167.

10.6 END-OF-LIFE ISSUES

1. Definition: End of life occurs when the physical body ceases all function as a result of acute illness, trauma, or chronic deterioration related to HIV or other chronic illness. End-of-life, or palliative, care is the multidisciplinary approach to terminal illness and the dying process that focuses on symptom management rather than cure or prolonging life (Billings, 1998). End-of-life care in children is not as well developed as adult care, because society expects children to reach adulthood (American Academy of Pediatrics, 2000).

2. Disclosure of diagnosis to dying child
   a. Diagnosis disclosure and need for palliative care to children should be based on their developmental age, their previous knowledge and exposure to death and dying, and should include honest explanations. Reactions to their diagnosis and the dying process will also be influenced by developmental age (Ethier, 2007).
   b. Disclosure of HIV: Some children die without knowing that their illness is related to HIV. Although disclosure of HIV status to the child is often described as preferable, some parents and caregivers do not choose this option (De Santis & Colin, 2005). In working with children, it is possible to discuss dying without discussing HIV status. Often caregivers will allow discussion of organ failure (e.g., "Your heart is not working well"). If there are more questions, it is important to work with the family to formulate answers that are as truthful as possible (Ethier, 2007).

3. Assessment of child and family need regarding unfinished tasks
   a. When appropriate, discuss with the family and child the level of comfort with death.
   b. The child may need to write a will. The child may have specific toys or items he or she wishes to leave to someone specific. If the child is afraid of being forgotten, he or she can be given control of memories that will be left behind.
   c. The family may need assistance in deciding how they want to say good-bye. It can be helpful to explore their unfinished business.

4. Interventions for dying child: All interventions should be family centered, culturally appropriate, and multidisciplinary in focus (Ethier, 2007).
   a. Decision making

Do not resuscitate (DNR) versus medical interventions: Some people believe that discussing end-of-life decisions will hasten death. It may be helpful if the practitioner discusses death as part of the natural course of life. For those children and adolescents mature enough to do so, living wills can be a helpful tool in deciding the child's and family's wishes.

It is important to clarify what the medical staff is telling the child and family.

Clarify staff, family, and the child's beliefs regarding the child's condition and whether or not it can be reversed with interventions.

If the family or child disagrees with the healthcare provider, explore the basis for the alternate viewpoint (e.g., previous experiences, health belief, and culture).

Parent and child disagreement on healthcare issues may require the intervention of the healthcare team.

An ethics committee intervention may be warranted if there is a disagreement. These meetings can be helpful for practitioners to work through their own thoughts regarding the situation.

b. Home hospice versus institutional care

   i) Hospice

      Some families are unable to have the child die at home. Previous experiences with death are a common reason for this. Some may be afraid of the reactions of the other children or people in the home. Counseling regarding fears and expectations of what death may look like can be helpful as knowledge can decrease fear.

      Explore whether area hospice agencies have experience with children who are dying. If they do not, the family may need more support from the HIV care provider regarding issues specific to children.

      A home assessment by a hospice provider is often useful to determine whether the home is adaptable for a terminally ill person.

      If the family's support network is not in agreement with this plan, arrangements can be made that are not disruptive to the process.

   ii) Hospital, nursing home, or other institution

      (1) If a family decides that the child cannot die at home, plans can be put in place for a peaceful death in an institution.

      (2) Hospice care can be provided in an institution, if acceptable by that institution.

      (3) Discussions regarding invasive procedures and DNRs need to be conducted early in the process. This is often helpful in reducing the child's and the family's chance of the choice becoming a crisis. However, it is important for families to know that up until the time of death, there is always the possibility of changing one's mind. Some families may decide to take their loved one home right before death. Others may choose to bring their loved one into the hospital. Flexibility is helpful in assisting with the dying process. Although there are guidelines, very rarely are two deaths the same. Children and families are as different as their unique life experiences.

5. Comfort care

  a. Complementary therapies: These techniques may be learned by the practitioner, or other professionals may be called in to assist the child. They may also be helpful to the child's caregivers as routes of support and coping mechanisms. It is imperative that those who provide these therapies are appropriately trained.

b. Pain management: Pharmacological pain management may be used in conjunction with alternative therapies.

c. Behavioral health services: It is helpful to assess how the child and caregivers view behavioral health services and what types of providers may be acceptable to them. Sometimes home services may be more appropriate, depending on the family situation. Some families may prefer to have a social worker visit their home; they may not want to attend therapy. This will depend on the individualized goals for the child and family.

d. Other common symptoms that warrant intervention include dyspnea, agitation, nausea, vomiting, depression, anxiety, and grief (American Academy of Pediatrics, 2000).

REFERENCES

American Academy of Pediatrics. (2000). Palliative care for children. *Pediatrics, 106*(2), 351–357.

Billings, J. A. (1998). What is palliative care? *Journal of Palliative Medicine, 1*(1), 73–81.

De Santis, J. P., & Colin, J. M. (2005). Don't ask don't tell? The ethics of disclosure of HIV-status to perinatally-infected children. *Brazilian Journal of Sexually Transmitted Diseases, 17*(3), 181–188.

Ethier, A. M. (2007). Family-centered end-of-life care. In M. J. Hockenberry & D. Wilson (Eds.), *Wong's nursing care of infants and children* (8th ed., pp. 957–988). St. Louis, MO: Mosby-Elsevier.

CHAPTER 11

Nursing Management Issues

11.1 CASE MANAGEMENT

1. Definitions of case management
   a. "A process of consumer support in which clients are assisted in negotiating for the services and supports they want for themselves" (Anthony, Cohen, Farkas, & Cohen, 1988, p. 220)
   b. Based on the recognition that a trusting and empowering direct relationship between the client and the case manager is essential to expedite the client's use of services along a continuum of care and to restore or maintain the client's independent functioning to the fullest extent possible (Sowell & Meadows, 1994)
   c. A service delivered by a discipline-specific provider with knowledge and experience that enables patients to have available options and services needed to meet their physical, mental, and emotional health needs (National Case Management Task Force, Case Management Society of America, 1995)
   d. A dynamic and systematic collaborative approach to providing and coordinating healthcare services to a defined population; a participative process to identify and facilitate options and services for meeting individuals' health needs, while decreasing fragmentation and duplication of care and enhancing quality, cost-effective clinical outcomes; uses a framework consisting of five components: assessment, planning, implementation, evaluation, and interaction (ANA, 1988)
   e. A collaborative process that assesses, plans, implements, coordinates, monitors, and evaluates the options and services required to meet an individual's health needs, using communication and available resources to promote quality, cost-effective outcomes (Commission for Case Manager Certification, 1996)
2. Case management practice
   a. A case manager is someone who has knowledge of the disease process, human nature, and the healthcare delivery system (U.S. Department of Health and Human Services, Health Resources and Services Administration, HIV/AIDS Bureau, 2001).
   b. The practice of case management spans the entire healthcare spectrum, including pre-acute, acute, and post-acute settings, and the involvement of varied care providers, including nurses, social workers, rehabilitation counselors, physicians, and other health professionals (Tahan, 2006).
3. Case management models

a. Nursing model
   i)   Nursing case management uses the nursing process and an RN as the case manager; the RN functions as the facilitator, coordinator, and manager of patient care services and expected outcomes. Rather than providing direct patient care, the RN focuses on using assessment skills and disease-specific knowledge to plan care according to the identified patient needs (Cesta, Tahan, & Fink, 1998).
   ii) Nursing case management uses a holistic approach to planning care for the patient, the significant other, and the family—as well as their interaction in the community—and is used in the following settings: ambulatory care, acute care, home care, long-term care, rehabilitation, and managed care.
   iii) Nursing case management leads to a decrease in duplication of services and an increase in economic savings and extensions of available benefits over the disease continuum.
b. Medical model
   i)   The medical model uses a medical provider (e.g., a physician, advanced nurse practitioner, or physician assistant) as the coordinator/gatekeeper of patient care services (medical care).
   ii) Potential deficiencies of this model are fragmentation of care and duplication of services. Additionally, because this model is provider driven, aspects of care other than the presenting medical problem may not be addressed due to a lack of knowledge of available services and resources.
c. Community-based/public health model
   i)   These models are focused on primary care and primary prevention and are predominantly focused on well and at-risk individuals or those who have a potential need for healthcare services.
   ii) Goals of these models are to support individuals to minimally maintain their present physical condition through use of disease-prevention methods and to empower them to maximize their optimal level of wellness through use of community resources.
d. Diagnosis-related/population-based model
   i)   This model focuses on a group of patients with a specific diagnosis. The management of the selected diagnosis may need improvement in the areas of cost and quality of care, or it may be at high risk for financial loss or have potential for revenue.
   ii) Criteria to be considered when deciding which population to case manage could include volume of the patient population, cost and complexity of care, the need for multiple services, and length of stay in an acute care facility (Tahan & Cesta, 1995).
e. Psychosocial model
   i)   Social work case management is a method of providing services whereby a professional social worker assesses the needs of the client and the client's family, when appropriate, and arranges, coordinates, monitors, evaluates, and advocates for a package of multiple services to meet the specific client's complex needs (Case Management Standards Work Group, National Association of Social Workers, 1992). Services provided may include the following:
        (1) Assessing housing and food needs of the client
        (2) Assisting the client in preparing a DNR, medical power of attorney, durable power of attorney, and advance directives

   (3) Investigating all sources of funding for medical care and entitlement programs that may provide coverage for medications, such as AIDS drug assistance programs (ADAP), drug studies, and vendor drug and compassionate use programs

4. Benefits of case management in the HIV epidemic
 a. Access to care
  i) Definition: ability and ease of patients to obtain health care when needed
  ii) A variety of issues are involved with access and quality of care, such as the following:
   (1) Locating quality case management that is also convenient for the service user
   (2) Maintaining a central location, with both private and public transportation access
   (3) Creating one system that provides both medical and psychosocial case managers
   (4) Providing specific cultural needs, such as translation
   (5) Providing staff members of both genders who are ethnically diverse
 b. Continuity of care
  i) Definition: seamless system of care, over the disease continuum, that supports the best patient outcomes
  ii) Involves use of an interdisciplinary team approach, including medical providers, nurses, social workers, nutritionists, pharmacists, client advocates, pastoral care, and others as needed. The primary goal of the team is to evaluate the effectiveness of a patient-supported plan of care. The team approach allows for communication exchanges among disciplines to appropriately evaluate and update the care plan as needed, without missing important data.
 c. Decreased fragmentation of care and decreased duplication of services
  i) With continual assessment of the patient's plan of care, the case manager is able to observe the progress of the plan and, with the patient, decide when the patient is ready to access services; with the patient in agreement, the possibility of a positive outcome is increased.
  ii) Communication is a tool used by the case manager to involve clients in the plan of care and allow them to decide which outcomes are appropriate for them.
 d. Support
  i) Many locales have established specific HIV support groups. However, because needed services may not be directly related to the HIV diagnosis, clear goals of care are necessary to address areas of the patient's life that require support. With a holistic approach to care, assessment helps determine the type of support needed and allows the case manager to appropriately direct care and resources.
  ii) Follow-up is necessary to ensure that the patient has followed through and actually accessed the service; the case manager provides encouragement and referral to services as new needs are identified.
 e. Education
  i) Education and knowledge empower clients and allow them to be active participants in their own plan of care.
  ii) Client education is often needed on the following topics:
   (1) Adherence techniques to enhance outcomes of drug regimens and medical treatment
   (2) Nutritional assessment and dietary counseling on implications of increased caloric requirements and on potential food-drug interactions

      (3) Effective navigation of the healthcare delivery system

      (4) Eligibility requirements for entitlement programs

      (5) Other needs, such as visual screening, stress management, and self-care and wellness strategies

5. Limitations of case management

   a. Access and quality of care issues

      i) Barriers to care may include difficulty in finding an educated provider; issues related to funding sources (e.g., third-party source/insurance, Medicare/Medicaid, managed care or public funding) or the healthcare delivery system; and social stigmatization.

6. Development of standards and protocols for case managers

   a. Education level and experience are key to quality of care for patients.

   b. Case managers should identify both strengths and weaknesses of the systems within their service area.

   c. Development and ongoing evaluation of all external referral sources across a wide network of services and providers should be conducted.

REFERENCES

American Nurses Association (ANA). (1988). *American Nurses Association Task Force on Case Management*. Kansas City, MO: Author.

Anthony, W. A., Cohen, M., Farkas, M., & Cohen, B. F. (1988). The chronically mental ill case management—More than a response to a dysfunctional system. *Community Mental Health Journal, 24*(3), 219–228.

Case Management Standards Work Group, National Association of Social Workers. (1992). *NASW standards for social work case management*. Washington, DC: Author. Retrieved April 1, 2009, from http://www.socialworkers.org/practice/standards/sw_case_mgmt.asp#intro

Cesta, T. G., Tahan, H. A., & Fink, L. F. (Eds.). (1998). *The case manager's survival guide: Winning strategies for clinical practice*. St. Louis, MO: Mosby.

Commission for Case Manager Certification. (1996). *CCM certification guide*. Rolling Meadows, IL: Author.

National Case Management Task Force, Case Management Society of America. (1995). *Standards of practice for case management*. Little Rock, AR: Author.

Sowell, R., & Meadows, T. (1994). An integrated case management model: Developing standards, evaluation, and outcomes. *Nursing Administration Quarterly, 18*(2), 53–64.

Tahan, H. A., & Cesta, T. G. (1995). Developing case management plans using a quality improvement model. *Journal of Nursing Administration, 24*(12), 49–58.

U.S. Department of Health and Human Services, Health Resources and Services Administration, HIV/AIDS Bureau. (2001). *Outcomes evaluation technical assistance guide: Case management outcomes, Titles I and II of the Ryan White CARE Act*. Washington, DC: Author.

11.2 ETHICAL AND LEGAL CONCERNS

1. Since the early days of the HIV/AIDS epidemic, ethical and legal issues have raised questions and concerns in relation to HIV/AIDS care; these issues have been due, in part, to the characteristics of HIV disease, the nature of the epidemic, and the nature of the populations infected with and affected by HIV.

2. Four principles are commonly used by healthcare professionals in dealing with ethical and legal issues in HIV care (Beauchamp & Childress, 2009):

   a. Nonmaleficence: avoiding harm or injury to others
   b. Beneficence: promoting the good or welfare of others
   c. Respect for autonomy: respecting the liberty, privacy, and self-determination of others
   d. Justice: treating others fairly
3. Other relevant principles include fidelity (keeping promises, contracts) and veracity (telling the truth).
4. Nurses caring for HIV-positive people and others affected by HIV must be aware of these ethical principles when evaluating their actions and the actions of others. Decision making is also guided by state and federal laws; thus, ethical and legal issues are closely related and often interrelated.
5. Other common approaches to ethical decision making in health care have been described (Lo, 2005) and include the following:
   a. Consequentialist approach: Actions are judged by the rightness or wrongness of their consequences (also described as utilitarian approach).
   b. Deontological approach: Actions in and of themselves may be wrong, regardless of the outcome (e.g., lying, breaching confidentiality).
   c. Case-based approach (casuistry): This involves comparing a current case to exemplar or paradigmatic ethical cases.
   d. Care-based ethics: Originally described by feminist ethicists and espoused by nurses, this ethical approach seeks to look beyond abstract, ethical principles and takes into account relationships and attempts to avoid interpersonal conflict.
6. Specific ethical issues in HIV care
   a. Individual choice: autonomy and self-determination
      i)   Individual choice is based on the ethical principle of respect for autonomy; autonomy deals with one's right to self-determination (Beauchamp & Childress, 2001; Lo, 2005).
      ii)   Autonomy incorporates the concepts of confidentiality, informed consent, the right to accept and to refuse medical treatment, privacy, and disclosure.
      iii) Autonomous individuals are free to choose and to self-govern.
      iv)   Within the context of health care, informed consent assists a person to voluntarily choose a course of action.
      v)   Other elements of informed consent require that the person understands the information, mutually participates in the decision making and does not merely sign the form, and accepts the plan for care freely and without coercion.
      vi)   Autonomy requires a person to be competent to have decision-making capacity.
      vii) Healthcare providers are obligated to protect persons with diminished capacity, as well as those who have never had the capacity for decision making.
   b. Inequitable access to care
      i)   Disparity has been noted in the United States in relation to access to health care, research participation, and experimental therapies.
      ii)   Many HIV-infected patients rely on Medicaid; others have no healthcare insurance, which has a major impact on their ability to get necessary care and therapies.
      iii) Managed care may also complicate the ability of patients who need complex or expensive treatment to get adequate care.

iv) All states participate in AIDS Drug Assistance Programs (ADAPs), which provide healthcare services, including medications, to patients; nurses are in an excellent position to advocate for access to these entitlements (see http://www.atdn.org/access/states/index.html for individual state resources).

v) Nurses should also advocate for their patients' access to clinical trials (see http://www.aidsinfo.nih.gov/ClinicalTrials and http://www.cpcra.org).

vi) People of color and women in the United States have been documented as not having equal access to HIV therapy and clinical drug trials (Cargill, 2006; Cargill, Stone, & Robinson, 2004; Krawczyk, Funkhouser, Kilby, & Vermund, 2006).

vii) Ninety-five percent of people with HIV/AIDS live in developing countries; HIV/AIDS is the leading cause of death in sub-Saharan Africa and the fourth cause of death worldwide; only 23% of people in the world who need HIV antiretroviral treatment currently receive it (UNAIDS, 2006).

viii) HIV has placed an additional financial burden on economically deficient healthcare systems in underdeveloped countries. It has taken 25 years to mount a significant global response to the HIV epidemic (UNAIDS, 2006).

ix) Antiretroviral therapy is extremely expensive, and global issues remain significant regarding cost and access to HIV therapy.

c. Privacy, confidentiality, and disclosure

i) Protecting the privacy of patients and safeguarding information that should remain confidential is central to maintaining autonomy and nonmaleficence.

ii) The following questions are designed to help healthcare providers consider the best ways to strike an appropriate balance among beneficence, nonmaleficence, justice, and autonomy (Green, Derlega, Yep, & Petronio, 2003):

(1) What approaches to teaching risk reduction or avoidance behavior respect the patient's autonomy and privacy?

(2) Does anyone besides the person being tested have a right or need to know the results?

(3) How does one reconcile the duty to warn with the duty to maintain privacy and confidentiality?

(4) Should results be disclosed only with the consent of the person being tested?

(5) What criteria are used for overriding confidentiality? (Not all ethical models will support all criteria.)

(6) What safeguards protect the confidentiality of patient information?

(7) How does a healthcare worker maintain privacy within the context of third-party notification policies? Mandatory testing? Mandatory names reporting laws? Partner notification requirements?

(8) What ethical models/principles can be used to establish that partners have a right to information about a person's HIV status if the infected person doesn't want them to know?

(9) What ethical models/principles would make it difficult to establish such rights?

(10) How is partner notification accomplished?

(11) How does duty to warn compare with privilege to warn? (Consequences of warning others may include violence.)

(12) How does disclosure violate the principle of justice in these situations?

(13) How can the healthcare worker assist patients in making disclosure decisions?

d. Discrimination and worker protection

    i)   The incidence of HIV/AIDS is disproportional among minority and disenfranchised groups.

    ii)   HIV/AIDS still carries a stigma not attached to many other serious diseases.

    iii)   To protect against or minimize discrimination, nurses must be aware of persons and groups that remain most vulnerable to obvious forms of discrimination.

    iv)   Nurses must consider the following about groups of HIV-infected patients:

        (1)   Which groups are most likely to suffer a significant loss of autonomy in the healthcare system?

        (2)   Which remain the most vulnerable to discrimination and thus the injustices involving privacy and confidentiality?

        (3)   Which are most likely to face significant discrimination in the workplace?

e. Estate, will, and advance care planning

    i)   Planning for the future entails attending to one's future healthcare needs, to a time when autonomous decision making is no longer possible, as well as to the care of one's dependent minor children, and disposition of one's tangible assets.

    ii)   Estate and will planning are appropriately carried out with the assistance of an attorney. Planning should happen early in the illness trajectory and be delayed until the patient is near to death.

    iii)   Future care of dependent children needs advance consideration, standby guardianship and custody arrangements for minors require legal proceedings, and some patients may need volunteer legal services if unable to afford legal costs. Again, planning should ideally begin early because hospitalization may occur urgently, with no time for making these legal arrangements.

    iv)   Advance care planning, enabled by the Patient Self-Determination Act of 1991, describes the process of making advance directives (Colby, 2006; Meisel & Cerminara, 2004).

    v)   Advance directives may include assigning a surrogate decision maker for healthcare decisions, called a *healthcare proxy* or *durable power of attorney for health care*, as well as providing directions for types of care desired (treatment directives), called a *living will* or *do not resuscitate (DNR) order* (Fins, 2006; Ulrich, 1999).

    vi)   Some states require that a person provide specific advance instructions (also referred to as "clear and convincing evidence") about withholding or withdrawing artificial food and hydration; a proxy decision maker in these states may not make decisions about these medical treatments.

    vii)   Living wills are not recognized in all states but may suffice to provide the "clear and convincing evidence" needed in a court proceeding.

    viii)   A DNR order is another form of treatment directive, one that authorizes withholding cardiopulmonary resuscitation (CPR) in the event of cardiopulmonary arrest.

    ix)   In many terminally ill AIDS patients, a DNR order is completely appropriate, and a focus on comfort care and palliation of symptoms is often desired by patients and families at the end of life.

    x)   HIV patients may be wary of signing advance directives because of a mistrust of the medical system (Jones, Messmer, Charron, & Parns, 2002).

    xi)   Other researchers have described situations in which patients may specifically *not* want someone to act as their surrogate decision maker. These antiproxies were often legal next of kin (Martin, Thiel, & Singer, 1999).

f. Ethical issues and the public health

    i)   The goal of prevention and public health campaigns includes HIV-positive and HIV-negative persons and focuses on keeping the whole community healthy. When considering public health interventions, one must ask the following:

        (1)   What approaches to teaching risk reduction or avoidance behavior respects autonomy and privacy?

        (2)   What ethical reasoning is used to support the provision of clean needles to drug users or condoms to teenagers?

        (3)   What ethical reasoning is used to oppose such programs?

        (4)   What are the issues that face risk reduction programs for children?

        (5)   What risk reduction approaches are supported by research?

    ii)   Nurses and other healthcare professionals may encounter HIV-infected individuals who continue with unsafe behaviors:

        (1)   How should healthcare professionals respond to those who practice unsafe behaviors that put others in jeopardy?

        (2)   How can respecting autonomy and culture be used to justify a minimalist approach to intervention?

        (3)   How can the utilitarian framework ("the rightness of an action based on consequences") be used to justify a more interventionist approach?

        (4)   Is there a role for compulsory testing for those who engage in unsafe behaviors? When might compulsory testing be protective of public health? What are the negative implications of this? In what instances is it more political than scientific?

    iii)   Testing of childbearing women and newborn infants

    iv)   Reasoned ethical positions can produce contradictory answers to questions.

    v)   What information and which ethical model/principles support your positions on the following questions? What information and which ethical model/principles would support contrary positions?

        (1)   What advice should an HIV-infected woman receive about pregnancy?

        (2)   With data that demonstrate the effectiveness of prenatal AZT in reducing the rate of transmission of HIV from mother to fetus, should all pregnant women be HIV-antibody tested?

        (3)   Should HIV testing be mandatory or voluntary?

        (4)   If the HIV antibody test is positive, is there an obligation to provide the patient with access to AZT?

        (5)   Is there an obligation for a mother to take AZT?

g. Ethical issues related to clinical trials

    i)   Disparity has been noted in access to research participation and experimental therapies.

ii)   People with HIV infection are often willing to take the risks of unproven therapies, including participation in underground buyers' clubs, expanded access programs, and clinical trials.

iii)   The exclusion of certain groups from research has been seen as discrimination rather than protection; access to clinical trials is generally seen as a benefit.

iv)   AIDS activists have challenged attitudes and some regulations regarding research participation and access to experimental therapies as too restrictive and discriminatory.

v)   Nurses are in an excellent position to advocate for access to care and to clinical trials for their patients.

vi)   In addition, trial design, rigid exclusion criteria, the use of placebos, double blinding, and clinical endpoints have been challenged by AIDS activists, researchers, alternative practitioners, and some pharmaceutical companies.

vii)   Scientific conflicts of interest, scientific integrity, competition in HIV research, and the role of economics in research have become important areas of concern.

viii)   The demand for quicker results, more effective clinical trials, and scientific integrity have led to stricter oversight by safety monitoring boards.

ix)   Community representatives have become more involved in decisions about research through community advisory boards.

x)   The right for people with terminal diagnoses to access investigational drugs has not been sustained by the courts (Abigail Alliance, 2008; Moller, 2006).

h. Obligation to provide care

    i)   According to the American Nurses Association's (ANA's) first provision of the *Code of Ethics for Nurses,* "The nurse, in all professional relationships, practices with compassion and respect for the inherent dignity, worth and uniqueness of every individual, unrestricted by consideration of social or economic status, personal attributes, or the nature of health problems" (2001, p. 7).

    ii)   An ethic of care emphasizes caring for others and their significant relationships and recognizing the special obligations toward and a willingness to act on behalf of people with whom one has a relationship (Gordon, Benner, & Noddings, 1996).

i. Protecting healthcare workers

    i)   If standards of practice include universal precautions, are healthcare workers protected by knowledge of a patient's HIV status?

    ii)   What changes in purchasing practices would better protect healthcare workers from occupational exposure to infections?

    iii)   What infectious agents are most responsible for occupational morbidity and mortality among healthcare workers?

j. Euthanasia, assisted suicide, and suicide

    i)   Euthanasia refers to the deliberate administration of medication to end a life (Quill, 2001).

    ii)   Suicide refers to the deliberate taking of one's own life.

    iii)   Euthanasia (except in the situation of capital punishment) and suicide are illegal acts in the United States, except assisted suicide in Oregon.

    iv)   Assisted suicide concerns providing patients with the means to end their life should they choose to do so (King & Jordan-Welch, 2003).

v)   Assisted suicide has been a passionately debated topic in recent years and is currently legal in the United States only in Oregon and Washington State; the right to die is not guaranteed by the U.S. Constitution (Vacco v. Quill, 1997) but may be authorized by individual states.

vi)   The ANA condones neither active euthanasia (1994a) nor assisted suicide (1994b).

vii)   ANAC's "Scope and Standards of Practice" definitively endorses palliative care "throughout the course of the [HIV] disease state" (2007b, p. 22) but does not have an explicit position on assisted suicide.

viii)   Voluntarily ceasing intake of hydration and nutrition has been described as an alternative to assisted suicide (Harvath et al., 2004; Schwarz, 2004).

ix)   Both ANA and ANAC wholeheartedly encourage pursuit of palliative care practices, which include aggressive attention to pain management, psychosocial, and spiritual care (ANAC, 2006, 2007a, 2007b; see also Ferrell & Coyle, 2001).

x)   Expert, compassionate care at the end of life is now recognized as a critical component of the wellness–illness continuum (Lynn, Schuster, & Kabcenell, 2000).

xi)   Although palliative care is increasingly recognized as a standard of care throughout the trajectory of the illness for patients with many chronic diseases, people with HIV/AIDS are still significantly undertreated with regard to pain and symptom management (ANAC, 2007b; Harding et al., 2005).

xii)   ANAC's position statement on palliative care endorses the following tenets (2006, para. 1):

(1)   Palliative care should be part of the comprehensive care of all patients with HIV/AIDS.

(2)   Palliative care should be integrated into the standard of care for patients with HIV/AIDS and their families from the first diagnosis of HIV until death.

(3)   Every provider should be able to provide or refer patients for palliative care, while simultaneously providing therapeutic treatment.

(4)   Palliative care should be integrated into education about HIV/AIDS for all providers.

(5)   Insurance plans, including Medicaid and Medicare, should eliminate any barriers to obtaining palliative care.

(6)   Research in this area is lacking and should be supported and encouraged.

REFERENCES

Abigail Alliance for Better Access to Developmental Drugs. (2008). *Organizational website.* Retrieved March 4, 2009, from http://www.abigail-alliance.org/

American Nurses Association (ANA). (1994a). *Position Statement: Active euthanasia.* Silver Spring, MD: Author.

American Nurses Association (ANA). (1994b). *Position Statement: Assisted suicide.* Silver Spring, MD: Author.

American Nurses Association (ANA). (2001). *Code of ethics for nurses with interpretive statements.* Silver Spring, MD: Author.

Association of Nurses in AIDS Care (ANAC). (2008, August). *Position Statement: Palliative care.* Retrieved March 4, 2009, from http://www.nursesinaidscare.org/i4a/pages/index.cfm?pageid=3300

Association of Nurses in AIDS Care (ANAC). (2007a). *HIV/AIDS nursing: Scope and standards of practice.* Silver Spring, MD: American Nurses Association.

Association of Nurses in AIDS Care (ANAC). (2007b). *Position statement: Pain management for persons living with HIV/AIDS.* Retrieved October 16, 2007, from http://www.anacnet.org/media/pdfs/PS_ANAC_Pain_Management_Rev_01_2007.pdf

Beauchamp, T. L., & Childress, J. F. (2009). *Principles of biomedical ethics* (6th ed.). New York: Oxford University Press.

Cargill, V. A. (2006). Management of women with HIV infection. *Advanced Studies in Medicine, 6*(3A), S130–S137, S145–S147.

Cargill, V. A., Stone, V. E., & Robinson, M. R. (2004). HIV treatment in African Americans: Challenges and opportunities. *Journal of Black Psychology, 30*(1), 24–39.

Colby, W. H. (2006). *Unplugged: Reclaiming our right to die in America.* New York: American Management Association.

Ferrell, B. R., & Coyle, N. (2001). *Textbook of palliative nursing.* New York: Oxford University Press.

Fins, J. J. (2006). *A palliative ethic of care: Clinical wisdom at life's end.* Sudbury, MA: Jones and Bartlett.

Gordon, S., Benner, P. E., & Noddings, N. (1996). *Caregiving: Readings in knowledge, practice, ethics, and politics.* Philadelphia: University of Pennsylvania Press.

Green, K., Derlega, V. J., Yep, G. A., & Petronio, S. (2003). *Privacy and disclosure of HIV in interpersonal relationships: A sourcebook for researchers and practitioners.* Mahwah, NJ: Lawrence Erlbaum Associates.

Harding, R., Easterbrook, P., Higginson, I. J., Karus, D., Raveis, V. H., & Marconi, K. (2005). Access and equity in HIV/AIDS palliative care: A review of the evidence and responses. *Palliative Medicine, 19*(3), 251–258.

Harvath, T. A., Miller, L. L., Goy, E., Jackson, A., Delorit, M., & Ganzini, L. (2004). Voluntary refusal of food and fluids: Attitudes of Oregon hospice nurses and social workers. *International Journal of Palliative Nursing, 10*(5), 236–241.

Jones, S. G., Messmer, P. R., Charron, S. A., & Parns, M. (2002). HIV-positive women and minority patients' satisfaction with inpatient hospital care. *AIDS Patient Care and STDs, 16*(3), 127–134.

King, P., & Jordan-Welch, M. (2003). Nurse-assisted suicide: Not an answer in end-of-life care. *Issues in Mental Health Nursing, 24*(1), 45–57.

Krawczyk, C., Funkhouser, E., Kilby, J. M., & Vermund, S. (2006). Delayed access to HIV diagnosis and care: Special concerns for the Southern United States. *AIDS Care: Psychological & Socio-Medical Aspects of AIDS/HIV, 18*(Suppl. 1), S35–S44.

Lo, B. (2005). *Resolving ethical dilemmas: A guide for clinicians* (3rd ed.). Philadelphia: Lippincott Williams & Wilkins.

Lynn, J., Schuster, J. L., & Kabcenell, A. (2000). *Improving care for the end of life: A sourcebook for health care managers and clinicians.* New York: Oxford University Press.

Martin, D. K., Thiel, E. C., & Singer, P. A. (1999). A new model of advance care planning: Observations from people with HIV. *Archives of Internal Medicine, 159*(1), 86–92.

Meisel, A. & Cerminara, K. L. (2004). *The right to die: The law of end-of-life decisionmaking* (3rd ed.). New York: Aspen.

Moller, M. (2006, May 9). Scrutinizing the rights of the terminally ill. *The Washington Post.* Retrieved May 20, 2009, from http://www.washingtonpost.com/wp=dyn/content/article/2006/05/08/AR2006050801131.html

Quill, T. E. (2001). *Caring for patients at the end of life: Facing an uncertain future together.* New York: Oxford University Press.

Schwarz, J. K. (2004). Responding to persistent requests for assistance in dying: A phenomenological inquiry. *International Journal of Palliative Nursing, 10*(5), 225-235.

Ulrich, L. P. (1999). *The Patient Self-Determination Act: Meeting the challenges in patient care.* Washington, DC: Georgetown University Press.

UNAIDS. (2006). *2006 Report on the global AIDS epidemic.* Retrieved April 2, 2009, from http://www.unaids.org/en/KnowledgeCentre/HIVData/GlobalReport/2006/default.asp

Vacco v. Quill, 117 S. Ct. 2293 (1997). Retrieved March 4, 2009, from http://supct.law.cornell.edu/supct/html/95-1858.ZO.html

11.3 PREVENTING TRANSMISSION OF HIV IN PATIENT CARE SETTINGS

1. Infection control
   a. Infection control is necessary to help ensure a safe environment for patients and healthcare workers (HCWs).

   b. When caring for patients, infection control practitioners recommend a two-tier system of isolation precautions, using both standard precautions and transmission-based precautions.

     i)   Standard precautions

        (1) All body fluids to be treated as if potentially infectious with HIV, hepatitis B (HBV), and hepatitis C (HCV)

        (2) Emphasizes use of appropriate hand-washing techniques, barrier equipment, and engineering controls or devices to reduce blood-borne pathogen transmission to HCWs from clients.

        (3) Used in situations in which exposure to blood or potentially infectious body fluids is anticipated; may be combined with transmission-based precautions (see below) if the hospitalized patient has or is suspected of having a highly transmissible disease.

     ii)   Transmission-based precautions

        (1) Designed to care for patients with known or suspected infections that can be transmitted by airborne, droplet, or contact modes

          (a) Droplet precautions: used when organism is transmitted by infected droplets that could come in contact with HCW's eyes or mucous membranes; HCWs are to wear gloves, regular mask and gown.

          (b) Airborne precautions: used to prevent transmission from airborne infectious agents, such as tuberculosis (TB), and require patient placement in a private room with negative air flow; HCWs must wear particulate respirator masks.

          (c) Contact precautions: used when organism is transmitted by direct contact; requires patient placement in a private room with disposable medical supplies; HCWs should wear gloves, mask, and gowns.

   c. Hand washing is one of the most effective methods to prevent transmission of blood-borne pathogens.

2. Postexposure prophylaxis

   a. Transmission of blood-borne pathogens, especially HIV, HBV, and HCV, is a concern for HCWs and patients; the diseases differ in modes of transmission, development of disease, and disease progression.

   b. All hospitals should have procedures for HCWs to report occupational exposures to blood and other body fluids. These procedures should include counseling and testing for potentially infectious diseases and, when appropriate, offering medications for the disease.

   c. Transmission of HIV, HBV, and HCV

     i)   Risk of transmission of HIV, HBV, and HCV from a hollow bore needle to HCW is 0.3%, 6–30%, and 1.8%, respectively (CDC, 2001).

     ii)   In the United States there have been a relatively small number of documented HIV infections from occupationally related injuries (CDC, 2001; Panlilo, Cardo, Grohskopf, Heneine, & Ross, 2005).

     iii) Factors that assist in determining risk of an injury include mode of transmission (whether the injury occurred with a percutaneous device or with a sharp or blunt instrument) and contact with skin or mucous membrane.

     iv) Assessment of percutaneous/sharp injury risk includes the following:

        (1) Determining the quantity of blood involved, the type of needle or sharp instrument (hollow bore/solid/size), and the depth of puncture

        (2) Establishing patient factors, including ascertaining whether the device came from use in a vein or artery, whether the source patient is in early HIV seroconversion or has advanced AIDS, and the patient's most recent viral load. The patient's most recent viral load will be useful to guide treatment for the HCW.

    v) Contact to non-intact skin exposures has not been documented with precise transmission estimates.

    vi) Risk following mucous membrane exposure is estimated to be 0.09%.

  d. Considerations and recommendations for post-exposure prophylaxis (PEP) for HIV:

    i) Early pathogenesis of HIV infection may theoretically be prevented by the administration of antiretroviral therapy within a few hours following exposure.

    ii) The risks and benefits of PEP must be thoroughly explained to the HCW. The use of PEP after an occupational exposure is not 100% effective in preventing HIV infection (CDC, 2001; Panlilo et al., 2005).

    iii) Antiretroviral therapy: All classes of antiretroviral medications could potentially be used to treat occupational exposure. Drug selection depends on several factors: the type of injury and device, the source patient's HIV viral load, and, when possible, the source patient's past and current regimens and resistance tests.

    iv) Nearly 50% of HCWs taking PEP have experienced adverse symptoms, and about 33% stop taking PEP because of adverse symptoms; a higher discontinuation rate was associated with triple combination therapy versus a two-drug regimen; reported symptoms included nausea, malaise, anorexia, and headache (CDC, 2001; Panlilo et al., 2005).

    v) PEP may be prescribed to pregnant women, except for efavirenz (Sustiva) because of its teratogenic effects.

    vi) The use of rapid testing of the source patient's blood (which will yield results in 15 minutes) helps inform the decision of PEP initiation and prevents unnecessary side effects from drug therapy (Panlilo et al., 2005).

3. OSHA regulations

  a. The incidence of occupationally acquired HIV infection created a need for the government to mandate safety programs in medical settings to protect HCWs and patients. In 1991, OSHA required all hospitals and medical facilities in the private setting to develop a blood-borne pathogen plan to educate HCWs about transmission of blood-borne pathogens, to communicate to HCWs how to avoid exposure, to use protective equipment, to introduce and evaluate engineering controls, and to provide medical care and follow-up for an injured employee.

  b. Blood-borne pathogen plans include engineering controls (devices and instruments) and work practice controls (policies and procedures) to reduce exposures.

    i) Engineering controls: personal protective equipment (PPE) must be made available, including gloves, gowns, and eye and foot protection to help prevent exposures. PPE must be the proper size for the employee. Particulate respirator masks must be worn in areas where TB is presumed or diagnosed.

    ii) Work practice controls are written policies and procedures that inform an HCW as to what type of PPE should be worn and the type of device necessary to perform care duties.

    iii) Sharp disposal units must be puncture resistant, labeled with the biohazard logo, and placed in convenient locations for HCWs. It is recommended that all boxes be no higher than 51 inches from the ground, within 6 feet of the treatment area, stabilized to prevent falling over, and replaced when three-fourths full.

iv) Patient placement is based on patient diagnosis. HIV/AIDS diagnosis by itself is not reason for isolation or placement in a private room; patients with communicable diseases, such as TB, require a private room with negative air flow. Table 11.3a details precautions for HIV-infected clients based on clinical syndromes.

v) There are no restrictions for food delivery to patients' rooms; reusable dishes and silverware can be used; however, appropriate washing and drying of dishes should be performed to kill any pathogens.

vi) Laboratory specimens should be placed in plastic tubes and containers and then placed in a labeled, biohazard, plastic leakproof bag. Minimal handing of specimens is recommended. During transportation to the lab, specimens should be placed in a covered leakproof container.

vii) Cleaners and disinfectants should be Environmental Protection Agency (EPA) approved and should be bactericidal, fungicidal, and tuberculocidal. In the home setting, patients may use diluted bleach or over-the-counter cleansing agents.

viii) Medical waste is disposed differently from general waste; depending upon state regulations, medical waste should be placed in a red bag with the biohazard symbol; these bags are designed to be thicker for protection against splitting.

ix) Biohazard labels must be placed on containers of blood, utility room doors, waste containers, and any other area or containers that contain blood or body fluids.

x) Linens are treated as infectious. Gloves must be worn while changing linen; linens are then placed in an impervious laundry bag. Industrial washing will remove potentially infectious material.

xi) Medical emergencies should be assessed, documented, and treated by the employer; PEP may be necessary, as well as HBV vaccine and immunoglobins; and policies and procedures for patient and employee serial testing should be implemented. The employer is responsible for payment for HCW and patient testing.

xii) Employers will educate their staff initially, and then annually, regarding the bloodborne pathogen plan and newly approved engineering controls and work practice controls. Employees hired into a position that places them in direct or indirect care of patients or body fluids must be offered the HBV vaccine within 10 days of employment (OSHA, 2006).

Table 11.3a Type of Precaution by Clinical Syndrome in HIV-Infected Patients

Clinical Syndrome	Precaution Required
Diarrhea	Contact
Respiratory with TB signs and symptoms	Airborne
Diagnosed with *S. pneumoniea, H. influenza,* influenza, or varicella zoster	Droplet and contact
Draining wounds, ulcers, and so forth	Contact

Source: Adapted from Sande, Eliopoulos, Moellering, & Gilbert, 2005.

REFERENCES

Centers for Disease Control and Prevention (CDC). (2001). Updated U.S. Public Health Service guidelines for the management of occupational exposures to HBV, HCV, and HIV and recommendations for postexposure prophylaxis. *Morbidity and Mortality Weekly Report, 50*(RR-11), 1–42.

Panlilo, A. L., Cardo, D. M., Grohskopf, L. A., Heneine, W., & Ross, S. C. (2005). Updated U.S. Public Health Service guidelines for the management of occupational exposures to HIV and recommendations for post-exposure prophylaxis. *Morbidity and Mortality Weekly Report, 54*(RR-09), 1–17.

Occupational Safety and Health Administration (OSHA). (2006). *Bloodborne pathogens 1910.1030.* Retrieved February 1, 2008, from http://www.osha.gov/pls/oshaweb/owadisp.show_document?p_table=STANDARDS&p_id=10051

Sande, M. E., Eliopoulos, G. M., Moellering, R. C., & Gilbert, D. N. (2005). *The Sanford guide to HIV/AIDS therapy.* (14th ed.). Sperryville, VA: Antimicrobial Therapy, Inc.

Selected Lab Values

Type of Test	Normal Value/Range	Comments
Tests of HIV-1		
Enzyme Immunoassay (EIA or ELISA) for HIV Antibodies	Nonreactive	• The test has sensitivity and specificity rates of > 98%. • HIV-antibody screening test; if positive, is confirmed with Western Blot • False negatives are usually due to testing in the window period; the interval from infection to reactive EIA averages 10–14 days. • Seroconversion may take 3 to 4 weeks, but virtually all individuals with HIV seroconvert within 6 months.
Western Blot (WB)	Negative: No bands	• HIV-antibody test used to confirm a reactive EIA; a positive WB shows reactivity to bands gp41+ gp120/160 or p24 + gp120/160. • An indeterminate test occurs when there is the presence of any band pattern that does not meet criteria for positive results (see previous discussion). • "False" positive EIA and WB in low-prevalence populations are very rare and are most often due to technical errors.
Rapid HIV Antibody Screening Tests		
Oral Fluids and Blood OraQuick Advance Rapid HIV-1/2 AntibodyTest Orasure Technologies, Inc.	Nonreactive	• OraQuick first received FDA approval 11/2002 as a rapid point-of-care test for use on fingerstick blood samples; designed to detect antibodies to HIV-1 within 20 minutes; later received FDA approval for venipuncture whole blood and

Type of Test	Normal Value/Range	Comments
		plasma; in 2004 OraQuick Advance received FDA approval for use with oral fluid and for detection of HIV-1 and HIV-2.
		• Has reported sensitivity of 99.6% and specificity of 100% using fingerstick whole-blood specimens; reported sensitivity of 99.3% and specificity of 99.8% using oral fluid.
		• Reactive (preliminary positive) must be confirmed.
		• Estimated time to set up and conduct test = < 5 minutes (< 10 min. for plasma) plus 20-minute wait time; window period for reading results (from last step of testing process) 20–40 minutes.
		• For oral fluid testing, the oral fluid sample is collected by swabbing the gums with the paddle-shaped device; test device is then added to the developer vial.
		• A red line at both the test and control locations indicates a valid reactive test result; a red line in only the control location indicates a valid negative test result; if no line appears at the control location or if lines appear outside the areas indicated by triangles, the test is invalid and should be repeated with a new device.
Blood (fingerstick, venipuncture) **Uni-Gold Recombigen HIV** Trinity Biotech	Nonreactive	• FDA approval 12/2003
		• Has reported sensitivity of 100% and specificity of 99.7% using fingerstick or venipuncture whole-blood specimens; reported sensitivity of 100% and specificity of 99.8% using serum or plasma.
		• Estimated time to set up and conduct test = < 5 minutes plus 10-minute wait time; window period for reading results (from last step of testing process) 10–12 minutes
		• Procedure: One drop of the patient blood sample is added to the device, followed by four drops of the wash solution; wait 10 minutes.

Type of Test	Normal Value/Range	Comments
		• A line in both the test and control regions indicates a reactive test; a line in only the control region indicates a negative test. • When used with whole blood, the test is valid only if the control line is present and the sample well is red, indicating that an adequate blood sample has been added.
Reveal G-3 Rapid HIV-1 Antibody Test MedMira, Inc.	Nonreactive	• FDA approval 4/2003 • Has reported sensitivity of 99.8% and specificity of 99.1% using serum; reported sensitivity of 99.8% and specificity of 98.6% using plasma. • Estimated time to set up and conduct test = 3–5 minutes; no additional wait time; results must be read immediately. • Considered reactive if both red control line and central red test dot appear; nonreactive if only control line appears; invalid if the control line does not appear.
MultiSpot HIV-1/ HIV-2 Rapid Test BioRad Laboratories	Nonreactive	• FDA approval 11/2004 • Has reported sensitivity of 100% and specificity of 99.93% using serum; reported sensitivity of 100% and specificity of 99.91% using plasma. • Estimated time to set up and conduct test = 10–15 minutes; no additional wait time; results can be read immediately or anytime up to 24 hours. • For interpretation of test results, consult manufacturer's package insert.
Clearview HIV-1/2 STAT-PAK Clearview COMPLETE HIV-1/2 Inverness Medical Professional Diagnostics	Nonreactive	• FDA approval 5/2006 • Has reported sensitivity of 99.7% and specificity of 99.9% using fingerstick or venipuncture whole-blood specimens; reported sensitivity of 100% and specificity of 99.91% using serum and plasma. • Sample collection: For serum, collect specimen in a tube without anticoagulant; for plasma, collect in a tube containing citrate, heparin, or EDTA; for whole blood (either through venipuncture or fingerstick), fill the sample loop provided in the kit.

Type of Test	Normal Value/Range	Comments
		• Estimated time to set up and conduct test = < 5 minutes plus 15-minute wait time; window period for reading results (from last step of testing process) 15–20 minutes • For interpretation of test results, consult manufacturer's package insert.
URINE **Maxim HIV-1** **Urine EIA** Maxim Biomedical	Nonreactive	• Only FDA approved screening EIA for urine • Before a determination of HIV-1 status can be made, specimens that are repeatedly reactive using this test should be further tested, only using the additional, more specific Cambridge Biotech Western Blot Kit.
HOME TESTING KIT **Home Access HIV-1** **Test System** Home Access Health Corp	Nonreactive	• FDA approved 7/1996; only product currently approved by FDA and legally sold in the United States as a "home" testing system for HIV. • Marketed as a kit called either "The Home Access HIV-1 Test System" or "The Home Access Express HIV-1 Test System." Can be purchased at pharmacies, by mail order, or online. • The kit is a home collection test system that requires users to collect a blood specimen at home. Using a personal identification number (PIN), they then mail the sample anonymously to a laboratory for testing. The PIN can then be used to obtain results. • The Home Access System offers users pre- and post-test, anonymous and confidential counseling through both printed material and telephone interaction; also provides the user with an interpretation of the test result. • At this time, there are no FDA-approved test kits that allow consumers to interpret test results at home.
PBMC (peripheral blood mononuclear cell culture)	Negative	• Measures infectious, cell-associated virus • Expensive, labor-intensive process that lasts 28 days

Type of Test	Normal Value/Range	Comments
		• Sensitivity between 95% and 100%
		• Quantitative results correlate with stage of HIV disease.
QUANTITATIVE PLASMA HIV RNA (VIRAL LOAD) FDA-approved tests include (but are not limited to) the following tests/ companies: • **RT-PCR;** Roche; Initial FDA approval 3/1999 • **Standard:** Amplicor 1.0 and 1.5; 400 to 750,000 copies/ml • **Ultrasensitive:** 50 to 75,000 copies/ml • **Versant HIV-1 RNA bDNA;** Bayer —Signal amplification nucleic acid probe; FDA approval 9/2002 —75 to 500,000 copies/ml • **Nuclisens HIV-1 QT**; bioMerieux, Inc; initial FDA approval 11/2001 —176 to 3,470,000 (IU/mL; 1 copy of HIV-1 RNA equals 1.7 International Units, WHO 1st International Standard for HIV-1 RNA for Nucleic Acid-Based Techniques)	Undetectable	• Quantitative measure of HIV viral load in plasma • Useful in the diagnosis of acute HIV infection, predicting progression in chronically infected individuals, risk of transmission with nearly any type of exposure, and for therapeutic monitoring • Assays should be obtained at times of clinical stability, at least 4 weeks after immunizations or intercurrent infections, and with use of the same lab and same technology. • In PCR-based assays, HIV RNA is converted into DNA by reverse transcription followed by PCR amplification of the DNA. The PCR product is detected by hybridization with an enzyme-conjugated probe specific for HIV-1, and quantified by reacting bound probe with a substrate that undergoes a color change, as in an ELISA. • The branched DNA assay uses nonenzymatic means to amplify the signal from HIV RNA; viral RNA is "captured" by hybridization to complementary oligonucleotides that are bound to the wells of a microtiter plate; the captured viral RNA target is then hybridized to branched oligonucleotides (hence the name *branched* DNA assay), which in turn are hybridized to enzyme-conjugated oligonucleotides that can be quantified as above.

Type of Test	Normal Value/Range	Comments
• **RealTime HIV-1**; Abbott —40 to 1 million copies/ml —FDA approval 5/2007 • **Cobas AmpliPrep/ Cobas TaqMan HIV Test;** Roche —40 to 10,000,000 copies/ml —FDA approval 5/2007		
HIV SURVEILLANCE BED HIV-1 Capture EIA Assay Calypte Biomedical Corporation	• Recently infected = a confirmed HIV-1 positive specimen is reactive on the standard sensitive EIA and has a normalized optical density of < 0.8 on the BED assay.	• Used for routine surveillance applications; assay used with the serologic testing algorithm for recent HIV seroconversion (STARHS) to estimate incidence of HIV in the U.S. population • The assay detects levels of anti-HIV IgG relative to total IgG and is based on the observation that the ratio of anti-HIV IgG to total IgG increases with time after HIV infection. • The BED in combination with the appropriate estimator is the preferred approach to calculating incidence of HIV infection in the United States and may be used in conjunction with information from additional sources (triangulation studies) to corroborate findings. • The assay is not for diagnosis of HIV infection.

PROGNOSTIC INDICATORS: Staging HIV and Therapeutic Management

CD4 CELL COUNT	Normal adult values are 800 to 1050/ml, with a range representing 2 standard deviations of about 500 to 1400/µl.	• CD4 cells are a primary target of HIV infection and decline progressively as HIV infection advances. • Test is used to stage the disease, provide guidelines for differential diagnosis of patient complaints, and dictate therapeutic decisions about antiviral treatment and prophylaxis of opportunistic disease. It is a prognostic indicator and complements the viral load assay.

Type of Test	Normal Value/Range	Comments
		• Individual variability of up to 15% can be seen in the course of 1 day. Small variations in the number of WBCs or in the percentage of lymphocytes greatly influence CD4 counts. Additional factors affecting CD4 cell count include: seasonal and diurnal variation, corticosteroid use, intercurrent illness, HTLV-1 coinfection, and inter- and intra-laboratory variation.
CD4 LYMPHOCYTE PERCENTAGE	> 29%	• Measures the percentage of total lymphocytes with the CD4 marker • Subject to variation based on CBC and differential; preferred measure of degree of immunosuppression • A CD4 % < 20 correlates with immunosuppression. • A CD4 % < 14 meets criteria for an AIDS diagnosis.

Tests for Therapeutic Management of HIV
RESISTANCE TESTING
• **Genotypic assays**
• **Phenotypic assays**
		• An in vitro method of measuring resistance to antiretroviral agents
		• Aids in the selection of antiretroviral drugs
		• Limitations:
		  • Measures only the dominant species at the time the test was performed, therefore resistant variants that may comprise less than 20% of the total viral population may not be detected due to being in reservoirs (CNS, latent CD4 cells, genital tract, lymph nodes)
		  • Individual must have a sufficient viral load to do the test (≥500–1000 copies/ml).
		  • Genotypic assays are hard to interpret because multiple mutations are required for individual ARV agent resistance and cross-resistance.
		  • Phenotypic assays are hard to interpret due to the thresholds used to define susceptibility.
		  • Individuals must be tested while on the ARV agents being evaluated.

Type of Test	Normal Value/Range	Comments
Genotypic assays		• Methodology involves: (1) amplification of gene for reverse transcriptase (RT), protease (Pr), or both by RT PCR; (2) DNA sequencing of amplicons generated for the dominant species; and (3) reporting of the mutations for each gene using a letter–number–letter standard.
Phenotypic assays		• This assay is comparable to conventional in vitro tests of antimicrobial sensitivity, in which the microbe is grown in serial dilutions of antiviral agents. • The RT and Pr genes from the patient's strain are inserted into the backbone of the laboratory clone by cloning or by recombination. • Replication is monitored at various drug concentrations and compared to a reference wild-type virus. • Results are reported as the IC50 for the test strain relative to that of the reference or wild-type strain.
ABACAVIR HYPER-SENSITIVITY (ABC HSR) HLA-B*5701	Negative	• Susceptibility to abacavir hypersensitivity (ABC HSR) is strongly associated with alleles carried on the 57.1 ancestral haplotype including HLA-B*5701 and Hsp70 Hom M493T. • In one study, prospective testing for HLA-B*5701 and exclusion of individuals carrying this allele from receiving abacavir substantially lowered the incidence of ABC HSR to 0% (95% confidence interval 0–0.075%). • 2008 DHHS guidelines recommend that HLA-B*5701 testing be performed before initiating abacavir. • The presence of HLA-B*5701 is usually detected by standard serological tests (which cannot discriminate between HLA-B57 subtypes) and by molecular genetic methods such as sequence-based typing (SBT), which is expensive.

Type of Test	Normal Value/Range	Comments
CORECEPTOR TROPISM ASSAY **Trofile** Monogram Biosciences, Inc.		• CCR5 inhibitors work by binding to CCR5 receptors. • 2008 DHHS HIV guidelines for adults and adolescents recommend that a coreceptor tropism assay should be performed whenever the use of a CCR5 inhibitor drug is being considered; might also be considered for patients who exhibit virologic failure on a CCR5 inhibitor drug. • Coreceptor tropism of the patient-derived virus is confirmed by testing viral susceptibility to specific CCR5 or CXCR4 inhibitors. • Takes about 2 weeks to perform • Requires plasma viral load at or above 1,000 copies/mL
Lactate	17 years of age and older: 0.5–2.2 mmol/L	• Lactic acidosis is an elevated venous lactate level. • A confirmed lactate level above 5 mmol/L in the presence of signs and symptoms associated with lactic acidemia should be used to diagnosis NRTI-associated lactic acidemia.
Glucose-6-phosphate dehydrogenase (G-6-PD)	4.6–13.5 U/g hemoglobin (Hgb)	• G-6-PD deficiency is a genetic condition that predisposes individuals to hemolysis following exposure to oxidant drugs, especially dapsone, primaquine, and sulfonamides. • Routine screening for G-6-PD deficiency is recommended in patients with specific genetic background, including men of the following ancestral backgrounds: African American, Italian, Sephardic Jew, Arab, and those from India and Southeast Asia.

Tests for Comorbid Conditions and Opportunistic Infections (OI)

SYPHILIS SEROLOGY VDRL or RPR	• Nonreactive • Weakly reactive • Reactive N.B.: Weakly reactive and reactive results are titered.	• 2008 DHHS HIV guidelines for adults and adolescents recommend that testing for *Treponema pallidum* be performed for each new patient during initial patient visit. • HIV-1 infection appears to alter the diagnosis, natural history, management, and outcome of *T. pallidum* infection.

Type of Test	Normal Value/Range	Comments
		• False-negative serologic tests have been reported among HIV-1–infected patients with documented *T. pallidum* infection; the 2004 CDC guidelines recommend that if the clinical suspicion of syphilis is high and serologic tests do not confirm the diagnosis, other diagnostic procedures (e.g., biopsy, darkfield examination, or direct fluorescent antibody staining of lesion material) should be pursued.
TUBERCULOSIS Tuberculosis Skin Testing (TST; PPD SKIN TEST)	No induration detected or induration < 5 mm	• 2004 CDC guidelines recommend routine testing with the TST using the Mantoux method of 5 TU units purified protein derivative for all HIV-infected individuals.
• Annual testing should be considered for those at high risk for TB.
• HIV-uninfected persons with a positive tuberculin skin test (TST) result have a 5–10% lifetime risk for developing TB, compared with a 7–10% annual risk in the HIV-1 infected person with a positive TST result.
• Routine anergy testing is no longer recommended due to its variability, poor predictive value, and because prophylaxis in anergic individuals has shown little efficacy in prevention of TB cases.
• A positive TST > 5 mm induration.
• HIV-1–infected pregnant women who do not have documentation of a negative TST result during the preceding year should be tested during pregnancy.
• The CDC 2004 HIV guidelines recommend susceptibility testing for first-line agents (isoniazid [INH], rifampin [RIF], and ethambutol [EMB]), regardless of the source of the specimen, for all patients with TB. Pyrazinamide (PZA) susceptibility testing should be performed on initial isolate if there is high prevalence of PZA resistance in the community.

Type of Test	Normal Value/Range	Comments
QuantiFERON-TB Gold Test (QFT-G)	Positive result indicates presence of IFN-gamma, which suggests that *M. tuberculosis* infection is likely. Negative result suggests that infection is unlikely. Indeterminate result suggests QFT-G results cannot be interpreted as a result of low mitogen response or high background response.	• FDA-approved (2005) whole-blood test to aid diagnosis of *Mycobacterium tuberculosis* infection, including latent tuberculosis infection (LTBI) and tuberculosis (TB) disease. • 2008 DHHS HIV guidelines for adults and adolescents recommend that the QFT TB test be performed for each new patient during the initial patient visit, unless the patient has a history of prior tuberculosis or a positive TST or QFT-G result. • A sample of whole blood is drawn from patient into a tube with heparin anti-clotting agent (per manufacturer's instructions). • Blood sample is mixed with antigens (mixtures of synthetic peptides representing two *M. tuberculosis* proteins (ESAT-6 and CFP-10) and controls. After incubation for 16 to 24 hours, the amount of interferon-gamma (IFN-gamma) is measured. • If the patient is infected with *M. tuberculosis*, the white blood cells will release IFN-gamma in response to contact with the TB antigens. The QFT-G results are based on the amount of IFN-gamma that is released in response to the antigens. • Clinical evaluation and additional tests (chest X-ray, sputum smear, and culture) are needed to confirm the diagnosis of LTBI or TB disease. • Prior BCG (bacille Calmette-Guérin) vaccination does not affect results. • Blood samples must be processed within 12 hours post-collection while WBCs are still viable. • Data are limited on the use of QFT-G in children younger than 17 years of age, among persons recently exposed to *M. tuberculosis*, and in immunocompromised persons.

Type of Test	Normal Value/Range	Comments
Toxoplasmosis gondii **Antibodies, IgG**	Negative antibodies = no latent infection. Positive antibodies = latent infection.	• In the United States, the greatest risk for *Toxoplasmosis gondii* encephalitis is among patients with a CD4$^+$ T lymphocyte count <50 cells/μL. • HIV-1–infected patients with *T. gondii* encephalitis are almost uniformly anti-toxoplasma IgG antibody seropositive; absence of IgG antibody makes toxoplasmosis diagnosis unlikely but not impossible.
Cytomegalovirus antibodies, IgG	Negative antibodies = no latent infection. Equivocal = repeat testing. Positive antibodies = latent infection.	• A negative IgG antibody level indicates that CMV is unlikely to be the cause of the disease process being investigated; certain patients with advanced immunosuppression might serorevert from antibody positive to antibody negative; as a result, a negative CMV IgG antibody test does not definitively eliminate the possibility of CMV disease.
HBV SEROLOGY HBcAb: Hepatitis B core antibody	Nonreactive (no core antibodies detected)	• 2008 DHHS HIV guidelines for adults and adolescents recommend hepatitis A, B, and C serologies for all new patients during initial visit. • HIV-1 infection is associated with an increased risk for the development of chronic hepatitis B after HBV exposure; limited data indicate that coinfected patients with chronic hepatitis B infection have higher HBV DNA levels and are more likely to have detectable hepatitis Be antigen (HBeAg), accelerated loss of protective hepatitis B surface antibody (anti-HBs), and an increased risk for liver-related mortality and morbidity.
HBsAb antibody	Nonreactive (no surface antibodies detected)	• Chronic hepatitis B is defined as detection of HBsAg for ≥ 6 months. • 2004 CDC guidelines recommend chronic HBV-infected patients be tested for HBeAg and antibody to HBeAg (anti-HBe). • CDC recommends that susceptible HIV-1–infected persons at risk for HBV infection should receive the hepatitis B vaccine series.

Type of Test	Normal Value/Range	Comments
HCV serology	Negative	• 2004 CDC HIV guidelines for treatment of opportunistic infections recommend testing of all HIV-1–infected patients for evidence of chronic HCV infection. • Initial testing for HCV should be performed using the most sensitive immunoassays licensed for detection of antibody to HCV in blood. • If serologic test results are indeterminate, testing for HCV RNA should be performed.
Anti-HCV EIA	Nonreactive (no antibodies detected)	• To confirm the presence of chronic infection, persons positive for antibody to HCV should be tested for HCV RNA by a qualitative HCV RNA assay with a lower limit of detection of $\leq$ 50 IU/mL.
HCV RIBA Recombinant immunoblot assay	Negative	• Used to confirm anti-HCV positive result • 2004 CDC HIV guidelines for treatment of opportunistic infections recommend more specific anti-HCV testing by a recombinant immunoblot assay (RIBA) for patients with a positive anti-HCV result by immunoassay and a negative test for HCV RNA.
RT-PCR for HCV RNA	Negative	• Used to confirm anti-HCV positive result • HCV RNA (quantitative or qualitative) is required to confirm chronic HCV infection. • A single positive qualitative HCV RNA result is sufficient to confirm the diagnosis of active HCV infection. • A negative result cannot exclude viremia because RNA levels might transiently decline below the limit of detection in persons with active infection. A repeat qualitative assay can be performed to confirm the absence of active infection.
Quantitative HCV PCR	Negative	• Substantial variability exists among available assays, and if serial values are required to evaluate disease or monitor antiviral therapy, continued use of the same quantitative assay for all assessments is recommended.

Type of Test	Normal Value/Range	Comments
		• HCV viral load does not correlate with degree of histologic injury observed on liver biopsy and does not serve as a surrogate for measuring disease severity; it provides prognostic information about response to antiviral therapy. • Quantitative HCV RNA is also useful for monitoring response to therapy.
HCV Genotype	HCV is grouped into six major genotypes, which are subtyped according to sequence characteristics and are designated as 1a, 1b, 1c, 2a, 2b, 2c, 3a, 3b, 4a–h, 5a, and 6a.	• Genotype assay identifies 6 genotypes and > 90 subtypes. • Up to 80% of patients with HCV genotype 2 or 3 disease respond favorably to antiviral therapy.

SELECTED REFERENCES

Benson, C. A., Kaplan, J. E., Masur, H., Pau, A., & Holmes, K. K. (2004). Treating opportunistic infections among HIV-infected adults and adolescents: Recommendations from CDC, the National Institutes of Health, and the HIV Medicine Association/Infectious Diseases Society of America. *Morbidity and Mortality Weekly Report, 53*(RR15), 1–112. Retrieved March 1, 2009, from http://www.cdc.gov/mmwr/preview/mmwrhtml/rr5315a1.htm

Centers for Disease Control and Prevention (CDC). (2007, October). *QuantiFERON-TB Gold test fact sheet.* Retrieved March 1, 2009, from http://www.cdc.gov/tb/pubs/tbfactsheets/QFT.htm

Centers for Disease Control and Prevention (CDC). (2007, October). *Using the BED HIV-1 Capture EIA Assay to estimate incidence using STARHS in the context of surveillance in the United States.* Retrieved March 1, 2009, from http://www.cdc.gov/hiv/topics/surveillance/resources/factsheets/BED.htm

Centers for Disease Control and Prevention (CDC). (2008, February 4). *FDA-approved rapid HIV antibody screening tests.* Retrieved March 1, 2009, from http://www.cdc.gov/hiv/topics/testing/rapid/rt-comparison.htm

Greenwald, J. L., Burstein, G., Pincus, J., & Branson, B. (2006). A rapid review of rapid HIV antibody tests. *Current Infectious Disease Reports, 8*(2), 125–131. Retrieved March 1, 2009, from http://www.cdc.gov/hiv/topics/testing/resources/journal_article/pdf/rapid_review.pdf

Martin, A. M., Nolan, D., & Mallas, S. (2005). HLA-B*5701 typing by sequence-specific amplification: Validation and comparison with sequence-based typing. *Tissue Antigens, 65*(6), 571–574.

U.S. Department of Human and Health Services (DHHS). Panel on Antiretroviral Guidelines for Adults and Adolescents. (2008, November 3). *Guidelines for the use of antiretroviral agents in HIV-1-infected adults and adolescents.* Retrieved March 1, 2009, from http://aidsinfo.nih.gov/contentfiles/AdultandAdolescentGL.pdf

APPENDIX B

Case Studies and Quiz Questions

SECTION 1. PATHOPHYSIOLOGY

Case Study 1: Patient D.S.

Present Health: D.S. is a 67-year-old male and a new patient at the outpatient infectious diseases clinic where you are a staff nurse. The patient was diagnosed with HIV disease 3 weeks ago at a large tertiary care center in another state. D.S. tells you that he has been very ill, lost "a lot" of weight, can't remember all that has happened in the last few weeks, and that he feels overwhelmed. At this time he has nausea, vomiting, diarrhea, and a very poor appetite. Also, his legs hurt and he feels weak and sleeps most of the time.

Past Health History: D.S. has had numerous upper respiratory infections and "walking" pneumonias for the last 10 years. These infections have been treated on an outpatient basis by his general practitioner. About 25 years ago, D.S. had a laryngectomy for cancer and he has fully recovered. Just prior to D.S.'s HIV diagnosis, he was admitted to a regional hospital for a hernia repair. After the hernia repair, he developed pneumonia. His pneumonia did not improve after multiple antibiotic courses at the regional hospital. Because he did not improve, two of his friends took him to the large tertiary care center, where he was diagnosed with bilateral *Pneumocystis* pneumonia (PCP; *Pneumocystis jiroveci* pneumonia), HIV, and AIDS. He had a negative TB skin test last year and had his hepatitis B vaccine series several years ago.

Social History: D.S. is a nonsmoker, does not use alcohol, and has no history of intravenous drug use. He lives alone. He has not been sexually active for 10 years. In the past he has been sexually active with men and with women. D.S. is a healthcare worker and has sustained multiple needle-sticks "over the years." Only two friends know about his HIV diagnosis, and both friends have "disowned" him. He has not told his family about his condition except that he has a "bad" pneumonia. He is worried because he has a $4,000 cap on his medication coverage. He lives in a very small town and is worried that if he fills prescriptions at the town pharmacy, "everyone will find out" about his HIV.

Allergies: Clindamycin

Medications: Bactrim daily; Mepron 15 cc daily; Zithromax 1200 mg once weekly; Diflucan 200 mg daily; Nystatin oral rinse daily; Zofran prn, Lomotil prn, Loperamide prn (has not been started on antiretroviral treatment)

Medical Diagnoses:
HIV disease
Pneumocystis pneumonia
Tinea of groin, rectum, and upper thighs
Diarrhea
Nausea
Oral candidiasis

Lab Values:
HIV-1 RNA by PCR: 76,400
CD4: 18/3%
Hemoglobin: 11.6
WBC: 2.5

Case Study Questions

1. Identify at least two possible HIV transmission risk factors in this case.
   Bisexuality; possibility of unprotected sex; high number of sexual partners; occupational exposure
2. List at least three signs and symptoms that may be clinically related to HIV disease.
   Weight loss; changes in mental status; feelings of anxiety; GI problems; pain in legs; malaise
3. What information from the patient's past health history might be related to HIV disease?
   Pneumonia

Pharmacology Quiz Questions

1. Which of the following drugs is indicated for both treatment and prophylaxis therapy for *Pneumocystis* pneumonia (PCP; *Pneumocystis jiroveci* pneumonia)?
   a. Zofran
   b. Lomotil
   c. Bactrim (TMP-SMX; Septra)
   d. Loperamide
2. Which of the following drugs is indicated for both treatment and prophylaxis therapy for oropharyngeal candidiasis (thrush)?
   a. Diflucan (fluconazole)
   b. Bactrim (TMP-SMX)
   c. Lomotil
   d. Pentamidine
3. Topical solutions used to treat oropharyngeal candidiasis (thrush) include:
   a. pentamidine
   b. nystatin
   c. acyclovir
   d. liquid nitrogen
4. The most common adverse effect to Bactrim (TMP-SMX) is:
   a. headache
   b. hypomagnesia
   c. rash
   d. hypokalemia
5. Lomotil (diphenoxylate/atropine) and Imodium (loperamide) are commonly used in HIV to treat:
   a. fever
   b. diarrhea
   c. nausea
   d. peripheral neuropathy

Pathophysiology Quiz Questions

1. Pathogenesis of HIV includes the origin of this disease. Where is HIV thought to have originated?
   a. United States
   b. France
   c. Africa
   d. South America
2. The transmission source(s) for HIV include(s):
   a. blood
   b. vaginal fluids and semen
   c. breastmilk
   d. all of the above

3. The progression of HIV to AIDS is defined as:
   a. HIV is the viral cause of a syndrome characterized by a progressive, ongoing, and disabling deterioration of the human immune system.
   b. HIV is the same as AIDS.
   c. HIV is the bacterial cause of a syndrome characterized by a progressive, ongoing, and disabling deterioration of the human immune system.
   d. AIDS is the viral cause of the syndrome of HIV.
4. Opportunistic infections associated with HIV disease are:
   a. bacterial and viral infections
   b. fungal infections
   c. protozoan infections
   d. all of the above
5. Opportunistic malignancies associated with HIV disease are:
   a. Kaposi's sarcoma
   b. Bell's palsy
   c. Non-Hodgkin's lymphoma
   d. a and c
6. The type of HIV most commonly found in the United States is:
   a. HIV-2
   b. HIV-1
   c. HIV-1 and HIV-2 are equally distributed in the United States
   d. None of the above
7. HIV-2 is most commonly found in:
   a. West Africa
   b. United States
   c. France
   d. South America
8. The etiology of AIDS is simply stated as:
   a. AIDS is caused by a bacteria.
   b. AIDS is caused by TB.
   c. AIDS is caused by CMV.
   d. AIDS is caused by HIV.
9. HIV is:
   a. a parasite
   b. a retrovirus
   c. a lentivirus
   d. all of the above
10. The *most* common route of HIV transmission is:
    a. needle-stick
    b. sexual contact
    c. breastmilk
    d. intravenous drug use

SECTION 2. MEDICAL-SURGICAL CARE

Case Study 2A: Patient Tim L.

Tim L., aged 22, presents to you in the college student health center with complaints of feeling tired and achy for the past few weeks. He also states that he had a sore throat a few weeks ago and that the lymph nodes in his groin "feel a little bigger than normal" but are not painful to touch. His vital signs are stable, although his pulse and blood pressure are slightly elevated. During his health history, he becomes very nervous. In a halting manner, and with shaky speech, he states that he has had several episodes of unprotected sex with different male partners over the last 2 years, and he is afraid that he may "have AIDS." Although he appears extremely apprehensive, he allows you to complete the health history and physical examination.

Case Study Questions

1. Based on the client's health history, is this client at risk for HIV infection?
   Yes, due to high-risk unprotected sexual encounters
2. Should this client be advised to have an HIV screening exam?
   Yes
3. What counseling and teaching should this client receive regarding HIV screening and diagnostic tests?
   Rapid HIV testing via oral swab can be done as a screening test, with screening results available in less than twenty minutes; if test results are positive, will require further testing to confirm HIV diagnosis; if negative, work with client to develop an action plan to eliminate or decrease high-risk behaviors

Medical-Surgical Quiz Questions

1. Clinical signs and symptoms of initial HIV infection include:
   a. weakness and paralysis of the arms and legs
   b. flulike symptoms
   c. headaches and seizures
   d. nonproductive cough and fever
2. A reactive HIV screening test means that the client has:
   a. HIV
   b. AIDS
   c. antibodies to HIV
   d. antigens to HIV
3. The HIV-positive client must be closely assessed for opportunistic infections when the:
   a. ELISA test is reactive
   b. Western Blot test is positive
   c. OraQuick Rapid Test is negative
   d. CD4 cell count is 200 or below

4. What should be included in the teaching plan to young adults about the spread of AIDS?
   a. Heterosexual transmission of HIV is on the rise.
   b. HIV in children is increasing.
   c. The greatest increase of HIV infection is by homosexual transmission.
   d. Transmission of HIV by IV drug users is prominent even when clean needles and sterile equipment are used.

5. Which statement, from a participant attending a class on HIV prevention, indicates an understanding of how to reduce transmission of HIV?
   a. "All women, even those who are HIV-positive, should breastfeed their babies because breastmilk is superior to cow's milk, and will help strengthen the baby's immune system."
   b. "Although I am faithful to my partner, I am afraid that he has been cheating on me, so I am going to tell him that we need to use condoms when we have sex."
   c. "If a girl doesn't have an orgasm during sex, she won't get HIV."
   d. "It's okay to use natural skin condoms instead of latex condoms because natural skin condoms are more environmentally friendly."

6. Which statement made by the client you are teaching about condom use indicates a need for clarification?
   a. "I will use a new condom each time I have intercourse."
   b. "I will wash the condom out with soap and water before I use it again."
   c. "I will always use a latex condom rather than a natural membrane condom."
   d. "When intercourse is over, I will keep the condom on my penis until it is out of the vagina."

Case Study 2B. Patient Mrs. P.

Mrs. P. comes to the clinic for her scheduled 3-month follow-up visit. She is a 42-year-old African American woman who has been HIV-positive for the past 10 years. She has been adherent to her prescribed HIV medications, and has been on the same prescription for the past 2 years. Her CD4 count remains within normal limits, and her viral load is undetectable. She is scheduled for clinic visits every 3 months to check her lab work and monitor her progress.

Today Mrs. P. states that she "just isn't feeling right." She reports that since her last appointment she has had increasing fatigue and at times "just feels all tuckered out." This has affected her activities of daily life (ADLs). She relates that she is not able to do her usual weekly grocery shopping, "it's just too tiring," and instead has been getting food items at the convenience store 1 block away from her apartment when she has the energy. Her daily exercise consists of walking up the stairs to her second-floor apartment. For the past 2 weeks she has not felt up to doing this, and has been using the elevator.

Clinical assessment reveals that Mrs. P.'s oral temperature is 97.2° F, pulse is 60, respirations are 16, and blood pressure is 116/78. Her height is 5 feet, 5 inches, and she weighs 115 pounds, a

5-pound weight loss in the last 3 months. Her skin is slightly paler than normal. Her SaO_2 level, assessed using a portable pulse oximeter and fingertip electrode, shows a decrease to 96% from her usual baseline level of 99%.

Case Study Questions

1. Based on assessment findings, what is happening with this patient? What further data (health history, physical examination, or diagnostic tests) are needed?
   May be suffering from anemia; check the CBC, hemoglobin and hematocrit, reticulocyte count
2. What nursing and medical interventions would you anticipate? What is the rationale for these interventions?
   Determine cause of anemia; if anemia is severe, the patient may need to have a blood transfusion; may be started on epoetin alfa (Epogen, Procrit)
3. What patient teaching is needed for this patient? What follow-up care planning would you anticipate for this patient?
   Patient education to recognize and report early signs of anemia, such as fatigue and shortness of breath; may need referral for dietary counseling and potential nutritional counseling

Medical-Surgical Quiz Questions

1. Which of the following is *not* a common HIV-related symptom?
   a. fever
   b. diarrhea
   c. shortness of breath
   d. anemia
2. Cryptosporidiosis in the HIV-positive patient can cause:
   a. severe diarrhea
   b. CNS lymphoma
   c. generalized lymphadenopathy
   d. visual changes
3. Histoplasmosis is a form of which type of infection?
   a. viral
   b. fungal
   c. bacterial
   d. protozoal
4. The client has tested positive on two different laboratory tests measuring antibodies to the human immunodeficiency virus (HIV). What is your interpretation of these test results?
   a. The client is at increased risk for the development of opportunistic infections.
   b. The client has been infected with the human immunodeficiency virus (HIV).
   c. The client is immune to the human immunodeficiency virus.
   d. The client has AIDS.

5. Bacterial opportunistic infections include:
   a. cytomegalovirus (CMV)
   b. bartonellosis
   c. cryptosporidiosis
   d. microsporidiosis
6. Classic signs of *Toxoplasmosis gondii* (*T. gondii*) in HIV/AIDS patients include:
   a. respiratory problems
   b. cardiac irregularities
   c. headache, confusion, motor weakness
   d. peripheral neuropathy
7. Viral opportunistic infections include:
   a. Kaposi's sarcoma
   b. cytomegalovirus (CMV)
   c. *Pneumocystis* pneumonia (PCP)
   d. *salmonella*
8. Nursing care planning includes protecting the immunodeficient patient from what potentially fatal complication?
   a. anaphylaxis
   b. infection
   c. autoimmune disease
   d. coronary artery disease
9. The client with AIDS and a CD4+ count of 100 is admitted with a compound fracture of the left leg. In addition, the client has a productive cough, fever, chills, and a history of night sweats. The client's PPD test is negative. What is your best action?
   a. Use standard precautions alone because the client does not have tuberculosis.
   b. Use airborne precautions alone because the client is taking appropriate therapy for HIV.
   c. Use standard precautions and airborne precautions because the client has tuberculosis.
   d. Think TB: Use standard precautions and airborne precautions until a chest X-ray film shows the client does NOT have TB.
10. Which of the following sputum exams are done to test for the presence of *Mycobacterium tuberculosis* (TB)?
    a. culture and sensitivity
    b. Gram stain
    c. acid-fast bacilli stain
    d. cytology tests

SECTION 3. PHARMACOLOGY

Case Study 3: Patient Mr. C.

Mr. C. is a 69-year-old African American male who was diagnosed with HIV in 1988. His past medical history includes HIV/AIDS, chronic hepatitis C virus, substance abuse, hypertension, history of a + PPD, and chronic pain related to an old injury. He is disabled and lives on SSI. He does not own a car, and lives about 50 miles from the clinic. He lives in a single room occupancy (SRO) apartment where other people frequently come in and out. His last CD4 cell count was 34 and viral load was > 350,000. He is nonadherent with all meds, and has difficulty keeping appointments for HIV and specialty clinics. His current medications include the following:

- Nelfinavir 250 mg 5 tabs po bid
- AZT 100 mg 3 tabs po bid
- Zerit 40 mg 1 tab po bid
- Bactrim DS 1 tab po qd
- Azithromycin 600 mg 2 tabs po every week on Monday
- Atenolol 50 mg 1 tab po qd
- Lasix 20 mg 1 tab po qd
- Tylenol 3 with codeine 1–2 tabs po q 6 h prn pain
- Metoprolol 100 mg 1 tab po qd
- Zolpidem 10 mg 1 po qhs

You see him today in clinic, and his BP is 190/102. He has lost 8 pounds since his last clinic visit 4 months ago. He says he has not been eating because his SSI check got lost in the mail or stolen and he has not had money for food. You review his med list with him, and he is not able to recall the correct name or dosing of his medications. He thinks he may not have even gotten them all in the mail last month. Mentally you add up the number of pills he should take each day. To take the medications properly, he would take 13 pills in the morning and 10 pills in the evening for a total pill burden of at least 23 pills a day. This does not include the Tylenol # 3 prn for pain or the azithromycin 1200 mg once weekly for mycobacterium avium complex (MAC) prophylaxis. You realize that before you can expect to make changes in the way he takes medication you will have to help him develop a plan to meet his basic needs of food, shelter, and transportation.

Shelter: You explain that it is important to have regular clinic visits and to be in touch with clinic staff when problems arise. He says his mother and daughter live near the clinic and he would be willing to move, if he could find a place to stay, so that he could be closer to them and the clinic. You know a community-based organization that has funds to help people relocate. He calls them and makes an appointment from your office for tomorrow. He seems hopeful, and has a good attitude about moving.

Food: Mr. C. says that he has gone to the local food pantries, but each provided only enough food to last 2–3 days and visits are limited to once a month. He does not qualify for food stamps. He has had to rely on family and friends for food for almost a month. He does not like to ask for handouts. Because of his age, he is eligible for a program that provides home-delivered meals in his community. He would like to enroll in the program, and you call to make the referral before he leaves. He will begin to receive meals within several days.

Transportation: It is difficult for Mr. C. to keep appointments because of his financial situation and the distance from the clinic. You assure him that if he moves closer, there is a program for discounted bus passes that will make getting around much easier.

Next you look at his medication list. You realize that if you take advantage of the new once-daily dosing options, it will greatly simplify his regimen. Because he has not taken his ART consistently there is a chance that he may already have resistance to his current medications. You suggest the following medications, and the provider agrees:

AM	**PM**
Metoprolol 100 mg qd	Sustiva 600 mg 1 tab po qhs
Atenolol 50 mg qd	Videx EC 1 tab po qhs
Bactrim DS 1 po qd	Epivir 300 mg 1 tab po qhs
<u>Lasix 20 mg qd</u>	<u>Zolpidem 10 mg 1 tab po qhs</u>
Total 4 pills q am	4 pills q pm

To further increase the chance of adherence, you offer to pour enough pills in 4 med boxes for him to last until his next monthly appointment and he agrees. You also provide a written list of medications for him to carry in his wallet.

Several months later you see Mr. C. in clinic again. He is excited to tell you how well he is doing. He was able to find housing within walking distance from the clinic, and has not missed an appointment for labs, specialists, or HIV clinic since his move. He claims not to miss any doses of medication since he has been coming in for monthly medication pours. He was also able to transfer to a home-delivered meal program at his new location. In addition, there are many more lunch and food pantry programs that he can use.

He is involved in a community-based program for people with HIV and is involved with a support group and a program that helps fund expenses for his dog. Although he continues to have numerous serious medical problems, his mood is positive and he seems hopeful. His CD4 count today is 168, and viral load is undetectable. He has gained about 18 pounds in the past 4 months. His BP is 117/80.

Case Study Questions

1. What are assessment clues that indicate a patient is having problems taking his medications as prescribed?
   There are several clues that a patient is having trouble being adherent to his medications:
   a. Look at the CD4 count and VL. If there has been a significant change in either, the nurse should ask nonjudgmental, open-ended questions about the patient's ability to take medications correctly. Phrase questions that allow the patient to tell you in his or her own words what he or she has difficulty with. For example, ask "How often do you miss a dose of your medication?" and "Why do you think that happens?" rather than " You didn't miss any doses of your medications, did you?"
   b. Patients who repeatedly refill prescriptions late often have problems with adherence. The nurse should try to find out why this is happening and what can be done to help. Some solutions are suggesting a source for mail order prescriptions for people who have transportation problems, pouring medications in pillboxes, or providing education about why adherence is important and what problems can stem from non-adherence.

2. Discuss how working with the patient to meet basic needs—food, shelter, transportation—can help improve medication adherence.

   Without a stable living situation adherence is difficult to maintain. Not having a safe place to keep medications and having uninvited people in and out of the living space can result in the loss or theft of medications and/or non-adherence for fear of someone finding medications and discovering the status of the patient. Proper nutrition is an essential component of health and can lead to increased wasting, poor absorption of medications, gastrointestinal disorders (nausea, diarrhea), and fatigue. Finally, transportation is necessary to obtain groceries, make medical appointments, and socialize.

3. Why is it important for patients to take their HIV medications as prescribed? What can happen if the patient is nonadherent?

   It is important for patients to take their HIV medications as prescribed. All medication dosages are based on a calculation of how long they remain in the bloodstream before being eliminated, and how much is needed to obtain the desired effect. With HIV medications, it is especially important to keep a "steady state" of drugs in the body to avoid viral resistance development. Once developed, resistance can result in the inability of entire classes of medications to be effective against the virus. Eventually the patient would not have any treatment choices and progress more rapidly to severe immune suppression and AIDS.

Pharmacology Quiz Questions

1. You are caring for a patient with HIV/AIDS who calls to report a new rash on his arm. You should:
   a. advise him to stop taking his ART immediately
   b. review his medication list and advise him to stop all NRTIs
   c. assess the extent and appearance of the rash before making a decision
   d. encourage him to go to the emergency department immediately
2. When discussing adherence with a patient, the nurse should:
   a. ask about his housing situation
   b. discuss proper dosing and specific dietary requirements
   c. provide a written list of medications and proper dosing times
   d. discuss all of the above
3. Protease inhibitors:
   a. compete for binding site on the surface of the CD4 cell
   b. work at the viral replication stage of reverse transcription
   c. are used as a prophylaxis for opportunistic infections
   d. act at the site of cleavage and assembly of new virions
4. Lipodystrophy syndromes involve:
   a. the redistribution of fat
   b. abdominal pain and distension
   c. paresthesias of the hands and feet
   d. weight loss

5. The patient you are caring for has a rise in liver function tests (LFTs) that are about 3 times the normal value. You suspect he may have:
   a. hyperlipidemia
   b. lipodystrophy
   c. hepatotoxicity
   d. insulin resistance

6. The most common adverse side effects of ART are:
   a. rash, weight loss, abdominal pain
   b. nausea, vomiting, diarrhea
   c. anorexia, bloating, diarrhea
   d. weight loss, nausea, rash

7. Medications from which of the following drug classes were the first class of drugs approved by the FDA for treatment of HIV/AIDS?
   a. Protease inhibitors (PI)
   b. Nonnucleoside reverse inhibitors (NNRTI)
   c. Nucleoside reverse transcriptase inhibitors (NRTI)
   d. Fusion inhibitors (FI)

8. When providing education to patients with hyperlipidemia, it is important to stress:
   a. the need for a low-fat diet and exercise
   b. changing ART as soon as possible
   c. alcohol can be consumed in moderate amounts
   d. the need for weekly weight monitoring

9. The term *adherence* means:
   a. taking medications most of the time
   b. doing what the healthcare provider tells you to do
   c. sticking to a care plan agreed upon by patient and provider
   d. having medications filled on time

10. The goal of ART is to:
    a. restore the immune system to a pre-infection level
    b. provide the lowest dose of the safest medication to achieve viral suppression
    c. maintain LFTs at a normal and safe level for each patient
    d. use medications from one class at a time to preserve other classes for later use

11. Which of the following medications is from the HIV entry and fusion inhibitor category?
    a. tipranavir (Aptivus)
    b. nevirapine
    c. saquinavir (Fortovase)
    d. maraviroc (Selzentry)

12. Which of the following medications is a nonnucleoside reverse transcriptase inhibitor (NNRTI)?
    a. zidovudine (AZT)
    b. etravirine (Intelence)
    c. emtricitabine (Emtriva)
    d. enfuvirtide (Fuzeon)

13. Which of the following medications is from the drug category integrase inhibitor?
    a. raltegravir (Isentress)
    b. tenofovir (Viread)
    c. saquinavir (Fortovase)
    d. atazanavir (Reyataz)
14. Which of the following medications is from the drug category protease inhibitors (PIs)?
    a. raltegravir (Isentress)
    b. etravirine (Intelence)
    c. darunavir (Prezista)
    d. maraviroc (Selzentry)
15. For patients with G-6-PD deficiency, the most common adverse effect(s) of dapsone or primaquine is/are:
    a. hypokalemia
    b. hyperchloremia
    c. jaundice
    d. methemoglobinemia and hemolysis
16. A medication regiment composed of drugs such as INH, rifambin or rifabutin, PZA, and ethambutol would be used to treat:
    a. CMV
    b. TB
    c. PCP
    d. cryptosporidiosis
17. Which of the following combination drugs contains efavirenz (Sustiva), emtricitabine (Emtriva), and tenofovir disoproxil fumarate (tenofovir DF or Viread)?
    a. Combivir
    b. Truvada
    c. Atripla
    d. Epzicom

SECTION 4. PSYCHIATRIC ISSUES

Case Study 4A: Patient L.J. (Adjustment Disorder)

L.J. is a 20-year-old African American male in his first year of college. He found out he was HIV+ 8 weeks ago through a routine screening for blood donation, and was shocked with these results. Since this time, he reports being anxious, having difficulty sleeping, feeling overwhelmed, and having vague fleeting thoughts of suicide. He says he would never act on these thoughts and would like to have all of these symptoms resolved so that he can concentrate on his studies. L.J.'s girlfriend of 10 months accompanies him on his first visit to the mental health clinical nurse specialist (CNS). Since finding out about his HIV diagnosis, L.J.'s girlfriend has tested negative and they are practicing safer sex.

L.J. was seen weekly by both the mental health CNS and clinic psychiatrist. L.J. is diagnosed with adjustment disorder with anxiety and depressed mood. He refused any psychotropic medications, stating that he was trying to adjust to taking all of the antiretroviral medications and just did not want to add to that burden at this time.

Over the course of the 3 months L.J. was seen for mental health in the HIV clinic, he reported relief from some of the anxiety, mild suicidal ideation, and feelings of being overwhelmed. His sleep has improved, and he reports overall feeling better able to handle his HIV illness.

Case Study Questions

1. What information is necessary to collect during the intake assessment interview?
    a. Suicidal ideation. Rationale: Addressing potentially life-threatening behaviors takes precedence, and a clinician needs to determine the severity and lethality of suicidal ideation.
    b. Areas of L.J.'s life that are adversely affected (school, relationships, work, etc.). Rationale: Adjustment disorder is characterized by significant impairment in usual functioning and marked distress that exceeds what is often seen with exposure to the stressor.
    c. Current stressors in all aspects of L.J.'s life. Timeline for when he found out he was HIV+ and the onset of symptoms. Detailed symptoms and severity of these symptoms. Rationale: Adjustment disorder is a response to stressors, and occurs within 3 months of the presenting stressor(s) and is resolved by 6 months.
    d. Assess for concurrent depression and anxiety. Rationale: Adjustment disorder is often seen with depressed mood, with anxiety, or with mixed anxiety and depressed mood.
2. List at least three nursing diagnoses for L.J.
    Impaired adjustment, ineffective coping, risk for suicide, disturbed sleep pattern, anxiety, spiritual distress
3. List at least three nursing interventions in working with L.J.
    a. Supportive psychotherapy (both individual and group) with focus on stress reduction and enhanced coping.
    b. Consider short-term antidepressant use.
    c. Help patient set realistic short-term goals.
    d. Teach relaxation skills.

Case Study 4B: Patient Larry (Depression)

Larry is a 45-year-old gay man diagnosed with HIV infection in 1987. He has a college degree and has been employed in a variety of jobs reflecting his educational preparation and intellect. He has not had an opportunistic infection, but is experiencing wasting and depletion of his CD4 count along with high viral loads. He has failed all HAART regimens and is increasingly angry and despondent over his future. His anger is frequently directed at the clinic staff and healthcare team, and he verbalizes anger at his physician for discussing end of life planning with him.

Larry has been with the same male partner for over 10 years, and they have had a history of couples therapy and individual therapy in order to address some of Larry's anger issues.

Larry has stopped engaging in activities he used to enjoy, such as creative writing, and is unable to do other activities from which he received tremendous personal satisfaction (hiking, swimming, and reading). He reports that he has no appetite, cannot sleep, feels depressed and sad all of the time, thinks occasionally about suicide, and has withdrawn from his usual circle of friends and support. He spends his days and nights sitting in a reclining chair in front of the television.

Larry has been followed by psychiatry and sees his mental health CNS frequently at the clinic. He is diagnosed with depression. He is on bupropion, sequential trials of different SSRIs, and zolpidem to treat his depression and sleep disorder. He reports some relief from his symptoms, which he attributes to the medication. In sessions with Larry, he is able to develop insight into his feelings and able to engage in care planning. His continues to experience exacerbations of his depression, usually accompanied by anger.

Case Study Questions

1. What information is necessary to collect during the intake assessment interview?
    a. History of psychiatric illnesses/diagnoses. Rationale: patient with anger, despondency, advanced HIV/AIDS, and occasional suicidal ideation requires frequent monitoring and follow-up.
    b. Symptoms of depression (depressed mood, anhedonia, guilt, suicidal ideation, sleep disturbance, appetite/weight changes, difficulty concentrating, energy level changes, psychomotor disturbance). Rationale: Clinical depression is the most commonly diagnosed mental health problem with HIV+ patients.
    c. Adherence to medication and treatment plan. Rationale: In order to experience therapeutic benefits from treatment plan, patient must participate in the plan. Often, a change in treatment adherence is a behavioral indicator of depression in HIV+ patients.
2. List at least three nursing diagnoses for Larry.
    Consider: Ineffective coping, powerlessness, hopelessness, anticipatory grieving, social isolation, disturbed sleep pattern
3. List at least three nursing interventions in working with Larry.
    a. Monitor for potential side effects from psychotropic medications
    b. Psychoeducation regarding depression, sleep, hygiene, and medications
    c. Supportive individual psychotherapy focusing on anger issues, skill-building for empowerment, grief, and development of insight
    d. Group therapy to address social isolation and development of insight
    e. Coordinate treatment plan with entire treatment team, with input from patient

Case Study 4C: Patient J.O. (Suicide)

J.O. is a 57-year-old gay Hispanic male living in a rural area. He has been HIV-infected for 10 years, and lost his lifelong partner to HIV several years ago. He has had no opportunistic infections and is fairly stable in his HIV illness. He is extremely bright, engaging, and a model patient concerning adherence to treatment regimens, clinic appointments, and participation in care planning. He is a clinic "favorite," known and liked by all of the staff and treatment team.

J.O. is terrified that he will develop HIV dementia. He worries constantly that the everyday for-getfulness that everyone experiences is actually the beginnings of his cognitive decline. In order to keep his mind alert and stimulated, he reads constantly, quizzes himself about TV shows, and keeps detailed notes about daily events. He confides his fears only to a close friend.

J.O. is found dead by an intentional overdose of medications. The HIV clinic staff are shocked and upset to learn of his death by suicide.

Case Study Questions

1. What nursing interventions would be appropriate in helping the clinic staff work through this trauma?
   a. Crisis debriefing: Suicide/loss debriefing is a structured group process that helps sur-vivors manage their responses to a suicide or other traumatic loss.
   b. Grief counseling: Persons working in HIV often experience multiple unresolved types of grief (chronic, absent, delayed, distorted).
   c. Establish a mechanism to acknowledge and memorialize the deaths of patients: Simple exercises, such as the reading the names of patients who have died during each staff meeting, can foster a sense of community and enhance perceptions of social support.
2. List at least three nursing diagnoses you would have given J.O.
   Fear, ineffective coping, risk for suicide, anxiety, social isolation, hopelessness, and spiritual distress
3. List three nursing interventions in working with J.O.
   a. Annual and PRN mental health screenings.
   b. Supportive individual and group psychotherapy for social support and development of insight.
   c. Psychoeducation re: anxiety, dementia, depression, and suicidal ideation

Case Study 4D: Patient Tracy (Multiple Diagnoses)

Tracy is a 25-year-old African American female with a history of crack cocaine abuse, schizo-phrenia, mild mental retardation, and HIV infection. She has two children, both of whom have been removed from the home by child protective agencies. She frequently engages in sex-for-drug exchanges and currently resides in public housing with her boyfriend, who has just been re-leased from prison on drug-related charges. The psychiatric home health nurse had to discharge Tracy from follow-up visits due to the presence of used needles in the house. Tracy is well known to the local community mental health clinics, who try to work in concert with the HIV clinic in meeting Tracy's needs. This is your first meeting with Tracy and you have been as-signed as her nurse in the clinic.

Case Study Questions

1. What information is necessary to collect during the intake assessment interview?

    a. History of mental illness including positive and negative symptoms of psychosis and cognitive symptoms: Identify positive and negative symptoms to aid in psychotropic treatment determination.

    b. Mental retardation severity: Cognitive symptoms may result from mental retardation.

    c. Substance abuse history: Substance use disorders occur frequently with severe and persistently mentally ill and may cause or exacerbate psychosis.

2. List at least three nursing diagnoses for Tracy.

Consider: ineffective coping, impaired parenting, risk for infection, deficient knowledge, noncompliance/nonadherence, impaired social interaction, disturbed thought processes, impaired verbal communication, and self-care deficit (grooming/dressing).

3. List at least three nursing interventions in working with Tracy.

    a. Attempt to engage patient in "partnership" of care (be straightforward, create structured environment, etc.)

    b. Initiate intensive counseling regarding safer sex, clean needle use, and other risk reduction, and medication adherence

    c. Offer drug rehabilitation services

    d. Coordinate psychiatric and primary care for HIV treatment

    e. Refer the patient to a social worker for assistance with housing, food stamps, and other services to reduce sex-for-drug exchange

Psychiatric Issues Quiz Questions

1. Suicide risk in persons with HIV/AIDS is
    a. not associated with co-morbid depression
    b. alleviated with cognitive decline
    c. no higher than in persons with other chronic medical conditions
    d. highest in the presence of concurrent mental health and substance use disorders

2. HIV is neurotropic. This implies that
    a. altered mental status is very common
    b. some opportunistic infections common in HIV involve the CNS
    c. all HIV-infected patients will have a mental health disorder
    d. the positive symptoms of schizophrenia respond to psychotropic treatment

3. Strategies to maintain the chronic, severely, and persistently mentally ill patient in HIV care include all of the following *except:*
    a. Maintain a separate file for all mental health diagnoses and medical data, assessments and plans
    b. Engage the patient in care by being honest and direct with information and answers to questions
    c. Contact patient in between visits by phone for follow-up
    d. Assess ARV adherence potential based on mental status at each visit

4. The most common mental health diagnosis for persons with HIV/AIDS is
   a. anxiety
   b. adjustment disorder
   c. dementia
   d. depression

5. Many somatic symptoms of depression for the HIV-infected patient are the same as for the non-HIV-infected patient. However, many HIV-infected patients may not report or acknowledge symptoms and may present with behavioral changes indicative of an underlying depression. An example of this type of symptom is:
   a. depressed mood
   b. anhedonia
   c. change in treatment adherence
   d. sleep disturbance

6. Certain factors that may present crises for HIV-infected patients include:
   a. adherence to both HIV medications and psychotropic medications
   b. coordination of care between medical and psychiatric clinicians/practitioners
   c. intensive case management
   d. progression of HIV disease

7. HIV-infected patients often experience worry, tension, fear, and nervousness, all common symptoms of anxiety. A frequent anxiety disorder that is diagnosed in HIV-infected patients is
   a. panic disorder
   b. insomnia
   c. dizziness
   d. diaphoresis

8. The early, mild stage of dementia is often indistinguishable from
   a. PTSD
   b. mild depression
   c. increased viral load
   d. anemia

9. Strategies to work with active HIV-infected substance users include
   a. mandating treatment for substance use problems
   b. apply a standardized set of interventions
   c. encourage harm-reduction techniques
   d. constantly and consistently emphasize the problems associated with substance use

10. Injection drug users who are HIV infected may also have a maladaptive personality disorder. The two most commonly diagnosed personality disorders among HIV infected patients are:
    a. narcissistic and antisocial
    b. dependent and histrionic
    c. borderline and antisocial
    d. depressed and anxious

11. A 55-year-old HIV+ male was told that he no longer has a job due to the agency making budget cuts. His initial response was anger and disbelief. He walks around for several days

after this news in a dazed state, has not slept, and has stopped eating. He is displaying features of:

    a. depression

    b. mania

    c. panic disorder

    d. normal grief reaction

12. A critical aspect of assessment for mood disorders is:

    a. a change in usual pattern of functioning

    b. the presence of anxiety

    c. the support systems available

    d. the ability to sleep

13. Since her diagnosis of HIV infection two weeks ago, Ms. P. paces constantly and talks about feeling hopeless. Which response would be helpful in establishing a therapeutic relationship with Ms. P.?

    a. smile at her as she walks by

    b. invite her to lunch

    c. use empathy when talking with her

    d. focus the interactions on treatment options

14. When recovering from a severe depression:

    a. the patient no longer needs counseling treatment

    b. the patient is unlikely to experience an exacerbation of depression

    c. the patient is considered less of a suicidal risk than when in a severe depression

    d. the patient is considered more of a suicidal risk than when in a severe depression

15. Which of the following is considered psychiatric management priority?

    a. attending to the patient's safety

    b. establishing and maintaining a therapeutic alliance

    c. determining medication options

    d. developing a treatment plan with the patient

SECTION 5. PEDIATRICS

Case Study 5: Patient Abby

A 3-year-old female Caucasian child was taken into care at 1 week of age and later adopted by her foster mother. The child, Abby, has been healthy and well. The adoptive mother teaches school. The child is in the 5th percentile for both height and weight but otherwise developmentally appropriate. The state has called the adoptive mother to notify her that this child's biological mother has tested positive for HIV and recommends the child be tested. The child's pediatrician feels that because the child has been so healthy, she does not need to be tested. The adoptive mother insists on the test, which turns out to be positive. The child is referred to a pediatric HIV clinic for care. On careful history, the child was noted to have had the mumps even though she was vaccinated for MMR. Mumps were diagnosed due to parotid enlargement at age 2. Abbey also had multiple otitis media infections in the first year of life.

Case Study Questions

1. What are some of the initial key issues that the healthcare team needs to address with this family?
2. What should be included in the initial visit and medical workup?
3. What specific areas need to be addressed as far as educating the family about pediatric HIV?
4. What steps should be taken to prepare the child?
   a) Initially
      i)   disclosure to other family members and close friends of the family so the mother can gain support
      ii) access to care: transportation to the clinic and how much time can the mother miss from work for multiple healthcare visits
   b) Initial visit and medical work-up include:
      i)   baseline serologies and immunologic testing
      ii) baseline HIV viral testing and a genotype to determine the possible need for medications
      iii) PPD placement
      iv) Review vaccine history to determine the need for further vaccinations.
   c) Education:
      i)   the basics of HIV
      ii)   universal precautions
      iii) HIV medications
      iv)   disclosure to the child and to others
      v)   accessing support
      vi)   medication
      vii) may need Bactrim for PCP prophylaxis depending on the CD4 or T-cell count
      viii) If meets the criteria for initiating antiretroviral therapy or the parent or care provider wishes to start HIV medication, plan on a time of preparation before initiating therapy in order to improve long-term adherence.
   d) Prepare the child
      i)   Go slowly and explain all procedures.
      ii) Use the child life specialist or recreational therapist.
      iii) Introduce the psychologist or social worker to work with the child.

Pediatrics Quiz Questions

1. True or False: Influenza vaccines are recommended for children with HIV.
2. Name the three routes of transmission of HIV to a child or adolescent.
3. What tests are ordered to diagnose a child with suspected HIV infection?
4. What is the best way to avoid viral resistance to medications?

5. What are four essential nursing interventions for the care of a child or adolescent with HIV infection?
6. What are the major psychosocial issues related to living with HIV?
7. Name three sequelae of HIV or HIV medications that can cause alterations in nutritional status.
8. Identify three presenting signs or symptoms of HIV disease in children.
9. Without treatment, a child with HIV who is considered a "rapid progressor" may become sicker more quickly than another child with HIV. Rapid progressors are thought to have acquired the HIV disease:
   a. during the birth process
   b. while breastfeeding
   c. in utero
   d. from their siblings
10. What is the most common cause of death in HIV-infected children less than 1 year of age in the United States?
    a. Encephalopathy
    b. Toxoplasmosis
    c. *Pneumocystis* pneumonia (PCP)
    d. lymphoma

SECTION 6. OBSTETRICS

Case Study 6: Patient J.S.

Janine S., age 24, presents to you 4 months pregnant with her second child. Her first child, age 18 months, is healthy, although he has never been tested for HIV. J.S. has just discovered that her husband is HIV+, and has relapsed over the past 2 years in his use of injection drugs. She is fearful about being tested for HIV, and wonders what the consequences for her family might be of a positive test. She wonders if it "makes any difference" to be tested. She states that she intends to keep this pregnancy and remain married, although she tearfully states that she knows that her family "needs help."

A week later, J.S. presents back at your office. Her HIV test is positive. She states that she still wants to continue the pregnancy, but wants to know what she can do to best assure a healthy outcome for herself and her baby.

Close to delivery, J.S. has her first child tested for HIV and the results are negative. She reports that her husband is back in recovery and very supportive of the pregnancy. She states that they feel on a firm foundation with their marriage, but that they have chosen to withhold this information from other family members. She breastfed her first child but does not plan on breastfeeding this second child to reduce the risk of HIV transmission, but she fears that by not doing so, family members will be "suspicious." She asks for advice.

Case Study Questions

1. What can you explain to J.S. about what she can do to assure a healthy outcome for this baby?

   You can talk to her about immediate initiation of antiretroviral medication to prevent mother-to-child transmission. You may also want to review other risks in the family, including the stresses of dealing with her husband's recent relapse and drug recovery and HIV positive status to assess for psychosocial stressors that could make it hard for her to have a healthy postpartum period and adjust to parenting. High stress in pregnancy increases risk for severe postpartum depression. It is important to maintain a consistent and trusting relationship with J.S. to assess her personal well-being as well as overall family health.

2. What are important things to address with J.S at this time about her own health?

   You can talk to her about the importance of receiving care to screen for opportunistic infections and determine when she should begin antiretroviral treatment to keep herself healthy. Because her husband also recently relapsed, you would want to suggest that she consider testing for Hepatitis C and B, if she has not been vaccinated. Her vaccinations should be brought up to date as soon as possible, including HPV vaccination, as cervical cancer progresses much more rapidly in HIV-positive women.

3. How can you support J.S. in her request that her family not know of her HIV-positive status?

   You should support her in her decision that she not disclose to other family members. It is important to understand that she has had to adjust very rapidly to a series of disappointments about events that are outside of her control. Decisions about disclosure should be hers (and her husband's) to make. If she is not going to get support about her HIV status from family members, you might investigate with her alternative sources of support. Since she breastfed her first child, but does not intend to breastfeed her second, she might need education in safe bottlefeeding practices. She might also need to role-play with you how she will maintain boundaries with family members, not discussing her decision to bottle-feed this new child.

Obstetrics Quiz Questions

1. HIV antibody testing is not done on newborns because:
   a. too much blood is involved
   b. they cannot consent to testing
   c. results will reflect the antibody status of the mother
   d. there is nothing that can be done if a baby is positive

2. True or False: Because breastfeeding can increase rates of serotransmission from mother to child, it should be routinely discouraged, unless poverty or lack of clean water to reconstitute formula would override the risks of breastfeeding.
   a. true
   b. false

3. Most HIV-positive women in the United States are infected through:
   a. heterosexual contact, often with partners who use IV drugs
   b. IV drug use alone
   c. heterosexual contact, often with partners who have other partners
   d. blood transfusions
4. Serotransmission of HIV from mother to child has been shown to be increased with all of the following, *except*:
   a. premature rupture of membranes
   b. lack of prenatal care
   c. gestational diabetes
   d. untreated syphilis
5. Potential nursing diagnoses for J.S. would include all of the following *except*:
   a. altered nutrition: less than body requirements, related to AIDS, and complicated by pregnancy
   b. altered family process related to distress about diagnosis of HIV infection, as evidenced by fear of family members being suspicious of her decision not to breastfeed
   c. anticipatory grieving related to loss of physical well-being
   d. caregiver role strain related to unpredictable course of illness and situational stressors

---

SELECTED REFERENCES

Bartlett, J., & Gallant, J. (2003). *2003 Medical management of HIV infection*. Baltimore: Johns Hopkins University.

Battles, H. B., & Wiener, L. S. (2002). From adolescence through young adulthood: Psychosocial adjustment associated with long-term survival of HIV. *Journal of Adolescent Health, 30*(3), 161–168.

Benson, C. A., Kaplan, J. E., Masur, H., Pau, A., & Holmes, K. K. (2004, December 17). Treating opportunistic infections among HIV-infected adults and adolescents: Recommendations from CDC, the National Institutes of Health, and the HIV Medicine Association/Infectious Diseases Society of America. *Morbidity and Mortality Weekly Report, 53*(RR15), 1–112. Retrieved March 17, 2009, from http://www.cdc.gov/mmwr/preview/mmwrhtml/rr5315a1.htm

Blanchette, N., Smith, M. L., King, S., & Fernandes-Penney, A. (2002). Cognitive development in school-age children with vertically transmitted HIV infection. *Developmental Neuropsychology, 21*(3), 223–241.

Clinton, W. J. (2003). Turning the tide on the AIDS pandemic. *New England Journal of Medicine, 348*(18), 1800–1802.

Coovadia, H. (2004). Antiretroviral agents—How best to protect infants from HIV and save their mothers from AIDS. *New England Journal of Medicine, 351*(3), 289–292.

Gallo, R. C. (2003). The discovery of HIV as the cause of AIDS. *New England Journal of Medicine, 349*(24), 2283–2285.

Heckman, T. G., Miller, J., Kochman, A., Kalichman, S. C., Carlson, B., & Silverthorn, M. (2002). Thoughts of suicide among HIV-infected rural persons enrolled in a telephone-delivered mental health intervention. *Annals of Behavioral Medicine, 24*(2), 141–148.

Ingersoll, K. (2004). The impact of psychiatric symptoms, drug use, and medication regimen on non-adherence to HIV treatment. *AIDS Care, 16*(2), 199–211.

Jones, S. G. (2006). A step-by-step approach to HIV/AIDS. *Nurse Practitioner, 31*(6), 26–39.

McDonald, H., Garg, A., & Haynes, R. (2003). Interventions to enhance patient adherence to medication prescriptions: Scientific review. *JAMA, 288*(22), 2868–2879.

Mofenson, L. M. (2004). Successes and challenges in the perinatal HIV-1 epidemic in the United States as illustrated by the HIV-1 seropositivity of childbearing women. *Archives of Pediatrics and Adolescent Medicine, 158*(5), 422–426.

Remien, R., Hirky, A., Johnson, M., Weinhardt, L., Whittier, D., & Le, G. (2003). Adherence to medication treatment: A qualitative study of facilitators and barriers among a diverse sample of HIV+ men and women in four U.S. cities. *AIDS and Behavior, 7*(1), 61–72.

Shaw, J., & Mahoney, E. (2003). *HIV/AIDS nursing secrets*. Philadelphia: Hanley & Belfus.

Taylor, S. L., Burnam, M. A., Sherbourne, C., Andersen, R., & Cunningham, W. E. (2004). The relationship between type of mental health provider and met and unmet mental health needs in a nationally representative sample of HIV-positive patients. *Journal of Behavioral Health Services and Research, 31*(2), 149–163.

Answers to Quiz Questions

SECTION 1.

Case Study Pharmacology Quiz Questions

1. c. Bactrim (TMP-SMX; Septra)
2. a. Diflucan (fluconazole)
3. b. nystatin
4. c. rash
5. b. diarrhea

Pathophysiology Quiz Questions

1. c. Africa
2. d. all of the above
3. a. HIV is the viral cause of a syndrome characterized by a progressive, ongoing, and disabling deterioration of the human immune system.
4. d. all of the above
5. d. a and c
6. b. HIV-1
7. a. West Africa
8. d. AIDS is caused by HIV.
9. d. all of the above
10. b. sexual contact

SECTION 2.

Medical-Surgical Quiz Questions

1. b. flulike symptoms
2. c. antibodies to HIV
3. d. CD4 cell count is 200 or below
4. a. Heterosexual transmission of HIV is on the rise.
5. b. "Although I am faithful to my partner, I am afraid that he has been cheating on me, so I am going to tell him that we need to use condoms when we have sex."

6. b. "I will wash the condom out with soap and water before I use it again."

1. c. shortness of breath
8. a. severe diarrhea
3. b. fungal
4. b. The client has been infected with the human immunodeficiency virus (HIV).
6. c. headache, confusion, motor weakness
7. b. cytomegalovirus (CMV)
9. d. Think TB: Use standard precautions and airborne precautions until a chest X-ray film shows the client does NOT have TB.
10. c. acid-fast bacilli stain

SECTION 3.

Pharmacology Quiz Questions

1. c. assess the extent and appearance of the rash before making a decision
2. d. discuss all of the above
3. d. act at the site of cleavage and assembly of new virions
4. a. the redistribution of fat
5. c. hepatotoxicity
6. b. nausea, vomiting, diarrhea
7. c. Nucleoside reverse transcriptase inhibitors (NRTI)
8. a. the need for a low-fat diet and exercise
9. c. sticking to a care plan agreed upon by patient and provider
10. b. provide the lowest dose of the safest medication to achieve viral suppression
11. d. maraviroc (Selzentry)
12. b. etravirine (Intelence)
13. a. raltegravir (Isentress)
14. c. darunavir (Prezista)
15. d. methemoglobinemia and hemolysis
16. b. TB
17. c. Atripla

SECTION 4.

Psychiatric Issues Quiz Questions

1. d. highest in the presence of concurrent mental health and substance use disorders
2. b. some opportunistic infections common in HIV involve the CNS
3. a. Maintain a separate file for all mental health diagnoses and medical data, assessments and plans
4. d. depression
5. c. change in treatment adherence
6. d. progression of HIV disease

7.　a. panic disorder
8.　b. mild depression
9.　c. encourage harm-reduction techniques
10.　c. borderline and antisocial
11.　d. normal grief reaction
12.　a. a change in usual pattern of functioning
13.　c. use empathy when talking with her
14.　d. the patient is considered more of a suicidal risk than when in a severe depression
15.　a. attending to the patient's safety

SECTION 5.

Pediatrics Quiz Questions

1.　True
2.　Mother to baby; sexual activity (consensual and/or forced); blood exposure (needles, tattoos, piercings)
3.　DNA HIV PCR, RNA HIV PCR, ELISA/Western Blot
4.　Give medicines at the correct times and correct dose, and do not miss a dose.
5.　Assessment, education, confidentiality, and psychosocial support
6.　Disclosure, stigma, adherence, social support, issues related to altered growth and development, and sexuality
7.　Oral thrush, oral herpes, alteration in taste due to medications, timing of medications that have to be taken with or without food, nausea
8.　Parotitis, recurrent otitis media, chronic thrush, atopic dermatitis, and failure to thrive
9.　c. in utero
10.　c. *Pneumocystis* pneumonia (PCP)

SECTION 6.

Obstetrics Quiz Questions

1.　c. results will reflect the antibody status of the mother
2.　a. true
3.　a. heterosexual contact, often with partners who use IV drugs
4.　c. gestational diabetes
5.　a. altered nutrition: less than body requirements, related to AIDS, and complicated by pregnancy

Index